T,

AF782638

May 2002.

Penni

Hope that this may be of real use for you

Tim.

Chronic Myeloid Leukaemia

Chronic Myeloid Leukaemia
Biology and Treatment

Edited by

ANGELO M CARELLA, MD
Division of Hematology and Stem Cell Transplantation Unit
Ospedale 'Casa Sollievo della Sofferenza'-IRCCS
San Giovanni Rotondo, Italy

GEORGE Q DALEY, MD, PhD
Whitehead Institute
Cambridge, MA, USA

CONNIE J EAVES, PhD
Terry Fox Laboratory
BC Cancer Agency
Vancouver, BC, Canada

JOHN M GOLDMAN, DM, FRCP, FRCPath
Hammersmith Hospital
Department of Haematology
Imperial College School of Medicine
London, UK

RÜDIGER HEHLMANN, MD
III Medizinische Klinik Mannheim
Universität Heidelberg
Mannheim, Germany

MARTIN DUNITZ

First published in the United Kingdom in 2001 by
Martin Dunitz Ltd
The Livery House
7–9 Pratt Street
London NW1 0AE

Tel:	+44-(0)20-7482-2202
Fax:	+44-(0)20-7267-0159
E-mail:	info.dunitz@tandf.co.uk
Website:	http://www.dunitz.co.uk

A CIP catalogue record for this book is available from the British Library

ISBN 1-85317-890-X

Distributed in the USA by
Fulfilment Center
Taylor & Francis
7625 Empire Drive
Florence, KY 41042, USA
Toll Free Tel: 1-800-634-7064
Email: cserve@routledge nv.com

Distributed in Canada by
Taylor & Francis
74 Rolark Drive
Scarborough
Ontario M1R 4G2, Canada
Toll Free Tel: 1-877-226-2237
Email: tal fran@istar.ca

Distributed in the rest of the world by
ITPS Limited
Cheriton House
North Way, Andover
Hampshire SP10 5BE, UK
Tel: +44 (0)1264 332424
Email: reception@itps.co.uk

Composition by Wearset, Boldon, Tyne and Wear
Printed and bound in Spain by Grafos S.A.

Contents

Preface vii

Contributors ix

Part 1 Molecular biology of chronic myeloid leukaemia

1. *BCR/ABL* gene structure and BCR function *Nora Heisterkamp, John Groffen* 3

2. BCR/ABL protein domain function and signaling *Ann Marie Pendergast* 19

3. Abnormalities in hematopoietic progenitor adhesion *Ravi Bhatia, Catherine Verfaillie* 41

4. Functional complementation of cytokine receptor signaling by BCR/ABL *Eugene Y Koh, George Q Daley* 55

5. Progenitor cell dynamics *Connie J Eaves, Allen C Eaves* 73

6. Animal models of Philadelphia-positive leukemia *Richard A Van Etten* 101

Part 2 Conventional treatment for chronic myeloid leukaemia

7. Biology of interferon *Thomas Fischer, Moshe Talpaz* 135

8. Interferon-α dosage regimens *Patricia CA Shepherd* 149

9. Chemotherapy versus interferon: Long-term effects *Andreas Hochhaus, Rüdiger Hehlmann* 165

10. Chemotherapy *Bengt Simonsson* 181

11. Interferon-α and Ara-C *Gianantonio Rosti, Elena Trabacchi, Francesca Bonifazi, Antonio de Vivo, Simona Bassi, Sante Tura* 191

12. Prognostic factors *Joerg Hasford, Markus Pfirrmann, Rüdiger Hehlmann, Patricia CA Shepherd, François Guilhot, François X Mahon, Josef Thaler, Juan L Steegmann, Hanneke C Kluin-Nelemans, Andries Louwagie, Kazunori Ohnishi, Otto Kloke* 205

13. Evidence-based guidelines for the treatment of chronic-phase chronic myeloid leukemia *Richard T Silver* 225

Part 3 Allogeneic haematopoietic stem cell transplantation for chronic myeloid leukaemia

14. Donor selection in allogeneic bone marrow transplantation *Andrea L Pay, Ann-Margaret Little, J Alejandro Madrigal* 241

15. Risk assessmant for allogeneic transplantation *Alois Gratwohl* 251

16. The decision whether to allograft a patient with CML *John M Goldman* 263

17. Conditioning regimens and T-cell depletion *Charles Craddock* 273
18. Blood versus marrow stem cells *Peter Dreger, Norbert Schmitz* 287
19. HLA-identical sibling transplantation *David G Savage* 303
20. Results with alternative donors *Jane F Apperley* 323
21. Patient monitoring after allogeneic stem cell transplantation or interferon-α therapy *Andreas Hochhaus* 339
22. Recommendations for assessment and definitions of response and relapse in CML: A report from the Chronic Leukemia Working Committee of the IBMTR *Sergio A Giralt, John M Goldman, Claudio Anasetti, Francisco Cervantes, Richard Champlin, Nicholas Cross, Andreas Hochhaus, John P Klein, Esperanza Papadopoulos, Kathleen Sobocinski, Daniel Weisdorf, Mary Horowitz on behalf of the Chronic Leukemia Working Committee of the IBMTR* 357
23. Basis of GVL *John M Barrett* 369
24. Donor lymphocyte infusions *Francesco Dazzi, Hans J Stauss* 385
25. Late complications, including late relapse *Gérard Socié, Rochelle E Curtis, John P Klein* 401

Part 4 Autografting in chronic myeloid leukaemia

26. Autografting with unmanipulated stem cells: The European experience *Arnaud Pigneux, Eduardo Olavarria, François X Mahon, Josy Reiffers* 421
27. Autografting with cultured marrow *Michael J Barnett, Connie J Eaves, Allen C Eaves* 431
28. Autografting with Ph-negative haematopoietic progenitor cells *Angelo M Carella* 445
29. Autologous hematopoietic stem cell transplantation: Experience at the University of Minnesota *Philip McGlave* 457
30. What role for autografting? A personal view *Stephen G O'Brien* 465

Part 5 Target-directed therapies: Chronic myeloid leukaemia as a paradigm for oncology

31. Gene therapy *Alan M Gewirtz* 475
32. Target-directed therapies *Mikhail L Gishizky* 485
33. Development of kinase inhibitors *Enrica Lerma, Toa Wang, Takuma Fujii, Victor Chang, David Austin, Albert A Deisseroth* 495
34. STI571 as a therapeutic agent *Michael E O'Dwyer, Michael J Mauro, Brian J Druker* 501
35. Immunotherapeutic strategies *Kathleen NS Cathcart, Javier Pinilla, David A Scheinberg* 507

Index 521

Preface

Much has changed in the field of chronic myeloid leukaemia (CML), particularly during the past decade. New advances in therapy and great achievements in cellular biology, molecular biology, and chemotherapy, coupled with the development of tyrosine kinase inhibitors, have all radically changed the clinical and basic approaches to the therapy of this disease. The chapters in this book reflect these changes, and each includes new data made available via the great advances in research into these topics, which have added so much to our understanding of this complex disease.

It is a pleasure to acknowledge the many obligations incurred in the preparation of this book. We are grateful to all the scientists who agreed to contribute to this work; without their willingness and enthusiasm, it would not have been possible to put together up-to-date reviews of the variety of biologic and therapeutic methods available today. We hope that the reader will benefit from this book, which should be suitable for specialists and postgraduate physicians in training as well as for undergraduate teaching in haematology.

AM Carella
GQ Daley
CJ Eaves
JM Goldman
R Hehlmann

Contributors

Claudio Anasetti, MD
Division of Clinical Research
Fred Hutchinson Cancer Research Center
1100 Fairview Avenue North
Seattle, WA 98109-1024
USA

Jane F Apperley, MD
Department of Haematology
Hammersmith Hospital
Imperial College School of Medicine
Du Cane Road
London W12 0NN
UK

David Austin, PhD
Department of Chemistry
Yale University
New Haven, CT 06115
USA

Michael J Barnett, BM
Leukemia/Bone Marrow Transplantation
Program of British Columbia
910 West 10th Avenue
Vancouver, BC V5Z 4E3
Canada

John M Barrett, MD
National Institutes of Health National Heart
Lung & Blood Institute
BMT Unit – RM 7N248
9000 Rockville Pike
Bethesda, MD 20892
USA

Simona Bassi, MD
Istituto di Ematologia e Oncologia Medica
"Lorenzo e Ariosto Seràgnoli"
Via G. Massarenti 9
40138 Bologna
Italy

Ravi Bhatia, MD
Department of Hematology & BMT
City of Hope National Medical Center
1500 East Duarte Road
Duarte, CA 91010
USA

Francesca Bonifazi, MD
Istituto di Ematologia e Oncologia Medica
"Lorenzo e Ariosto Seràgnoli"
Via G. Massarenti 9
40138 Bologna
Italy

Angelo M Carella, MD
Division of Hematology and Stem Cell Transplantation Unit
Casa Sollievo della Sofferenza-IRCS
Viale Cappuccini 86
71013 San Giovanni Rotondo
Italy

Kathleen NS Cathcart, MD
Department of Medicine
Memorial Sloan-Kettering Cancer Center
1275 York Avenue
New York, NY 10021
USA

Francisco Cervantes, MD
Postgraduate School of Hematology
Department of Hematology
Hospital Clinic
Villarroel 170
08036 Barcelona
Spain

Richard E Champlin, MD
Department of Blood and Marrow Transplantation
UT MD Anderson Cancer Center
1515 Holcombe Blvd., Box 423
Houston, TX 77030
USA

Victor Chang, MD
Yale University School of Medicine
333 Cedar Street
New Haven, CT 06520-8032
USA

Charles Craddock, MRCP, MRCPath
Department of Haematology
University of Birmingham NHS Trust
Queen Elizabeth Medical Center
Vincent Drive
Edgbaston
Birmingham B15 2TH
UK

Nicholas Cross, PhD
Hammersmith Hospital
Department of Haematology
Imperial College School of Medicine
Du Cane Road
London W12 0NN
UK

Rochelle E Curtis, MA
Division of Cancer Epidemiology & Genetics
National Cancer Institute
Bethesda, MD 20892
USA

George Q Daley, MD, PhD
Division of Hematology/Oncology
Massachusetts General Hospital, Boston
Whitehead Institute
9 Cambridge Center
Cambridge, MA 02142
USA

Francesco Dazzi, MD
Leukaemia Unit
Department of Haematology and Immunology
Hammersmith Hospital, ICSM
Du Cane Road
London W12 0NN
UK

Albert A Deisseroth, MD
Yale University School of Medicine
333 Cedar Street
New Haven, CT 06520-8032
USA

Antonio de Vivo, MD
Istituto di Ematologia e Oncologia Medica
"Lorenzo e Ariosto Seràgnoli"
Via G. Massarenti 9
40138 Bologna
Italy

Peter Dreger, MD
Second Department of Medicine
Christian-Albrechts Universität Kiel
D-24116 Kiel 1
Germany

Brian J Druker, MD
Division of Hematology & Medical Oncology
Department of Medicine
Oregon Health Sciences University, L592
3181 SW Sam Jackson Park Road
Portland, OR 97201-3098
USA

Allen C Eaves, MD, PhD
Terry Fox Laboratory
BC Cancer Agency
601 West 10th Avenue
Vancouver, BC V5Z 1L3
Canada

Connie J Eaves, PhD
Terry Fox Laboratory
BC Cancer Agency
601 West 10th Avenue
Vancouver, BC V5Z 1L3
Canada

Takuma Fujii, PhD, MD
Yale University School of Medicine
333 Cedar Street
New Haven, CT 06520-8032
USA

Thomas Fischer, MD
III Medical Department
Hematology/Oncology
Johannes Gutenberg-Universität
Langenbeckstr. 1
55101 Mainz
Germanny

Alan M Gewirtz, MD
University of Pennsylvania
School of Medicine
422 Curie Boulevard
Room 513b, BRB1
Philadelphia, PA 19104-6140
USA

Sergio Giralt, MD
Department of Blood and Marrow
Transplantation
UT MD Anderson Cancer Center
1515 Holcombe Blvd., Box 423
Houston, TX 77030
USA

Mikhail L Gishizky, PhD
Sugen, Inc
230 East Grand Avenue South
San Francisco, CA 94080
USA

John M Goldman, DM, FRCP, FRCPath
Hammersmith Hospital
Department of Haematology
Imperial College School of Medicine
Du Cane Road
London W12 0NN
UK

Alois Gratwohl, MD, PhD
Division of Hematology
Department of Internal Medicine
Kantonsspital
Petersgraben 4
4031 Basel
Switzerland

John Groffen, PhD
Section of Molecular Carcinogenesis
Division of Hematology/Oncology, MS#54
Childrens Hospital of Los Angeles
4650 Sunset Blvd
Los Angeles, CA 90027
USA

François Guilhot, MD
Department of Haematology & Medical
Oncology
Centre Hospitalier Universitaire de Poitiers
350 Avenue Jacques Coeur
86021 Poitiers
France

Joerg Hasford, MD, PhD
IBE, University of Munich
Marchioninstrasse 15
81377 Munich
Germany

Rüdiger Hehlmann, MD
III Medizinische Klinik Mannheim
Universität Heidelberg
Wiesbadener Strasse 7-11
68305 Mannheim
Germany

Nora Heisterkamp, PhD
Section of Molecular Carcinogenesis
Division of Hematology/Oncology, MS 54
Childrens Hospital of Los Angeles
4650 Sunset Blvd
Los Angeles, CA 90027
USA

Andreas Hochhaus, MD
III Medizinische Klinik Mannheim
Univeristät Heidelberg
Wiesbadener Strasse 7-11
68305 Mannheim
Germany

Mary M Horowitz, MD, MS
IBMTR/ABMTR
Medical College of Wisconsin
8701 Watertown Plank Road
Milwaukee, WI 53226
USA

John P Klein, PhD
Division of Biostatistics
Medical College of Wisconsin
8701 Watertown Plank Road
Milwaukee, WI 53226
USA

Hanneke C Kluin-Nelemans, MD
Department of Hematology
Groningen University Hospital
Hanzeplein 1
9713 GZ Groningen
The Netherlands

Otto Kloke, MD
Abteilung Innere Medizin/Krebszentrum
Universitätsklinikum Essen
Hufelandstrasse 55
45122 Essen
Germany

Eugene Y Koh, PhD
Whitehead Institute
9 Cambridge Center
Cambridge, MA 02142
USA

Enrica Lerma, MD
Yale University School of Medicine
333 Cedar Street
New Haven, CT 06520-8032
USA

Ann-Margaret Little, BSc, PhD
The Anthony Nolan Research Institute
The Royal Free Hospital
Pond Street
London NW3 2QG
UK

Andries Louwagie, MD
Department of Hematology
AZ St. Jan Ruddershove 10
8000 Brugge
Belgium

J Alejandro Madrigal, MD, PhD, FRCP, MRCPath
The Anthony Nolan Research Institute
The Royal Free Hospital
Pond Street
London NW3 2QG
UK

Michael J Mauro, MD
Division of Hematology & Medical Oncology
Department of Medicine
Oregon Health Sciences University, OP28
3181 SW Sam Jackson Park Road
Portland, OR 97201
USA

François-Xavier Mahon, MD
Laboratoire de Greffe de Moelle
UMR CNRS 5540
Université Victor Segalen Bordeaux 2
146 rue Léo Saignat
33076 Bordeaux Cedex
France

Philip McGlave, MD
Division of Hematology, Oncology and Transplantation
University of Minnesota
Mayo Building
420 Delaware Street SE
Minneapolis, MN 54455-0374
USA

Stephen G O'Brien, PhD, MRCP (UK), MRCPath
Department of Haematology
University of Newcastle
Royal Victoria Infirmary
Newcastle-upon-Tyne
NE1 4LP
UK

Michael E O'Dwyer, MD
Division of Hematology & Medical Oncology
Department of Medicine
Oregon Health Sciences University, OP28
3181 SW Sam Jackson Park Road
Portland, OR 97201
USA

Kazunori Ohnishi, MD
Internal Medicine III
Hamamatsu University, School of Medicine
3600 Handa-cho
Hamamatsu 431-31
Japan

Eduardo Olavarria, MD
Haematology Department
Hammersmith Hospital, ICSM
Du Cane Road
London W12 0NN
UK

Esperanza B Papadopoulos, MD
Department of Medicine
Memorial Sloan-Kettering Cancer Center
1275 York Avenue
New York, NY 10021
USA

Andrea L Pay, BSc
The Anthony Nolan Research Institute
The Royal Free Hospital
Pond Street
London NW3 2QG
UK

Ann Marie Pendergast, PhD
Department of Pharmacology & Cancer Biology
Duke University Medical Center, Box 3813
Durham, NC 27710
USA

Markus Pfirrmann, MSc
IBE, University of Munich
Marchioninistrasse 15
81377 Munich
German

Arnaud Pigneux, MD
Service d'Hématologie
Hôpital du Haut-Lévêque
Centre François Magendie
Avenue de Magellan
33604 Pessac
France

Javier Pinilla, MD, PhD
Department of Medicine
Memorial Sloan-Kettering Cancer Center
1275 York Avenue
New York, NY 10021
USA

Josy Reiffers, MD
Groupe Hospitalier Sud
Centre François Magendie
Avenue de Magellan
33604 Pessac
France

Gianantonio Rosti, MD
Istituto di Ematologia e Oncologia Medica
"Lorenzo e Ariosto Seràgnoli"
Via G. Massarenti 9
40138 Bologna
Italy

David G Savage, MD
Blood & Marrow Stem Cell Transplantation
Hematology-Oncology Division
Columbia-Presbyterian Medical Center
177 Fort Washington Avenue
New York, NY 10032
USA

David A Scheinberg, MD, PhD
Department of Medicine
Memorial Sloan-Kettering Cancer Center
1275 York Avenue
New York, NY 10021
USA

Norbert Schmitz, MD
Second Department of Medicine
Christian-Albrechts-Universität
Chemnitzstr 33
D-24116 Kiel
Germany

Patricia CA Shepherd, MRCP, FRCPath
Department of Haematology
Western General Hospital
Edinburgh, EH4 2XU
UK

Richard T Silver, MD
Department of Hematology & Oncology
NY Presbyterian Hospital
Weill Cornell Medical Center
525 East 68th Street
New York, NY 10021
USA

Bengt Simonsson, MD, PhD
Department of Internal Medicine
Section of Hematology
University Hospital
S-75185 Uppsala
Sweden

Kathleen Sobocinski, MS
IBMTR/ABMTR
Medical College of Wisconsin
8701 Watertown Plank Road
Milwaukee, WI 53226
USA

Gérard Socié, MD, PhD
D'Hématologie Greffe de Moelle
Hôpital St Louis
1 Avenue Claude Vellefaux
75475 Paris, Cedex 10
France

Hans J Stauss
Department of Haematology and Immunology
Hammersmith Hospital, ICMS
Du Cane Road
London W12 0NN
UK

Juan Luis Steegmann, MD
Hospital Universitario de la Princesa
Servicio de Hematología
C/. Diego de León
28006 Madrid
Spain

Moshe Talpaz, MD
Department of Bioimmunotherapy
MD Anderson Cancer Center
1515 Holcombe Blvd.
Houston, TX 77030
USA

Josef Thaler, MD
Universitätsklinik für Innere Medizin
Anichstraße 35
6020 Innsbruck
Austria

Elena Trabacchi, MD
Istituto di Ematologia e Oncologia Medica
"Lorenzo e Ariosto Seràgnoli"
Via G. Massarenti 9
40138 Bologna
Italy

Sante Tura, MD
Istituto di Ematologia e Oncologia Medica
"Lorenzo e Ariosto Seràgnoli"
Via G. Massarenti 9
40138 Bologna
Italy

Richard A Van Etten, MD, PhD
Center for Blood Research
Harvard Medical School
200 Longwood Avenue
Boston, MA 02115-5717
USA

Catherine Verfaillie, MD
Stem Cell Institute
Moos Tower 14-287A
University of Minnesota Health Center
420 Delaware St, SE
Minneapolis, MN 55455
USA

Tao Wang
Yale University School of Medicine
333 Cedar Street
New Haven, CT 06520-8032
USA

Daniel Weisdorf, MD
Adult Blood & Marrow Transplantation
Program
University of Minnesota
516 Delaware Street SE
Minneapolis, MN 55455
USA

Part 1

Molecular biology of chronic myeloid leukaemia

1

BCR/ABL gene structure and BCR function

Nora Heisterkamp, John Groffen

CONTENTS • *BCR*, *ABL*, and the Ph chromosome on a genomic level • BCR protein and function • The whole BCR protein in vivo • Conclusions and perspectives

BCR, *ABL*, AND THE PH CHROMOSOME ON A GENOMIC LEVEL

Genomic history of the Ph chromosome

Nowell and Hungerford[1] discovered the first consistent chromosome abnormality in human cancer in 1960. They identified a small abnormal chromosome in chronic myeloid leukemia (CML), and named it the Philadelphia (Ph) chromosome after the city in which it was discovered. The exact origin of this minute chromosome was unclear at that point in time.

Later technical improvements allowed for a better identification of individual chromosomes, and in 1973 Rowley[2] reported that the Ph chromosome represented a translocation between chromosomes 9 and 22 with breakpoints in the long arms at q34 and q11 respectively. In the years that followed, molecular biology took off, leading to the first cloning of mammalian homologues of the transforming sequences transduced by type C RNA viruses. In 1983, overlapping segments of exons 2–11 of the human *ABL* tyrosine kinase proto-oncogene were cloned from a cosmid library using Abelson murine leukemia virus acquired cellular sequences as a probe.[3] Around that time, somatic cell hybrids were being developed, which retained a limited number of human chromosomes and allowed one to deduce the chromosomal location of a gene. Using this technology, the human *ABL* gene was localized to chromosome 9.[4]

Investigators in the Department of Cell Biology and Genetics at the Erasmus University in the Netherlands were focused on identification of the molecular basis of the Ph chromosome. They had derived somatic cell hybrids that contained the Ph chromosome. In a collaborative effort, a human *ABL* probe was hybridized to DNA of such somatic cell hybrids, leading to the surprising discovery that *ABL* had been translocated from chromosome 9 and was now present on the Ph chromosome.[5] This showed for the first time that the t(9;22) is reciprocal, since the segment that moved from chromosome 9 to 22 was too small to be easily visualized cytogenetically.

Although neither the orientation nor the distance of *ABL* to the breakpoint at q34 on chromosome 9 were known, we undertook to clone more 5' sequences of the *ABL* locus. Because DNA isolated from involved spleens of CML patients was readily available (in the past, splenectomy was used to reduce the tumor burden of patients), each region that we cloned was examined for abnormalities in the patient samples. Fortunately, the first breakpoint discovered[6] was situated at a relatively small distance from *ABL* exon 1a – we now know that *ABL* contains a 175 kb first intron,[7] and if breakpoints had been clustered in its 5' end, we would not have discovered them: the region between exons 1b and 1a proved to be very difficult to clone, and we abandoned attempts to fully clone it several years later. Currently, t(9;22) breakpoints on chromosome 9 in a larger number of patients have been analyzed. The vast majority of breakpoints are found between *ABL* exons 1b, 1a, and exon 2, with occasional exceptions (for detailed reviews, see Melo[8,9]). Importantly, all contain an intact ABL tyrosine kinase domain. The tyrosine kinase activity of ABL in the deregulated BCR/ABL fusion protein is central to its leukemogenic activity.

Cloning of the 22/9 breakpoint fragment provided chromosome 22 sequences, which led to the isolation of the breakpoint cluster region (*BCR*) gene on chromosome 22.[10,11] The deduced amino acid sequence of this gene provided no clues whatsoever regarding its function, but the amount of proteins sequenced and the number of structural or functional domains recognized in proteins in general were quite limited at the time. As discussed below, a much more detailed picture of the BCR protein is currently emerging.

What about the ABL/BCR reciprocal translocation product?

As noted above, the Ph translocation is reciprocal, so that, in general, the 3' end of the *BCR* gene ends up on chromosome 9 behind the *ABL* promoter(s) and exon 1b or 1a. Depending upon the exact locations of the breakpoints in *ABL* and *BCR*, different products can be expected, and reverse-transcriptase polymerase chain reaction (RT-PCR) has in fact demonstrated that such products exist in patient material.[8,12,13]

These chimeric mRNAs can be translated into proteins. The reciprocal ABL/BCR product of the p210 BCR/ABL-generating translocation would consist of ABL exon 1b-encoded sequences fused in-frame to the BCR GTPase-activating (GAP) domain (more about this domain below). ABL contains an N-terminal myristoylation site, which could cause an abnormal membrane association of the GAP, since BCR does not contain a myristoylation site. Thus the ABL/BCR protein could have an abnormal biological activity. To investigate this, we have generated a p210-reciprocal *ABL/BCR* DNA construct and used it to make transgenic mice (JW Voncken and N Heisterkamp, unpublished results). One line of mice was followed for several years, but no specific disease developed, although we could show *ABL/BCR* mRNA in the peripheral blood of these animals using RT-PCR. Therefore, the effect of the reciprocal translocation product on leukemogenesis in humans, if any, is likely to be very modest.

BCR gene intron–exon organization and breakpoints

The *BCR* gene is also relatively large – around 135 kb. It has been entirely cloned and sequenced.[14,15] In total, there are 23 exons, with exon 1 around 71.5 kb upstream from exon 2. There is a clear preference for breakpoints to occur in certain regions and less frequently in others – hence the name breakpoint cluster region gene. The vast majority of breakpoints are found in major and minor breakpoint cluster regions (M-*bcr* and m-*bcr*), located between exons 13–16 and exons 1–2, respectively. Apart from these, sporadic cases of breakpoints in different introns have been reported. A major area of controversy throughout the years has been whether the exact location of the breakpoint has any effect on the type of leukemia or on disease outcome.[8,9] In theory, an effect could be possible, since the alternative breakpoints result in the production of BCR/ABL proteins including different BCR domains (also see below).

The most clear-cut differences appear to be produced by breakpoints in the major versus the minor breakpoint cluster regions. Breakpoints in the M-*bcr* produce the 'classical' BCR/ABL p210 protein, which is typical of CML and a percentage of Ph-positive acute

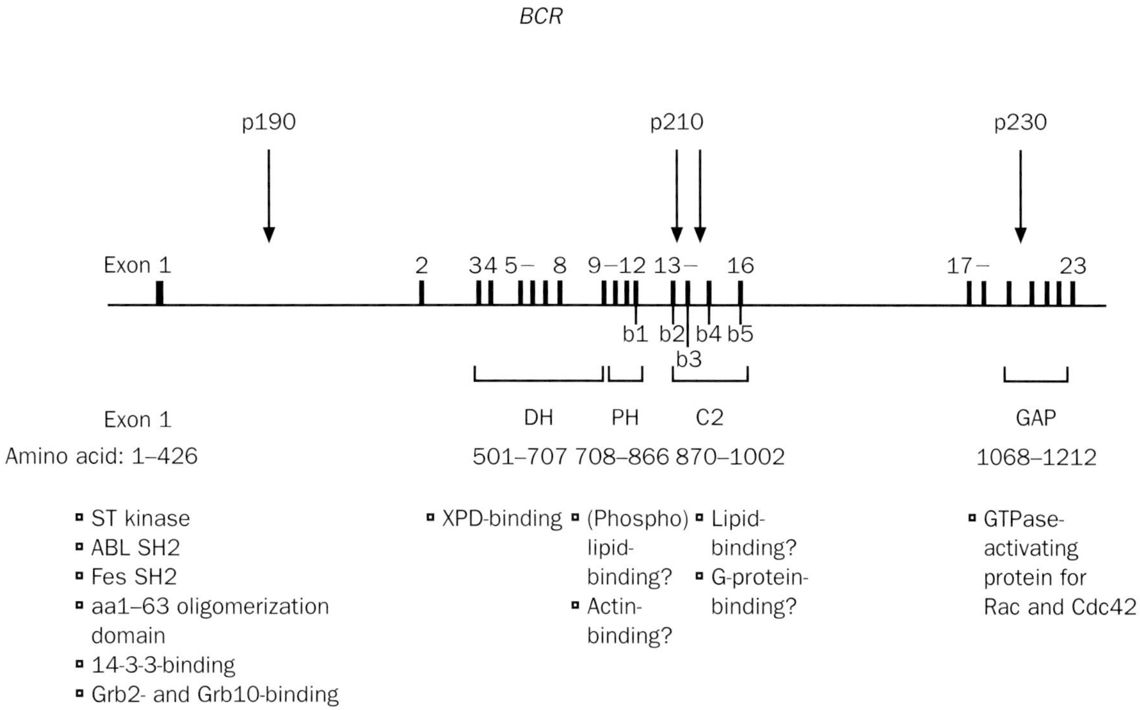

Figure 1.1 Schematic overview of the *BCR* gene. See text for the abbreviations used.

lymphoblastic leukemia (ALL). A p190 protein is produced by translocated chromosomes with a breakpoint in m-*bcr* (see Figure 1.1). This fusion protein is found in Ph-positive ALL, especially in children.[8,9] The association of p190 with a more aggressive type of disease is supported by the higher tyrosine kinase activity of this protein and experiments in model systems including mice and transfected cells.[16–21] However, sensitive RT-PCR techniques have detected p190 mRNA in CML patients who express a p210 protein. Also, as mentioned, a subgroup of ALL patients express the p210 that is associated with chronic disease in CML. Therefore, the association of either type of BCR/ABL fusion protein with chronic or acute disease, or with lymphoid versus myeloid leukemia, is not absolute.[8,9]

p210 and p190 differ in a large region of the BCR protein, which includes two distinct domains: the Dbl homology and pleckstrin homology domains. A third, rare variant encoding a p230 (see Figure 1.1) was reported to be associated with a more benign type of disease in humans.[22,23] Li et al[21] showed that this protein had a lower intrinsic kinase activity than p190 and p210, but all three forms of BCR/ABL induced an identical CML-like disease in mice. However, p190 was more potent in inducing B-lineage lymphoid leukemia than p210 or p230.

A difference in outcome between patients who express p210 BCR/ABL proteins that differ only in the presence or absence of 25 amino acid residues encoded by exon 14 has been a long-standing controversy, which seems to have evolved towards the viewpoint that no clear differences exist.[8,9] The possible significance of these domains in BCR to the different BCR/ABL proteins will be discussed below.

Cause of the generation of the *BCR/ABL* chimeric gene

A question that has fascinated most investigators from the beginning is why this translocation occurs with such specificity. Obviously, *BCR/ABL* fusions that do not produce a functional protein would not be expected to lead to leukemogenesis. But, as described below, there are other genes that can provide the necessary ingredients to deregulate ABL and that make it oncogenic. Why then are no glutathione-S-transferase/ABL or EpoR/ABL chimeric proteins found in human leukemia?

A series of interesting experiments may shed some light on this matter. Two studies by the same group showed that in total bone marrow and human lymphocytes, *BCR* and *ABL* genes in the nucleus were found closer together than would be expected by chance.[24–26] Subsequently, Neves and colleagues[26] measured the distance between *BCR* and *ABL* in hematopoietic cells of different lineages and at different stages of the cell cycle using 3-D preserved cells, non-isotopic in situ hybridization, and confocal microscopy. This analysis showed that *BCR* and *ABL* become closely associated at the transition of late S to G_2 in all cell types analyzed. However, the control β-globin gene was also found in close proximity to *ABL* in some cells, indicating that the close proximity of *ABL* and *BCR* cannot be the only factor responsible for the high degree of recombination between these loci.

BCR PROTEIN AND FUNCTION

Sizes

The BCR protein has a 160 kDa molecular mass. Although other-sized proteins have been detected with different antisera,[27,28] their origin has remained unclear. Similarly, in humans, there are two mRNA species, of 7 and 4.3 kb, with the 4.3 kb product containing all known sequences necessary to encode the p160 protein.[29] Curiously, mice only express a 7 kb species, suggesting that the larger mRNA may contain more 5' or 3' untranslated sequences than the 4.3 kb product.[30]

In some tissues and after certain stimuli, the p160 protein is found to migrate as a doublet. Phosphorylation is one type of post-translational modification that is known to modify BCR and account for mobility shifts. In lymphomas of BCR/ABL p190 transgenic mice, the endogenous murine Bcr protein migrates as a doublet,[31] probably because of its tyrosine phosphorylation by BCR/ABL.[32] Phosphorylated Bcr protein is also detectable in several areas of the brain after subjection of mice to cold stress (JW Voncken and N Heisterkamp, unpublished). As described below, the BCR protein itself is a serine/threonine kinase and can autophosphorylate. In addition, it is a substrate for several tyrosine kinases, including (BCR/)ABL, Fes, and Hck in vivo.[33–35]

N-terminal oligomerization domain

The very N-terminal part of p160 including amino acid residues 1–63 contains an oligomerization domain.[36] This α-helical coiled-coil region, which is also present in all BCR/ABL proteins, mediates homodimerization between individual BCR/ABL proteins and is required for activation of the ABL kinase and of its actin-crosslinking activity.[36–38] Its function within the BCR protein itself is presently unclear: no studies have been reported that investigate whether this region is necessary for activation of the BCR serine/threonine kinase or for activation of other functions.

The key feature of this region for BCR/ABL is not its specific sequence, but rather its ability to cause oligomerization of BCR/ABL. Replacement of this domain by the leucine zipper of the yeast transcription factor GCN4 yielded a fusion protein that showed many of the features of BCR/ABL.[39] Similarly, substitution of this region by glutathione-S-transferase, which has dimerization capability, produced a fusion protein that retained some of the transforming properties of BCR/ABL.[40] When the extracellular ligand-binding domain of the erythropoietin receptor (EpoR) was fused to ABL, ABL activation and transformation occurred after addition of erythropoietin.[41] Finally, rare cases of human acute lymphoblastic leukemia express TEL/ABL fusion proteins, in which ABL is activated.[42,43] Tyrosine phosphorylation of substrates was found to be very similar in cells transfected by BCR/ABL and by TEL/ABL.[44] The role of BCR sequences in transformation by BCR/ABL is also discussed in Chapter 2.

The BCR serine/threonine kinase

Initial analysis of the p160 showed that it had an intrinsic or associated serine/threonine (S/T) kinase activity.[45] A detailed study subsequently demonstrated that the activity was intrinsic, and delineated the kinase domain.[46] Somewhat surprisingly, this domain is unrelated to any other kinase isolated to date, and has an unusual nucleotide-binding domain that contains paired cysteine residues.[46] Extensive efforts to identify related sequences in genomic or cDNA libraries failed to demonstrate the existence of any (distantly) related kinase domains (T Fioretos, N Heisterkamp, and J Groffen, unpublished). Even the ABR protein, which is closely related to BCR in structure over its entire length, lacks this domain.[47,48] The function of the S/T kinase is not known, and it appears to be constitutively active. Mutation of cysteine residue C332→L abolishes the kinase activity.[46,49] The sites of S/T autophosphorylation or the effect, if any, on the BCR S/T kinase itself or GAP activity have not been determined.

Similarly, few physiological substrates for the kinase have been identified, with the exception of BAP-1, one of the 14-3-3 family members, which are widely expressed and bind to phosphoserine residues.[49,50] 14-3-3 proteins are abundant, small proteins that exist as dimers in the cytosol. They can bind to different signal transduction molecules such as the serine/threonine kinases Raf and protein kinase C. Dimeric 14-3-3 was shown to maintain Raf in an inactive state in the absence of GTP-bound Ras, whereas it appears to stabilize the active conformation of Raf after its in vivo activation.[51] In contrast, protein kinase C is inhibited by 14-3-3 binding.[52]

Braselmann and McCormick[49] identified 14-3-3$_{\beta}$ as one of 18 different targets using full-length BCR in the yeast two-hybrid system. Using a similar screen, we have also identified 14-3-3 as one of 12 different positives, which also included BCR itself and the XPB/ERCC-3 protein (A Reichert, N Heisterkamp, and J Groffen, unpublished).

Braselmann and McCormick[49] delineated the interacting region as residues 295–413, containing the S/T-rich 'B box' in the kinase domain of BCR. BCR can phosphorylate the 14-3-3 protein.[50] The binding of 14-3-3 to BCR also mediated complex formation between BCR and active, membrane-associated Raf, but complex formation did not influence Raf activation of the MAP kinase pathway, and nor were any other biological effects of complex formation evident.[49] Therefore, the significance of this interaction for the BCR S/T kinase activity or for Raf remains undefined.

Tyrosine phosphorylation of BCR

Although the function of the S/T kinase domain is not known, a number of studies have examined its regulation by tyrosine phosphorylation. The BCR/ABL protein tyrosine-phosphorylates residues Y177, Y283, Y328, and Y360 in BCR, which are all located in the region encoded by the first *BCR* exon. BCR mutants of tyrosine residue Y360 have reduced *trans*-S/T-phosphorylation activity, but still autophosphorylate, whereas Y328/Y360 double mutants lack both *trans*- and autophosphorylation activity. These data show that tyrosine phosphorylation regulates the ability of BCR to S/T-phosphorylate itself as well as other, exogenous, substrates.[53,54] Using baculovirus-expressed proteins, we have examined whether the tyrosine phosphorylation of BCR by BCR/ABL had any effect on the GTPase activating activity of the BCR C-terminal domain, but both tyrosine-phosphorylated and non-phosphorylated BCR stimulated GTP hydrolysis of Rac equally well.[31]

Three tyrosine kinases of the extended Src family have been shown to tyrosine-phosphorylate residues in BCR. These include normal ABL,[33] Fes, and Hck.[34,35] It is unknown whether BCR reciprocally S/T-phosphorylates any of these tyrosine kinases. The interaction between ABL and BCR is unusual, in that the ABL SH2 domain is capable of binding to a region encoded by *BCR* exon 1 in a phosphotyrosine-independent manner with a relatively low affinity.[55] In addition, non-tyrosine-phosphorylated BCR protein expressed in baculovirus bound to bacterially expressed SH2 domains of phospholipase C_γ (PLC_γ) (C-terminal + N-terminal SH2), Ras GAP (N-terminal SH2) and Shc.[56] However, Li and Smithgall[57] could detect no binding of the ABL SH2 domain to baculovirus-produced BCR in vitro, whereas tyrosine phosphorylation of BCR by Fes caused an association between the ABL SH2 domain and BCR. Apart from the ABL SH2 domain, the C-terminal $p85_\alpha$ phosphatidylinositol 3'-kinase (PI3-K) subunit SH2 domain also bound to phosphotyrosine residues in BCR. Thus it appears that although some SH2 domains can interact with the BCR protein in the absence of phosphotyrosine on the latter, binding is clearly enhanced by its presence.

Although Hck was shown to phosphorylate BCR tyrosine residue 177, it is unknown to what part of BCR/ABL it binds.[35] Fes phosphorylates residues Y177 and Y246 and one of the Y279/283/289 cluster of residues, all located in the region encoded by *BCR* exon 1. Similar to the effect of ABL, tyrosine phosphorylation of BCR by Fes suppresses the BCR S/T kinase activity towards the 14-3-3/BAP-1 protein in vitro.[57,58] As mentioned above, the binding of tyrosine-phosphorylated BCR to the SH2 domain of ABL was enhanced, as was the in vitro binding to the SH2 domains of Grb2 (also see below), ABL, Src, RasGAP, PLC_γ, and the $p85_\alpha$ subunit of PI3-K.[58] Binding of Fes to BCR was mediated by the Fes SH2 domain, which bound as efficiently as the ABL SH2 domain to BCR, and by an N-terminal domain of Fes including amino acid residues 1–347.[34] Co-expression of BCR and Fes in transfected cells showed that Fes autophosphorylation was enhanced.[57]

These data are of interest in that Fes is a tyrosine kinase whose expression is restricted mainly but not exclusively to hematopoietic (myeloid) cell types.[59–62] Increased tyrosine phosphorylation of Fes has been found in primary leukemic cells and in p210-expressing cell lines.[63] The combined results described above could provide a mechanism for this. However, the biological significance in vivo of the interactions of BCR with ABL, Fes, and Hck have not been defined.

Grb2- and Grb10-binding sites

Tyrosine residue 177 described above, when it is phosphorylated, is a binding site for the SH2 domain of Grb2. Since Grb2 can form a complex with Sos, an exchange factor for Ras, tyrosine phosphorylation of BCR or BCR/ABL on Y177 can link these proteins for example to the Ras pathway.[64,65] Although Sos is the most intensively studied Grb2 SH3-binding protein, other alternative binding proteins exist, such as Socs1, a downstream component of the Kit receptor tyrosine kinase pathway. Since Socs1 SH2 domain binding to the Kit receptor suppresses the mitogenic activity of Kit,[66] it could be of interest to examine putative BCR/ABL–Grb2–Socs1–Kit receptor complex formation.

Ras activation was first demonstrated by measuring the levels of Ras–GTP in murine myeloid cells transfected by *BCR/ABL*.[67] Also, Ras was shown to be necessary for soft agar growth of fibroblasts transfected by *BCR/ABL* and for high-density outgrowth of pre-B cells in murine bone marrow infected with retroviruses expressing BCR/ABL with or without dominant-negative Ras GAP or Ras.[68] However, the physiological significance of this is presently not clear, and it should therefore be informative to determine whether Ras is activated in primary patient material. This should now be feasible using recently described methods to measure Ras–GTP.[69]

Using tyrosine-phosphorylated BCR/ABL as a bait in a so-called yeast two-hybrid screen, Bai and colleagues[70] isolated a new BCR/ABL-binding protein, the adapter Grb10. The SH2 domain of Grb10 binds to a region in BCR encompassing amino acid residues 242–446. It was shown that BCR/ABL and Grb10 co-immunoprecipitate in CML cells.[70] Grb10 consists of a proline-rich region, a central pleckstrin homology (PH, also see below) domain, and a C-terminal SH2 domain. It was initially identified as a protein that binds to the activated insulin-like growth factor receptor, and is involved in downregulation of its signal.[71] The Grb10 SH2 domain binds in a phosphotyrosine-independent manner to the Raf1 and MEK1 S/T kinases.[72] It will be of interest to see through which domain Grb10 binds to BCR, because this will have implications for other components of a putative multiprotein complex including BCR.

Dbl homology (DH) domain

The proteins described above all bind to or interact with residues encoded by *BCR* exon 1, a region encompassing 426 amino acid residues (see Figure 1.1). Exons 3–9 encode a domain of around 206 amino acid residues, which has homology to the *dbl* proto-oncogene.[73,74] *dbl* was recovered as a transforming oncogene.[75] It was generated by the truncation of a protein that has exchange factor activity for members of the Rho family of GTPases.[76,77] Rho family members include Rac1, Rac2, and Rac3, as well as Cdc42 and the Rho proteins, and are associated with processes related to actin reorganization.[78] However, these GTP-binding proteins have since been implicated in a wide variety of cellular processes, including cellular transformation and production of reactive oxygen species (ROS) (for a review, see Van Aelst et al[79]). As with the Ras–GTPases, Rho family members act as molecular switches that exist in an active, GTP-bound and an inactive, GDP-bound form. Dbl family members convert Rho family members into their active configurations by catalyzing the exchange of bound GDP for GTP. A large number of putative exchange factors that contain a Dbl-homology (DH) domain have been isolated, some as transforming oncogenes. A number were shown to have exchange factor activity. However, there are also DH-containing proteins for which such activity for Rho family members could not be demonstrated initially, or at all.[79] For example, Sos was identified as an exchange factor for Ras, but it also contains a DH domain. Interestingly, tyrosine phosphorylation of Sos activates the DH domain so that it can then act as an exchange factor for Rac.[80] Similarly, Vav needs tyrosine phosphorylation for activation of its DH domain as an exchange factor for Rac,[81,82] and the PI3-K product phosphatidylinositol-3,4,5-trisphosphate enhances this.[83] In contrast, the Dbl-homology domain in the Ras-specific exchange factors GRF1 and GRF2 appears to have a different function. It mediates oligomer formation between GRF1 and GRF2, and thereby stimulates downstream activation of Raf.[84]

BCR and the related ABR protein[47,48] both contain a Dbl-homology domain. However, in comparison with Dbl, the exchange factor activity of this isolated domain in vitro is very modest, and appears to be somewhat better for Rho than for Rac.[85] It is possible that in vivo, additional interactions and/or modifications are needed to stimulate this exchange factor activity. However, there are no data indicating that this domain actually functions as an exchange factor for Rac family members in vivo. The issue is of more than merely academic interest, since this region plus the PH and C2 domains are what constitute the difference between the p190 and p210 forms of the BCR/ABL protein. Possibly, this question can be resolved with the application of new techniques to better detect activation of small GTPases.

Binding partners of the Dbl-homology domain: XPB/ERCC-3 protein

Takeda et al[86] have investigated which protein(s) could bind to the DH region by screening a human placental library in yeast using amino acid residues 413–789 of BCR as bait. The sole positive obtained was the XPB/ERCC-3 protein, a DNA helicase that is part of the TFIIH multiprotein complex required for class II gene transcription and nucleotide excision repair. Apart from the TFIIH components, XPB was also reported to bind to a subunit of the proteasome.[87]

Overexpressed GST-tagged full-length XPB was able to co-precipitate p210 BCR/ABL in transfected cells, and was tyrosine-phosphorylated by BCR/ABL. It also bound to overexpressed and to endogenous BCR protein. Interestingly, the XPB protein contained phosphotyrosine in three CML cell lines.[86] However, it is not readily apparent how and when this protein, which is predominantly in the nucleus, would interact with BCR, which is a putative exchange factor for the Rho family and which is located in the cytoplasm. The functional significance of the interaction between the normal cellular BCR protein and the XPB protein is currently also not clear.

Pleckstrin homology domain

The pleckstrin homology (PH) domain of Bcr is located C-terminal to the DH domain, approximately from residues 708 to 866 (Figure 1.1). It is a domain that mediates protein–lipid interactions in other proteins, and is found in many of the Dbl-homologous exchange factors. PH domains can regulate the activity of the proteins that contain them by targeting the protein to lipids in the membrane. Alternatively, these domains can locally increase the concentration of the proteins that carry them, enabling oligomerization to take place, which can result in activation (for a review, see Songyang[88]). Recently, it was reported that some PH domains are able to bind to F-actin, thus localizing the proteins that contain them to the cytoskeleton.[89] For BCR, no experiments have been performed to elucidate the role of the PH domain in BCR protein function, for example by deleting this domain and investigating the S/T kinase activity or GAP activity of the mutant. With respect to the BCR/ABL fusion protein, it is of interest to note that increased actin-binding and crosslinking activity was described when the BCR/ABL protein was compared with normal ABL, which has an actin-binding domain.[37,39,90] A possible actin-binding function of the PH domain of BCR may contribute to the more acutely transforming properties of the p190, which lacks the PH domain, as compared with p210.

C2 domain

This domain was recognized as a lipid-binding domain present in a wide variety of proteins such as phospholipases C and D (PLC and PLD), protein kinase C and BCR.[91,92] Many C2 domains bind membranes in a calcium-dependent manner. Some penetrate the hydrophobic region of the membrane, whereas others bind electrostatically,[93] for example to phosphatidylserine. However, the C2 domains of PLCβ1 and PLCβ2 do not bind membranes, but instead bind to activated (GTP-bound) $G_{\alpha q}$ subunits, themselves components of heterotrimeric G proteins. In this context, it should be noted that PLCβ1 and PLCβ2 are activated by binding to activated heterotrimeric G proteins.[94]

The possible function of the C2 domain in BCR has not been explored, but the data described above suggest a number of possibilities. Most remarkably, this region is missing from p190 BCR/ABL, and it almost perfectly coincides with the polypeptide encoded by M-*bcr* exons b2–b5 (residues 870–1002; Figure 1.1). Thus, breakpoints within M-*bcr* will disrupt it. It is of interest that the p230 protein should contain an intact C2 domain, which could partially determine the subcellular location of the BCR/ABL protein, and because of this may influence the potency of the effect of the fusion protein.

GTPase-activating protein (GAP) domain

This region approximately encompasses amino acid residues 1068–1212 of the BCR protein and is encoded by exons 19–22 (Figure 1.1). Therefore it is absent from the BCR/ABL fusion proteins. The activity of this domain is the best understood in vivo biological function of the BCR protein. In 1991, Diekmann and colleagues[95] reported that the C-terminal end of BCR had homology to the newly sequenced Rho GAP protein, and demonstrated that this region in BCR showed GTPase activating activity in vitro towards Rac.

Rho GAP homologous regions have subsequently been identified in a large number of other proteins, establishing that mammalian cells express a variety of GAPs for small GTPases of the Rho family.[79] Some of these may be specific for one or more Rho family members, whereas others may be tissue-specific or may be expressed in certain subcellular locations, or at different time points during development.

In vitro, BCR acts as a GAP for Rac1, Rac2, Rac3, and Cdc42, but not for Rho.[95–97] Since these small GTPases have a very high rate of spontaneous GTP hydrolysis in vitro, one could question the need for a GTPase-activating protein to catalyze this conversion. In vivo however, Rac–GTP is likely to be complexed to other proteins, which could stabilize the GTP-bound form.[79] Indeed, the so-called CRIB domains of some Rho family member effectors retain these small GTPases in their GTP-bound form, which has resulted in their use as a tool to specifically detect the activated, GTP-bound form (see e.g. Benard et al[98]).

THE WHOLE BCR PROTEIN IN VIVO

Many of the results described above were obtained more or less in vitro. Because Ph-positive leukemia is a disease of hematopoietic cell types, it was of interest to examine the normal cellular function of the BCR protein in vivo in such cells. To this end, we used homologous recombination to generate a null mutant *bcr* mouse.[99]

These mice are viable and fertile, and because of this we were able to generate *bcr*-null animals also expressing BCR/ABL p190. The long-term follow-up of a cohort of these mice and of matched wild-type BCR/ABL p190 mice showed that the absence or presence of endogenous BCR had no effect on the latency or speed of leukemogenesis. This result indicates that although cellular BCR can form complexes with BCR/ABL via the BCR N-terminal oligomerization domain, this does not have a measurable effect on the speed with which leukemia develops in vivo.[31] However, other studies in cell lines suggest that BCR can act as a negative regulator of the BCR/ABL oncoprotein. Overexpression of the normal BCR protein in *BCR/ABL*-transfected cells was found to cause a decrease in the amount of cellular phosphotyrosine and in the transformation efficiency of BCR/ABL. The inhibitory effect of BCR was dependent upon achieving elevated levels of BCR expression relative to that of BCR/ABL.[100]

The *bcr*-null mutants were also tested for the function of their different hematopoietic compartments. A very clear difference with control wild-type mice was found in the oxidative burst, one function of professional phagocytes, which they utilize to kill microorganisms. *bcr*-null mutant neutrophils were shown to be more sensitive to priming stimuli than wild-type and to have more ROS production. In an experimental model for endotoxemia (septic shock), *bcr*-null mutants were found to be severely affected by doses of lipopolysaccharide that had very little effect on wild-type mice, but which even resulted in the death of some of the null mutants. This experiment and others showed that one function of BCR pertains to the regulation of the oxidative burst in macrophages and neutrophils. Since one of the regulators of the oxidative burst is Rac2 (for a recent review, see Baboir[101]), a possible substrate for BCR, the level of membrane-bound Rac2 was compared in null and wild-type neutrophils after stimulation of these cells to produce the oxidative burst. The increase of membrane-bound Rac2 in the null mutant confirmed that an important function of BCR in vivo in myeloid cells is to regulate GTP-bound levels of Rac2.[99] This result was also of interest in view of the leukemogenic properties of BCR/ABL in myeloid-lineage cells in CML.

Although not discussed above, BCR is not a hematopoietic-specific protein. In fact, it is ubiquitously expressed, albeit at different levels, with the highest overall levels detected in brain.[47,102–104] Thus, it was surprising that the phenotype of the *bcr*-null mutants was relatively mild. One other feature by which these mice distinguished themselves was by decreased body weight and markedly increased fighting behavior among males.

We explored this difference using several approaches, and concluded that the null mutants show a defect in the regulation of hormonal and behavioral stress response. Increased plasma glucocorticoid levels were found after physiological stress, as well as signs of consistently elevated catabolism in general. Therefore, it is likely that BCR downregulates some aspect of Rac function that is involved in mediating the effects of glucocorticoids.[105]

CONCLUSIONS AND PERSPECTIVES

More than 15 years have elapsed since the identification of the breakpoint cluster region gene. We now have a global understanding of one of the functions of one of the domains of this protein in hematopoietic cells: regulation of ROS production via the small GTPase Rac2. Extrapolating from what is currently known, it is possible that normal BCR functions to regulate ROS production in cell types other than professional phagocytes such as macrophages and neutrophils, since there is increasing evidence that other cell types use ROS as normal signaling mediators and that this may also be regulated by Racs.[106–108] Indeed, a homologue of the catalytic subunit of the superoxide-generating NADPH oxidase of phagocytes was recently isolated and found to be expressed in different tissues. Overexpression of this gene caused enhanced ROS production and transformation of fibroblasts.[109]

It remains to be seen if regulation of ROS production by Rac is the only function executed by the large, multidomain BCR protein, or whether BCR is also involved in other regulatory functions associated with Rac.[79] Apart from the GAP domain, there is no clear understanding of the function of the S/T kinase, DH, PH, and C2 domains within the BCR protein or in the cell. With the increasing knowledge of signal transduction processes and the domains that mediate the signals, it should be possible to design focused experiments to investigate this. Such information should be of value in view of the possible biological role of BCR in control of the oxidative burst; sepsis syndrome is the leading cause of death in adult non-coronary intensive care units.[110] Finally, an understanding of the functions of the different subdomains of BCR should certainly lead to improved insight into the role of these domains within the BCR/ABL protein.

ACKNOWLEDGEMENTS

This work was supported by PHS Grants CA47456 to JG and CA50248 to NH. An extensive body of literature has been published on *BCR/ABL* in the past 17 years, and unfortunately it is impossible to cite all the excellent original papers dealing with the topic covered by this chapter.

REFERENCES

1. Nowell P, Hungerford D, A minute chromosome in human granulocytic leukemia. *Science* 1960; **132:** 1497.
2. Rowley JD, A new consistent chromosomal abnormality in chronic myelogenous leukemia identified by quinacrine fluorescence and Giemsa staining. *Nature* 1973; **243:** 290–3.

3. Heisterkamp N, Groffen J, Stephenson JR, The human v-abl cellular homologue. *J Mol Appl Genet* 1983; **2:** 57–68.
4. Heisterkamp N, Groffen J, Stephenson JR et al, Chromosomal localization of human cellular homologues of two viral oncogenes. *Nature* 1982; **299:** 747–9.
5. de Klein A, Geurts van Kessel A, Grosveld G et al, A cellular oncogene is translocated to the Philadelphia chromosome in chronic myelocytic leukemia. *Nature* 1982; **300:** 765–7.
6. Heisterkamp N, Stephenson JR, Groffen J et al, Localization of the c-abl oncogene adjacent to a translocation breakpoint in chronic myelocytic leukemia. *Nature* 1983; **306:** 239–42.
7. Bernards A, Rubin CM, Westbrook CA et al, The first intron in the human c-abl gene is at least 200 kilobases long and is a target for translocations in chronic myelogenous leukemia. *Mol Cell Biol* 1987; **7:** 3231–6.
8. Melo JV, BCR–ABL gene variants. *Baillière's Clin Haematol* 1997; **10:** 203–22.
9. Melo JV, The diversity of BCR–ABL fusion proteins and their relationship to leukemia phenotype. *Blood* 1996; **88:** 2375–84.
10. Groffen J, Stephenson JR, Heisterkamp N et al, Philadelphia chromosomal breakpoints are clustered within a limited region, bcr, on chromosome 22. *Cell* 1984; **36:** 93–9.
11. Heisterkamp N, Stam K, Groffen J et al, Structural organization of the *bcr* gene and its role in the Ph' translocation. *Nature* 1985; **315:** 758–61.
12. Melo JV, Gordon DE, Cross NC, Goldman JM, The ABL–BCR fusion gene is expressed in chronic myeloid leukemia. *Blood* 1993; **81:** 158–65.
13. Melo JV, Gordon DE, Tuszynski A et al, Expression of the ABL–BCR fusion gene in Philadelphia-positive acute lymphoblastic leukemia. *Blood* 1993; **81:** 2488–91.
14. Heisterkamp N, Knoppel E, Groffen J, The first BCR gene intron contains breakpoints in Philadelphia chromosome positive leukemia. *Nucleic Acids Res* 1988; **16:** 10069–81.
15. Chissoe SL, Bodenteich A, Wang Y-F et al, Sequence and analysis of the human ABL gene, the BCR gene, and regions involved in the Philadelphia chromosomal translocation. *Genomics* 1995; **27:** 67–82.
16. McLaughlin J, Chianese E, Witte ON, Alternative forms of the BCR–ABL oncogene have quantitatively different potencies for stimulation of immature lymphoid cells. *Mol Cell Biol* 1989; **9:** 1866–74.
17. McLaughlin J, Chianese E, Witte ON, In vitro transformation of immature hematopoietic cells by the P210 BCR/ABL oncogene product of the Philadelphia chromosome. *Proc Natl Acad Sci USA* 1987; **84:** 6558–62.
18. Lugo TG, Pendergast AM, Muller AJ, Witte ON, Tyrosine kinase activity and transformation potency of bcr–abl oncogene products. *Science* 1990; **247:** 1079–82.
19. Kelliher M, Knott A, McLaughlin J et al, Differences in oncogenic potency but not target cell specificity distinguish the two forms of the BCR/ABL oncogene. *Mol Cell Biol* 1991; **11:** 4710–16.
20. Voncken JW, Kaartinen V, Germeraad WTV et al, BCR/ABL p210 and p190 cause distinct leukemia in transgenic mice. *Blood* 1995; **86:** 4603–11.
21. Li S, Ilaria RL Jr, Million RP et al, The p190, P210, and P230 forms of the BCR/ABL oncogene induce a similar chronic myeloid leukemia-like syndrome in mice but have different lymphoid leukemogenic activity. *J Exp Med* 1999; **189:** 1399–412.
22. Saglio G, Guerrasio A, Rosso C et al, New types of Bcr/Abl junction in Philadelphia chromosome-positive chronic myelogenous leukemia. *Blood* 1990; **76:** 1819–24.
23. Pane F, Frigeri F, Sindona M et al, Neutrophilic-chronic myeloid leukemia: a distinct disease with a specific molecular marker. *Blood* 1996; **88:** 2410–14.
24. Kozubek S, Lukasova E, Ryznar L et al, Distribution of ABL and BCR genes in cell nuclei of normal and irradiated lymphocytes. *Blood* 1997; **89:** 4537–45.
25. Lukasova E, Kozubek S, Kozubek M et al, Localization and distance between ABL and BCR genes in interphase nuclei of bone marrow cells of control donors and patients with chronic myeloid leukaemia. *Hum Genet* 1997; **100:** 525–35.
26. Neves H, Ramos C, da Silva MG et al, The nuclear topography of ABL, BCR, PML, and RARalpha genes: evidence for gene proximity in specific phases of the cell cycle and stages of hematopoietic differentiation. *Blood* 1999; **93:** 1197–207.
27. Li WJ, Dreazen O, Kloetzer W et al,

Characterization of bcr gene products in hematopoietic cells. *Oncogene* 1989; **4:** 127–38.
28. Dhut S, Chaplin T, Young BD, BCR–ABL and BCR proteins: biochemical characterization and localization. *Leukemia* 1990; **4:** 745–50.
29. Hariharan IK, Adams JM, DNA sequence for human bcr, the gene that translocates to the abl oncogene in chronic myeloid leukaemia. *EMBO J* 1987; **6:** 115–19.
30. Zhu QS, Heisterkamp N, Groffen J, Unique organization of the human BCR gene promoter. *Nucleic Acids Res* 1990; **18:** 7119–25.
31. Voncken JW, Kaartinen V, Groffen J, Heisterkamp N, Bcr/Abl associated leukemogenesis in bcr null mutant mice. *Oncogene* 1998; **16:** 2029–32.
32. Liu J, Campbell M, Guo JG et al, Bcr–Abl tyrosine kinase is autophosphorylated or transphosphorylates p160 BCR on tyrosine predominantly within the first BCR exon. *Oncogene* 1993; **8:** 101–9.
33. Ma G, Lu D, Wu Y et al, Bcr phosphorylated on tyrosine 177 binds Grb2. *Oncogene* 1997; **14:** 2367–72.
34. Maru Y, Peters KL, Afar DEH et al, Tyrosine phosphorylation of BCR by FPS/FES protein-tyrosine kinases induces association of BCR with GRB-2/SOS. *Mol Cell Biol* 1995; **15:** 835–42.
35. Warmuth M, Bergmann M, Priess A et al, The Src family kinase Hck interacts with Bcr–Abl by a kinase-independent mechanism and phosphorylates the Grb2-binding site of Bcr. *J Biol Chem* 1997; **272:** 33260–70.
36. McWhirter JR, Galasso DL, Wang JY, A coiled-coil oligomerization domain of Bcr is essential for the transforming function of Bcr–Abl oncoproteins. *Mol Cell Biol* 1993; **13:** 7587–95.
37. McWhirter JR, Wang JY, Activation of tyrosinase kinase and microfilament-binding functions of c-abl by bcr sequences in bcr/abl fusion proteins. *Mol Cell Biol* 1991; **11:** 1553–65.
38. McWhirter JR, Wang JY, Effect of Bcr sequences on the cellular function of the Bcr–Abl oncoprotein. *Oncogene* 1997; **15:** 1625–34.
39. McWhirter JR, Wang JY, An actin-binding function contributes to transformation by the Bcr–Abl oncoprotein of Philadelphia chromosome-positive human leukemias. *EMBO J* 1993; **12:** 1533–46.
40. Maru Y, Afar DE, Witte ON, Shibuya M, The dimerization property of glutathione S-transferase partially reactivates Bcr–Abl lacking the oligomerization domain. *J Biol Chem* 1996; **271:** 15353–7.
41. Okuda K, D'Andrea A, Van Etten RA, Griffin JD, A chimeric receptor/oncogene that can be regulated by a ligand in vitro and in vivo. *J Clin Invest* 1997; **100:** 1708–15.
42. Papadopoulos P, Ridge SA, Boucher CA et al, The novel activation of ABL by fusion to an ets-related gene, TEL. *Cancer Res* 1995; **55:** 34–8.
43. Hannemann JR, McManus DM, Kabarowski JH, Wiedemann LM, Haemopoietic transformation by the TEL/ABL oncogene. *Br J Haematol* 1998; **102:** 475–85.
44. Okuda K, Golub TR, Gilliland DG, Griffin JD, p210BCR/ABL, p190BCR/ABL, and TEL/ABL activate similar signal transduction pathways in hematopoietic cell lines. *Oncogene* 1996; **13:** 1147–52.
45. Stam K, Heisterkamp N, Reynolds FHJ, Groffen J, Evidence that the Ph[1] gene encodes a 160,000-dalton phosphoprotein with associated kinase activity. *Mol Cell Biol* 1987; **7:** 1955–60.
46. Maru Y, Witte ON, The BCR gene encodes a novel serine/threonine kinase activity within a single exon. *Cell* 1991; **67:** 459–68.
47. Heisterkamp N, Kaartinen V, van Soest S et al, Human ABR encodes a protein with GAPrac activity and homology to the DBL nucleotide exchange factor domain. *J Biol Chem* 1993; **268:** 16903–6.
48. Tan E-C, Leung T, Manser E, Lim L, The human active breakpoint cluster region-related gene encodes a brain protein with homology to guanine nucleotide exchange proteins and GTPase-activating proteins. *J Biol Chem* 1993; **268:** 27291–8.
49. Braselmann S, McCormick F, BCR and RAF form a complex in vivo via 14-3-3 proteins. *EMBO J* 1995; **14:** 4839–48.
50. Reuther GW, Fu H, Cripe LD et al, Association of the protein kinases c-BCR and Bcr–Abl with proteins of the 14-3-3 family. *Science* 1994; **266:** 129–33.
51. Tzivion G, Luo Z, Avruch J, A dimeric 14-3-3 protein is an essential cofactor for Raf kinase activity. *Nature* 1998; **394:** 88–92.
52. Hausser A, Storz P, Link G et al, Protein kinase C mu is negatively regulated by 14-3-3 signal transduction proteins. *J Biol Chem* 1999; **274:** 9258–64.
53. Liu J, Wu Y, Ma GZ et al, Inhibition of Bcr serine kinase by tyrosine phosphorylation. *Mol Cell Biol* 1996; **16:** 998–1005.

54. Wu Y, Liu J, Arlinghaus RB, Requirement of two specific tyrosine residues for the catalytic activity of Bcr serine/threonine kinase. *Oncogene* 1998; **16:** 141–6.
55. Pendergast AM, Muller AJ, Havlik MH et al, BCR sequences essential for transformation by the BCR–ABL oncogene bind to the ABL SH2 regulatory domain in a non-phosphotyrosine-dependent manner. *Cell* 1991; **66:** 161–71.
56. Muller AJ, Pendergast A-M, Havlik MH et al, A limited set of SH2 domains binds BCR through a high-affinity phosphotyrosine-independent interaction. *Mol Cell Biol* 1992; **12:** 5087–93.
57. Li J, Smithgall TE, Co-expression with BCR induces activation of the FES tyrosine kinase and phosphorylation of specific N-terminal BCR tyrosine residues. *J Biol Chem* 1996; **271:** 32930–6.
58. Peters KL, Smithgall TE, Tyrosine phosphorylation enhances the SH2 domain-binding activity of Bcr and inhibits Bcr interaction with 14-3-3 proteins. *Cell Signal* 1999; **11:** 507–14.
59. MacDonald I, Levy J, Pawson T, Expression of the mammalian c-fes protein in hematopoietic cells and identification of a distinct fes-related protein. *Mol Cell Biol* 1985; **10:** 2543–51.
60. Feldman RA, Gabrilove JL, Tam JP et al, Specific expression of the human cellular fps/fes-encoded protein NCP92 in normal and leukemic myeloid cells. *Proc Natl Acad Sci USA* 1985; **82:** 2379–83.
61. Ferrari S, Torelli U, Selleri L et al, Expression of human c-fes onc-gene occurs at detectable levels in myeloid but not in lymphoid cell populations. *Br J Haematol* 1985; **59:** 21–5.
62. Haigh J, McVeigh J, Greer P, The fps/fes tyrosine kinase is expressed in myeloid, vascular endothelial, epithelial, and neuronal cells and is localized in the trans-Golgi network. *Cell Growth Differ* 1996; **7:** 931–44.
63. Ernst TJ, Slattery KE, Griffin JD, p210Bcr/Abl and p160v-Abl induce an increase in the tyrosine phosphorylation of p93c-Fes. *J Biol Chem* 1994; **269:** 5764–9.
64. Pendergast AM, Quilliam LA, Cripe LD et al, BCR–ABL-induced oncogenesis is mediated by direct interaction with the SH2 domain of the GRB-2 adaptor protein. *Cell* 1993; **75:** 175–85.
65. Puil L, Liu J, Gish G et al, Bcr–Abl oncoproteins bind directly to activators of the Ras signalling pathway. *EMBO J* 1994; **13:** 764–73.
66. De Sepulveda P, Okkenhaug K, Rose JL et al, Socs1 binds to multiple signalling proteins and suppresses steel factor-dependent proliferation. *EMBO J* 1999; **18:** 904–15.
67. Mandanas RA, Leibowitz DS, Gharehbaghi K et al, Role of p21 RAS in p210 bcr–abl transformation of murine myeloid cells. *Blood* 1993; **82:** 1838–47.
68. Sawyers CL, McLaughlin J, Witte ON, Genetic requirement for Ras in the transformation of fibroblasts and hematopoietic cells by the Bcr–Abl oncogene. *J Exp Med* 1995; **181:** 307–13.
69. De Rooij J, Bos JL, Minimal Ras-binding domain of Raf1 can be used as an activation-specific probe for Ras. *Oncogene* 1997; **14:** 623–5.
70. Bai RY, Jahn T, Schrem S et al, The SH2-containing adapter protein GRB10 interacts with BCR–ABL. *Oncogene* 1998; **17:** 941–8.
71. Morrione A, Valentinis B, Li S et al, Grb10: a new substrate of the insulin-like growth factor I receptor. *Cancer Res* 1996; **56:** 3165–7.
72. Nantel A, Mohammad-Ali K, Sherk J et al, Interaction of the Grb10 adapter protein with the Raf1 and MEK1 kinases. *J Biol Chem* 1998; **273:** 10475–84.
73. Ron D, Zannini M, Lewis M et al, A region of proto-dbl essential for its transforming activity shows sequence similarity to a yeast cell cycle gene, CDC24, and the human breakpoint cluster gene, bcr. *New Biol* 1991; **3:** 372–9.
74. Adams JM, Houston H, Allen J et al, The hematopoietically expressed vav proto-oncogene shares homology with the dbl GDP–GTP exchange factor, the bcr gene and a yeast gene (CDC24) involved in cytoskeletal organization. *Oncogene* 1992; **7:** 611–18.
75. Eva A, Aaronson SA, Isolation of a new human oncogene from a diffuse B-cell lymphoma. *Nature* 1985; **316:** 273–5.
76. Hart MJ, Eva A, Zangrill D et al, Cellular transformation and guanine nucleotide exchange activity are catalyzed by a common domain on the *dbl* oncogene product. *J Biol Chem* 1994; **269:** 62–5.
77. Hart MJ, Eva A, Evans T et al, Catalysis of guanine nucleotide exchange on the CDC42Hs protein by the dbl oncogene product. *Nature* 1991; **354:** 311–14.
78. Hall A, Rho GTPases and the actin cytoskeleton. *Science* 1998; **279:** 509–13.
79. Van Aelst L, D'Souza-Schorey C, Rho GTPases and signalling networks. *Genes Dev* 1997; **11:** 2295–322.

80. Nimnual AS, Yatsula BA, Bar-Sagi D, Coupling of Ras and Rac guanosine triphosphates through the Ras exchanger Sos. *Science* 1998; **279:** 560–6.
81. Crespo P, Schuebel KE, Ostrom AA et al, Phosphotyrosine-dependent activation of Rac-1 GDP/GTP exchange by the vav proto-oncogene product. *Nature* 1997; **385:** 169–72.
82. Han J, Das B, Wei W et al, Lck regulates Vav activation of members of the Rho family of GTPases. *Mol Cell Biol* 1997; **17:** 1346–53.
83. Han J, Luby-Phelps K, Das B et al, Role of substrates and products of PI 3-kinase in regulating activation of Rac-related guanosine triphosphatases by Vav. *Science* 1998; **279:** 558–60.
84. Anborgh PH, Qian X, Papageorge AG et al, Ras-specific exchange factor GRF: oligomerization through its Dbl homology domain and calcium-dependent activation of Raf. *Mol Cell Biol* 1999; **19:** 4611–22.
85. Xu X, Chuang T-H, Kaartinen V et al, Abr and Bcr are multifunctional proteins which regulate the Rho family GTP-binding proteins. *Proc Natl Acad Sci USA* 1995; **92:** 10282–6.
86. Takeda N, Shibuya M, Maru Y, The BCR–ABL oncoprotein potentially interacts with the xeroderma pigmentosum group B protein. *Proc Natl Acad Sci USA* 1999; **96:** 203–7.
87. Weeda G, Rossignol M, Fraser RA et al, The XPB subunit of repair/transcription factor TFIIH directly interacts with SUG1, a subunit of the 26S proteasome and putative transcription factor. *Nucleic Acids Res* 1997; **25:** 2274–83.
88. Songyang Z, Recognition and regulation of primary-sequence motifs by signaling modular domains. *Prog Biophys Mol Biol* 1999; **71:** 359–72.
89. Yao L, Janmey P, Frigeri LG et al, Pleckstrin homology domains interact with filamentous actin. *J Biol Chem* 1999; **274:** 19752–61.
90. Van Etten RA, Jackson P, Baltimore D, The mouse type IV c-abl gene product is a nuclear protein, and activation of transforming ability is associated with cytoplasmic localization. *Cell* 1989; **58:** 669–78.
91. Ponting CP, Parker PJ, Extending the C2 domain family: C2s in PKCs delta, epsilon, eta, theta, phospholipases, GAPs, and perforin. *Protein Sci* 1996; **5:** 162–6.
92. Nalefski EA, Falke JJ, The C2 domain calcium-binding motif: structural and functional diversity. *Protein Sci* 1996; **5:** 2375–90.
93. Davletov B, Perisic O, Williams RL, Calcium-dependent membrane penetration is a hallmark of the C2 domain of cytosolic phospholipase A2 whereas the C2A domain of synaptotagmin binds membranes electrostatically. *J Biol Chem* 1998; **273:** 19093–6.
94. Wang T, Pentyala S, Elliott JT et al, Selective interaction of the C2 domains of phospholipase C-beta1 and -beta2 with activated galphaq subunits: an alternative function for C2-signaling modules. *Proc Natl Acad Sci USA* 1999; **96:** 7843–6.
95. Diekmann D, Brill S, Garrett MD et al, Bcr encodes a GTPase-activating protein for p21rac. *Nature* 1991; **351:** 400–2.
96. Chuang TH, Xu X, Kaartinen V et al, Abr and Bcr are multifunctional regulators of the Rho GTP-binding family. *Proc Natl Acad Sci USA* 1995; **92:** 10282–6.
97. Haataja L, Fioretos T, Groffen J, Heisterkamp N, Characterization of Rac3, a novel member of the Rho family. *J Biol Chem* 1997; **272:** 20384–8.
98. Benard V, Bohl BP, Bokoch GM, Characterization of Rac and Cdc42 activation in chemoattractant-stimulated human neutrophils using a novel assay for active GTPases. *J Biol Chem* 1999; **274:** 13198–204.
99. Voncken JW, van Schaik H, Kaartinen V et al, Increased neutrophil respiratory burst in bcr-null mutants. *Cell* 1995; **80:** 719–28.
100. Wu Y, Ma G, Lu D et al, Bcr: a negative regulator of the Bcr–Abl oncoprotein. *Oncogene* 1999; **18:** 4416–24.
101. Baboir BM, NADPH oxidase: an update. *Blood* 1999; **93:** 1464–76.
102. Collins S, Coleman H, Groudine M, Expression of bcr and bcr–abl fusion transcripts in normal and leukemic cells. *Mol Cell Biol* 1987; **7:** 2870–6.
103. Lifshitz B, Fainstein E, Marcelle C et al, Bcr genes and transcripts. *Oncogene* 1988; **2:** 113–17.
104. Fioretos T, Voncken JW, Baram TZ et al, Regional localization and developmental expression of the *BCR* gene in rodent brain. *Cell Mol Biol Res* 1995; **41:** 97–102.
105. Voncken JW, Baram TZ, Gonzales-Gomez I et al, Abnormal stress response and increased fighting behavior in mice lacking the bcr gene product. *Int J Mol Med* 1998; **2:** 577–83.
106. Sundaresan M, Yu ZX, Ferrans VJ et al, Regulation of reactive-oxygen-species generation in fibroblasts by Rac1. *Biochem J* 1996; **318:** 379–82.
107. Irani K, Xia Y, Zweier JL et al, Mitogenic signal-

ing mediated by oxidants in Ras-transformed fibroblasts. *Science* 1997; **275:** 1649–52.
108. Joneson T, Bar-Sagi D, A Rac1 effector site controlling mitogenesis through superoxide production. *J Biol Chem* 1998; **273:** 17991–4.
109. Suh Y-A, Arnold RS, Lassegue B et al, Cell transformation by the superoxide-generating oxidase Mox1. *Nature* 1999; **401:** 79–82.
110. Schoenberg MH, Weiss M, Radermacher O, Outcome of patients with sepsis and septic shock after ICU treatment. *Langenbecks Arch Surg* 1998; **383:** 44–8.

2

BCR/ABL protein domain function and signaling

Ann Marie Pendergast

CONTENTS • Introduction • *BCR/ABL* and human leukemias: diverse BCR/ABL chimeric proteins give rise to distinct disease phenotypes • Involvement of specific BCR/ABL sequences in oncogenic transformation • Signaling pathways downstream of BCR/ABL • Conclusions and future directions

INTRODUCTION

Studies carried out over 20 years ago first linked the ABL kinases to the development of cancer.[1] Oncogenic activation of c-*ABL* was initially shown to occur as a result of structural alterations of the c-ABL protein. Four naturally occurring c-*ABL*-derived oncogenes have been identified to date. They are the v-*abl* oncogene of the Abelson murine leukemia virus (A-MuLV),[2] the v-*abl* oncogene of the Hardy–Zuckerman-2 feline sarcoma virus (HZ2-FSV),[3] the *BCR/ABL* chimeric oncogene of Philadelphia chromosome positive human leukemias,[4,5] and the *TEL/ABL* chimeric oncogene associated with acute lymphoblastic and myeloid human leukemias.[6,7] The BCR/ABL and TEL/ABL proteins arise as a consequence of chromosomal translocation events that fuse N-terminal sequences from the *BCR* and *TEL* genes, respectively, to sequences upstream of the second exon of c-*ABL*.[4,5,7] The N-terminal sequences derived from the BCR and TEL proteins provide oligomerization domains and other sequences important for the oncogenicity of the chimeric proteins. Interestingly, unlike the normal c-ABL protein, which localizes to nuclear and cytosolic compartments, the majority of the oncogenic ABL proteins localize predominantly to the cytoplasm.[8,9] This chapter will focus primarily on our current understanding of the contribution of specific domains in BCR/ABL to oncogenesis and the identification of signaling pathways employed by BCR/ABL to transform cells.

BCR/ABL AND HUMAN LEUKEMIAS: DIVERSE BCR/ABL CHIMERIC PROTEINS GIVE RISE TO DISTINCT DISEASE PHENOTYPES

The *BCR/ABL* oncogene arises as a result of a chromosomal translocation event between human chromosomes 9 and 22, designated as the Philadelphia chromosome (Ph) or t(9;22)(q34;q11).[10] The translocation produces at least three distinct chimeric *BCR/ABL* oncogenes, which are associated with several forms of human leukemia.[5] Over 95% of patients with chronic myeloid leukemia (CML) have the Ph and express a *BCR/ABL* chimeric gene in their leukemic cells.[11,12] CML was the first disease linked to a specific chromosomal abnormality that was later shown to involve the activation of a specific oncogene. The t(9;22)(q34;q11) translocation is also found in 10–20% of adults and 2–5% of children with acute lymphoblastic leukemia (ALL), some cases of acute myeloid leukemia (AML), lymphoma, myeloma, and more recently, Ph-positive chronic neutrophilic leukemia (CNL).[5,13,14] The most compelling evidence implicating the *BCR/ABL* oncogenes as the causative elements in Ph-positive CML and ALL is their ability to induce leukemias in mice.[15–21]

The translocation between chromosomes 9 and 22 juxtaposes variable sequences from the *BCR* (breakpoint cluster region) gene on chromosome 22 to the majority of the c-*ABL* gene on chromosome 9. The breakpoint in chromosome 9 usually occurs upstream of exon 2 of c-*ABL*, and therefore the chimeric proteins contain the ABL SH3 domain and all the ABL sequences downstream of this domain[4,5] (Figure 2.1). In contrast, the breakpoints in *BCR* usually occur within one of three regions, designated the major breakpoint cluster region (M-*bcr*), the minor breakpoint cluster region (m-*bcr*), and a breakpoint located in the 3′ end of the gene (μ-*bcr*) (Figure 2.1). The hybrid genes generate three distinct transcripts and corresponding protein products designated p185, p210, and p230, which are associated with the m-*bcr*, M-*bcr*, and μ-*bcr* breakpoints, respectively (Figure 2.1).

A correlation exists between the structure of the chimeric BCR/ABL proteins and the various hematological malignancies associated with their expression. The smaller p185 BCR/ABL (also known as p190 BCR/ABL) is associated primarily with ALL, p210 BCR/ABL is primarily associated with CML and some cases of ALL, and p230 BCR/ABL is mainly linked to CNL. CML is a clonal myeloproliferative disorder that results from neoplastic transformation of the primitive hematopoietic stem cell.[22] The disease is characterized by an initial chronic phase lasting for 3–5 years and leading to a blastic phase. The blastic phase resembles an acute leukemia, and is generally fatal. During the initial chronic phase of CML, myeloid progenitor cells retain their ability to differentiate and increase in number. Progression of the disease is associated with accelerated growth of immature myeloid or lymphoid cells that lose their capacity to differentiate.[4,5] Thus, expression of p210 BCR/ABL appears to have a subtle effect on the growth of multipotent hematopoietic progenitor cells, and does not block their ability to differentiate. Use of in vitro cell culture systems has confirmed that expression of p210 BCR/ABL in bone-marrow-derived multipotent progenitor cells results in the growth of mixed-lineage colonies that are growth-factor-dependent and retain their ability to differentiate.[23] In contrast, expression of p185 BCR/ABL is most commonly associated with ALL[24] and AML,[25] highly aggressive malignancies that involve the proliferation of early lymphoid and myeloid precursors that fail to differentiate.[26] More recently, a novel chimeric *BCR/ABL* fusion gene was identified that encodes the majority of the *BCR* gene and is associated with the μ-*bcr* breakpoint. The protein product of the translocation was predicted to be a 230 kDa protein. This chimeric BCR/ABL molecule is associated with CNL, a rare myeloproliferative disorder characterized by a mild hematological phenotype and a low tendency to acute blastic transformation.[13,14] Cells expressing this novel chimeric p230 BCR/ABL fusion appear to have a limited proliferative advantage, and exhibit little disruption in the normal process of granulocytic differentiation compared with those cells expressing the p210 BCR/ABL protein associated with CML.[13] Indeed, CNL is characterized by the presence of large numbers of mature neutrophils and an indolent or benign clinical course. However, a few patients with typical CML have been reported to have the μ-*bcr* breakpoint that generates p230 BCR/ABL.[27–29]

The inclusion or exclusion of specific BCR sequences in the various BCR/ABL chimeras may determine the disease phenotype. In general, the smaller the amount of BCR sequence

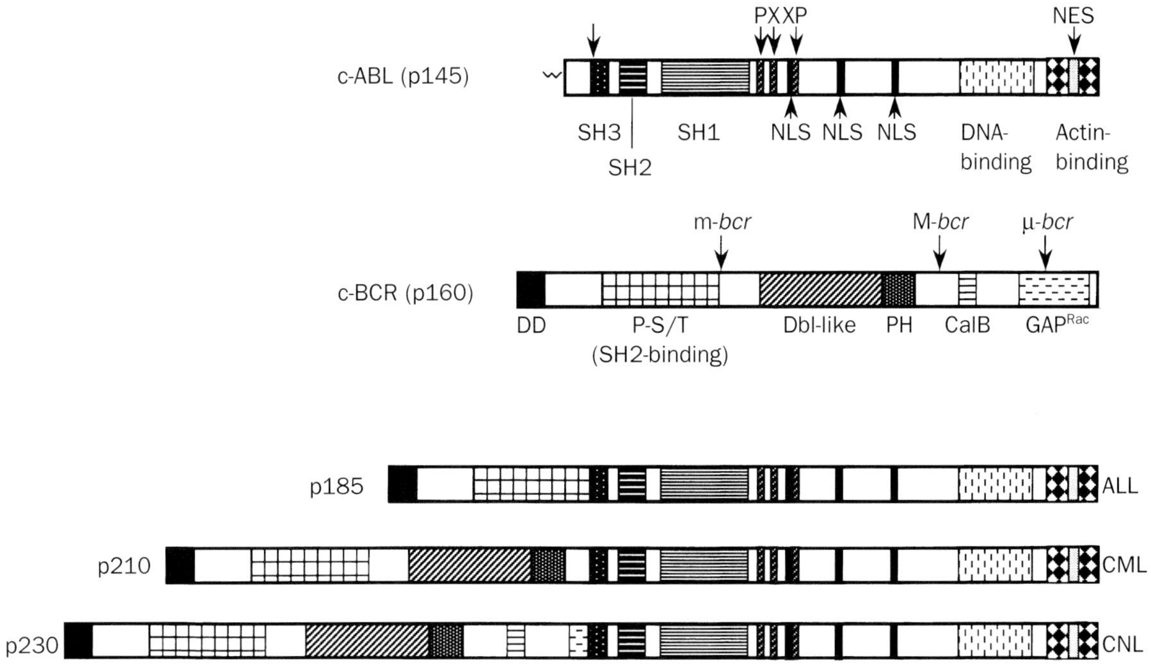

Figure 2.1 Structural features of c-ABL, c-BCR, and BCR/ABL. The structures of c-ABL (p145), c-BCR (p160), and the three BCR/ABL fusion proteins are shown. The p185 BCR/ABL protein is primarily associated with ALL, p210 BCR/ABL with CML, and p230 BCR/ABL with CNL. Structural domains in c-BCR are the dimerization domain (DD), the proline-, serine-, threonine-rich domain that binds SH2 domains in a phosphotyrosine-independent manner, the Dbl-like domain, the pleckstrin homology (PH) domain, the calcium-phospholipid-binding (CalB) domain, and the GTPase-activating protein for $p21^{Rac}$ domain (GAP^{Rac}). Structural domains in c-ABL are the SH3, SH2, and SH1 (tyrosine kinase) domains, proline-rich sequences that contain PXXP motifs for SH3 domain binding, three nuclear localization signals (NLS), the DNA-binding domain, the actin-binding domain, and the nuclear export signal (NES). The arrows indicate the positions of the breakpoints in c-ABL and c-BCR.

retained in a chimeric BCR/ABL protein, the more aggressive is the phenotype of the leukemia associated with its expression. This correlation has also been observed for p185 and p210 BCR/ABL following their expression in transgenic mice.[18] Mice expressing p210 BCR/ABL developed leukemia of myeloid and B- and T-lymphoid origin after a relatively long latency period. In contrast, the p185 BCR/ABL transgenic mice developed exclusively leukemias of B-cell origin with a relatively short latency.[18] Thus, in this murine transgenic model, comparable expression of p210 and p185 BCR/ABL oncoproteins results in biologically distinct phenotypes that mirror the clinical presentation of the human leukemias associated with their expression. The molecular basis for the distinct pathologies associated with p210 and p185 may be due to differences in their structural and functional properties (see below) or to the presence or absence of specific transcriptional regulatory elements within *BCR* intronic sequences.[30] In naturally occurring human leukemias, another possibility is that specific breakpoints may be preferentially generated in different cell types. It has been proposed that the rarity of p185 BCR/ABL in CML patients may be due to restriction of the m-*bcr* breakpoint to progenitor cells committed to the lymphoid lineage.[31] However, this explanation is inconsistent with the frequent occurrence of Ph-positive granulocytic and erythroid colonies in the marrow, and of Ph-positive granulocytes in the blood, of patients with Ph-positive ALL.[32–34] These findings suggest that a multipotential target cell, possibly the stem cell, is involved in the development of p185-positive ALL.

Comparison of the biological properties of p185, p210, and p230 BCR/ABL in two different studies has produced data to support two alternative models for the association of different BCR/ABL proteins with leukemias that are phenotypically distinct. Indirect support for the hypothesis that *BCR* intron 1 breakpoints (m-*bcr*) are more common in lymphoid precursors, while breakpoints downstream in *BCR* (M-*bcr* and μ-*bcr*) occur more often in myeloid precursors, was provided in one study.[31] It was shown that all three forms of BCR/ABL induce an identical CML-like syndrome in mice receiving transduced bone marrow from 5-fluorouracil-pretreated donors.[31] In contrast, a second study showed that under similar experimental conditions, p230 BCR/ABL induced a myeloproliferative disease with a much longer latency (up to 27 weeks) compared with that induced by p185 and p210 BCR/ABL (4–5 weeks).[35] Future studies are required to directly address the nature of the cell of origin for the various BCR/ABL-induced leukemias.

An alternative model to explain the association of the three forms of BCR/ABL with different disease spectra proposes that the various BCR/ABL proteins have different intrinsic leukemogenic activities, which result in the promotion of lymphoid versus myeloid differentiation. Support for this model was provided by the finding that in primary mouse bone marrow cultures, p210 and p230 are impaired in their ability to produce cytokine-independent pre-B cells compared with p185.[35] p185 BCR/ABL is very efficient at driving lymphoid expansion, even under conditions that favor myeloid growth. Both p210 and p230 BCR/ABL proteins generate cells of the myeloid/monocyte lineage under these conditions.[35]

Under different cell culture conditions, additional differences were observed among the three BCR/ABL forms. Expansion of primary mouse bone marrow cells transduced with retroviruses containing each of the various BCR/ABL tyrosine kinases, in the presence of cytokines but without stroma, revealed that p230-expressing cells require cytokines for optimal growth, while p185- and p210-expressing cells are growth-factor-independent.[35] Direct comparison of the proliferative properties of p210- and p230-transduced primary mouse bone marrow cells in the absence of cytokines and stroma showed a 40-fold greater expansion for the p210-expressing cells compared with the p230-expressing cells.[35] The presence of different amounts of BCR sequence in the three BCR/ABL tyrosine kinases may account for their distinct biological properties. In support of this possibility, comparison of the leukemogenic activity of p210 BCR/ABL with that of an activated ABL kinase lacking BCR sequences showed that the latter induced only lymphoid malignancies in mice and did not stimulate the growth of myeloid colonies in vitro.[36] In contrast, p210 BCR/ABL efficiently induced a CML-like disease in mice and stimulated the growth of myeloid cells in vitro.[36] These findings strongly support the notion that BCR sequences modulate the induction of different forms of leukemia when fused to the ABL tyrosine kinase.

INVOLVEMENT OF SPECIFIC BCR/ABL SEQUENCES IN ONCOGENIC TRANSFORMATION

Assays for BCR/ABL-mediated transformation

Structural analysis of the BCR/ABL molecule has revealed that multiple domains in BCR/ABL act in concert to activate the oncogenic potential of the chimeric tyrosine kinase. Examination of the transforming properties of wild-type and mutant forms of BCR/ABL has been carried out in diverse cell types and model systems. These include analysis of BCR/ABL transformation in NIH-3T3 fibroblasts, Rat-1 fibroblasts, growth-factor-dependent hematopoietic cells, primary mouse bone marrow cells, and murine models of BCR/ABL-induced leukemias. Several laboratories have shown that NIH-3T3 fibroblasts are not transformed by BCR/ABL under conditions where these cells are readily transformed by v-Abl.[37] The difference in the transforming activities between BCR/ABL and v-Abl in NIH-3T3 cells has been ascribed to their different subcellular localizations. The v-Abl protein is myristoylated and associates with the plasma membrane, and membrane localization is critical for its transforming activity.[37] In contrast, BCR/ABL localizes to actin filaments and is not associated with the plasma membrane.[38,39]

While NIH-3T3 cells are not readily transformed by BCR/ABL, expression of BCR/ABL in Rat-1 fibroblasts elicits distinct morphological changes, anchorage-independent growth, and tumorigenicity in nude mice.[40] The Rat-1 fibroblast system has proven to be extremely useful for the identification of oncogenes and normal cellular genes that cooperate with BCR/ABL to transform cells.[40,41] A major limitation in employing fibroblasts to study the transforming properties of BCR/ABL is that these cells are not the targets of BCR/ABL transformation in vivo. Thus, a number of hematopoietic cell lines of myeloid and lymphoid origin have been employed for the analysis of BCR/ABL transformation.[42–48] BCR/ABL expression in interleukin-3 (IL-3)-dependent hematopoietic cells such as the lymphoblastoid Ba/F3 and the 32D myeloid progenitor cell lines renders these cells independent of IL-3 for growth and tumorigenic in nude mice. These findings indicate that distinct structural and functional domains are required for transformation of fibroblasts and hematopoietic cells by activated ABL proteins.

While hematopoietic cell lines have been useful in the identification of signaling pathways downstream of BCR/ABL, these cells are not the best system for comparing the leukemogenic properties of the various BCR/ABL isoforms.[31,35] Expression of p185, p210, and p230 in 32D myeloid cells produces very similar phenotypes with regard to cytokine-independent growth and tumor formation after injection in mice. Lineage-restricted myeloid or lymphoid cell lines carry a variable number of mutations, and may be easily transformed by forms of BCR/ABL that are weakly leukemogenic. Therefore, primary bone marrow cells constitute a better system for analysis and comparison of the oncogenicity of the various BCR/ABL forms. Earlier studies showed that infection of primary bone marrow cells with p185 and p210 BCR/ABL-containing retroviruses resulted in the clonal outgrowth of early B-lymphoid cells, even under conditions that favored myeloid cell expansion.[49,50] The BCR/ABL-transformed B-lymphoid cells were tumorigenic in mice. More recently, using different culture and infection conditions, it was shown that infection of lineage-unrestricted primary mouse bone marrow cells with retroviruses encoding different BCR/ABL forms results in the expansion of cells of the myeloid/monocyte lineage by p210 and p230 BCR/ABL, while p185 BCR/ABL induces the expansion of lymphoid cells.[35] These findings indicate that primary bone marrow cells are a better system to compare the biological properties of the BCR/ABL isoforms, or to compare wild-type and mutated forms of BCR/ABL.

Among the best systems for testing the tumorigenicity of wild-type and mutant forms of BCR/ABL are the murine models for CML and ALL. Several murine models for BCR/ABL-induced leukemias have been employed. Use of these systems has provided compelling evidence for the causative role of BCR/ABL in the induction of leukemias, and they are currently being employed for analysis of the role of the various BCR/ABL domains in leukemogenesis. An excellent discussion of the use of various mouse models for the study of BCR/ABL-induced leukemias can be found in Chapter 6.

Role of BCR sequences

A molecular understanding of the contribution of the BCR sequences to the oncogenicity of BCR/ABL and to the diverse phenotypes associated with expression of the p185, p210, and p230 BCR/ABL proteins has begun to emerge. Direct demonstration that the BCR sequences were required for the transforming activity of BCR/ABL was first provided by analyzing the effects of deletions and substitutions in the BCR component of the BCR/ABL chimera on the ability of the fusion proteins to transform fibroblasts and hematopoietic cells.[38,39,51,52] Two distinct regions of BCR were shown to be important for BCR/ABL transformation: BCR N-terminal amino acids (amino acids 1–63 in one study or 3–39 in another report) and a BCR central region (encompassing amino acids 176–242 or 176–426).[38,39,51] Both BCR regions were shown to be required for transformation of Rat-1 fibroblasts and primary mouse bone marrow cells.[38,39,51] However, only the first 63 amino acids of BCR were required for abrogation of cytokine-dependent growth of the BaF3 lymphoblastoid cell line.[39] The central region of BCR encompassing amino acids 176–426 is dispensable for IL-3-independent growth of BaF3 cells, but deletion of this region of BCR markedly inhibits the ability of 32D myeloid cells to proliferate without growth factor and to form tumors in mice.[45] Thus, these findings indicate that the structural requirements for BCR/ABL transformation are cell-context-dependent.

What properties are conferred by specific BCR sequences to activate the transforming potential of BCR/ABL? Analysis of the BCR protein has revealed the presence of multiple functional and structural domains (Figure 2.1). Among these are an N-terminal dimerization domain (DD) comprising the first 63 amino acids of BCR,[39] a serine/threonine-rich region (P-S/T) that binds to SH2 domains in a phosphotyrosine-independent manner,[52] an intrinsic serine/threonine protein kinase activity encoded by the first exon of *BCR*,[53] a region of homology to Dbl, a guanine nucleotide exchange factor for the Rho family of GTPases (Dbl-like),[54] a pleckstrin homology (PH) domain,[54] a calcium-dependent membrane/phospholipid (CalB) domain,[55] and a GTPase-activating protein activity for the Rac GTPase (GAP^{Rac}).[56] The existence of these various domains within a single polypeptide suggests that BCR may function as a point of crosstalk among multiple intracellular signaling pathways. Analysis of *bcr*-null mutant mice has shown that BCR regulates Rac-mediated superoxide production in vivo during neutrophil activation.[57]

The first 63 amino acids of BCR comprise a dimerization/oligomerization domain that is required for the formation of BCR homotetramers.[39] These results are consistent with the observation that p210 BCR/ABL elutes from gel filtration columns with an apparent molecular mass of about 800 kDa, which corresponds to the elution of BCR/ABL tetramers.[58] An intact oligomerization domain in BCR/ABL is required not only for the activation of its transforming activity but also for activation of the tyrosine kinase and F-actin-binding activities of BCR/ABL.[38,39] Oligomerization has been shown to be an important mechanism for activating the kinase activities of receptor and non-receptor protein tyrosine kinases.[59,60] In BCR, the oligomerization function is dependent on a coiled-coil domain.[39]

The second region in *BCR* shown to be required for transformation corresponds to amino acids 176–426.[51] This region encodes a serine-rich sequence important for binding to SH2 domains in a phosphotyrosine-independent manner,[52] and also contains binding sites for at least two proteins implicated in signaling pathways. The Grb2 adaptor protein binds to a phosphorylated tyrosine at position 177 in the region encoded by the *BCR* first exon,[61,62] and the 14-3-3 proteins bind to amino acids 299–385 within the serine-rich region of BCR.[63,64] While the role of 14-3-3 proteins in BCR/ABL transformation remains to be defined, binding of the Grb2 adaptor to the phosphorylated tyrosine 177 in BCR/ABL is required for transformation of Rat-1 fibroblasts.[41,48,61] However, the Grb2-

binding site is not required for abrogation of cytokine-dependent growth of hematopoietic cell lines by BCR/ABL.[45,48] The appearance of outgrowths of transformed B-lymphoid cells following retroviral infection of mouse bone marrow with a BCR/ABL mutant deficient in Grb2 binding was shown to be impaired compared with wild-type BCR/ABL in one study,[61] but not in another.[48] Differences in the cells employed for the preparation of the helper-free retroviral stocks, the levels of BCR/ABL protein expressed in the target cells, or other technical factors may account for the different results in the two studies. Recently, using an optimized murine bone marrow transduction/transplantation system, Million and Van Etten[65] have shown that the Grb2-binding site is required for the induction of CML-like disease by BCR/ABL in mice. Mutation of tyrosine 177 to phenylalanine in p210 BCR/ABL severely compromises the ability of the tyrosine kinase to induce CML-like disease in mice, and instead the mice develop B- and T-lymphoid leukemias of longer latency. Similar results have been reported by others.[66] Taken together, these findings strongly support a requirement for the Grb2-binding site in BCR/ABL for efficient induction of CML-like disease.

The sequences encoded by the first exon of *BCR* are sufficient to activate the tyrosine kinase and transforming properties of ABL in the BCR/ABL chimera. However, it is becoming apparent that the inclusion or exclusion of specific BCR domains in the known BCR/ABL fusion proteins correlates with the development of distinct disease phenotypes.[5,35] p185 BCR/ABL retains only the *BCR* first-exon sequences that include the oligomerization domain, Grb2-binding site, and serine-rich sequences (Figure 2.1). p210 BCR/ABL contains, in addition to the sequences encoded by the *BCR* first exon, the Dbl homology domain and the PH domain (Figure 2.1). It is unclear whether the reduced transforming potency and distinct disease phenotype associated with p210 BCR/ABL expression are due to its decreased tyrosine kinase activity compared with p185 BCR/ABL,[67] or to the presence of novel functions associated with the retention of the Dbl-like and PH domains in p210 BCR/ABL. The PH domain together with the Dbl-like domain may allow for interaction of p210 BCR/ABL with specific cellular targets in multipotent progenitor cells or lymphoid-committed cells that may alter their growth and differentiation properties.

The p230 BCR/ABL protein associated with CNL retains over 90% of the BCR amino acids in the fusion product (Figure 2.1). In addition to the BCR sequences present in p210 BCR/ABL, p230 retains the CalB domain and the N-terminal portion of the GTPase-activating protein domain (GAP^{Rac}). CalB is a conserved domain present in various calcium-responsive signaling proteins and in p120 GAP. The CalB motif confers Ca^{2+}-dependent interactions with cellular membranes, and binds to phospholipids.[55] It remains to be determined whether p230 BCR/ABL has GAP^{Rac} activity. p230 has reduced tyrosine kinase activity compared with the p185 and p210 BCR/ABL proteins.[31] The presence of distinct structural and functional domains in p230 BCR/ABL, or its lower kinase activity, may account for the limited proliferative advantage of the cells where it is expressed. Future studies will test these possibilities.

Role of ABL sequences

In addition to the contribution of BCR sequences to the transforming activity of BCR/ABL, specific ABL functions are essential for BCR/ABL-mediated transformation. Primary among these is the ABL tyrosine kinase activity. A tyrosine-kinase-defective BCR/ABL molecule that contains a single point mutation (lysine to arginine) in the ABL ATP-binding site fails to transform Rat-1 fibroblasts and hematopoietic primary bone marrow cells.[68] Also, a kinase-defective BCR/ABL is unable to elicit cytokine-independent growth of hematopoietic cells.[45] Thus, the presence of BCR sequences alone is not sufficient to induce transformation, and a functional ABL tyrosine kinase is essential for BCR/ABL-induced transformation.

Activation of the ABL tyrosine kinase in the BCR/ABL chimera results in autophosphorylation at multiple tyrosines. One of the autophosphorylated sites is tyrosine 1294 in the tyrosine kinase domain of p210 BCR/ABL,[68] which corresponds to tyrosine 793 in p185 BCR/ABL or tyrosine 412 in c-*ABL* type 1b. This tyrosine in ABL is positioned in the activation loop of the tyrosine kinase domain. The crystal structure of the insulin receptor[69] and the c-Src kinase domains[70] revealed the importance of this tyrosine for kinase activation. The activation-loop tyrosine of several protein tyrosine kinases is required for their biological and biochemical activities. In BCR/ABL, replacement of the activation-loop tyrosine with phenylalanine greatly diminishes its ability to transform Rat-1 fibroblasts.[48,68] Interestingly, overexpression of the *myc* gene partially rescues the transforming capacity of this BCR/ABL autophosphorylation mutant.[41,68] However, the activation-loop tyrosine is not required for abrogation of cytokine-dependent growth of hematopoietic cell lines by BCR/ABL.[45,48,68] In contrast, mice inoculated with growth-factor-independent lymphoid cells expressing the p210 BCR/ABL (Y1294F) autophosphorylation mutant display a less malignant phenotype and distinct pathology than those injected with growth-factor-independent cells expressing the wild-type p210 BCR/ABL protein.[68] Conflicting results exist regarding the ability of the BCR/ABL autophosphorylation mutant to transform murine bone marrow cells following infection with retroviruses encoding the BCR/ABL molecules. In one study, the p210 BCR/ABL (Y1294F) mutant was impaired in its ability to transform bone marrow cells.[68] In contrast, a different study using the p185 BCR/ABL (Y793F) autophosphorylation mutant reported that this mutant transforms bone marrow cells with only slightly reduced efficiency compared with the wild-type p185 BCR/ABL protein.[48] It is not clear whether differences in retroviral titers, the form of BCR/ABL employed, or other variations can account for the disparate results. Future studies that test the leukemogenic potential of the autophosphorylation mutant of BCR/ABL in mouse models of CML and ALL will be required to establish the relevance of this phosphorylation site to BCR/ABL-mediated transformation.

Other ABL sequences have been reported to play a role in the transforming activity of BCR/ABL. They are the SH2, SH3, and actin-binding domains. Deletion of the SH2 domain or mutation of the arginine within the conserved FLVRES motif of the ABL SH2 domain markedly decreases the transforming activity of BCR/ABL in Rat-1 fibroblasts.[38,41,48] Mutation of the arginine in the FLVRES motif abolishes the ability of the SH2 domain to bind to tyrosine-phosphorylated proteins.[71] Interestingly, overexpression of myc in Rat-1 cells expressing the SH2 domain-defective p185 BCR/ABL (R552L) protein restores transforming activity to levels comparable to that of the wild-type BCR/ABL as measured in a soft agar growth assay.[41] However, BCR/ABL proteins that lack a functional SH2 domain are as efficient as wild-type BCR/ABL in eliciting cytokine-independent growth of factor-dependent hematopoietic cells.[38,45,48,72–74] Deletion of the SH2 domain in BCR/ABL has been shown to render the IL-3-dependent FDCP-1 myeloid cells growth-factor-independent.[73] Interestingly, unlike the wild-type BCR/ABL protein, the SH2 domain-deleted BCR/ABL did not secrete IL-3. In contrast, BCR/ABL renders 32D myeloid cells and BaF3 lymphoid cells growth-factor-independent without autocrine stimulation by secreted growth factors.[45] Thus, BCR/ABL can abrogate the growth factor dependence of cells by more than one mechanism.

Mutation of the SH2 domain does not affect the ability of BCR/ABL to transform primary bone marrow cells in vitro.[48] However, tumorigenicity by BCR/ABL in vivo requires an intact SH2 domain.[48,75] Injection of bone marrow cells transformed by a p185 BCR/ABL SH2 (R552L) mutant into CB-17 *scid/scid* mice results in the development of tumors with a fourfold lower frequency and fivefold longer latency period compared with those obtained with cells transformed with wild-type BCR/ABL.[48] Similarly, a p210ΔSH2 BCR/ABL protein is impaired in its ability to induce leukemia in *scid* mice compared with wild-type p210 BCR/ABL.[75] In contrast, using a well-characterized murine bone marrow infection/transplantation model of CML-like leukemia,[19,31] it was shown that the SH2 domain is not required for induction of B-lymphoid leukemia by p185 BCR/ABL, but it is required for efficient induction of CML-like disease by p210 BCR/ABL.[76] These results indicate that there is a differential requirement for the ABL SH2 domain for the induction of B-lymphoid or CML-like leukemias.

The role of the ABL SH3 domain in the development of BCR/ABL-induced leukemias remains unclear. One report showed that deletion of the SH3 does not affect the ability of BCR/ABL to protect cells from apoptosis, induce cytokine-independent proliferation, and transform primary bone marrow cells in vitro.[77] However, leukemic growth in *scid* mice induced by 32D cells expressing a BCR/ABL protein lacking the SH3 domain (BCR/ABLΔSH3) was delayed two- to fourfold compared with wild-type BCR/ABL-expressing 32D cells.[77] The homing capacity of 32D cells expressing BCR/ABLΔSH3 was two- to threefold lower than that of wild-type BCR/ABL-expressing 32D cells.[77] In addition, cells expressing BCR/ABLΔSH3 displayed reduced invasive potential in vitro and showed decreased adhesion to stroma compared with cells expressing wild-type BCR/ABL.[77] Deletion of the BCR/ABL SH3 domain is not as deleterious as deletion of the SH2 domain or Grb2-binding site for in vivo leukemogenesis, but its loss may affect the severity of the disease. In contrast, a recent report showed that the ABL SH3 domain is either not required or redundant for BCR/ABL-induced myeloproliferative disease using the mouse model for CML.[36] A clear conclusion of both studies is that the SH3 domain is not required for leukemogenesis of either 32D cells or primary bone marrow cells expressing BCR/ABL. These results are consistent with the finding that rare p210 BCR/ABL chimeric molecules lacking a functional SH3 domain have been detected in a few CML patients.[5,78]

A role of the ABL actin-binding domain in transformation by BCR/ABL has been described.[38] Mutations in BCR/ABL that abolish binding to F-actin reduce the ability of BCR/ABL to transform Rat-1 fibroblasts and to abrogate the IL-3-dependent growth of Ba/F3 cells. Reports from several laboratories suggest that a link exists between BCR/ABL expression and defective adhesion in leukemia (see below). Thus, it is of importance to analyze the leukemogenic properties of a BCR/ABL protein lacking a functional F-actin-binding domain in the murine models of BCR/ABL-induced leukemias.

SIGNALING PATHWAYS DOWNSTREAM OF BCR/ABL

A large number of proteins have been identified that associate with BCR/ABL, are phosphorylated by the BCR/ABL tyrosine kinase, or are induced/activated by BCR/ABL expression. Among these are adaptor proteins, receptors, enzymes (kinases, phosphatases, GTPases), transcription factors, and cytoskeletal proteins (Figure 2.2). Only a few of these potential BCR/ABL downstream targets have been shown to be required for BCR/ABL transformation.

The Ras pathway

The Ras pathway is absolutely required for transformation by BCR/ABL. Expression of BCR/ABL results in the accumulation of the active, GTP-bound form of Ras.[45,46,79] Ras activity is regulated by the opposing actions of GTPase-activating proteins (GAPs) and guanine nucleotide exchange factors (GEFs). Activation of Ras by BCR/ABL has been proposed to occur via regulation of both GAPs and GEFs. Downregulation of BCR/ABL expression in CML cells with antisense oligonucleotides specific for BCR/ABL inhibited Ras activation and stimulated p120 Ras GAP activity.[80] Co-expression of BCR/ABL with the catalytic domain of

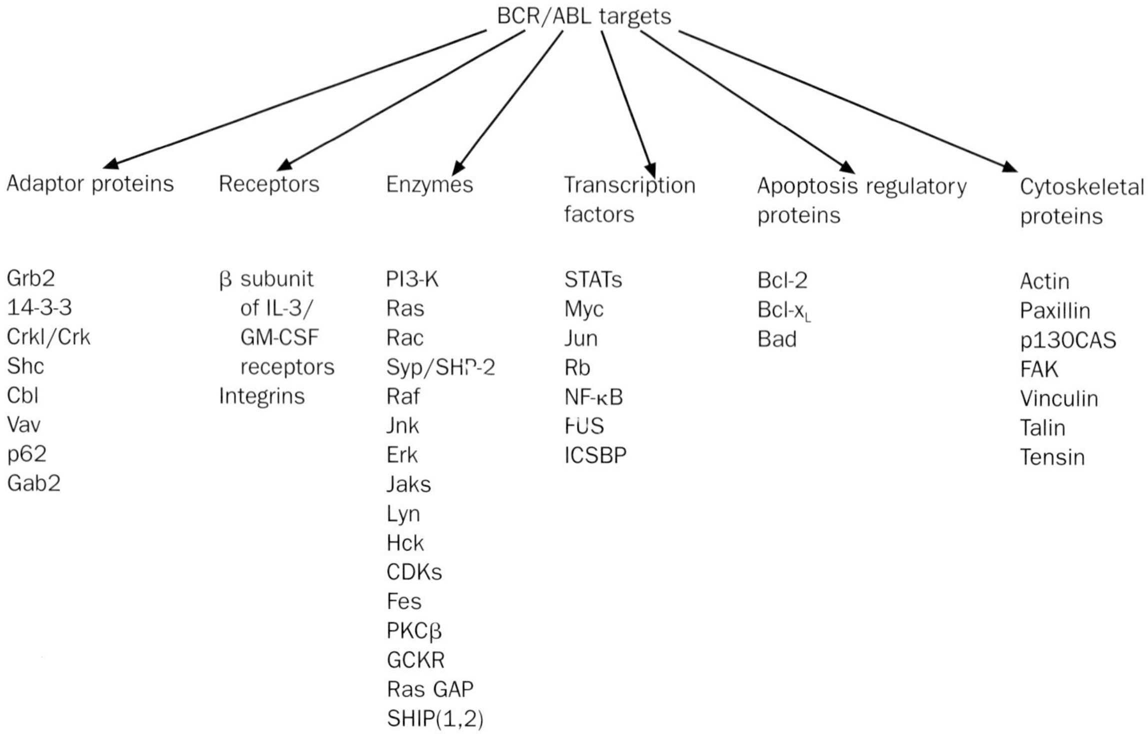

Figure 2.2 Targets of the BCR/ABL tyrosine kinase. Listed are adaptor proteins, receptors, enzymes, transcription factors, apoptosis regulatory proteins, and cytoskeletal proteins. Some of the proteins bind to BCR/ABL, others are phosphorylated by BCR/ABL, and others are upregulated or downregulated in BCR/ABL-expressing cells.

p120 Ras GAP reduced BCR/ABL transformation.[81] It has been reported that p210 BCR/ABL may inhibit p120 Ras GAP through phosphorylation of p62 Dok, a scaffold protein that is tyrosine-phosphorylated in BCR/ABL-transformed cells.[82,83] The p62 Dok protein binds to p120 Ras GAP, but only when p62 Dok is tyrosine-phosphorylated. It was shown that tyrosine-phosphorylated p62 Dok inhibits Ras GAP activity.[84] This finding suggests that p210 BCR/ABL may activate the Ras pathway, in part by inhibiting Ras GAP, a key downregulator of Ras signaling. This model suggests that p62 Dok plays a positive role in the activation of the Ras–MAP kinase (Ras–Erk) cascade in BCR/ABL-transformed cells. However, recent work has shown that p62 Dok is a negative regulator of MAP kinase (Erk) and cell proliferation upon crosslinking of the B-cell receptor.[85] The p62 Dok protein may have different effects on Ras signaling in normal and transformed cells. A definition of the role of p62 Dok in BCR/ABL signaling awaits the use of p62 Dok-deficient cells as targets of BCR/ABL transformation.

Activation of Ras by BCR/ABL is also mediated by activation of GEFs such as Sos. The first link between BCR/ABL and GEFs was provided by the finding that BCR/ABL binds directly to the Grb2 adaptor protein.[61,62,86] Grb2 is a 26 kDa protein comprising a single SH2 domain flanked by two SH3 domains.[87] Grb2 links activated tyrosine kinases to the Ras pathway via the Sos GEF.[87] The Grb2 SH2 domains binds to specific tyrosine-phosphorylated sites in the activated protein tyrosine kinases, while the Grb2 SH3 domains bind to proline-rich sequences in Sos. Grb2 binds to BCR/ABL via direct interaction of the GRB2 SH2 domain with phosphorylated tyrosine 177 of BCR/ABL.[61,62] Mutation of the Grb2-binding site in BCR/ABL results in a dramatic decrease in Ras activation, and BCR/ABL-mediated transformation in fibroblasts.[61] Furthermore, an intact Grb2-binding site is required for the induction of CML myeloproliferative syndrome in mice.[65,66] The existence of a BCR/ABL–Grb2–Sos complex is supported by the finding that Sos co-immunoprecipitates with BCR/ABL.[62]

Additional evidence to support a requirement for Ras function in BCR/ABL transformation was provided by the use of dominant interfering mutants of Ras and Grb2. The asparagine 17 (N17) Ras mutant protein neutralizes normal Ras function by competing with normal Ras for binding to GEFs. N17 Ras suppresses normal growth upon constitutive expression. Therefore, inducible expression of N17 Ras was used to show that blocking Ras function in BCR/ABL-expressing hematopoietic cells induces cell death by an apoptotic mechanism.[47] Similarly, expression of Grb2 mutant proteins lacking the SH3 domains inhibits BCR/ABL-induced Ras activation and dramatically decreases BCR/ABL-mediated transformation of fibroblasts and hematopoietic cells in vitro and formation of tumors in mice.[88] Taken together, these findings show that Ras is a required component for BCR/ABL-transformation. However, we have identified a BCR/ABL mutant protein, BCR/ABLΔ176–427, that has impaired transforming activity in myeloid progenitor cells, and activates Ras.[45] Thus, while Ras is required for BCR/ABL-mediated transformation, it is not sufficient.

Multiple routes to Ras activation by BCR/ABL have been described. The BCR/ABL Y177F protein deficient in Grb2 binding activates Ras in 32D myeloid cells to levels similar to those obtained with wild-type BCR/ABL.[45] Furthermore, loss of the Grb2-binding site in BCR/ABL does not affect the anti-apoptotic and transforming properties of BCR/ABL in hematopoietic cells.[45,48] BCR/ABL activates Ras in the absence of direct Grb2 binding in these cells. Among candidate proteins that function to recruit Grb2 and activate Ras in cells expressing BCR/ABL are the Shc adaptor protein and the SHP-2 protein tyrosine phosphatase. Increased tyrosine phosphorylation of Shc and association of Shc with Grb2 is detected in BCR/ABL-expressing cells.[62,86] Although complexes of Shc with BCR/ABL have been detected, it is unknown whether the interaction of Shc with BCR/ABL is direct or indirect.[62,86,89] Regardless, tyrosine-phosphorylated Shc may provide for an alternative route, linking BCR/ABL to Ras. A role for Shc in BCR/ABL transformation was suggested by the enhanced efficiency of fibroblast and hematopoietic transformation obtained by increasing the dosage of Shc in cells that express wild-type or mutant forms of BCR/ABL.[48] However, demonstration of a direct requirement for Shc in BCR/ABL signaling and transformation will require the use of Shc dominant-negative mutants in cells expressing BCR/ABL.

The SHP-2 phosphotyrosine phosphatase (previously known as Syp) is constitutively tyrosine-phosphorylated in BCR/ABL-expressing cells and forms stable complexes with Grb2.[90] It is not yet known whether SHP-2 is required for BCR/ABL-dependent Ras activation and transformation. Use of SHP-2-null mutant proteins that function as dominant negatives will be needed to determine whether SHP-2 plays a role in BCR/ABL transformation and signaling to Ras. Signaling proteins other than Shc and SHP-2 may function to recruit and activate Grb2–Sos complexes in cells expressing BCR/ABL. The BCR protein has been reported to become tyrosine-phosphorylated in BCR/ABL-expressing cells.[91] Tyrosine-phosphorylated BCR may recruit Grb2 and contribute to RAS activation and transformation. Interestingly, a recent report has shown that endogenous BCR is not required for the induction of B-cell ALL in chimeric mice expressing p185 BCR/ABL.[92] Regardless of the signaling complexes employed by BCR/ABL to activate Ras, it is clear that activation of Ras is critical for the transforming and anti-apoptotic properties of BCR/ABL.

Activated Ras elicits the activation of downstream signaling proteins such as Raf-1,[93] Erk,[46,77] and Jnk[46,77,94] (Figure 2.2). The activation of Erk (MAP kinase) by BCR/ABL is critically dependent on the levels of BCR/ABL protein expressed.[46] In cells where BCR/ABL is expressed at approximately similar levels as the endogenous c-ABL, no detectable increase in Erk activity is observed.[44,46] Higher levels of BCR/ABL expression result in significantly increased Erk activity.[46,77] Downregulation of Raf-1 expression or activity inhibits BCR/ABL-dependent proliferation of hematopoietic cells.[93] Similarly, dominant-negative mutants of c-Jun, which is a target of Jnk, impair BCR/ABL transforming activity.[94] Taken together, these findings show that multiple components of the Ras pathway are required for BCR/ABL transformation.

The PI3-K–Akt pathway

BCR/ABL activates phosphatidylinositol 3'-kinase (PI3-K), a lipid kinase that phosphorylates phosphoinositols at the D-3' position of the inositol ring.[95] PI3-K is a heterodimer that consists of an 85 kDa (p85) regulatory subunit and a 110 kDa (p110) catalytic subunit. Multiple growth factors induce activation of PI3-K through various mechanisms. Activation of PI3-K may occur as a consequence of binding of the two SH2 domains in p85 to tyrosine-phosphorylated sites in growth factor receptor tyrosine kinases,[96] leading to activation of the p110 lipid kinase subunit. Alternatively PI3-K may become activated by binding of proline-rich sequences in p85 to SH3 domains of Src-family tyrosine kinases.[97] PI3-K may also be activated by direct binding of activated Ras to the p110 catalytic subunit.[98] The mechanism employed by BCR/ABL to activate PI3-K remains unclear. BCR/ABL tyrosine kinase activity is required for PI3-K activation, but direct binding of p85 to BCR/ABL is not.[99] However, PI3-K activation by BCR/ABL is dependent on complex formation between p85 and BCR/ABL, as detected by co-immunoprecipitation of BCR/ABL with anti-p85 antibodies.[75] Association of BCR/ABL with PI3-K may be indirect, and is likely to be mediated by adaptor proteins such as Cbl,[100,101] SHC,[89] or SHP-2.[102]

One study reported that activation of PI3-K by BCR/ABL requires an intact BCR/ABL SH2 domain.[75] The BCR/ABL SH2 domain mutant proteins formed a complex with p85 but failed to stimulate PI3-K catalytic activity in 32Dcl3 myeloid cells.[75] In contrast, a second study showed that PI3-K activity was not impaired in hematopoietic cell lines and primary malignant lymphoblasts expressing the BCR/ABL SH2 mutant proteins, and that the levels of PI3-K activation in these cells were comparable to those observed in the cells expressing wild-type BCR/ABL.[76] The reasons for the contradictory results in the two studies are unclear, and additional work is required to examine the mechanisms of PI3-K activation by BCR/ABL. Activation of PI3-K by BCR/ABL was reported to be independent of Ras activation and to be upstream of the Akt serine kinase,[75] in agreement with reports linking the two signaling proteins.[103] Akt activity was shown to be essential for BCR/ABL-mediated leukemogenesis in vitro and in vivo.[75]

What is the contribution of the PI3-K–Akt pathway to BCR/ABL-mediated transformation? Similar to the Ras pathway,[45–47] the PI3-K pathway appears to be required for both the proliferation and survival of BCR/ABL-expressing cells.[75,95] PI3-K and Akt activities were shown to be required for the proliferation of BCR/ABL-expressing cells.[75,95] Furthermore, co-expression of a dominant-negative form of Akt with wild-type BCR/ABL suppressed the induction of c-Myc, a transcription factor required for cell proliferation, and of Bcl-2, a cell survival protein induced by BCR/ABL and growth factors.[75] Interestingly, a BCR/ABL mutant that lacks the SH2 domain was shown to be deficient in the induction of Bcl-2, and modestly deficient in c-Myc induction, compared with wild-type BCR/ABL.[75] These results link the PI3-K–Akt pathway to the proliferative and cell survival effects associated with BCR/ABL expression.

The anti-apoptotic effects of BCR/ABL appear to be mediated by multiple pathways. Some of these pathways are dependent on the activation of the PI3-K–Akt pathway, while others may be independent. It has been proposed that susceptibility to cell death is regulated by the relative levels and interactions of anti-apoptotic (Bcl-2, Bcl-x_L) and pro-apoptotic (Bad, Bax) members of the Bcl-2 protein family.[103] BCR/ABL expression results in enhanced expression of Bcl-2 and/or Bcl-x_L, depending on the cell type.[104–106] Survival and oncogenic stimuli affect not only the expression but also the subcellular localization and phosphorylation status of Bcl-2 family members. BCR/ABL expression elicits the phosphorylation of the pro-apoptotic Bad protein.[106–108] Phosphorylation of Bad on serines 112 and 136 results in its sequestration in the cytoplasm by binding to 14-3-3 proteins. In contrast, unphosphorylated Bad binds to Bcl-2 and Bcl-x_L proteins localized in the mitochondrial membrane, thus blocking their cell survival effects.[103] Two BCR/ABL-activated protein kinases have been implicated in the phosphorylation of Bad: Akt[75] and Raf.[107,108] Activated Akt phosphorylates serine 136, while serine 112 is phosphorylated by PKA and p90 RSK.[103] Recently, the p21-activated protein kinase PAK1 was shown to phosphorylate Bad in vitro and in vivo on serines 112 and 136.[109] It remains to be established whether phosphorylation of Bad in BCR/ABL-expressing cells is also mediated by PAK1. Interestingly, BCR/ABL activates the Rac-GTPase, an upstream activator of the PAK1 serine kinase.[110]

In addition to Bad, Akt has been shown to phosphorylate caspase 9, a cysteine protease that functions as an initiator caspase upstream of effector caspases such as caspase 3. The latter cleave cellular substrates important in the apoptotic program.[103] Phosphorylation of caspase 9 by Akt blocks cytochrome-*c*-mediated activation of caspase 9.[103] Interestingly, BCR/ABL has been shown to delay apoptosis upstream of procaspase 3 activation.[111–113] While most reports have linked BCR/ABL to the block of apoptotic events upstream of cytochrome *c* release, active Akt in BCR/ABL-expressing cells may also function downstream of cytochrome *c* release by blocking caspase 9 activation.

The Jak–STAT pathway

The Janus kinase (Jak) family of protein tyrosine kinases and the signal transducer and activator of transcription (STAT) family of latent transcription factors are critical mediators of cytokine and growth factor signaling.[114] Cytokines and growth factors activate Jak protein tyrosine kinases, which in turn phosphorylate one or more STAT transcription factors. The activated STATs dimerize, translocate to the nucleus, and bind to specific sequences in DNA, thereby activating transcription of target genes.[114] The 185 and p210 forms of BCR/ABL have been shown to induce tyrosine phosphorylation and transcriptional activation of STAT5.[115–118] In addition to STAT5, STAT1 and -3 are activated by BCR/ABL expression.[115,116] While some reports indicate that STAT activation by BCR/ABL does not involve Jak activation,[115,116] others have shown that BCR/ABL activates Jaks, which may in turn activate the STATs.[117]

Regardless of whether BCR/ABL activates STATs through Jak-dependent or Jak-independent pathways, activation of STAT5 by BCR/ABL may play a role in the proliferation and viability of BCR/ABL-expressing cells. Expression of a dominant-negative mutant of STAT5 in 32Dcl3 myeloid cells that express wild-type BCR/ABL inhibited the anti-apoptotic, proliferative, and leukemogenic activities of BCR/ABL.[118] Furthermore, activation of STAT5 by BCR/ABL required the SH2 and SH3 domains of BCR/ABL.[118] The STAT5-activation-deficient BCR/ABLΔSH3ΔSH2 mutant activated Ras but did not protect 32Dcl3 cells from apoptosis following withdrawal of cytokine and serum, and did not induce leukemias in mice. A dominant-active form of STAT5 restored anti-apoptotic and proliferative activities to the BCR/ABLΔSH3ΔSH2 mutant protein.[118] A second study showed that inducible expression of a dominant-negative form of STAT5 in BaF3 cells expressing p210 BCR/ABL inhibited the growth of these cells, without causing cell cycle arrest.[119] The STAT5 dominant-negative decreased the viability of p210/BaF3 cells and increased the sensitivity of these cells to cytotoxic agents. The reduction in the growth rate of p210/BaF3 cells co-expressing the STAT5 dominant-negative was due to the decreased viability of the cells.[119] Taken together, these findings support a role for STAT5 in BCR/ABL signaling and transformation. However, direct proof of the relevance of STAT5 activation to BCR/ABL-dependent leukemogenesis awaits the use of mice deficient for STAT5, which are now available[120] and can be used as targets of BCR/ABL-mediated transformation.

The relevant downstream targets of STAT5 that contribute to BCR/ABL-dependent transformation remain to be defined. Among the known targets of STAT5 is the Bcl-x_L anti-apoptotic protein.[121] However, expression of Bcl-x_L was independent of STAT5 in BaF3 cells expressing BCR/ABL.[119] The targets of STAT5 that may play a role in BCR/ABL-mediated leukemogenesis remain to be identified.

Transcription factors

Among the transcription factors shown to be important for BCR/ABL transformation are c-Jun,[94] c-Myc,[40,41,122] and NF-κB[123,124] (Figure 2.2). Dominant-negative mutants of c-Jun impair BCR/ABL transforming activity in Rat-1 fibroblasts,[94] in agreement with reports that the Ras pathway and downstream targets such as Jnk/c-Jun are important for BCR/ABL transformation. Similarly, dominant-negative mutant c-Myc proteins suppressed transformation of fibroblasts and primary bone marrow pre-B cells by BCR/ABL.[122] While the domains involved in c-Myc induction by BCR/ABL remain to be established, it is clear that c-Myc is required for BCR/ABL transformation.

More recently, it was shown that p185 and p210 BCR/ABL proteins activate the NF-κB transcription factor in hematopoietic cells.[123,124] Activation of NF-κB by BCR/ABL is dependent on BCR/ABL tyrosine kinase activity, and is partially dependent on Ras.[123] BCR/ABL expression induces nuclear translocation of NF-κB and enhances the transactivation function of the Rel A/p65 subunit of NF-κB. The latter effect is partially dependent on a functional Ras protein.[123] Downregulation of the p65 subunit of NF-κB with antisense oligonucleotides in DA1 hematopoietic cells expressing p210 BCR/ABL resulted in failure to survive after removal of IL-3 and produced growth inhibition in one study.[124] A second study showed that BCR/ABL does not require NF-κB to protect 32D myeloid cells from apoptosis following IL-3 withdrawal.[123] However, NF-κB was required for BCR/ABL-mediated tumorigenicity in mice, and for transformation of primary bone marrow cells by BCR/ABL.[123] NF-κB may play different roles in the anti-apoptotic and proliferative pathways downstream of BCR/ABL, depending on the target cell type. A role for NF-κB in cell adhesion in BCR/ABL-expressing cells remains to be investigated. In this regard, it has been shown that NF-κB induces tumor regression by downregulating cell adhesion molecules.[125]

Other pathways downstream of BCR/ABL

Among other signaling proteins important for BCR/ABL transformation is the Rac-GTPase.[110] Rac plays critical roles in the regulation of cell migration, as well as in cell survival and mitogenesis. Rac is activated in cells expressing kinase-active BCR/ABL.[110] Inhibition of Rac activity in cells expressing BCR/ABL did not affect cell survival, and caused a modest decrease in proliferation.[110] However, inhibition of Rac function impaired the invasive and leukemogenic activities of BCR/ABL.[110] The mechanism employed by BCR/ABL to activate Rac is unclear, and it is not known whether PI3-K is upstream or downstream of Rac in this pathway.

The non-receptor tyrosine kinases Hck and Fes have also been implicated as downstream targets of BCR/ABL.[126,127] The Hck tyrosine kinase binds to and is activated by BCR/ABL. A kinase-defective Hck suppresses the growth of DAGM cells expressing BCR/ABL in the absence of cytokines, but kinase-defective Hck does not affect proliferation in response to IL-3.[126] In contrast, the wild-type form of the Fes protein tyrosine kinase has been shown to suppress cytokine-independent outgrowth of myeloid cells by BCR/ABL.[127] The Fes tyrosine kinase associates with BCR/ABL and is phosphorylated by it, which correlates with stimulation of Fes tyrosine kinase activity. Thus, while Fes activation suppresses BCR/ABL signaling, the Hck tyrosine kinase may be required for BCR/ABL transformation.

The SH2-containing phosphatidylinositol-3,4,5-trisphosphate 5-phosphatases SHIP1 and SHIP2 have been implicated as downstream targets of BCR/ABL. Both SHIP1 and SHIP2 are constitutively tyrosine-phosphorylated in CML primary hematopoietic progenitor cells.[128] Interestingly, BCR/ABL inhibits expression of SHIP1. Inhibition of BCR/ABL tyrosine kinase activity with STI571 caused re-expression of SHIP1.[129] Downregulation of SHIP1 by BCR/ABL was caused by a decrease in the half-life of SHIP1 protein in BCR/ABL-positive cells, and by a decrease in SHIP1 mRNA.[129] The reduction of SHIP1 in cells expressing BCR/ABL suggests that SHIP1 plays a negative role in leukemogenesis. This conclusion is consistent with the finding that targeted disruption of SHIP1 in the mouse elicits a myeloproliferative syndrome.[130] Loss of SHIP1 function may be a component of the progression of CML.

Similarly, downregulation of the ICSBP (interferon consensus sequence binding protein) is observed in BCR/ABL-induced CML-like disease.[131] ICSBP overexpression inhibits BCR/ABL-induced CML-like disease.[131] Interestingly, overexpression of ICSBP does not inhibit, but rather enhances, BCR/ABL-induced B-lymphoid leukemias in mice.[131] This finding suggests that ICSBP may play distinct roles in the development of myeloid and lymphoid leukemias. Consistent with this possibility, ICSBP-deficient mice develop a CML-like syndrome.[132]

BCR/ABL also elicits the downregulation of the Abi adaptor proteins.[133] These were initially identified as binding partners for the c-Abl tyrosine kinase.[134,135] More recently, the Abi adaptors have been implicated as linkers between the Ras- and Rac-GTPases.[136] Abi proteins are degraded by BCR/ABL via the ubiquitin-dependent proteasome machinery, through a Ras-independent pathway.[133] Abi proteins are lost in cell lines and primary bone marrow cells isolated from patients with aggressive BCR/ABL-positive leukemias. The role of Abi proteins in BCR/ABL-mediated transformation remains to be defined, but it may be important for Rac-dependent processes such as cell adhesion and migration.

CONCLUSIONS AND FUTURE DIRECTIONS

While great progress has been made in the identification of functional domains in BCR/ABL that are important for leukemogenesis and the definition of signaling pathways activated by BCR/ABL, many unanswered questions remain. Among these is the nature of the target cell for the various forms of BCR/ABL (p185, p210, and p230) associated with distinct forms of human leukemia. Also, the role of many signaling proteins that are phosphorylated, activated, or downregulated following BCR/ABL expression remains to be determined. In particular, it is important to understand the link between tyrosine phosphorylation of cytoskeletal proteins and changes in cell adhesion and migration of the BCR/ABL-expressing cells. Little information exists regarding the crosstalk among survival and mitogenic pathways, with pathways that control cell adhesion and migration of BCR/ABL-positive cells. The identification of pathways that are critical for BCR/ABL transformation, such as the Ras and PI3-K pathways, has provided novel targets for the treatment of BCR/ABL-positive leukemias. Elucidation of the additional pathways required for BCR/ABL leukemogenesis will provide alternative targets for the development of anti-leukemic drugs.

ACKNOWLEDGEMENTS

Research in the author's laboratory was supported by grants from the NCI (CA61033 and CA70940) and the Leukemia Society of America.

REFERENCES

1. Rosenberg N, Witte ON, The viral and cellular forms of the Abelson (abl) oncogene. *Adv Virus Res* 1988; **35:** 39–81.
2. Goff SP, Gilboa E, Witte ON, Baltimore D, Structure of the Abelson murine leukemia virus genome and the homologous cellular gene: studies with cloned viral DNA. *Cell* 1980; **22:** 777–85.
3. Bergold PJ, Blumenthal JA, D'Andrea E et al, Nucleic acid sequence and oncogenic properties of the HZ2 feline sarcoma virus v-abl insert. *J Virol* 1987; **61:** 1193–202.
4. Kurzrock R, Gutterman JU, Talpaz M, The molecular genetics of Philadelphia chromosome-positive leukemias. *N Engl J Med* 1988; **319:** 990–8.
5. Melo JV, The diversity of BCR–ABL fusion proteins and their relationship to leukemia phenotype. *Blood* 1996; **7:** 2375–84.
6. Papadopoulos P, Ridge SA, Boucher CA et al, The novel activation of ABL by fusion to an *ets*-related gene, TEL. *Cancer Res* 1995; **55:** 34–8.
7. Golub TR, Goga A, Barker GF et al, Oligomerization of the ABL tyrosine kinase by the ets protein TEL in human leukemia. *Mol Cell Biol* 1996; **16:** 4107–16.
8. Van Etten RA, Jackson P, Baltimore D, The mouse type IV c-abl gene product is a nuclear protein, and activation of transforming ability is associated with cytoplasmic localization. *Cell* 1989; **58:** 669–78.
9. Wetzler M, Talpaz M, Van Etten RA et al, Subcellular localization of Bcr, Abl, and Bcr–Abl proteins in normal and leukemic cells and correlation of expression with myeloid differentiation. *J Clin Invest* 1993; **92:** 1925–39.
10. Rowley JD, A new consistent chromosomal abnormality in chronic myelogenous leukemia identified by quinacrine fluorescence and Giemsa staining. *Nature* 1973; **243:** 290–3.
11. Klein A, van Kessel AG, Grosweld G et al, A cellular oncogene is translocated to the Philadelphia chromosome in chronic myelocytic leukemia. *Nature* 1982; **300:** 765–7.
12. Bartram CR, de Klein A, Hagemeijer A et al, Translocation of c-abl oncogene correlates with the presence of a Philadelphia chromosome in chronic myelocytic leukemia. *Nature* 1983; **306:** 277–80.
13. Pane F, Frigen F, Sindona M et al, Neutrophilic-chronic myeloid leukemia: a distinct disease with a specific molecular marker (BCR/ABL with C3/A2 junction). *Blood* 1996; **88:** 2410–14.
14. Saglio G, Guerrasio A, Rosso C et al, New type of Bcr/Abl junction in Philadelphia chromosome-positive chronic myelogenous leukemia. *Blood* 1990; **76:** 1819–24.
15. Daley GQ, Van Etten RA, Baltimore D, Induction of chronic myelogenous leukemia in mice by the P210 *bcr/abl* gene of the Philadelphia chromosome. *Science* 1990; **247:** 824–30.
16. Kelliher MA, McLaughlin J, Witte ON, Rosenberg N, Induction of a chronic myelogenous leukemia-like syndrome in mice with *v-abl* and *BCR/ABL*. *Proc Natl Acad Sci USA* 1990; **87:** 6649–53.
17. Gishizky ML, Johnson-White J, Witte ON, Efficient transplantation of BCR–ABL-induced chronic myelogenous leukemia-like syndrome in mice. *Proc Natl Acad Sci USA* 1993; **90:** 3755–9.
18. Voncken JW, Kaartinen V, Pattengale PK et al, BCR/ABL p210 and p190 cause distinct leukemia in transgenic mice. *Blood* 1995; **86:** 4603–11.
19. Pear WS, Miller JP, Xu L et al, Efficient and rapid induction of a chronic myelogenous leukemia-like myeloproliferative disease in mice receiving p210 bcr/abl-transduced bone marrow. *Blood* 1998; **92:** 3780–92.
20. Zhang X, Ren R, Bcr–Abl efficiently induces a myeloproliferative disease and production of excess interleukin-3 and granulocyte–macrophage colony-stimulating factor in mice: a novel model for chronic myelogenous leukemia. *Blood* 1998; **92:** 3829–40.
21. Huettner CS, Zhang P, Van Etten RA, Tenen DG, Reversibility of acute B-cell leukaemia

induced by BCR-ABL1. *Nature Genet* 2000; **24:** 57–60.

22. Fialkow PJ, Jacobsen RJ, Papayannopoulou T, Chronic myelocytic leukemia: clonal origin in a stem cell common to granulocyte, erythrocyte, platelet and monocyte/macrophage. *Am J Med* 1977; **63:** 125–30.
23. Gishizky ML, Witte ON, Initiation of deregulated growth of multipotent progenitor cells by bcr–abl in vitro. *Science* 1992; **256:** 836–9.
24. Clark SC, McLaughlin J, Timmons M et al, Expression of a distinctive BCR–ABL oncogene in Ph[1]-positive acute lymphocytic leukemia (ALL). *Science* 1988; **239:** 775–7.
25. Kurzrock R, Shtalrid M, Romero P et al, A novel c-abl protein product in Philadelphia-positive acute lymphoblastic leukaemia. *Nature* 1987; **325:** 631–5.
26. Ribeiro RC, Abromowitch M, Raimondi SC et al, Clinical and biological hallmarks of the Philadelphia chromosome in childhood acute lymphoblastic leukemia. *Blood* 1987; **70:** 948–53.
27. Mittre H, Leymarie P, Macro M, Leporrier M, A new case of chronic myeloid leukemia with c3/a2 BCR–ABL junction: Is it really a distinct disease? *Blood* 1997; **89:** 4239–40.
28. Briz M, Vilches C, Cabrera R et al, Typical chronic myelogenous leukemia with e19a2 junction BCR/ABL transcript. *Blood* 1997; **90:** 5024–5.
29. Wilson G, Frost L, Goodeye A et al, Bcr–Abl transcript with an e19a2 (c3a2) junction in classical chronic myelogenous leukemia. *Blood* 1997; **89:** 3064.
30. Stewart MJ, Cox G, Reifel-Miller A et al, A novel transcriptional suppressor located within a downstream intron of the *BCR* gene. *J Biol Chem* 1994; **269:** 10820–9.
31. Li S, Ilaria RL Jr, Million RP et al, The p190, p210 and p230 forms of the BCR/ABL oncogene induce a similar chronic myeloid leukemia-like syndrome in mice but have different lymphoid leukemogenic activity. *J Exp Med* 1999; **189:** 1399–412.
32. Tachibana N, Raimondi SC, Lauer SJ et al, Evidence for a multipotential stem cell disease in some childhood Philadelphia chromosome-positive acute lymphoblastic leukemia. *Blood* 1987; **70:** 1458–61.
33. Dow L, Tachibana N, Raimondi SC et al, Comparative biochemical and cytogenetic studies of childhood acute lymphoblastic leukemia with the Philadelphia chromosome and other 22q11 variants. *Blood* 1989; **73:** 1291–7.
34. Schenk T, Keyhani A, Bottcher S et al, Multilineage involvement of Philadelphia chromosome positive acute lymphoblastic leukemia. *Leukemia* 1998; **12:** 666–74.
35. Quackenbush RC, Reuther GW, Miller JP et al, Analysis of the biologic properties of p230 Bcr–Abl reveals unique and overlapping properties with the oncogenic p185 and p210 Bcr–Abl tyrosine kinases. *Blood* 2000; **95:** 2913–21.
36. Gross AW, Zhang X, Ren R, Bcr–Abl with an SH3 deletion retains the ability to induce a myeloproliferative disease in mice, yet c-Abl activated by an SH3 deletion induces only lymphoid malignancy. *Mol Cell Biol* 1999; **19:** 6918–28.
37. Daley GQ, McLaughlin J, Witte ON, Baltimore D, The CML-specific P210 bcr/abl protein, unlike v-abl, does not transform NIH/3T3 fibroblasts. *Science* 1987; **237:** 532–5.
38. McWhirter JR, Wang JY, An actin-binding function contributes to transformation by the Bcr–Abl oncoprotein of Philadelphia chromosome-positive human leukemias. *EMBO J* 1993; **12:** 1533–46.
39. McWhirter JR, Galasso DL, Wang JYJ, A coiled-coil oligomerization domain of bcr is essential for the transforming function of bcr–abl oncoproteins. *Mol Cell Biol* 1993; **13:** 7587–95.
40. Lugo TG, Witte ON, The BCR-ABL oncogene transforms Rat-1 cells and cooperates with *v-myc*. *Mol Cell Biol* 1989; **9:** 1263–70.
41. Afar DEH, Goga A, McLaughlin L et al, Differential complementation of Bcr–Abl point mutants with c-Myc. *Science* 1994; **264:** 424–6.
42. Daley GQ, Baltimore D, Transformation of an interleukin 3-dependent hematopoietic cell line by the chronic myelogenous leukemia-specific p210 BCR/ABL protein. *Proc Natl Acad Sci USA* 1988; **85:** 9312–16.
43. Carlesso N, Griffin JD, Druker BJ, Use of a temperature-sensitive mutant to define the biological effects of the p210 BCR–ABL tyrosine kinase on proliferation of a factor-dependent murine myeloid cell line. *Oncogene* 1994; **9:** 149–56.
44. Kabarowski JHS, Allen PB, Wiedemann L, A temperature sensitive p210 BCR–ABL mutant defines the primary consequences of BCR–ABL tyrosine kinase expression in growth factor dependent cells. *EMBO J* 1994; **13:** 5887–95.

45. Cortez D, Kadlec L, Pendergast AM, Structural and signaling requirements for BCR–ABL mediated transformation and inhibition of apoptosis. *Mol Cell Biol* 1995; **15:** 5531–41.
46. Cortez DG, Reuther G, Pendergast AM, The Bcr–Abl tyrosine kinase activates mitogenic signaling pathways and stimulates G1-to-S phase transition in hematopoietic cells. *Oncogene* 1997; **15:** 2333–42.
47. Cortez D, Stoica G, Pierce JH, Pendergast AM, The BCR–ABL tyrosine kinase inhibits apoptosis by activating a Ras-dependent signaling pathway. *Oncogene* 1996; **13:** 2589–94.
48. Goga A, McLaughlin J, Afar DE et al, Alternative signals to RAS for hematopoietic transformation by the BCR–ABL oncogene. *Cell* 1995; **82:** 981–8.
49. McLaughlin J, Chianese E, Witte ON, In vitro transformation of immature hematopoietic cells by the p210 BCR/ABL oncogene product of the Philadelphia chromosome. *Proc Natl Acad Sci USA* 1987; **84:** 6558–62.
50. Young JC, Witte ON, Selective transformation of primitive lymphoid cells by the BCR/ABL oncogene expressed in long-term lymphoid or myeloid cultures. *Mol Cell Biol* 1988; **8:** 4079–87.
51. Muller AJ, Young JC, Pendergast AM et al, BCR first exon sequences specifically activate the BCR/ABL tyrosine kinase oncogene of Philadelphia chromosome-positive human leukemias. *Mol Cell Biol* 1991; **11:** 1785–92.
52. Pendergast AM, Muller AJ, Havlik MH et al, BCR sequences essential for transformation by the BCR–ABL oncogene bind to the ABL SH2 regulatory domain in a non-phosphotyrosine-dependent manner. *Cell* 1991; **66:** 161–71.
53. Maru Y, Witte ON, The *bcr* gene encodes a novel serine/threonine kinase activity within a single exon. *Cell* 1991; **67:** 459–68.
54. Aelst LV, D'Souza-Schorey C, Rho GTPases and signaling networks. *Genes Dev* 1997; **11:** 2295–322.
55. Gawler DJ, Zhang L-J, Reedijk M et al, CaLB: a 43 amino acid calcium-dependent membrane/phospholipid binding domain in p120 Ras GTPase-activating protein. *Oncogene* 1995; **10:** 817–25.
56. Diekmann D, Brill S, Garrett MD et al, *Bcr* encodes a GTPase-activating protein for $p21^{rac}$. *Nature* 1991; **351:** 400–2.
57. Voncken JW, van Schaick H, Kaartinen V et al, Increased neutrophil respiratory burst in *bcr*-null mutants. *Cell* 1995; **80:** 719–28.
58. Pendergast AM, Clark R, Kawasaki ES et al, Baculovirus expression of functional p210 BCR–ABL oncogene product. *Oncogene* 1989; **4:** 759–66.
59. Heldin C-H, Dimerization of cell surface receptors in signal transduction. *Cell* 1995; **80:** 213–23.
60. Weiss A, Schlessinger J, Switching signals on or off by receptor dimerization. *Cell* 1998; **94:** 277–80.
61. Pendergast AM, Quilliam LA, Cripe LD et al, BCR–ABL-induced oncogenesis is mediated by direct interaction with the SH2 domain of the GRB-2 adaptor protein. *Cell* 1993; **75:** 175–85.
62. Puil L, Liu J, Gish G et al, Bcr–Abl oncoproteins bind directly to activators of the Ras signalling pathway. *EMBO J* 1994; **13:** 764–73.
63. Reuther GW, Fu H, Cripe LD et al, Association of c-BCR and BCR–ABL with 14-3-3 family proteins. *Science* 1994; **266:** 129–33.
64. Braselmann S, McCormick F, BCR and RAF form a complex in vivo via 14-3-3 proteins. *EMBO J* 1995; **14:** 4839–48.
65. Million RP, Van Etten RA, The Grb2 binding site is required for induction of chronic myeloid leukemia-like disease in mice by the Bcr/Abl tyrosine kinase. *Blood* 2000; **96:** 664–70.
66. Pear WS, Miller J, Xu LW et al, Murine models for studying the pathogenesis of chronic myelogenous leukemia. *Blood* 1997; **90:** 393a.
67. Lugo TG, Pendergast A, Muller AJ, Witte ON, Tyrosine kinase activity and transformation potency of bcr-abl oncogene products. *Science* 1990; **247:** 1079–82.
68. Pendergast AM, Gishizky ML, Havlik MK, Witte ON, SH1 domain autophosphorylation of p210 BCR/ABL is required for transformation but not growth factor independence. *Mol Cell Biol* 1993; **13:** 1728–36.
69. Hubbard SR, Wei L, Ellis L, Hendrickson WA, Crystal structure of the tyrosine kinase domain of the human insulin receptor. *Nature* 1994; **372:** 746–54.
70. Xu W, Doshi A, Lei M et al, Crystal structures of c-Src reveal features of its autoinhibitory mechanism. *Mol Cell* 1999; **3:** 629–38.
71. Mayer BJ, Jackson PK, Van Etten RA, Baltimore D, Point mutations in the *abl* SH2 domain coordinately impair phosphotyrosine binding in vitro and transforming activity in vivo. *Mol Cell Biol* 1992; **12:** 609–18.
72. Oda T, Tamura S, Matsuguchi M et al, The SH2

domain of ABL is not required for factor-independent growth induced by BCR–ABL in a murine myeloid cell line. *Leukemia* 1995; **9:** 295–301.

73. Anderson SM, Mladenovic J, The BCR/ABL oncogene requires both kinase activity and *src*-homology 2 domain to induce cytokine secretion. *Blood* 1996; **87:** 238–44.
74. Ilaria RL, Van Etten RA, The SH2 domain of $P210^{BCR/ABL}$ is not required for transformation of hematopoietic factor-dependent cells. *Blood* 1995; **86:** 3897–904.
75. Skorski T, Bellacosa A, Nieborowska-Skorska M et al, Transformation of hematopoietic cells by BCR/ABL requires activation of a PI-3K/Akt-dependent pathway. *EMBO J* 1997; **16:** 6151–61.
76. Ilaria RL, De Aos IE, Roumiantsev S et al, The SH2 domain of BCR/ABL is required for induction of CML-like disease in mice but not for activation of phosphatidylinositol 3-kinase. *Blood* 1998; **92:** 92a.
77. Skorski T, Nieborowska-Skorska M, Wlodarski P et al, The SH3 domain contributes to BCR/ABL-dependent leukemogenesis in vivo: role in adhesion, invasion and homing. *Blood* 1998; **91:** 406–18.
78. Polak JZ, Zemanova K, Michalova H et al, A new case of chronic myeloid leukemia (CML) in myeloid blast crisis with an atypical (b3/a3) junction of the BCR/ABL gene. *Leukemia* 1998; **12:** 250.
79. Mandanas RA, Leibowitz DS, Gharehbaghi K et al, Role of p21 RAS in p210 bcr–abl transformation of murine myeloid cells. *Blood* 1993; **82:** 1838–47.
80. Skorski T, Kanakaraj P, Ku D-H et al, Negative regulation of p120GAP GTPase promoting activity by $p210^{bcr/abl}$: implication for RAS-dependent Philadelphia chromosome positive cell growth. *J Exp Med* 1994; **179:** 1855–65.
81. Sawyers CL, McLaughlin J, Witte ON, Genetic requirements for Ras in the transformation of fibroblasts and hematopoietic cells by the Bcr–Abl oncogene. *J Exp Med* 1995; **181:** 307–13.
82. Carpino N, Wisniewski D, Strife A et al, $p62^{dok}$: a constitutively tyrosine-phosphorylated, GAP-associated protein in chronic myelogenous leukemia progenitor cells. *Cell* 1997; **88:** 197–204.
83. Yamanashi Y, Baltimore D, Identification of the Abl- and rasGAP-associated 62 kDa protein as a docking protein, dok. *Cell* 1997; **88:** 205–11.
84. Kashige N, Carpino N, Kobayashi R, Tyrosine phosphorylation of $p62^{dok}$ by $p210^{bcr-abl}$ inhibits RasGAP activity. *Proc Natl Acad Sci USA* 2000; **97:** 2093–8.
85. Yamanashi Y, Tamura T, Kanamori T et al, Role of the rasGAP-associated docking protein $p62^{dok}$ in negative regulation of B cell receptor-mediated signaling. *Genes Dev* 2000; **14:** 11–16.
86. Tauchi T, Boswell HS, Leibowitz D, Broxmeyer HE, Coupling between p210bcr–abl and Shc and Grb2 adaptor proteins in hematopoietic cells permits growth factor receptor-independent link to Ras activation pathway. *J Exp Med* 1994; **179:** 167–75.
87. Schlessinger J, How receptor tyrosine kinases activate Ras. *Trends Biochem Sci* 1993; **18:** 273–5.
88. Gishizky ML, Cortez D, Pendergast AM, Mutant forms of growth factor-binding protein-2 reverse BCR–ABL-induced transformation. *Proc Natl Acad Sci USA* 1995; **92:** 10889–93.
89. Harrison-Findik D, Susa M, Varticovski L, Association of phosphatidylinositol 3-kinase with SHC in chronic myelogenous leukemia cells. *Oncogene* 1995; **10:** 1385–91.
90. Tauchi T, Feng G-S, Shen R et al, SH2-containing phosphotyrosine phosphatase Syp is a target of p210bcr–abl tyrosine kinase. *J Biol Chem* 1994; **269:** 14381–7.
91. Liu J, Wu Y, Ma GZ et al, Inhibition of Bcr serine kinase by tyrosine phosphorylation. *Mol Cell Biol* 1996; **16:** 998–1005.
92. Castellanos A, Pintado B, Weruaga E et al, A *BCR–ABL p190* fusion gene made by homologous recombination causes B-cell acute lymphoblastic leukemias in chimeric mice with independence of the endogenous bcr product. *Blood* 1997; **90:** 2168–74.
93. Skorski T, Nieborowska-Skorska M, Szczylik C et al, c-Raf-1 serine/threonine kinase is required in BCR/ABL-dependent and normal hematopoiesis. *Cancer Res* 1995; **55:** 2275–8.
94. Raitano AB, Halpern JR, Hambuch TM, Sawyers CL, The Bcr–Abl leukemia oncogene activates Jun kinase and requires Jun for transformation. *Proc Natl Acad Sci* 1995; **92:** 11746–50.
95. Skorski T, Kanakaraj P, Nieborowska-Skorska M et al, Phosphatidylinositol-3 kinase activity is regulated by BCR/ABL and is required for the growth of Philadelphia chromosome-positive cells. *Blood* 1995; **86:** 726–46.
96. Carpenter CL, Auger KL, Chanudhuri M et al, Phosphatidylinositol 3-kinase is activated by

phosphopeptides that bind to the SH2 domains of the p85 kD subunit. *J Biol Chem* 1993; **268:** 9478–83.
97. Pleiman CM, Hertz WM, Cambier JC, Activation of phosphatidylinositol-3' kinase by Src-family kinase SH3 binding to the p85 subunit. *Science* 1994; **263:** 1609–12.
98. Rodriguez-Viciana P, Warne PH, Dhand R et al, Phosphatidylinositol-3-OH kinase as a direct target of Ras. *Nature* 1994; **370:** 527–32.
99. Jain SK, Susa M, Keeler ML et al, PI 3-kinase activation in BCR/abl-transformed hematopoietic cells does not require interaction of p85 SH2 domains with p210 BCR/abl. *Blood* 1996; **88:** 1542–50.
100. Sattler M, Salgia R, Okuda K et al, The proto-oncogene produce p120CBL and the adaptor proteins CRKL and c-CRK link c-ABL, p190BCR/ABL and p210BCR/ABL to the phosphatidylinositol 3'-kinase pathway. *Oncogene* 1996; **12:** 839–46.
101. Jain SK, Langdon WY, Varticovski L, Tyrosine phosphorylation of p120^{cbl} in BCR/abl transformed hematopoietic cells mediates enhanced association with phosphatidylinositol 3-kinase. *Oncogene* 1997; **14:** 2217–28.
102. Tauchi T, Miyazawa K, Feng G-S et al, A coiled-coil tetramerization domain of BCR–ABL is essential for the interactions of SH2-containing signal transduction molecules. *J Biol Chem* 1997; **272:** 1389–94.
103. Datta SR, Brunet A, Greenberg ME, Cellular survival: a play in three Akts. *Genes Dev* 1999; **13:** 2905–27.
104. Sanchez-Garcia L, Grutz G, Tumorigenic activity of the BCR–ABL oncogenes is mediated by BCL2. *Proc Natl Acad Sci USA* 1995; **92:** 5287–91.
105. Amarante-Mendes GP, McGahon AJ, Nishioka WK et al, Bcl-2-independent Bcr–Abl-mediated resistance to apoptosis: protection is correlated with up regulation of Bcl-x_L. *Oncogene* 1998; **16:** 1383–90.
106. Salomoni P, Condorelli F, Sweeney SM, Calabretta B, Versatility of BCR/ABL-expressing leukemic cells in circumventing proapoptotic BAD effects. *Blood* 2000; **96:** 676–84.
107. Salomoni P, Wasik MA, Riedel RF et al, Expression of constitutively active Raf-1 in the mitochondria restores antiapoptotic and leukemogenic potential of a transformation-deficient BCR/ABL mutant. *J Exp Med* 1998; **187:** 1–13.
108. Neshat MS, Raitano AB, Wang HG et al, The survival function of the Bcr–Abl oncogene is mediated by bad-dependent and -independent pathways: Roles for phosphatidylinositol 3-kinase and Raf. *Mol Cell Biol* 2000; **20:** 1179–86.
109. Schurmann A, Mooney AF, Sanders LC et al, p21-activated kinase 1 phosphorylates the death agonist bad and protects cells from apoptosis. *Mol Cell Biol* 2000; **20:** 453–61.
110. Skorski T, Wlodarski P, Daheron L et al, BCR/ABL-mediated leukemogenesis requires the activity of the small GTP-binding protein Rac. *Proc Natl Acad Sci USA* 1998; **95:** 11858–62.
111. Martins LM, Mesner PW, Kottke TJ et al, Comparison of caspase activation and subcellular localization in HL-60 and K562 cells undergoing etoposide-induced apoptosis. *Blood* 1997; **90:** 4283–96.
112. Amarante-Mendes GP, Kim CN, Liu L et al, Bcr–Abl exerts its antiapoptotic effect against diverse apoptotic stimuli through blockage of mitochondrial release of cytochrome C and activation of caspase-3. *Blood* 1998; **91:** 1700–5.
113. Dubrez L, Eymin B, Sordet O et al, BCR–ABL delays apoptosis upstream of procaspase-3 activation. *Blood* 1998; **91:** 2415–22.
114. Briscoe J, Kohlhuer F, Muller M, JAKs and STATs branch out. *Trends Cell Biol* 1996; **6:** 336–40.
115. Carlesso N, Frank DA, Griffin JD, Tyrosyl phosphorylation and DNA binding activity of signal transducers and activators of transcription (STAT) proteins in hematopoietic cell lines transformed by Bcr/Abl. *J Exp Med* 1996; **183:** 811–20.
116. Ilaria RL, Van Etten RA, p210 and p190$^{BCR/ABL}$ induce the tyrosine phosphorylation and DNA binding activity of multiple specific STAT family members. *J Biol Chem* 1996; **271:** 31704–10.
117. Shuai K, Halper J, ten Hoeve J et al, Constitutive activation of STAT5 by the BCR–ABL oncogene in chronic myelogenous leukemia. *Oncogene* 1996; **13:** 247–54.
118. Nieborowska-Skorska M, Wasik MA, Slupianek A et al, Signal transducer and activator of transcription (STAT)5 activation by BCR/ABL is dependent on intact Src homology (SH)3 and SH2 domains of BCR/ABL and is required for leukemogenesis. *J Exp Med* 1999; **189:** 1229–42.
119. Sillaber C, Gesbert F, Frank DA et al, STAT5 activation contributes to growth and viability in Bcr/Abl-transformed cells. *Blood* 2000; **95:** 2118–25.

120. Teglund S, McKay C, Schuetz E et al, Stat5 and Stat5b proteins have essential and nonessential, or redundant, roles in cytokine responses. *Cell* 1998; **93:** 841–50.
121. Socolovsky M, Fallon AEJ, Want S et al, Fetal anemia and apoptosis of red cell progenitors in Stat5a−/− 5b−/− mice: a direct role for Stat5 in Bcl-X_L induction. *Cell* 1999; **98:** 181–91.
122. Sawyers CL, Callahan W, Witte ON, Dominant negative MYC blocks transformation by ABL oncogenes. *Cell* 1992; **70:** 901–10.
123. Reuther JY, Reuther GW, Cortez D et al, Activation of NF-κB is required for Bcr-Abl-mediated tumorigenesis. *Genes Dev* 1998; **12:** 968–81.
124. Hamdane M, David-Cordonnier M-H, D'Halluin JC, Activation of p65 NF-κB protein by $p210^{BCR-ABL}$ in a myeloid cell line ($p210^{BCR-ABL}$ activated p65 NF-κB). *Oncogene* 1997; **15:** 2267–75.
125. Baldwin AS, The NF-kappa B and I-kappa B proteins: new discoveries and insights. *Annu Rev Immunol* 1996; **14:** 649–81.
126. Lionberger JM, Wilson MB, Smithgall TE, Transformation of myeloid leukemia cells to cytokine independence by Bcr–Abl is suppressed by kinase-defective Hck. *J Biol Chem* 2000; **275:** 18581–5.
127. Lionberger JM, Smithgall TE, The c-Fes protein-tyrosine kinase suppresses cytokine-independent outgrowth of myeloid leukemia cells induced by Bcr–Abl. *Cancer Res* 2000; **60:** 1097–103.
128. Wisniewski D, Strife A, Swendeman S et al, A novel SH2-containing phosphatidylinositol 3,4,5-trisphosphate 5-phosphatase (SHIP2) is constitutively tyrosine phosphorylated and associated with src homologous and collagen gene (SHC) in chronic myelogenous leukemia progenitor cells. *Blood* 1999; **93:** 2707–20.
129. Sattler M, Verma S, Byrne CH et al, BCR/ABL directly inhibits expression of SHIP, an SH2-containing polyinositol-5-phosphatase involved in the regulation of hematopoiesis. *Mol Cell Biol* 1999; **19:** 7473–80.
130. Helgason CD, Damen JE, Rosten P et al, Targeted disruption of SHIP leads to hemopoietic perturbations, lung pathology, and a shortened life span. *Genes Dev* 1998; **12:** 1610–20.
131. Hao SX, Ren R, Expression of interferon consensus sequence binding protein (ICSBP) is down-regulated in Bcr–Abl-induced murine chronic myelogenous leukemia-like disease, and forced coexpression of ICSBP inhibits Bcr–Abl-induced myeloproliferative disorder. *Mol Cell Biol* 2000; **20:** 1149–61.
132. Holtschke T, Lohler J, Kanno Y et al, Immunodeficiency and chronic myelogenous leukemia-like syndrome in mice with a targeted mutation of the ICSBP gene. *Cell* 1996; **87:** 307–17.
133. Dai Z, Quackenbush RC, Courtney KD et al, Oncogenic Abl and Src tyrosine kinases elicit the ubiquitin-dependent degradation of target proteins through a Ras-independent pathway. *Genes Dev* 1998; **12:** 1415–24.
134. Dai Z, Pendergast AM, Abi-2, a novel SH3-containing protein, interacts with the c-Abl tyrosine kinase and modulates c-Abl transforming activity. *Genes Dev* 1995; **9:** 2569–82.
135. Shi Y, Alin K, Goff SP, Abl-interactor-1, a novel SH3 protein binding to the carboxy-terminal portion of the Abl protein, suppresses v-abl transforming activity. *Genes Dev* 1995; **9:** 2583–97.
136. Scita G, Nordstrom J, Carbone R et al, EPS8 and E3B1 transduce signals from Ras to Rac. *Nature* 1999; **401:** 290–3.

3

Abnormalities in hematopoietic progenitor adhesion

Ravi Bhatia, Catherine Verfaillie

CONTENTS • Introduction • Abnormal adhesion of CML progenitors • Abnormal adhesion-mediated signaling in CML progenitors • Abnormal migration of CML progenitors on fibronectin • IFN-α restores normal integrin-mediated adhesion and motility of CML progenitors • Mechanism of abnormal integrin receptor function in CML cells • Potential BCR/ABL signaling pathways leading to abnormal integrin function • Conclusions

INTRODUCTION

Normal hematopoiesis is a highly regulated process that occurs in close proximity to the marrow stromal microenvironment. Survival, proliferation, and differentiation of normal hematopoietic progenitors are regulated by interactions with stromal-derived positive and negative regulatory growth factors and with adhesive ligands on stromal cells and stromal extracellular matrix components[1,2] (Figure 3.1). Adhesion of normal hematopoietic progenitors to stromal microenvironmental elements is mediated by multiple receptors, including $\alpha_4\beta_1$ and $\alpha_5\beta_1$ integrin receptors, CD44, and selectins. Progenitors adhere to cell-surface adhesive ligands such as VCAM-1 and ICAM-1, and extracellular matrix (ECM) components such as fibronectin, thrombospondin, and hyaluronic acid.[3–5] In addition to playing a role in anchoring hematopoietic progenitors to appropriate microenvironmental locations and in progenitor migration, homing, and mobilization,[6–9] adhesion receptors also play a direct role in the regulation of progenitor growth.[10–12]

The characteristic features of chronic myeloid leukemia (CML) include abnormal unregulated expansion of malignant BCR/ABL-positive progenitors and precursors as well as premature circulation of malignant progenitors and extramedullary hematopoiesis.[13] Abnormalities in adhesive interactions between CML hematopoietic progenitors and the marrow stromal microenvironment may play a role not only in their abnormal circulation but also in their unregulated growth.

ABNORMAL ADHESION OF CML PROGENITORS

Abnormal adhesion of CML progenitors to stroma

Gordon et al[14] made the original observation that CML hematopoietic progenitors have altered adhesive interactions with marrow stromal layers. They reported that CML blast colony-forming cells (Bl-CFC) demonstrated reduced adhesion to stromal layers. This

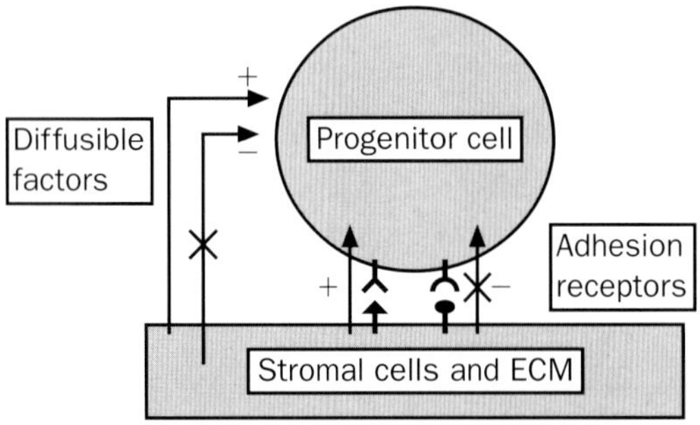

Figure 3.1 Microenvironmental regulation of hematopoietic progenitor growth. The marrow microenvironment regulates normal progenitor survival, proliferation, and differentiation. Normal hematopoietic progenitors adhere to stromal elements in a lineage- and maturation-specific manner. Stromal regulation of hematopoiesis occurs both through engagement of growth factor receptors on progenitor cells by stroma-derived positive and negative regulatory growth factors and through engagement of adhesion receptors by ligands on stromal cells and stromal extracellular matrix (ECM) components. Adhesion receptors, besides playing important roles in anchoring hematopoietic progenitors to appropriate microenvironmental locations and in progenitor migration, homing, and mobilization, also play a direct role in the regulation of progenitor growth. Lack of response to negative regulatory signals from the microenvironment transduced by adhesion receptors as well as receptors for humoral inhibitors may contribute to the unregulated growth of malignant hematopoietic progenitors in CML (×).

observation has been confirmed in subsequent studies, which showed that both malignant CFC and long-term culture-initiating cells (LTC-IC) from CML patients adhered less to stroma than did normal progenitors.[15] As described below, defective expression or function of several adhesion receptors has been described in CML progenitors. The most well-characterized is a defect in β_1 integrin adhesion receptors. However, defects in other receptors may also play a role in abnormal adhesion of CML progenitors to the marrow microenvironment.

Abnormal β_1 integrin-mediated adhesion to fibronectin

$\alpha_4\beta_1$ and $\alpha_5\beta_1$ integrin receptors play important roles in the adhesion and migration of normal hematopoietic progenitors to stroma. Normal primitive progenitors (LTC-IC) use both $\alpha_4\beta_1$ and $\alpha_5\beta_1$ integrins to adhere to fibronectin whereas committed progenitors adhere to fibronectin mainly through $\alpha_5\beta_1$ integrins.[3,4,8] $\alpha_4\beta_1$ integrin interaction with VCAM on the surface of stromal cells also plays a role in progenitor interactions with stroma.[3,16] Philadelphia chromosome (Ph)-positive CML CFC and LTC-IC, on the other hand, adhere significantly less to $\alpha_4\beta_1$- and $\alpha_5\beta_1$-binding fibronectin fragments than do benign primitive progenitors from CML or normal bone marrow.[15] They do, however, adhere to collagen type IV and laminin, ECM components of basement membranes. Evaluation of adhesion receptor expression demonstrates equal expression of fibronectin receptors (α_4, α_5, and β_1 integrins) on progenitors from normal and CML bone marrow. However, a fraction of CML progenitors express α_2 and α_6 receptors, associated with adhesion to laminin and collagen, whereas these receptors are absent from normal progenitors.[15] These observations suggest that the premature release of malignant Ph-positive progenitors into the circulation may be caused by loss of adhesive interactions with stroma and/or fibronectin and acquisition of adhesive interactions with basement membrane components.[15]

Abnormalities in CD44

CD44 is a cell-surface proteoglycan which is expressed at high levels on normal hematopoietic progenitors and which has been implicated in the regulation of normal hematopoiesis. In CML, a significantly greater proportion of circulating progenitors express very high levels of CD44. In addition, there is increased expression of the alternatively spliced exon v10, which is restricted to a small proportion of normal differentiated $CD34^-$ cells. These observations suggest that CD44 expression may be deregulated in CML.[17] Interestingly, activation of β_1 integrins with an activating anti-integrin antibody was found to upregulate CD44-mediated adhesion of CML progenitors to fibronectin, suggesting that altered β_1 integrin function may alter CD44 regulation of adhesion and proliferation in CML.[18]

Selectins

L-selectin is a leukocyte cell-surface glycoprotein that mediates adhesive interactions between circulating cells and vascular endothelium. The mean percentage of $CD34^+$ cells expressing L-selectin from untreated CML patients was significantly lower than that from normal controls. Decreased L-selectin expression could lead to homing defects of CML progenitors.[19]

LFA-3

The cytoadhesion molecule lymphocyte function antigen 3 (LFA-3, CD58) is expressed on normal hematopoietic progenitors. LFA-3 interaction with CD2 may be important for negative regulation of normal progenitor growth by T lymphocytes. Progenitor cells from untreated CML patients showed greatly reduced or absent LFA-3 expression, whereas progenitors from patients treated with interferon-α (IFN-α) in vivo or in vitro expressed surface LFA-3 at more normal levels. LFA-3-deficient CML progenitor cells were unable to stimulate normal regulatory proliferative responses in autologous T cells. LFA-3 deficiency may help explain adhesive abnormalities of CML progenitor cells and abnormal clonal proliferation in vivo.[20]

Deficient adhesion through a phosphatidylinositol-linked receptor

A phosphatidylinositol-anchored cell adhesion molecule involved in normal primitive progenitor (Bl-CFC) adhesion to stroma has also been reported to be deficient in CML. On the other hand, other phosphatidylinositol-linked receptors such as DAF were expressed normally on CML progenitors.[21]

ABNORMAL ADHESION-MEDIATED SIGNALING IN CML PROGENITORS

Continuous proliferation in stromal cultures

Cashman et al[22] showed that adherent progenitors in normal long-term culture are usually quiescent, suggesting that negative regulatory influences from the stromal adherent layer may inhibit normal progenitor proliferation. These may include diffusible factors such as transforming growth factor β (TGF-β) and hematopoietically active chemokines such as macrophage inflammatory protein 1α (MIP-1α).[23,24] In addition, engagement of adhesion receptors as a result of adhesion to stroma may also play a role in stromal regulation of progenitor proliferation. In contrast, CML progenitors in the adherent stromal fraction of long-term bone marrow cultures are continuously proliferating.[25] This suggests that CML progenitors are unresponsive to the growth-inhibitory influences mediated by stroma-derived negative regulatory factors. Although CML progenitors respond normally to the growth-inhibitory effects of TGF-β, some studies suggest that they may not respond to inhibitory chemokines, such as MIP-1α and macrophage chemotactic protein 1 (MCP-1). This may explain in part their continued proliferation even when in contact with stroma.[24,26]

Reduced adhesion-mediated proliferation inhibition

In addition to diffusible inhibitory factors, direct contact with stroma also contributes to inhibition of normal progenitor proliferation. Adhesion of normal $CD34^+$ cells, CFC or LTC-IC to metabolically inactivated stromal layers results in a reduction in the proportion of progenitors in S-phase. Similarly, adhesion to fibronectin and crosslinking of integrin receptors with anti-integrin antibodies also inhibits normal CD34$^+$ cells and CFC proliferation, suggesting that adhesion-mediated inhibition of proliferation may be mediated by transduction of inhibitory signals following engagement of β_1 integrin receptors.[11,27] In contrast CML CD34$^+$ cells or CFC are unresponsive to proliferation inhibition following co-culture with stroma or fibronectin or engagement of β_1 integrins directly with anti-integrin antibodies. This suggests that, in addition to impaired integrin-mediated adhesion, proliferation inhibitory signaling through integrin receptors is impaired in CML progenitors.[28]

This was confirmed further by studies demonstrating inhibition in G_1–S progression following integrin engagement on normal CD34$^+$ cells grown in 'physiological concentrations' of growth factors. This was associated with increased levels of p27^{Kip}, reduced cyclin E and A levels, and decreased cyclin-dependent kinase 2 (Cdk2) activity. Stimulation with high concentrations of interleukin-3 (IL-3) or stem cell factor (SCF) overrides the inhibitory effect of integrin stimulation, prevents inhibition of G_1–S progression and prevents p27^{Kip} elevation following integrin stimulation. In CML CD34$^+$ cells, on the other hand, adhesion resulted in only marginal reduction of the fraction of cells in S-phase compared with non-adherent cells, and levels of p27^{Kip} cyclin E and cyclin A were similar in adherent and non-adherent cells. Baseline levels of p27^{Kip} were significantly elevated in CML cells, suggesting that the mechanisms of suppression of integrin-mediated signaling by BCR/ABL may be different from that of IL-3.[29]

ABNORMAL MIGRATION OF CML PROGENITORS ON FIBRONECTIN

When placed on fibronectin-coated surfaces, CML progenitors produce more pseudopodia and display abnormally increased and persistent mobility.[30] CML CD34$^+$ cells also show increased spontaneous and vectorial mobility on fibronectin, but not on ICAM.[31] These abnormalities could be reversed after prolonged exposure to IFN-α. These studies indicate that, in contrast to reduced integrin-mediated adhesion to fibronectin, CML progenitors have enhanced mobility on fibronectin. Abnormal migration on fibronectin may contribute to the abnormal peripheral circulation of CML progenitors.

IFN-α RESTORES NORMAL INTEGRIN-MEDIATED ADHESION AND MOTILITY OF CML PROGENITORS

IFN-α treatment can restore normal hematopoiesis in a fraction of CML patients.[32] Although IFN-α treatment leads to partial inhibition of CML committed progenitor growth, especially late committed progenitor growth, it similarly inhibits normal committed progenitor growth, indicating that there must be an alternative mechanism underlying its ability to selectively suppress malignant progenitor growth.[33] Dowding et al[34] showed that treatment of stroma with IFN-α leads to increased attachment of CML progenitors, suggesting that IFN-α may reverse the abnormality in progenitor–stroma interactions seen in CML. It has also been shown that IFN-α treatment of CML progenitors results in dose- and time-dependent enhancement of adhesion of CML progenitors to stroma and fibronectin mediated via β_1 integrins.[35] No change in receptor expression was seen, suggesting that enhanced adhesion after IFN-α treatment was related to altered integrin receptor function. Treatment of normal stromal layers with IFN-α also resulted in enhanced adhesion of CML progenitors through β_1 integrins.[36] This effect may be mediated in part by enhanced stromal production of the chemokine MIP-1α that was capable of enhancing CML progenitor adhesion. In addition, IFN-α treatment restores normal motility of CML cells on fibronectin.[30,31] Further, IFN-α treatment can also restore inhibition of CML

CFC proliferation after contact with stroma and fibronectin and after integrin stimulation with antibody-mediated crosslinking.[28] These observations suggest that IFN-α can restore integrin-mediated adhesion, mobility, and proliferation-inhibitory signaling in CML progenitors, which may explain, at least in part, its efficacy in the treatment of CML.

MECHANISM OF ABNORMAL INTEGRIN RECEPTOR FUNCTION IN CML CELLS

Role of *BCR/ABL*

Several lines of experimental evidence suggest that abnormal integrin function in CML progenitors is related to the presence of the *BCR/ABL* gene. Exposure to antisense oligonucleotides (AS-ODNs) specific for *BCR/ABL* restores integrin-mediated adhesion of CML primary progenitors to stroma and fibronectin as well as integrin-mediated proliferation inhibition in CML progenitors after co-culture with stroma and fibronectin or after antibody-mediated integrin receptor crosslinking.[37] *BCR/ABL* AS-ODNs did not affect integrin function in normal progenitors. Tyrphostin (AG957), a tyrosine kinase inhibitor with anti-BCR/ABL kinase activity, also restored integrin-mediated adhesion and proliferation inhibition in CML progenitors, but did not affect integrin function in normal progenitors.[38] These observations suggest a role for BCR/ABL tyrosine kinase activity in abnormal integrin function in CML cells.

On the other hand, integrin-dependent cell binding to soluble and immobilized fibronectin in growth-factor-dependent hematopoietic cell lines was enhanced following *BCR/ABL* transfection when cells were assayed in the absence of growth factors.[39] In non-transfected cells, withdrawal of growth factor resulted in inhibition of adhesion, whereas exposure to growth factor rapidly enhanced their adhesion. The enhanced adhesion of BCR/ABL-containing cell lines to fibronectin may reflect the ability of BCR/ABL to replace growth factor as an adhesion-modulatory stimulus in growth-factor-dependent cell lines. Other studies indicate that the *BCR/ABL* gene abrogates the anchorage requirement for proliferation of fibroblastic cells, which requires integrin interaction with the extracellular matrix, but not the growth factor requirement.[40] These studies in cell lines provide further indication of the ability of *BCR/ABL* to modulate integrin function.

Abnormalities in integrin cytoskeletal interactions

Integrins are heterodimers of α and β subunits, each with a large extracellular ligand-binding domain, a single transmembrane domain, and a short cytoplasmic domain. Integrin stimulation leads to receptor clustering and formation of multimolecular focal adhesion complexes of integrins, cytoskeletal elements, and signaling proteins.[41] Interaction of the integrin cytoplasmic domain with cytoskeletal elements plays a role both in regulation of integrin binding to external ligands (inside-out signaling) and in transduction of signals into the cell following engagement of integrin receptors by ligand (outside-in signaling).[41,42] In CML cells, p210 BCR/ABL localizes primarily in the cytoplasm,[43] co-localizing with actin fibers, and in focal adhesion-like structures.[30,44] As discussed below, several prominent substrates for BCR/ABL are cytoskeletal proteins. Therefore, it is possible that abnormal integrin function in CML cells may be related to BCR/ABL-induced abnormalities in integrin–cytoskeletal interactions (Figure 3.2).

Cell lines in which *BCR/ABL* has been introduced demonstrate multiple cytoskeletal abnormalities, including increased membrane ruffling, filopodia formation, accelerated protrusion and retraction of pseudopodia, and continuous mobility on fibronectin-coated surfaces. Similar abnormalities are seen in CML $CD34^+$ cells.[30] In normal $CD34^+$ progenitors, antibody-mediated crosslinking of β_1 integrins results in their redistribution into caps via a process requiring receptor–cytoskeletal interactions.[27] In

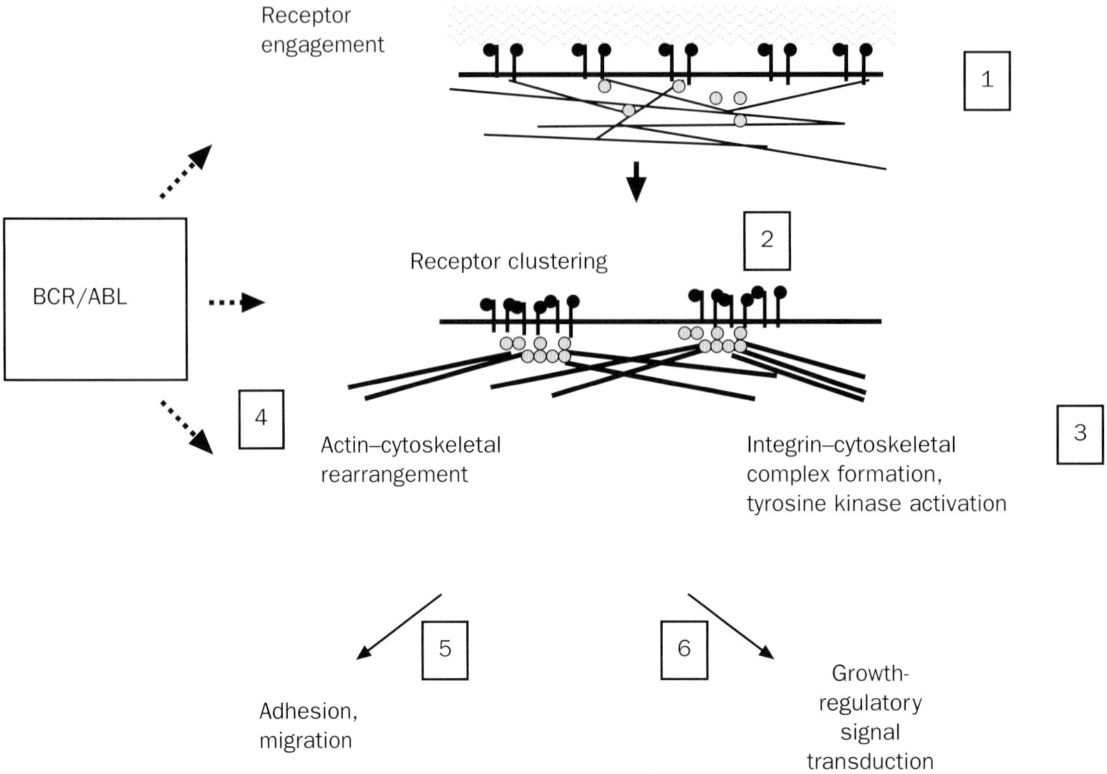

Figure 3.2 Abnormalities in integrin-mediated adhesion and signaling in CML. Integrins are heterodimers of α and β subunits, each with a large extracellular ligand-binding domain, a single transmembrane domain, and a short cytoplasmic domain. Interaction of the integrin cytoplasmic domain with cytoskeletal elements is important both for regulation of integrin binding to external ligands (inside-out signaling) and for transduction of signals into the cell following engagement of integrin receptors by ligand (outside-in signaling). Engagement by ligand leads to receptor clustering, formation of multimolecular complexes of integrins with cytoskeletal elements, and actin cytoskeletal rearrangements, all of which are important for adhesion. A number of adapter and signaling proteins, including tyrosine kinases, are recruited to integrin–cytoskeletal complexes, leading to transduction of signals affecting proliferation and differentiation. In CML, the presence of BCR/ABL leads to altered receptor affinity for ligand (1), abnormal receptor clustering (2), decreased integrin–cytoskeleton complex formation (3), abnormal actin polymerization and actin cytoskeleton organization (4), reduced adhesion (5), and impaired transfer of proliferation-regulatory signaling (6).

contrast, β_1 integrin capping is significantly impaired in CML CD34$^+$ cells, suggesting abnormalities in integrin–cytoskeletal interactions.[45] This appears to be related to the presence of the *BCR/ABL* gene, since capping is also impaired in *BCR/ABL*-transfected cell lines and reversed following exposure to anti-*BCR/ABL* antisense AS-ODNs. Defective receptor capping was not seen for non-integrin receptors. In addition, actin polymerization and actin cytoskeletal organization are abnormal in CML CD34$^+$ and M07e$^{BCR/ABL}$ cells. Further studies suggested that impaired β_1 integrin capping and defective integrin-mediated adhesion and proliferation inhibition in CML cells were related to abnormally enhanced integrin–

cytoskeletal association and restricted receptor mobility.[45] Finally, IFN-α, which restores integrin-mediated adhesion and signaling in CML progenitors, also enhanced integrin capping in CD34+ cells.[45] These studies suggest that p210 BCR/ABL induces abnormal association of integrin receptors with the cytoskeleton and restricted receptor mobility.

Alternative splicing of integrin receptors

The alternatively sliced β_{1b} integrin differs from the common β_{1a} form in the last 20 C-terminal amino acids.[46,47] Since β_{1b} integrins cannot interact with cytoskeletal proteins, increased β_{1b} levels prevent localization of β_{1a} integrins to focal contacts, resulting in dominant-negative effects on adhesion.[46,47] Increased levels of β_{1b} integrin are seen in CML CD34+ cells. Interestingly, expression of β_{1b} integrins is inhibited by IFN-α and AS-ODNs to *BCR/ABL*, suggesting that increased β_{1b} integrin levels may in part be responsible for defective integrin function in CML. The role of *BCR/ABL* in regulation of β_{1b} expression requires elucidation.[48]

Abnormal receptor affinity

Modulation of integrin receptor affinity by the activating antibody 8A2 resulted in increased $\alpha_5\beta_1$-dependent adhesion of K562 cells and CML CD34+ cells to fibronectin.[49] This suggests that decreased receptor affinity may contribute to abnormal integrin function in CML. Reduced integrin receptor affinity in CML may also be a consequence of abnormal receptor–cytoskeletal interactions, since receptor interaction with cytoskeletal elements may modulate affinity.[50]

POTENTIAL BCR/ABL SIGNALING PATHWAYS LEADING TO ABNORMAL INTEGRIN FUNCTION

There are several possible signaling mechanisms that can be activated by BCR/ABL that could potentially lead to induction of abnormal integrin function in CML cells (Figure 3.3). However, these signaling mechanisms have been identified in *BCR/ABL*-transfected cell lines, which usually highly overexpress BCR/ABL, and it remains to be determined whether these pathways are activated in primary CML cells and if they are directly involved in induction of abnormal integrin function in CML cells.

F-actin binding

The C-terminus of c-ABL contains distinct F- and G-actin-binding domains, which can cooperate to bundle actin filaments.[51] On adhesion to fibronectin, a transient recruitment of c-ABL to focal adhesions is seen, coincident with export from the nucleus, followed by return of activated c-ABL to the nucleus.[52] Therefore c-ABL appears to be activated by adhesion, and may transmit integrin signals to the nucleus. In contrast to c-ABL, which shows both nuclear and cytoplasmic localization, BCR/ABL shows increased actin binding and predominantly cytoplasmic localization.[43] Significantly, the actin-binding function of BCR/ABL contributes to its transforming activity.[53] BCR sequences in the BCR/ABL fusion protein, specifically an N-terminus coiled-coil oligomerization domain of BCR, activate the actin binding functions of c-ABL.[44] In addition, the BCR Dbl homology domain present in p210 BCR/ABL but not p190 BCR/ABL also contributes to stabilization of actin filaments by BCR/ABL.[54]

Activation of Crkl

Crkl, a 39 kDa adapter protein, is the major phosphorylated protein in primary CML cells.[55] Crkl directly binds BCR/ABL proline-rich regions via its SH3 domain. However, Crkl still complexes with BCR/ABL constructs with mutations in the proline-rich region, as a result of indirect interactions with BCR/ABL via other proteins such as Cbl.[56] Crkl forms a link

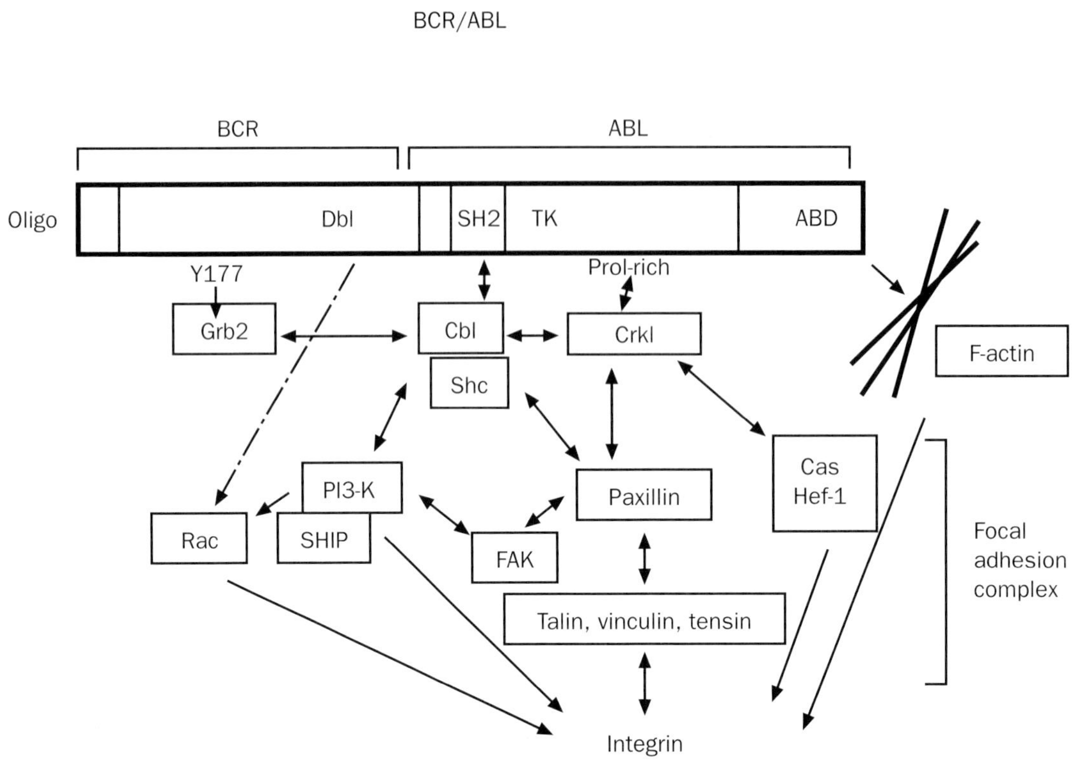

Figure 3.3 BCR/ABL signaling pathways that may lead to abnormal integrin function in CML cells. BCR/ABL can activate several possible signaling mechanisms that could potentially lead to induction of abnormal integrin function in CML cells. Increased activity of the ABL tyrosine kinase domain (TK), which is essential to BCR/ABL-induced transformation, plays an important role in abnormal integrin function in CML cells. BCR/ABL shows increased actin-binding activity via its C-terminus actin-binding domain (ABD) compared with c-ABL. BCR sequences, specifically an N-terminus coiled-coil oligomerization domain (Oligo), are required for the increased actin-binding activity of BCR/ABL. The adapter protein Crkl is the major phosphorylated protein in primary CML cells. Crkl directly binds BCR/ABL proline-rich regions (Prol-rich) via its SH3 domain and indirectly via other proteins such as Cbl. Crkl links BCR/ABL to several proteins that have important interactions with integrin receptors, such as paxillin, Cas, and Hef-1. Constitutive phosphorylation of the focal adhesion proteins paxillin, vinculin, talin, and tensin and the focal adhesion kinase (FAK), and association of FAK, vinculin, talin, and tensin in complexes with paxillin has been observed in BCR/ABL-transformed cell lines. The adapter proteins Cbl and Shc bind the SH2 domain of BCR/ABL directly, and also indirectly by forming complexes with the Crkl SH2 domain or Grb2 (which binds to a phosphotyrosine at position 177 (Y177) in the BCR-derived portion of the molecule). The p85 regulatory subunit of phosphatidylinositol 3′-kinase (PI3-K) is phosphorylated and shows increased association with Cbl and Shc in BCR/ABL-transformed cells, and abnormal constitutive activation of PI3-K is seen. The BCR Dbl homology (Dbl) domain is potentially capable of activating the small G proteins Rho. The related protein Rac complexes with BCR/ABL and shows enhanced activity in BCR/ABL-transformed cell lines. Since PI3-K, Rho, and Rac play important roles in the regulation of actin cytoskeletal rearrangement and integrin–cytoskeletal complex formation, their abnormal activation by BCR/ABL could contribute to abnormal integrin-mediated adhesion, migration, and signaling in CML cells.

between BCR/ABL and several proteins that have important interactions with integrin receptors, such as paxillin, Cas, and Hef-1.[57–60] In myeloid cells, integrin ligation induces Crkl to associate with tyrosine-phosphorylated Cbl.[61] Crkl overexpression in cell lines alters cell morphology and induces integrin-mediated adhesion to fibronectin.[62,63] Therefore, activation of Crkl signaling by BCR/ABL may play a role in alterations in focal adhesion proteins and abnormal integrin function in CML primary cells.

Alterations in focal adhesion proteins

Constitutive phosphorylation of the focal adhesion proteins paxillin, FAK, vinculin, talin, and tensin, and association of FAK, vinculin, talin, and tensin in complexes with paxillin, have been observed in BCR/ABL-transformed cell lines.[64,65]

Paxillin, a 68 kDa protein that localizes in focal adhesion, associates with BCR/ABL, Crkl and several other focal adhesion proteins in multimeric complexes.[66] In addition to binding Crkl, paxillin may also bind to BCR/ABL through Cbl. Paxillin may play a role in signal transduction from BCR/ABL and Crkl to the cytoskeleton and integrin receptors.

Cas, a 125 kDa protein seen in focal-adhesion-like structures, constitutively associates with the focal adhesion proteins tensin, Fak, and paxillin in normal cells, and is a mediator of FAK-promoted migration.[67] In CML cells, Cas is tyrosine-phosphorylated and constitutively associates with BCR/ABL and Crkl, and its normal interaction with tensin is disrupted.[58] Hef-1, a 110 kDa protein structurally similar to Cas, is also tyrosine-phosphorylated and is complexed to the Crkl SH2 domain in p190 BCR/ABL-transfected cells.[68] Therefore, as with paxillin, association of Cas and Hef-1 with BCR/ABL and Crkl may contribute to defective integrin receptor function.

Phosphatidylinositol signaling

Phosphatidylinositol 3'-kinase (PI3-K) plays an important role in the regulation of actin cytoskeletal rearrangement and integrin–cytoskeletal complex formation.[69–71] Abnormal constitutive activation of PI3-K is seen in BCR/ABL-transformed cells.[72] Activation of PI3-K and its downstream target Akt contributes to transformation of murine hematopoietic cells by BCR/ABL.[73]

The p85 regulatory subunit of PI3-K is phosphorylated and shows increased association with Cbl and Shc in BCR/ABL-transformed cells.[74–76] The adapter protein Cbl can link BCR/ABL to p85 via binding of the SH2 and SH3 domains of p85 to Cbl.[75,77] Phosphorylated Cbl directly binds the SH2 domain of BCR/ABL, and also binds BCR/ABL indirectly by forming complexes with the Crkl SH2 domain or Grb2.[59–77] Oncogenic forms of Cbl can abrogate the anchorage dependence but not the growth factor requirement for proliferation of adherent cells.[78] This is similar to what has been described for BCR/ABL, suggesting that abnormal activation of Cbl could play a role in the effects of BCR/ABL on adhesion-mediated signaling. This effect may be mediated via PI3-K-dependent or -independent mechanisms.

Further evidence for the importance of altered phosphatidylinositol metabolism in BCR/ABL-induced transformation comes from studies of the phosphatidylinositol 5-phosphatase SHIP. SHIP is involved in hematopoietic regulation, since targeted disruption leads to a myeloproliferative syndrome in mice. SHIP is complexed with SHP, a tyrosine phosphatase, in response to growth factor stimulation. SHP may negatively regulate SHIP by dephosphorylation. In BCR/ABL-transformed cells, SHIP is heavily phosphorylated and constitutively complexed with SHP, and SHIP levels are reduced. This suggests that the function of this complex may be altered with reduced SHIP activity and increased levels of 5-phosphate lipids. Inhibition of BCR/ABL tyrosine kinase activity restores SHIP expression, suggesting that BCR/ABL directly inhibits SHIP expression.[79]

Rac

Rho, Rac, and Cdc42 are small G proteins that act as molecular switches regulating actin cytoskeletal organization, integrin–cytoskeletal interactions, mobility, and invasiveness.[80] These proteins also interact with PI3-K, and activation of PI3-K by Rac and Cdc42 plays a critical role in alteration of actin organization, and promotes mobility and invasiveness.[81]

Rac activity has been reported to be enhanced in BCR/ABL-transformed cell lines. Transfection of dominant-negative Rac into these cells resulted in a marked reduction in invasiveness, whereas proliferation and susceptibility to apoptosis were less affected. In vivo, leukemogenesis was markedly impaired, with reduced homing of cells to marrow and spleen.[82]

In another study, introduction of constitutively activated Rho, Rac, and p110 PI3-K into myeloid cell lines resulted in increased motility and ruffling of cell membranes. Introduction of dominant-negative Rac and Cdc42 reversed hypermotility of BCR/ABL-transformed cells. It was further shown that Rac co-precipitates with BCR/ABL.[83] These observations suggest a role for Rac in abnormal motility of BCR/ABL-transformed cells.

CONCLUSIONS

BCR/ABL-induced abnormalities in adhesion, migration, and adhesion-mediated growth-regulatory signaling may contribute to abnormal circulation and proliferation of CML progenitors. Defects in β_1 integrin receptor function play a major role in these abnormalities, although abnormalities in the functions of other receptors may also be important. Studies in BCR/ABL-transformed cell lines suggest that multiple signaling mechanisms activated by BCR/ABL could potentially affect integrin-mediated adhesion and signaling in CML cells. Constitutive phosphorylation and recruitment to signaling complexes of several proteins that are involved in normal integrin-mediated inside-out and outside-in signaling are observed in these lines. Abnormal constitutive activation of components of signaling pathways responsible for physiological regulation of integrin function may impair normal, regulated activation of these signaling mechanisms, and may result in impaired integrin-mediated adhesion, motility, and signaling. The relevance of these various observations to CML is not clear at this time, since the disease arises in an early hematopoietic stem or progenitor cell for which existing cell lines are not adequate models. Future studies need to address which of these mechanisms are active in primary CML progenitors and are responsible for the observed defects in integrin function and other aspects of the transformed phenotype.

REFERENCES

1. Dexter TM, Coutinho LH, Spooncer E et al, Stromal cells in haemopoiesis. *Ciba Found Symp*, 1990: **148:** 76–95.
2. Zuckerman KS, Wicha MS, Extracellular matrix production by the adherent cells in long-term murine marrow cultures. *Blood* 1983; **61:** 540–56.
3. Teixido J, Hemler ME, Greenberger JS, Anklesaria P, Role of β1 and β2 integrins in the adhesion of human CD34^{hi} stem cells to bone marrow stroma. *J Clin Invest* 1992; **90:** 358–67.
4. Verfaillie CM, McCarthy JB, McGlave PB, Differentiation of primitive human multipotent hematopoietic progenitors into single lineage clonogenic progenitors is accompanied by alterations in their adhesion to fibronectin. *J Exp Med* 1991; **174:** 693–703.
5. Verfaillie C, Hurley R, Bhatia R, McCarthy JB, Role of bone marrow matrix in normal and abnormal hematopoiesis. *Crit Rev Oncol Hematol* 1994; **16:** 201–24.
6. Miyake K, Weissman IL, Greenberger JS, Kincade PW, Evidence for a role of the integrin VLA-4 in lympho-hemopoeisis. *J Exp Med* 1991; **173:** 599–607.
7. Prosper F, Stroncek D, McCarthy JB, Verfaillie CM, Mobilization and homing of peripheral blood progenitors is related to reversible down-regulation of alpha4 beta1 integrin expression and function. *J Clin Invest* 1998; **101:** 2456–67.

8. Williams DA, Rios M, Stephens C, Patel VP, Fibronectin and VLA-4 in hematopoietic stem cell-microenvironment interactions. *Nature* 1991; **352:** 438–41.
9. Papayannapoulou T, Priestly GV, Nakamoto B, Anti-VLA-4/VCAM-1-induced mobilization requires cooperative signaling through the kit/mkit pathway. *Blood* 1998; **91:** 2231–39.
10. Verfaillie CM, Cantanzaro P, Direct contact with stroma inhibits proliferation of human long-term culture initiating cells. *Leukemia* 1996; **10:** 498–504.
11. Hurley RW, McCarthy JB, Verfaillie CM, Direct adhesion to bone marrow stroma via fibronectin receptors inhibits hematopoietic progenitor proliferation. *J Clin Invest* 1995; **96:** 511–19.
12. Dao MA, Hashino K, Kato I, Nolta JA, Adhesion to fibronectin maintains regenerative capacity during ex vivo culture and transduction of human hematopoietic stem and progenitor cells. *Blood* 1998; **92:** 4612–21.
13. Sawyers CL, Chronic myeloid leukemia. *N Engl J Med* 1999; **340:** 1330–40.
14. Gordon MY, Dowding CR, Riley GP et al, Altered adhesive interactions with marrow stroma of hematopoietic progenitor cells in chronic myelogenous leukaemia. *Nature* 1984; **328:** 342–44.
15. Verfaillie CM, McCarthy JB, McGlave PB, Mechanisms underlying abnormal trafficking of malignant progenitors in chronic myelogenous leukemia: decreased adhesion to stroma and fibronectin but increased adhesion to the basement membrane components laminin and collagen type IV. *J Clin Invest* 1992; **90:** 1232–39.
16. Simmons PJ, Masinovsky B, Longenecker BM et al, Vascular cell adhesion molecule 1 is expressed by bone marrow stromal cells and mediates binding of hematopoietic cells. *Blood* 1992; **80:** 388–95.
17. Ghaffari S, Dougherty GJ, Lansdorp PM et al, Differentiation-associated changes in CD44 isoform expression during normal hematopoiesis and their alteration in chronic myelogenous leukemia. *Blood* 1995; **86:** 2976–85.
18. Lundell BI, McCarthy JB, Kovach NL, Verfaillie CM, Activation of beta1 integrins on CML progenitors reveals cooperation between beta1 integrins and CD44 in the regulation of adhesion and proliferation. *Leukemia* 1997; **11:** 822–9.
19. Kawaishi K, Kimura A, Katoh O et al, Decreased L-selectin expression in CD34-positive cells from patients with chronic myelogenous leukemia. *Br J Hematol* 1996; **93:** 367–74.
20. Upadhyaya G, Guba SC, Sih SA et al, Interferon-alpha restores the deficient expression of the cytoadhesion molecule lymphocyte function antigen-3 by chronic myelogenous leukemia progenitor cells. *J Clin Invest* 1991; **88:** 2131–6.
21. Gordon MY, Atkinson J, Clarke D et al, Deficiency of a phosphatidylinositol-anchored cell adhesion molecule influences haematopoietic progenitor binding to marrow stroma in chronic myelogenous leukemia. *Leukemia* 1991; **5:** 693–8.
22. Cashman J, Eaves AC, Eaves CJ, Regulated proliferation of primitive hematopoietic progenitors in long-term human marrow cultures. *Blood* 1985; **66:** 1002–5.
23. Cashman JD, Eaves AC, Raines EW et al, Mechanisms that regulate the cell cycle status of very primitive hematopoietic cells in long-term human marrow cultures. I. Stimulatory role of a variety of mesenchymal cell activators and inhibitory role of TGF-β. *Blood* 1990; **75:** 96–101.
24. Eaves CJ, Cashman JD, Wolpe SD, Eaves AC, Unresponsiveness of primitive chronic myeloid leukemia cells to macrophage inflammatory protein 1 alpha, an inhibitor of primitive normal hematopoietic cells. *Proc Natl Acad Sci USA* 1993; **90:** 12015–19.
25. Eaves AC, Cashman JD, Gaboury LA et al, Unregulated proliferation of primitive chronic myeloid leukemia progenitors in the presence of normal marrow adherent cells. *Proc Natl Acad Sci USA* 1986; **83:** 5306–10.
26. Cashman JD, Eaves CJ, Sarris AH, Eaves AC, MCP-1, not MIP-1alpha, is the endogenous chemokine that cooperates with TGF-beta to inhibit the cycling of primitive normal but not leukemic (CML) progenitors in long-term human marrow cultures. *Blood* 1998; **92:** 2338–44.
27. Hurley RW, McCarthy JB, Wayner EA, Verfaillie CM, Monoclonal antibody crosslinking of the alpha 4 or beta 1 integrin inhibits committed clonogenic hematopoietic progenitor proliferation. *Exp Hematol* 1997; **25:** 321–8.
28. Bhatia R, McCarthy JB, Verfaillie CM, Interferon-alpha restores normal beta 1 integrin-mediated inhibition of hematopoietic progenitor proliferation by the marrow microenvironment in chronic myelogenous leukemia. *Blood* 1996; **87:** 3883–91.
29. Jiang YH, Prosper F, Verfaillie CM, Opposing effect of integrin engagement and stimulation of

IL3 and SCF receptors on p27KIP level differentially regulate normal CD34+ cell cycle progression. *Blood* 1998; **92:** 673A.

30. Salgia R, Li J-L, Ewaniuk DS et al, BCR/ABL induces multiple abnormalities of cytoskeletal function. *J Clin Invest* 1997; **100:** 46–57.
31. Weber E, McCarthy JB, Verfaillie CM, CML CD34+ hematopoietic progenitor cells are hypermotile on fibronectin but not on ICAM-1. *Blood* 1998; **92:** 94A.
32. Talpaz M, Kantarjian H, Kurzrock R et al, Interferon-alpha produces sustained cytogenetic responses in chronic myelogenous leukemia. Philadelphia chromosome-positive patients. *Ann Intern Med* 1991; **114:** 532–8.
33. Galvani DW, Cawley JC, Mechanism of action of α-interferon in chronic granulocytic leukemia: evidence for preferential inhibition of late progenitors. *Br J Haematol* 1989; **73:** 475–9.
34. Dowding C, Guo A-P, Osterholz J et al, Interferon-α overrides the deficient adhesion of chronic myeloid leukemia primitive progenitor cells to bone marrow stromal cells. *Blood* 1991; **78:** 499–505.
35. Bhatia R, Wayner EA, McGlave PB, Verfaillie CM, Interferon-alpha restores normal adhesion of chronic myelogenous leukemia hematopoietic progenitors to bone marrow stroma by correcting impaired beta 1 integrin receptor function. *J Clin Invest* 1994; **94:** 384–91.
36. Bhatia R, McGlave PB, Verfaillie CM, Treatment of marrow stroma with interferon-alpha restores normal beta 1 integrin-dependent adhesion of chronic myelogenous leukemia hematopoietic progenitors. Role of MIP-1 alpha. *J Clin Invest* 1995; **96:** 931–9.
37. Bhatia R, Verfaillie CM, Inhibition of BCR–ABL expression with antisense oligonucleotides restores β1 integrin mediated adhesion and proliferation inhibition in chronic myelogenous leukemia hematopoietic progenitors. *Blood* 1998; **91:** 3414–22.
38. Bhatia R, Munthe HM, Verfaillie CM, Tyrphostin AG957, a tyrosine kinase inhibitor with anti-BCR/ABL tyrosine kinase activity restores β1 integrin mediated adhesion and inhibitory signaling in chronic myelogenous leukemia hematopoietic progenitors. *Leukemia* 1998; **12:** 1708–17.
39. Bazzoni G, Carlesso N, Griffin JD, Hemler ME, Bcr/Abl expression stimulates integrin function in hematopoietic cell lines. *J Clin Invest* 1996; **98:** 521–8.
40. Renshaw MW, McWhirter JR, Wang JYJ, The human leukemia oncogene bcr–abl abrogates the anchorage requirement but not the growth factor requirement for proliferation. *Mol Cell Biol* 1995; **15:** 1286–93.
41. Hynes RO, Integrins: versatility, modulation, and signaling in cell adhesion. *Cell* 1992; **69:** 11–25.
42. Clark EA, Brugge JS, Integrins and signal transduction pathways: the road taken. *Science* 1995; **268:** 233–39.
43. Weitzler M, Talpaz M, Van Etten RA et al, Subcellular localization of Bcr, Abl, and Bcr–Abl proteins in normal and leukemic cells and correlation of expression with myeloid differentiation. *J Clin Invest* 1993; **92:** 1925–39.
44. McWhirter JR, Wang JYJ, Activation of tyrosine kinase and microfilament-binding functions of c-abl by bcr sequences in bcr/abl fusion proteins. *Mol Cell Biol* 1991; **11:** 1553–65.
45. Bhatia R, Munthe HM, Verfaillie CM, Role of abnormal integrin–cytoskeletal interactions in impaired β1 integrin function in chronic myelogenous leukemia hematopoietic progenitors. *Exp Hematol* 1999; **27:** 1384–96.
46. Balzac F, Belkin AM, Koteliansky VE et al, Expression and functional analysis of a cytoplasmic domain variant of the beta 1 integrin subunit. *J Cell Biol* 1993; **121:** 171–8.
47. Zhao RCH, Tarone G, Verfaillie CM, Presence of the adhesion inhibitory β1b integrin isoform on CML but not normal progenitors is at least in part responsible for the decreased CML progenitor adhesion. *Blood* 1997; **90:** 393A.
48. Lundell BI, McCarthy JB, Kovach NL, Verfaillie CM, Activation-dependent alpha5beta1 integrin-mediated adhesion to fibronectin decreases proliferation of chronic myelogenous leukemia progenitors and K562 cells. *Blood* 1996; **87:** 2450–8.
49. Schwartz MA, Schaller MD, Ginsberg MH, Integrins: emerging paradigms of signal transduction. *Annu Rev Cell Dev Biol* 1995; **11:** 549–99.
50. Van Etten R, Jackson P, Baltimore D et al, The COOH terminus of c-Abl tyrosine kinase contains distinct F- and G-actin binding domains with bundling activity. *J Cell Biol* 1994; **124:** 325–40.
51. Lewis JM, Bhaskaran R, Taagepara S et al, Integrin regulation of c-Abl tyrosine kinase activity and cytoplasmic-nuclear transport. *Proc Natl Acad Sci USA* 1996; **93:** 15174–79.

52. McWhirter JR, Wang JYJ, An actin-binding function contributes to transformation by the BCR–ABL oncoprotein of Philadelphia chromosome-positive human leukemias. *EMBO J* 1993; **12:** 1533–46.
53. McWhirter JR, Wang JYJ, Effect of Bcr sequences on the cellular function of the Bcr–Abl oncoprotein. *Oncogene* 1997; **15:** 1625–34.
54. Oda T, Heaney C, Hagopian JR et al, Crkl is the major tyrosine-phosphorylated protein in neutrophils from patients with chronic myelogenous leukemia. *J Biol Chem* 1994; **269:** 22925–28.
55. Heaney C, Kolibaba K, Bhat A et al, Direct binding of CRKL to BCR–ABL is not required for BCR–ABL transformation. *Blood* 1997; **89:** 297–306.
56. Salgia R, Uemera N, Okuda K et al, CRKL links p210BCR/ABL with paxillin in chronic myelogenous leukemia cells. *J Biol Chem* 1995; **270:** 29145–50.
57. Salgia R, Pisick E, Sattler M et al, p130CAS forms a signaling complex with the adapter protein CRKL in hematopoietic cells transformed by the BCR/ABL oncogene. *J Biol Chem* 1996; **271:** 25198–203.
58. de Jong R, ten Hoeve J, Heisterkamp N, Groffen J, Crkl is complexed with tyrosine-phosphorylated Cbl in Ph-positive leukemia. *J Biol Chem* 1995; **270:** 21468–71.
59. Uemura N, Salgia R, Li J-L et al, The BCR/ABL oncogene alters interaction of the adapter proteins CRKL and CRK with cellular proteins. *Leukemia* 1997; **11:** 376–85.
60. Sattler M, Salgia R, Shrikhande G et al, Differential signaling after b1integrin ligation is mediated through binding of CRKL to p120CBL and p110HEF1. *J Biol Chem* 1997; **272:** 14320–26.
61. Arai A, Nosaka Y, Kohsaka H et al, Crkl activates integrin-mediated hematopoietic cell adhesion through the guanine exchange factor C3G. *Blood* 1999; **93:** 3713–22.
62. Uemura N, Salgia R, Ewaniuk DS, Little MT, Involvement of the adapter protein CRKL in integrin-mediated adhesion. *Oncogene* 1999; **18:** 3343–53.
63. Salgia R, Brunkhorst B, Pisick E et al, Increased tyrosine phosphorylation of focal adhesion proteins in myeloid cell lines expressing $p210^{BCR/ABL}$. *Oncogene* 1995; **11:** 1149–55.
64. Gotoh A, Miyazawa K, Ohyashiki K et al, Tyrosine phosphorylation and activation of focal adhesion kinase (p125FAK) by BCR–ABL oncoprotein. *Exp Hematol* 1995; **23:** 1153–9.
65. Salgia R, Li J-L, Lo SH et al, Molecular cloning of human paxillin, a focal adhesion protein phosphorylated by $P210^{BCR/ABL}$. *J Biol Chem* 1995; **270:** 5039–47.
66. Cary LA, Han DC, Polte TR et al, Identification of p130cas as a mediator of focal adhesion kinase-promoted cell migration. *J Cell Biol* 1998; **140:** 211–21.
67. de Jong R, van Wijk A, Haataja L et al, BCR/ABL-induced leukemogenesis causes phosphorylation of Hef1 and its association with Crkl. *J Biol Chem* 1997; **272:** 32649–55.
68. Shimizu Y, Mobley JL, Finkelstein LD, Chan ASH, A role for phosphatidylinositol 3-kinase in the regulation of beta-1 integrin activity by the CD2 antigen. *J Cell Biol* 1995; **131:** 1867–80.
69. Guinebault C, Payrastre B, Racaud-Sultan C et al, Integrin-dependent translocation of phosphoinositide 3-kinase to the cytoskeleton of thrombin-activated platelets involves specific interactions of p85α with actin filaments and focal adhesion kinase. *J Cell Biol* 1995; **129:** 831–42.
70. Rodriguez-Viciana P, Warne PH, Khwaja A et al, Role of phosphoinositide 3-OH kinase in cell transformation and control of the actin cytoskeleton by Ras. *Cell* 1997; **89:** 457–67.
71. Skorski T, Kanakaraj P, Nieborowska-Skorska M et al, Phosphatidylinositol-3 kinase activity is regulated by BCR/ABL and is required for the growth of Philadelphia chromosome-positive cells. *Blood* 1995; **86:** 726–36.
72. Skorski T, Bellacosa A, Nieborowska-Skorska M et al, Transformation of hematopoietic cells by BCR/ABL requires activation of a PI-3K/Akt-dependent pathway. *EMBO J* 1997; **16:** 6151–61.
73. Harrison-Findik D, Susa M, Varticovski L, Association of phosphatidylinositol 3-kinase with SHC in chronic myelogeneous leukemia cells. *Oncogene* 1995; **10:** 1385–91.
74. Sattler M, Salgia R, Okuda K et al, The proto-oncogene product $p120^{CBL}$ and the adapter proteins CRKL and c-CRK link c-ABL, $p190^{BCR/ABL}$ and $p210^{BCR/ABL}$ to the phosphoinositol-3′ kinase pathway. *Oncogene* 1996; **12:** 839–46.
75. Jain SK, Langdon WY, Varticovski L, Tyrosine phosphorylation of p120cbl in BCR/abl transformed hematopoietic cells mediates enhanced association with phosphatidylinositol 3-kinase. *Oncogene* 1997; **14:** 2217–28.
76. Bhat A, Kolibaba K, Oda T et al, Interactions of CBL with BCR–ABL and CRKL in BCR–ABL-

transformed myeloid cells. *J Biol Chem* 1997; **272:** 16170–5.
77. Ojaniemi M, Langdon WY, Vuori K, Oncogenic forms of Cbl abrogate the anchorage requirement but not the growth factor requirement for proliferation. *Oncogene* 1998; **16:** 3159–67.
78. Sattler M, Salgia R, Shrikhande G et al, The phosphatidylinositol polyphosphate 5-phosphatase SHIP and the protein tyrosine phosphatase SHP-2 form a complex in hematopoietic cells which can be regulated by BCR/ABL and growth factors. *Oncogene* 1997; **15:** 2379–84.
79. Hall A, Rho GTPases and the actin cytoskeleton. *Science* 1998; **279:** 509–19.
80. Kelly PJ, Westwick JK, Whitehead IP et al, Cdc42 and Rac1 induce integrin-mediated cell motility and invasiveness through PI(3)K. *Nature* 1997; **390:** 632–36.
81. Skorski T, Wlodarski P, Daheron L et al, BCR/ABL mediated leukemogenesis requires the activity of the small GRP-binding protein Rac. *Proc Natl Acad Sci USA* 1998; **95:** 11858–62.
82. Salgia R, Lin J, Narsimhan RP et al, Role of small GTPases and P13-kinase in controlling cell motility of untransformed and BCR/ABL transformed hematopietic cells. *Blood* 1998; **92:** 487A.

4

Functional complementation of cytokine receptor signaling by BCR/ABL

Eugene Y Koh, George Q Daley

CONTENTS • Introduction • Bone marrow samples from patients with MPDs reveal autonomous hematopoiesis, suggesting intrinsic cell defects in the cytokine receptor signaling circuitry • Expression of BCR/ABL in hematopoietic cells demonstrates direct and potent effects on cytokine-independent proliferation and survival • Complementation of cytokine receptor signaling by BCR/ABL: cell-intrinsic activation or autocrine stimulation, or both? • Mimicry at the molecular level • Oligomerization and localization: critical elements of BCR/ABL activation • Mitogenesis via activation of the Ras pathway and c-Myc • Enhanced cell survival activation of the PI3-K–Akt and Jak–STAT pathways • Conclusion: BCR/ABL – the ultimate oncoprotein

INTRODUCTION

Homeostasis within the hematopoietic system is tightly controlled by over a dozen hematopoietic growth factors, termed cytokines, that drive progenitor proliferation, facilitate differentiation, and enhance cell survival.[1,2] Under normal circumstances blood cell populations maintain a steady balance of production and turnover, but in response to hemorrhage, hypoxia, or infection, enhanced cytokine generation stimulates the bone marrow to boost blood cell production. Bone marrow pathology can be viewed as alterations of cell proliferation, differentiation, and death – processes intimately linked to cytokines. Understanding cytokine regulation is particularly pertinent to the myeloproliferative disorders (MPDs), an interesting class of bone marrow diseases characterized by massive expansion in blood cell numbers but relatively normal differentiation and cellular function. The molecular lesions in these disorders appear less disruptive to the overall program of hematopoiesis than do the mutations underlying the more aggressive acute leukemias, which have equally robust hyperproliferation but greatly compromised differentiation and marrow function. Understanding how cytokine regulation is altered in the MPDs may shed light on the molecular basis of hematopoietic homeostasis itself.

Chronic myeloid leukemia (CML) is the most widely studied of the human MPDs, a group of related diseases that includes polycythemia vera (PV), essential thrombocythemia (ET), and myeloid metaplasia/myelofibrosis (MMM). The hallmark of these disorders is multilineage myeloid hyperplasia – clinically marked by the expansion of white blood cells, red blood cells, and platelets, and revealed pathologically within the bone marrow as hyperplasia of myeloid, erythroid, and megakaryocytic progenitors. The histopathology of CML and the other MPDs resembles a pathological process of excessive cytokine production, but in virtually all cases cytokine production is normal and even suppressed. The pathology arises from intrinsic cellular defects that mimic activated cytokine receptor signaling. These diseases all demonstrate inappropriate cell growth (proliferative effect) and cell survival (anti-apoptotic effect), while differentiation is largely unaffected. Knowledge that the BCR/ABL oncoprotein is responsible for CML has provided an excellent opportunity to dissect how this protein alters hematopoietic cell dynamics and has become a paradigm for investigation of molecular mechanisms that might be common among the MPDs. In this chapter, we shall explore the notion that the CML-associated BCR/ABL oncoprotein disrupts the regulation of hematopoiesis through the inappropriate activation of cytokine receptor signal transduction pathways. This dysregulation of hematopoiesis is apparent from hematopoietic colony-forming assays of bone marrow from diseased patients, experimental transformation of cell lines and primary cells, and detailed molecular investigations. These data expose BCR/ABL as a complex and opportunistic oncoprotein that exploits existing pathways to drive hematopoietic proliferation, enhance cell survival, and induce cell transformation.

BONE MARROW SAMPLES FROM PATIENTS WITH MPDs REVEAL AUTONOMUS HEMATOPOIESIS, SUGGESTING INTRINSIC CELL DEFECTS IN THE CYTOKINE RECEPTOR SIGNALING CIRCUITRY

Hematopoietic progenitors from the marrow or peripheral blood of patients with primary MPDs proliferate and differentiate in a cell-autonomous manner when tested in colony formation assays. Cytokine-independent hematopoiesis has been most consistently demonstrated for erythroid progenitors, partly because of the unique and specific effect of erythropoietin (Epo) on the red blood cell lineage. Samples of bone marrow or blood taken from patients with MPDs yield erythroid colonies in methylcellulose (semisolid) cultures in the absence of Epo, which is strictly required for the terminal differentiation of normal progenitors. Autonomous erythropoiesis and megakaryopoiesis, when detected, can serve as diagnostic criteria for patients with PV and ET, and has been explored in CML patients to investigate how the BCR/ABL protein might account for cytokine-independent hematopoiesis in this disorder.

In bone marrow samples taken from patients with CML, Eaves and colleagues[3] first demonstrated autonomous erythropoiesis in cultures supplemented with serum only. More recent experiments have employed 'serum-free' media supplemented with insulin, bovine serum albumin, and transferrin only.[4] Under these defined conditions, addition of stem cell factor (SCF – the ligand for c-Kit) was required for erythroid colonies to develop from CML samples in the absence of Epo.[4] These data demonstrate that progenitor cells from CML patients escape the need for Epo in sustaining the proliferation and differentiation of the erythroid lineage, but also suggest that factors in serum cooperate with BCR/ABL to generate red blood cells. Thus, BCR/ABL provides some of the signals, but other factors, perhaps insulin or insulin-like growth factor I (IGF-I), are also required. The strict requirement for SCF under artificial serum-free conditions may not reflect an absolute necessity, since in more enriched bone marrow microenvironments and in serum-containing cultures, a combination of other factors may be sufficient.

Quantitative analyses of the cytokine responsiveness of erythroid and myeloid colonies from patient samples reveal altered dose–response relationships.[5–7] As in CML, the addition of SCF to cultures enhanced the formation of Epo-independent erythroid colonies in bone marrow samples from patients with PV.[6,7] Interleukin-3 (IL-3) was over 100-fold more potent in supporting erythroid progenitors from PV patients than those from controls.[5] This hypersensitivity to growth factors extended to other myeloid progenitors derived from PV samples. Granulocyte–macrophage colony-forming units (CFU-GM) were significantly more responsive to IL-3 and granulocyte–macrophage colony-stimulating factor (GM-CSF).[8] These data demonstrated that the abnormal myeloid progenitors were able to survive, proliferate, and differentiate in suboptimal concentrations of cytokines. Furthermore, these bone marrow culture assays reveal that hematopoietic progenitors in patients with MPDs respond abnormally to environmental cues from cytokines, as if an intrinsic 'rheostat' were programmed for an abnormally robust response. Plating hematopoietic progenitors in semisolid media allows one to study effects on single progenitors in isolation, thereby narrowing the possible interpretations of the mechanisms at work. Collectively, the data from these colony assays in semisolid media suggest strongly that the dysregulation in cytokine responsiveness is intrinsic to the hematopoietic progenitors themselves.

Interestingly, studies have not consistently observed altered cytokine responsiveness of all myeloid progenitors in the myeloproliferative disorders, including CML. Some but not all groups report spontaneous CFU-GM colonies,[4,9] and classic studies in CML suggested that a full complement of cytokines was required to sustain complete myeloid colony formation. The identification of SCF and the refinement of assay conditions with cloned growth factors led to the observation that SCF appears to vastly potentiate the outgrowth of CFU-GM in patients with CML, ET, and PV. Variation among patient samples and different in vitro culture conditions likely account for the discrepancies in the literature. Nevertheless, relaxed cytokine dependence of myelopoiesis in assays of hematopoietic colony formation has been a consistent hallmark of MPDs, and when detected can contribute valuable diagnostic information in patient evaluations. Over the past decade, the means by which BCR/ABL alters the hematopoietic cell response to cytokines have been extensively explored, and the molecular mechanisms to account for complementation of cytokine receptor signaling have emerged in detail.

EXPRESSION OF BCR/ABL IN HEMATOPOIETIC CELLS DEMONSTRATES DIRECT AND POTENT EFFECTS ON CYTOKINE-INDEPENDENT PROLIFERATION AND SURVIVAL

Experimental manipulation of BCR/ABL in primary bone marrow cells and hematopoietic cell lines in culture provides an opportunity to move beyond observational studies of patient bone marrow. To determine whether BCR/ABL can directly substitute for signaling by a cytokine receptor, Ghaffari and colleagues tested fetal liver cells from genetically engineered mice that lack the Epo receptor (EpoR).[10] The $EpoR^{-/-}$ red cell precursors cannot relay signals from Epo, and therefore fail to proliferate and are fated to apoptose. EpoR knockout mice ($EpoR^{-/-}$) die around embryonic day 12–14 of severe fetal anemia. Erythroid colony-forming cells (erythroid burst-forming units (BFU-E) and colony-forming units (CFU-E)) are present in the knockout mice and can be rescued by infection with a retrovirus carrying EpoR. Retroviral expression of BCR/ABL in the $EpoR^{-/-}$ fetal liver cells completely rescued erythroid colony formation, thereby demonstrating direct genetic complementation of cytokine receptor function.[11]

CML involves abnormal expansion not only of committed colony-forming cells but also of early, primitive hematopoietic progenitors (for a detailed discussion, see Chapter 5). To understand the role of BCR/ABL transformation in more primitive hematopoietic progenitors, several groups have analyzed long-term cultures of primary murine bone marrow cells transduced with BCR/ABL through retroviral infection.[12–15] Interestingly, bone marrow cells infected with BCR/ABL and propagated in culture generate clonal outgrowths of cytokine-independent immature B-lymphoid cells or occasionally mast cells, and not myeloid cell lines as might be predicted from the disease phenotype.[12–15] The difficulty in generating myeloid cell lines is striking; to date, culture conditions for generating BCR/ABL-transformed myeloid cells in vitro have not been established. Gishizky and Witte[15] attempted to transform myeloid progenitors by introducing BCR/ABL into bone marrow cultures, and noticed that with prolonged culturing in vitro (>6 weeks), the cells became cytokine-independent. The kinetics of the population outgrowth suggest that additional epigenetic or genetic events were necessary for the establishment of the immortalized, cytokine-independent cell lines. This observation raises several questions about the lineage specificity of the transforming ability of the *BCR/ABL* oncogene and the existence of other cooperating events in the pathogenesis of CML and Philadelphia chromosome (Ph)-positive lymphoid leukemia.

In the early stages of culture, BCR/ABL-infected bone marrow cells undergo an initial burst of proliferation – an event representing the stimulatory effects of BCR/ABL on committed progenitors (i.e. the colony-forming cells (CFCs)). Following prolonged liquid culture, the cell population weathers an apoptotic crisis before a clonal population emerges. Studies from Radfar et al[16] provide insight into the potential mechanisms needed to bypass this apoptotic crisis. Instead of the *BCR/ABL* oncogene, Radfar and colleagues investigated how the viral oncogene v-*abl* (a fusion between the retroviral *gag* gene and the murine c-*abl* gene) transformed murine bone marrow cells. Their experiments demonstrated that dysregulation of tumor suppressor pathways mediated by p53 and $p19^{Arf}$ was necessary to enable fully transformed cell lines to emerge in culture. To substantiate this conclusion, they introduced the v-*abl* retrovirus into murine bone marrow cells derived from $p53^{-/-}$ or $ink4a/Arf^{-/-}$ mice, and observed immediate cell transformation without any period of apoptotic crisis. Their work implies that loss of *p53* or *ink4A/Arf* locus function may be essential in allowing primary cells to adapt to the harsh conditions of the tissue culture environment (e.g. growth without supporting stromal cells, hyperoxic conditions, high serum concentrations). Future studies will establish whether inactivation of these loci is an obligatory step for generation of leukemia in vivo.

Transformation assays of primary murine bone marrow cells raise several questions about the lineage specificity of the transformation induced by the *BCR/ABL* oncogene. The ease in transforming the lymphoid lineage in vitro seems contrary to the nature of CML. Perhaps, the in vitro culturing conditions may not be permissive for early myeloid progenitors to grow. Alternatively, the inability to establish cytokine-independent myeloid cell lines in vitro may reflect toxicity from high-level expression of BCR/ABL by the retroviral promoter in early myeloid progenitors. The levels of BCR/ABL protein in artificial transformation assays do not reflect the levels detected in hematopoietic progenitors derived from CML patients.[17] The high levels of *BCR/ABL* oncogene obtained from the BCR/ABL retrovirus are apparently tolerated in primary CFCs and factor-dependent cell lines.[11,18–21] Cortez and colleagues[21] argued that a critical threshold level was needed before the *BCR/ABL* oncogene was able to render the 32D cell line cytokine-independent. Cambier and colleagues[20] used the *bcr* promoter to mimic more physiological expression levels of the *BCR/ABL* oncogene. Although the BCR/ABL protein was expressed at levels two- to eightfold lower than when driven by a retroviral promoter, the IL-3-dependent myeloid FDC-P1 cells were still rendered cytokine-independent. Interestingly, with low levels of BCR/ABL expression, these cytokine-independent cells were now hypersensitive to cytokines and grew at a faster rate when exogenous IL-3 was added. These findings suggest that there may be differential effects of the *BCR/ABL* oncogene based on varying levels of protein expression and that this observation must be taken into account when interpreting the results of experimental manipulations of BCR/ABL in primary hematopoietic cells and cell lines.

In addition, the time dependence of BCR/ABL-mediated transformation of primary bone marrow cells is a critical issue in understanding the pathogenesis of the disease. Central to this issue is the conundrum: Does the *BCR/ABL* oncogene represent the first and only step necessary in the pathogenesis of chronic-phase CML, or are other genetic or epigenetic events also required? To investigate this role of BCR/ABL in transforming hematopoietic tissue, several laboratories have employed cytokine-dependent hematopoietic cell lines. These results, however, must be interpreted with caution, because established cell lines carry genetic alterations that allow them to be immortal and survive under tissue culture conditions. Despite the fact that these cell lines have unknown genetic backgrounds, they have been enormously useful for studying the mechanisms of cytokine signaling and BCR/ABL transformation.

BCR/ABL expression is able to render cytokine-dependent murine and human cells completely cytokine-independent,[22–25] confirming that the BCR/ABL oncoprotein is alone sufficient to act as a replacement for certain cytokines. The transformation of these cytokine-dependent cell lines may functionally represent the transformation of late hematopoietic progenitors – the CFCs. The CFCs (i.e. BFU-E, CFU-E, and CFU-GM) are late myeloid progenitors that depend on serum and one cytokine (rather than a combination of cytokines) to survive, proliferate, and differentiate.[1,2]

Several groups have examined the kinetics of BCR/ABL-induced factor independence in cell lines, using inducible systems to turn on and off the *BCR/ABL* oncogene.[21,26,27] Kabarowski and Carlesso and colleagues[26,27] used a temperature-sensitive mutant of BCR/ABL (ts-p210), which was inactive at 38°C (non-permissive temperature) and active at 32°C (permissive temperature). In one study,[27] when IL-3-dependent pro-B lymphoid BaF3 cells expressing ts-p210 were placed at the permissive temperature in the absence of IL-3, a majority of cells underwent apoptosis (programmed cell death). Some cells survived, and within three to four weeks a clonal or oligoclonal population emerged. Kabarowski and colleagues concluded that the *BCR/ABL* oncogene does not provide an immediate survival and proliferative signal. Instead, sustained kinase activity over a prolonged time induced the eventual factor-independent outgrowth, suggesting that additional epigenetic or genetic events were required before a factor-independent population emerges. These results are reminiscent of the apoptotic crisis seen in BCR/ABL transformation of primary lymphoid cells. In contrast, Carlesso et al[26] and Cortez et al[21] introduced their respective inducible systems into the murine IL-3-dependent myeloid cell line 32D. Carlesso and colleagues found that upon IL-3 withdrawal at permissive temperature, 32D cells expressing ts-p210 were immediately rendered factor-independent. Cortez and colleagues used a glucocorticoid responsive promoter to induce the *BCR/ABL* oncogene at the transcriptional level. Upon glucocorticoid (dexamethasone) treatment and IL-3 withdrawal, the IL-3-dependent myeloid cells 32D accumulated functional BCR/ABL protein, which was also immediately sufficient to induce cell survival and proliferation.

Given the predominance of lymphoid transformation of primary bone marrow cells in culture, one might predict that the lymphoid cell line BaF/3 would be easier to transform than the myeloid cell line 32D. However, the Kabarowski paper suggests that BaF3 cells may need to adapt to the signals provided by the *BCR/ABL* oncogene and that BCR/ABL may not act as a direct and immediate surrogate of IL-3-mediated signaling. The BaF/3 cells may require additional epigenetic or genetic events in order to be transformed by BCR/ABL, while perhaps the 32D cells are perfectly competent to receive signals from BCR/ABL. The conflicting results may reflect lineage differences between lymphoid and myeloid cells, varying culture conditions, or different levels of BCR/ABL protein expression among the cell lines. These three experiments are difficult to reconcile, in part because of the unknown genetic differences between the BaF3 and 32D cell lines. Nevertheless, these data demonstrate the ability of BCR/ABL to complement cytokine signaling.

COMPLEMENTATION OF CYTOKINE RECEPTOR SIGNALING BY BCR/ABL: CELL-INTRINSIC ACTIVATION OR AUTOCRINE STIMULATION, OR BOTH?

The behavior of hematopoietic progenitors from patients with MPD clearly demonstrates that the molecular defects complement some aspects of cytokine signaling. For CML, the one case where the molecular lesion is known, at least two potential explanations for cytokine complementation by BCR/ABL have been suggested by previous data. Evidence that BCR/ABL can activate mitogenic signaling pathways shared by cytokine receptors argues that the BCR/ABL oncoprotein directly mimics cytokine receptor signaling.[1,11] Alternatively, BCR/ABL might stimulate progenitor cells to produce their own cytokines and thereby create an autocrine stimulation loop. In order to distinguish between the two hypotheses, many papers have examined this question through the transformation of cytokine-dependent cell lines, the generation of murine models of CML, and the in vitro culture of primary patient samples. When all data are taken into account, the most compelling explanation proves to be some combination of both mechanisms.

Cytokine-dependent cell lines derived from both human and murine sources have proven invaluable in defining the mechanisms of transformation by BCR/ABL. Numerous such cell lines have been isolated, including BaF3, 32D, FDC-P1, M-07e, and TF-1. Because the cells rapidly apoptose when deprived of cytokines and fail to form leukemias when injected into murine hosts, they have been widely employed as surrogates for primary hematopoietic tissue. When expressed at high levels, BCR/ABL can completely replace the requirement for the particular cytokine in the growth medium, but the transduced cells remain dependent on growth factors provided by serum.[22–25] BCR/ABL-mediated transformation of the murine IL-3-dependent pro-B-cell line BaF3 occurs with no evidence for autocrine stimulation, supporting the claim that BCR/ABL expression could entirely replace the signals emanating from the IL-3 receptor.[22]

In contrast to a direct proliferative effect of BCR/ABL, endogenous production of cytokines by BCR/ABL-transformed hematopoietic cells has been detected by several groups, implicating autocrine mechanisms in CML. Two groups expressed BCR/ABL in the murine IL-3-dependent myeloid cell line FDC-P1, and detected IL-3 production by the transformed cells.[23,25] Anderson and colleagues[25] defined the critical region of BCR/ABL that provoked autocrine IL-3 production as the Src-homology-2 (SH2) domain. This protein motif, found in many signaling molecules, binds phosphorylated tyrosine residues and allows for coupling to adapter proteins. Although deletion of the SH2 region eliminated the production of IL-3, this mutant of BCR/ABL was still able to render the cells factor-independent, suggesting that an autocrine loop was not necessary for the cytokine-independent growth of the BCR/ABL-transformed FDC-P1 cells. Sirard and colleagues[22] introduced the BCR/ABL oncogene into a distinct human myeloid cell line, M-07e, that was dependent on either IL-3 or GM-CSF for survival. Low levels of GM-CSF and IL-3 production were detected from the M-07e cells expressing BCR/ABL, and cell proliferation was compromised by incubation with neutralizing antibodies to GM-CSF and IL-3, demonstrating that the proliferation was dependent on the autocrine production of these two growth factors.

The apparent discrepancy between the results obtained with the BaF/3, FDC-P1, and M-07e cell lines may reflect lineage-specific effects of BCR/ABL. BCR/ABL may be unable to stimulate cytokine production in lymphoid progenitors such as BaF/3 cells. Young and colleagues[28] found that the *ABL* oncogenes – both v-*abl* and *BCR/ABL* – transformed primary pre-B cells without evoking an IL-7 autocrine/paracrine stimulation loop. These results suggest that the lymphoid lineage can be transformed in a completely cell-autonomous fashion. On the other hand, there is mounting evidence that expression of BCR/ABL may induce myeloid progenitors to produce low levels of cytokines, which may therefore play a role in stimulating proliferation. In one murine model of CML, retroviral transduction of *BCR/ABL* into bone marrow induced low-level expression of IL-3 and GM-CSF, potentially contributing to the development of the CML-like disease in mice by autocrine or paracrine stimulation.[29] This demonstration of cytokine production in primary cells expressing BCR/ABL argues that the autocrine mechanism may not be peculiar to cell lines in tissue culture. Nevertheless, the artificially high levels of BCR/ABL expression from the strong retroviral promoters employed for bone marrow expression probably do not reflect the endogenous levels of BCR/ABL seen in the human disease. Thus, overexpression of BCR/ABL may artifactually induce hematopoietic progenitors to produce cytokines, which may or may not play a central role in disease. Introduction of BCR/ABL into bone marrow cells that are genetically deficient in IL-3 production due to gene knockout induces an aggressive CML-like disease in transplanted mice.[30] This argues that autocrine production of IL-3 is not required to sustain the pathological expansion of myeloid cells in murine models of CML, although the formal possibility remains that BCR/ABL may stimulate the autocrine production of multiple redundant cytokines, any one of which might contribute to disease in humans. Again, the precise level of BCR/ABL expression may be critical to understanding CML pathogenesis. Bedi and colleagues[17] report that primitive CML progenitors express little *BCR/ABL* mRNA, while more differentiated progeny have increased levels of *BCR/ABL* message. This paper behooves caution in interpreting experiments using retroviruses to express the *BCR/ABL* oncogene in levels beyond physiological amounts.

To investigate the possibility of autocrine and paracrine cytokine production in human CML, several laboratories have eschewed cell lines and instead focused on primary patient samples. In one study, serum from patients with CML increased the number of colonies derived from normal bone marrow cultures by 500% when compared with serum from healthy patients, suggesting possible paracrine factors in CML pathogenesis.[31] However, Otsuka and colleagues[32] were unable to detect abnormal cytokine production in CML patient samples, using Northern blotting techniques. In a more recent study using a highly sensitive assay based on the reverse-transcriptase–polymerase chain reaction (RT-PCR), Eaves and colleagues[33] detected IL-3 and granulocyte colony-stimulating factor (G-CSF) production in primitive hematopoietic progenitors, but not in more differentiated progeny. They documented cytokine-independent proliferation of $CD34^+$ progenitors, which was largely blocked by neutralizing antibody to IL-3. Autocrine cytokine production disappeared in more committed hematopoietic cells, providing an explanation for why cytokines are required to score hematopoietic colonies in methylcellulose assays, and why previous studies might have underestimated the degree of autonomous progenitor proliferation in bone marrow samples. In a separate series of experiments, primitive CML cells were maintained in culture for up to three weeks without any exogenous cytokines, presumably because the cells were producing low amounts of their own factors that sustained proliferation in an autocrine fashion.[34] The detection of cytokine production in cells from CML patients, and the ability to block cytokine-independent cell proliferation with antibodies against IL-3, is compelling evidence that autocrine stimulation may play a role in CML. However, if IL-3 is secreted by leukemic progenitors in CML patients, we are left to explain why CML is a clonal disease and why normal progenitors are not also expanded by a paracrine effect. Perhaps the BCR/ABL-positive cells are also hypersensitive to cytokines, thereby creating a preferential expansion of CML progenitors over normal tissue with these low amounts of cytokines. The resolution of these apparent paradoxes must await further investigation.

MIMICRY AT THE MOLECULAR LEVEL

At a molecular level, BCR/ABL signaling closely mimics the signaling pathways of cytokine receptors. Both cytokine receptor activation and the BCR/ABL oncoprotein induce a tyrosine phosphorylation cascade, and numerous proteins are common substrates[26,35,36] (Figure 4.1). To date, the *BCR/ABL* oncogene has been shown to bind and phosphorylate several proteins: Crkl,[37–39] Cbl,[40] Grb2,[41] p62Dok,[42,43] Rin,[44] and Shc.[41] In addition to binding to these mediators of signal transduction, the *BCR/ABL* oncogene has been shown to associate with the B_c (beta-common) subunit of the IL-3 receptor and the c-Kit receptor.[45,46] Thus, the BCR/ABL oncoprotein interacts directly with the cytokine receptors and signaling pathway components to activate comparable programs. Therefore, understanding the specificity and redundancy of these networks should shed light on the molecular mechanisms of BCR/ABL transformation.

Cytokine receptors are proteins that mediate hematopoietic cell survival and proliferation through a number of mechanisms. Upon ligand (e.g. cytokine) binding, receptors recruit signaling and adaptor proteins that provide at least three critical signals for hematopoiesis: (1) mitogenesis, chiefly through Ras activation; (2) cell cycle progression, due to upregulation of c-Myc and activation of D-type cyclins; and (3) cell survival, through induction of Bcl-2 or Bcl-x_L.[47–49] Overexpression of c-Myc alone in the absence of an appropriate signal for cell survival (e.g. expression of a member of the Bcl-2

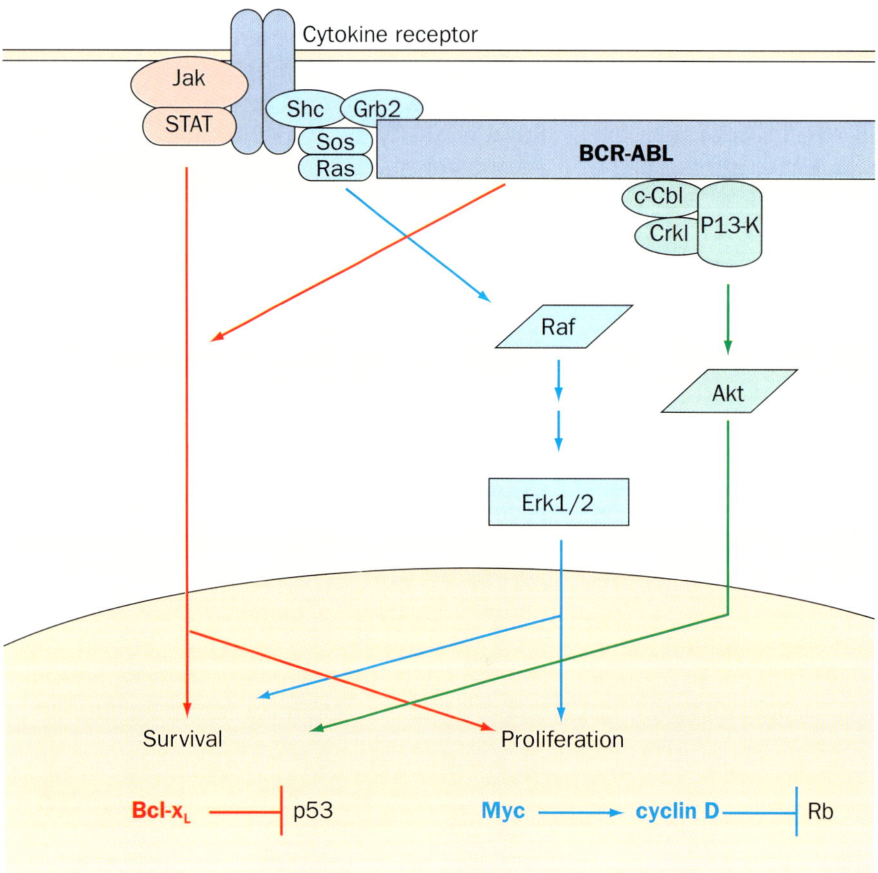

Figure 4.1 The BCR/ABL and cytokine signaling pathways overlap, activating numerous molecules to drive cell proliferation and induce cell survival. Critical to the oncogenic potential of BCR/ABL is the ability to bypass two key tumor suppressor pathways, Rb and p53, through the overexpression of cyclin D and Bcl-x_L, respectively.

family of anti-apoptotic proteins) will enhance cell apoptosis.[50] Moreover, expression of anti-apoptotic genes alone enable cells to survive cytokine withdrawal, but the cells fail to proliferate.[51–54] Therefore, all three mechanisms must be active for hematopoietic precursors to survive and proliferate. Interestingly, the BCR/ABL oncoprotein may be sufficient to accomplish all three of these tasks on its own. In doing so, BCR/ABL mimics cytokine receptor signaling and provides for cell-intrinsic, cytokine-independent hematopoietic cell survival, proliferation, and differentiation.

OLIGOMERIZATION AND LOCALIZATION: CRITICAL ELEMENTS OF BCR/ABL ACTIVATION

A common theme among membrane receptors is their activation by self-association, which is typically ligand-mediated. Depending upon the particular structure of the cytokine receptor, dimerization or oligomerization enables the activation of a tyrosine-specific kinase activity resident within the cytoplasmic signaling domain (e.g. c-Kit or c-Fms), or recruitment of tyrosine kinases such as Jak2 and the initiation of downstream signaling events. Likewise, oligomerization of BCR/ABL is critical for the autophosphorylation of the ABL kinase domain, thereby activating the kinase further and initiating the oncogenic signaling network. The BCR region is the critical domain that allows for oligomerization and activation of the fusion oncoprotein.[55] In addition to oligomerization, the ABL protein must be re-localized from the nucleus, where it normally resides, to the cytoplasm so that the BCR/ABL form can phosphorylate many of the cytoplasmic signaling substrates.[56] The actin-binding domain of the ABL region helps to bring the activated BCR/ABL kinase in close proximity to many of the protein substrates that mediate anti-apoptotic and proliferative signals.[57] Oligomerization of the ABL kinase by the amino-terminal coiled-coil domain of BCR provides for spontaneous and constitutive activation of kinase signaling and induces a cascade in hematopoietic cells that provides the functional equivalent of continuous occupancy of the cytokine receptor and constitutive cytokine receptor signaling.

MITOGENESIS VIA ACTIVATION OF THE Ras PATHWAY AND c-Myc

Cytokine receptors and many oncogenic tyrosine kinases activate the Ras signaling pathway.[58] Ras activation is facilitated by association with Sos, a guanine nucleotide exchange factor that helps to maintain Ras in its active GTP-bound state. Upon cytokine receptor activation, the adaptor proteins Grb2 and Shc relocate Sos to the membrane in close proximity to Ras. Nucleotide exchange ensues, and Ras becomes activated. Ras in turn stimulates many downstream targets, including Raf, a serine/threonine kinase that activates Erk (extracellular signal regulated kinase – also known as MAP kinase, MAPK).[59,60] The Erk signaling cascade plays a critical role in cell proliferation by inducing several immediate–early genes, including AP-1, a heterodimer of c-Jun and c-Fos.

Several laboratories have demonstrated that the *BCR/ABL* oncogene activates the Ras pathway in a manner strikingly similar to cytokine receptors.[61–65] Upon autophosphorylation, BCR/ABL recruits Grb2, Shc, and Sos in a signaling complex, thereby activating Ras and inducing a proliferative signal. The Ras signaling pathway is critical to cytokine-induced hematopoietic cell proliferation. Activated components of the Ras signaling cascade can fully or partially substitute for cytokine signaling in factor-dependent cell lines, and may participate in some leukemias. A constitutively active mutant of Raf can render two cytokine-dependent cell lines completely factor-independent.[66,67] Raf activation may have pleiotropic effects, providing both a proliferative and an anti-apoptotic signal.[68] In TF-1, a human myeloid GM-CSF-dependent cell line, ectopic expression of constitutive Raf mutants stimulates an autocrine/pararcine loop of GM-CSF production.[67] Raf may not provide the full complement of cytokine receptor signals, but circumvents this deficiency through the production of its own cytokines. In a similar fashion, production of IL-3 and G-CSF in early myeloid progenitors from CML patients may cooperate with BCR/ABL signal transduction.[33] Simple overexpression of the adaptor protein Shc rendered hematopoietic cell lines hypersensitive to the cytokine GM-CSF.[69] Likewise, hematopoietic cells with non-functional alleles of NF-1, which normally downregulates Ras signaling, are also hypersensitive to GM-CSF.[70–72] In humans, the loss of NF-1 function is associated with juvenile CML (JCML), an MPD that afflicts infants and is not associated with the Philadelphia chromosome. Although mutations in Ras are exceedingly common in cancers, there is a striking lack of Ras mutation in Ph^+ leukemias, suggesting that the *BCR/ABL* oncogene fulfills the role of Ras pathway activation.[73–75]

c-Myc activation provides a unique proliferative signal that is independent of the proliferation signals from the Ras pathway. The pleiotropic effects of c-Myc signaling are not well understood, and cannot be substituted by Ras or other signaling pathways.[76] In hematopoietic cells, cytokine receptor activation results in the upregulation of c-Myc.[77] Likewise, BCR/ABL can stimulate c-*myc* transcription.[78–81] The SH2 mutant of BCR/ABL has been studied extensively to elucidate the mechanism of c-Myc induction by the *BCR/ABL* oncogene.[79–81] Although these studies used the p185 form of BCR/ABL that is associated with acute lymphoblastic leukemia (ALL), results are likely comparable for the p210 form that is associated with CML. In assays of fibroblast transformation, Afar and colleagues[79–81] used the SH2 mutant of p185 to identify candidate genes that would complement the transformation deficiency of this SH2 mutant. They identified *cyclin D1* and c-*myc* as genes that rescued the deficiency of the SH2 mutant of p185 to transform fibroblasts. To validate that c-Myc was relevant and necessary to BCR/ABL signaling, Afar and colleagues[81] demonstrated that a dominant-negative form of c-*myc* blocked the ability of BCR/ABL to transform primary bone marrow cells. Cyclin D1, a mediator of cell cycle progression, is a downstream target of c-Myc induction, and may be responsible for BCR/ABL signaling in fibroblasts. In hematopoietic tissue, cyclin D2 may be the more relevant mediator of BCR/ABL-induced proliferation, since bone marrow cells from mice deficient in cyclin D2 fail to respond to BCR/ABL-mediated transformation.[82]

ENHANCED CELL SURVIVAL: ACTIVATION OF THE PI3-K–Akt AND Jak–STAT PATHWAYS

While the Ras signaling pathway provides a potent signal for cell proliferation, both cytokine receptors and the *BCR/ABL* oncogene activate anti-apoptotic signals through two mechanisms: the PI3-K–Akt pathway and the Jak–STAT pathway. Upon cytokine receptor activation, the phosphatidylinositol 3′-kinase (PI3-K) protein complex, a heterodimer of p85 and p110 subunits, associates with the cell membrane and induces a cascade of events, which includes the activation of Akt (protein kinase B) and the upregulation of anti-apoptotic genes, such as *bcl-2* and *bcl-*x_L.[83–86] Several laboratories have demonstrated that BCR/ABL mimics the activated cytokine receptor by recruiting the PI3-K protein complex through association with two adaptor proteins: c-Cbl and Crkl.[87–89] In addition to activating PI3-K through direct interaction, the *BCR/ABL* oncogene may activate PI3-K indirectly through activation of Ras.[90] Skorski and colleagues[18,19] found that activation of the PI3-K–Akt pathway was necessary for the *BCR/ABL* oncogene to transform myeloid cells.

Cytokine receptors that lack intrinsic kinase ability typically associate with the Janus family of non-receptor tyrosine kinases – Jaks.[91–93] Upon cytokine stimulation, the Jaks phosphorylate the receptor and several signaling proteins, including the STAT (signal transducer and activator of transcription) family of transcription factors. Tyrosine phosphorylation of the STATs induces homo- or heterodimerization of these proteins, allowing for nuclear translocation and the activation of transcription of several genes, including the anti-apoptotic genes *bcl-2* and *bcl-x_L*. Mimicking cytokine receptor signaling, the *BCR/ABL* oncogene can also phosphorylate and activate the STAT proteins (chiefly STAT5, but also STAT1 and 3), either through direct phosphorylation or through activation of the Jaks.[45,94–96] STAT5 activation seems to mediate the upregulation of the anti-apoptotic gene *bcl-x_L* in hematopoietic cells.[97] A dominant-negative form of STAT5 reduces the proliferation rate of the murine IL-3-dependent BaF/3 cells, presumably because the cells are undergoing apoptosis more frequently.[98] Traditionally, the Jak–STAT pathway has been interpreted as mediating an anti-apoptotic signal and not a proliferative signal. However, recent studies have demonstrated that STAT signaling can directly mediate the upregulation of c-Myc and cyclin D, both key mediators of cell cycle progression.[47,99,100] The integration of STAT signaling with Bcl-2 and c-Myc correlates perfectly with the known consequences of the *BCR/ABL* oncogene. Mutational analyses have shown that the SH3 and SH2 domains of the BCR/ABL oncogene are both critical for the activation of STAT5; the SH2 mutant of BCR/ABL in previous studies lacks the ability to upregulate Bcl-2 and c-Myc.[78] These observations validate the importance of the Jak–STAT pathway as a mediator of both anti-apoptosis and proliferation.

CONCLUSION: BCR/ABL – THE ULTIMATE ONCOPROTEIN

Rather than focusing on individual molecular mediators of BCR/ABL transformation, Hoover and colleagues[101] have examined the integration of signaling pathways. They demonstrated that the *BCR/ABL* oncogene activates the Ras, STAT, and Akt pathways to provide overlapping and redundant survival and proliferative signals to hematopoietic cells, thereby mimicking cytokine receptor signaling pathways. The *BCR/ABL* oncogene does not activate a single signaling pathway, but rather activates the multifaceted communication network of the cytokine system (Figure 4.1).

While BCR/ABL acts in part to mimic cytokine signaling, the abnormal behavior of CML cells suggests that BCR/ABL does much more. If the inappropriate activation of cytokine signaling were alone responsible for the pathogenesis of CML and other MPDs, then one might expect that mutations that activate cytokine overexpression or generate constitutive receptor signaling would result in primary MPD. Mutations in the Epo receptor have been identified in familial erythrocytosis, and mutations in the 5' untranslated region of thrombopoietin have been identified in familial thrombocythemia.[102–106] However, these diseases involve benign elevations in red blood cells and platelets respectively, and do not appear to carry the same risk of progression to malignant leukemia. While overexpression of IL-3 or GM-CSF in murine models results in a CML-like MPD, there is little evidence for monoclonality, and the predisposition of these disorders to evolve to blast crisis has never been established. Continuous stimulation of native polyclonal hematopoiesis does not appear to be associated with any appreciable increased risk of leukemic transformation. There are strikingly few mutations in cytokine receptors that are associated with malignant disease,[107–110] suggesting that leukemias result from more than just aberrant cytokine receptor signaling.

Most likely, the *BCR/ABL* oncogene is providing tumorigenic signals in addition to activating cytokine signaling pathways. Young and colleagues[28] demonstrated the ability of BCR/ABL to induce not only IL-7-independent growth, but also tumorigenic properties in pre-B cells transformed with the *BCR/ABL* oncogene. Interestingly, the overexpression of IL-7 in these pre-B cells was able to render the cells factor-independent, but not tumorigenic. Under a paradigm proposed by Weinberg and colleagues,[111] a limited number of genetic events is responsible for changing a primary cell into a malignant cell. These experiments identified four obligatory steps:

1. the inactivation of the *Rb* tumor suppressor gene (via large T);
2. the inactivation of the *p53* tumor suppressor gene (via large T);
3. the activation of a proliferative signal through Ras activation;
4. the maintenance of telomeres through the telomerase enzyme.

Stem cells maintain their telomeres through a low basal activity of the telomerase enzyme. Because CML is a disease of the hematopoietic stem cell, the telomerase enzyme is naturally active. As previously discussed, the *BCR/ABL* oncogene can activate Ras through its interaction with Grb2 or Shc. Through the activation of the PI3-K pathway and the Jak–STAT pathway, the *BCR/ABL* oncogene effectively blocks many apoptotic signals, which are often mediated by p53. Finally, the *BCR/ABL* oncogene overcomes the growth arrest mediated by the Rb tumor suppressor through the induction and subsequent overexpression of the cyclin D pathway, thereby bypassing the Rb-mediated block of cell cycle progression. In many respects, the *BCR/ABL* oncogene is the ultimate oncogene, activating the necessary pathways for tumorigenesis in one step.

The *BCR/ABL* oncogene has become a significant paradigm for understanding the molecular pathogenesis of hematopoietic malignancy. It causes the dysregulation of cytokine signaling, providing inappropriate signals for both cell survival and proliferation. Several other translocation products involved in human leukemias also complement for cytokine action: TEL/PDGFR in chronic myelomonocytic leukemia (CMML), TEL/ABL in acute myeloid leukemia (AML), and TEL/Jak in T-ALL.[112–120] The common feature of these translocation products is the activated tyrosine kinase, which provides proliferative signals through Ras and Myc, while also supplying anti-apoptotic signals through STAT and Akt. In MPDs with no known molecular basis, the phenomenon of cytokine-relaxed hematopoiesis is likely to involve common mechanisms that result in the inappropriate activation of cytokine receptor signaling pathways, enhanced cell survival, and constitutive cell proliferation. Our Whitehead laboratory has attempted functional cloning strategies to identify mutated signaling molecules that allow for cytokine-hypersensitive or cytokine-independent hematopoiesis.[66] While these dominantly acting (gain-of-function) mutations may point us toward the common pathways responsible for leukemia, inactivation of tumor suppressor genes may also contribute to MPD, as has been demonstrated by gene knockout models in mice (e.g. ICSBP$^{-/-}$ and NF-1$^{-/-}$ mice).[70,72,121] Clearly, despite our detailed knowledge of how the BCR/ABL oncoprotein functions in CML, much remains to be learned about the many distinct modes by which normal hematopoietic cells can become transformed.

ACKNOWLEDGEMENTS

GQD is the Birnbaum scholar of the Leukemia and Lymphoma Society of America and supported by grants from the Edward J Mallinckrodt, Jr Foundation, the Burroughs–Wellcome Fund, the Schering–Plough Research Institute, and the National Cancer Institute.

REFERENCES

1. Socolovsky M, Lodish HF, Daley GQ, Control of hematopoietic differentiation: lack of specificity in signaling by cytokine receptors. *Proc Natl Acad Sci USA* 1998; **95:** 6573–5.
2. Metcalf D, Hematopoietic regulators: redundancy or subtlety? *Blood* 1993; **82:** 3515–23.
3. Eaves AC, Eaves CJ, Abnormalities in the erythroid progenitor compartments in patients with chronic myelogenous leukemia (CML). *Exp Hematol* 1979; **7**(Suppl 5): 65–75.
4. Issaad C, Vainchenker W, Growth of erythroid colonies in chronic myelogenous leukemia is independent of erythropoietin only in the presence of steel factor. *Blood* 1994; **84:** 3447–56.
5. Dai CH, Krantz SB, Means RT Jr et al,

Polycythemia vera blood burst-forming units–erythroid are hypersensitive to interleukin-3. *J Clin Invest* 1991; **87:** 391–6.
6. Dai CH, Krantz SB, Green WF, Gilbert HS, Polycythaemia vera. III. Burst-forming units–erythroid (BFU-E) response to stem cell factor and c-kit receptor expression. *Br J Haematol* 1994; **86:** 12–21.
7. Muller EW, de Wolf JT, Hendriks DW et al, Recombinant human mast cell growth factor supports erythroid colony formation in polycythemia vera in the presence and absence of erythropoietin and serum. *Exp Hematol* 1993; **21:** 1353–7.
8. Dai CH, Krantz SB, Dessypris EN et al, Polycythemia vera. II. Hypersensitivity of bone marrow erythroid, granulocyte–macrophage, and megakaryocyte progenitor cells to interleukin-3 and granulocyte–macrophage colony-stimulating factor. *Blood* 1992; **80:** 891–9.
9. Siitonen T, Zheng A, Savolainen ER, Koistinen P, The effect of mast cell growth factor on peripheral blood granulocyte–macrophage colony-forming cells in methylcellulose in myeloproliferative disorders. *Eur J Haematol* 1995; **55:** 228–34.
10. Ghaffari S, Wu H, Gerlach M et al, BCR–ABL and v-SRC tyrosine kinase oncoproteins support normal erythroid development in erythropoietin receptor-deficient progenitor cells. *Proc Natl Acad Sci USA* 1999; **96:** 13186–90.
11. Wu H, Liu X, Jaenisch R, Lodish HF, Generation of committed erythroid BFU-E and CFU-E progenitors does not require erythropoietin or the erythropoietin receptor. *Cell* 1995; **83:** 59–67.
12. Young JC, Witte ON, Selective transformation of primitive lymphoid cells by the BCR/ABL oncogene expressed in long-term lymphoid or myeloid cultures. *Mol Cell Biol* 1988; **8:** 4079–87.
13. McLaughlin J, Chianese E, Witte ON, Alternative forms of the BCR–ABL oncogene have quantitatively different potencies for stimulation of immature lymphoid cells. *Mol Cell Biol* 1989; **9:** 1866–74.
14. McLaughlin J, Chianese E, Witte ON, In vitro transformation of immature hematopoietic cells by the P210 BCR/ABL oncogene product of the Philadelphia chromosome. *Proc Natl Acad Sci USA* 1987; **84:** 6558–62.
15. Gishizky ML, Witte ON, Initiation of deregulated growth of multipotent progenitor cells by bcr–abl in vitro. *Science* 1992; **256:** 836–9.
16. Radfar A, Unnikrishnan I, Lee HW et al, p19(Arf) induces p53-dependent apoptosis during abelson virus-mediated pre-B cell transformation. *Proc Natl Acad Sci USA* 1998; **95:** 13194–9.
17. Bedi A, Zehnbauer BA, Collector MI et al, BCR–ABL gene rearrangement and expression of primitive hematopoietic progenitors in chronic myeloid leukemia. *Blood* 1993; **81:** 2898–902.
18. Skorski T, Kanakaraj P, Nieborowska-Skorska M et al, Phosphatidylinositol-3 kinase activity is regulated by BCR/ABL and is required for the growth of Philadelphia chromosome-positive cells. *Blood* 1995; **86:** 726–36.
19. Skorski T, Bellacosa A, Nieborowska-Skorska M et al, Transformation of hematopoietic cells by BCR/ABL requires activation of a PI-3k/Akt-dependent pathway. *EMBO J* 1997; **16:** 6151–61.
20. Cambier N, Chopra R, Strasser A et al, BCR–ABL activates pathways mediating cytokine independence and protection against apoptosis in murine hematopoietic cells in a dose-dependent manner. *Oncogene* 1998; **16:** 335–48.
21. Cortez D, Reuther G, Pendergast AM, The Bcr–Abl tyrosine kinase activates mitogenic signaling pathways and stimulates G1-to-S phase transition in hematopoietic cells. *Oncogene* 1997; **15:** 2333–42.
22. Daley GQ, Baltimore D, Transformation of an interleukin 3-dependent hematopoietic cell line by the chronic myelogenous leukemia-specific P210bcr/abl protein. *Proc Natl Acad Sci USA* 1988; **85:** 9312–16.
23. Hariharan IK, Adams JM, Cory S, bcr–abl oncogene renders myeloid cell line factor independent: potential autocrine mechanism in chronic myeloid leukemia. *Oncogene Res* 1988; **3:** 387–99.
24. Sirard C, Laneuville P, Dick JE, Expression of bcr–abl abrogates factor-dependent growth of human hematopoietic M07E cells by an autocrine mechanism. *Blood* 1994; **83:** 1575–85.
25. Anderson SM, Mladenovic J, The BCR–ABL oncogene requires both kinase activity and src-homology 2 domain to induce cytokine secretion. *Blood* 1996; **87:** 238–44.
26. Carlesso N, Griffin JD, Druker BJ, Use of a temperature-sensitive mutant to define the biological effects of the p210BCR–ABL tyrosine kinase on proliferation of a factor-dependent murine myeloid cell line. *Oncogene* 1994; **9:** 149–56.

27. Kabarowski JH, Allen PB, Wiedemann LM, A temperature sensitive p210 BCR–ABL mutant defines the primary consequences of BCR–ABL tyrosine kinase expression in growth factor dependent cells. *EMBO J* 1994; **13:** 5887–95.
28. Young JC, Gishizky ML, Witte ON, Hyperexpression of interleukin-7 is not necessary or sufficient for transformation of a pre-B lymphoid cell line. *Mol Cell Biol* 1991; **11:** 854–63.
29. Zhang X, Ren R, Bcr–Abl efficiently induces a myeloproliferative disease and production of excess interleukin-3 and granulocyte–macrophage colony-stimulating factor in mice: a novel model for chronic myelogenous leukemia. *Blood* 1998; **92:** 3829–40.
30. Li S, Gillessen S, Dranoff G, Van Etten RA, Interleukin-3 and granulocyte–macrophage colony stimulating factor are not required for induction of chronic myeloid leukemia-like disease in mice by the p210 BCR/ABL oncogene. *Blood* 1999; **94**(Suppl 1): 2672a.
31. Brown RD, Yuen E, Kronenberg H, Rickard KA, Stimulation of persisting colonies in agar cultures by sera from patients with CML and AML. *Blood* 1986; **68:** 37–40.
32. Otsuka T, Eaves CJ, Humphries RK et al, Lack of evidence for abnormal autocrine or paracrine mechanisms underlying the uncontrolled proliferation of primitive chronic myeloid leukemia progenitor cells. *Leukemia* 1991; **5:** 861–8.
33. Jiang X, Lopez A, Holyoake T et al, Autocrine production and action of IL-3 and granulocyte colony-stimulating factor in chronic myeloid leukemia. *Proc Natl Acad Sci USA* 1999; **96:** 12804–9.
34. Maguer-Satta V, Burl S, Liu L et al, BCR–ABL accelerates C2-ceramide-induced apoptosis. *Oncogene* 1998; **16:** 237–48.
35. Matulonis U, Salgia R, Okuda K et al, Interleukin-3 and p210 BCR/ABL activate both unique and overlapping pathways of signal transduction in a factor-dependent myeloid cell line. *Exp Hematol* 1993; **21:** 1460–6.
36. Sattler M, Salgia R, Activation of hematopoietic growth factor signal transduction pathways by the human oncogene BCR/ABL. *Cytokine Growth Factor Rev* 1997; **8:** 63–79.
37. Oda T, Heaney C, Hagopian JR et al, Crkl is the major tyrosine-phosphorylated protein in neutrophils from patients with chronic myelogenous leukemia. *J Biol Chem* 1994; **269:** 22925–8.
38. Nichols GL, Raines MA, Vera JC et al, Identification of CRKL as the constitutively phosphorylated 39-kD tyrosine phosphoprotein in chronic myelogenous leukemia cells. *Blood* 1994; **84:** 2912–18.
39. ten Hoeve J, Arlinghaus RB, Guo JQ et al, Tyrosine phosphorylation of CRKL in Philadelphia+ leukemia. *Blood* 1994; **84:** 1731–6.
40. de Jong R, ten Hoeve J, Heisterkamp N, Groffen J, Crkl is complexed with tyrosine-phosphorylated Cbl in Ph-positive leukemia. *J Biol Chem* 1995; **270:** 21468–71.
41. Puil L, Liu J, Gish G et al, Bcr–Abl oncoproteins bind directly to activators of the Ras signalling pathway. *EMBO J* 1994; **13:** 764–73.
42. Yamanashi Y, Baltimore D, Identification of the Abl- and rasGAP-associated 62 kDa protein as a docking protein, Dok. *Cell* 1997; **88:** 205–11.
43. Carpino N, Wisniewski D, Strife A et al, p62(dok): a constitutively tyrosine-phosphorylated, GAP-associated protein in chronic myelogenous leukemia progenitor cells. *Cell* 1997; **88:** 197–204.
44. Afar DE, Han L, McLaughlin J et al, Regulation of the oncogenic activity of BCR–ABL by a tightly bound substrate protein RIN1. *Immunity* 1997; **6:** 773–82.
45. Wilson-Rawls J, Xie S, Liu J et al, P210 Bcr–Abl interacts with the interleukin 3 receptor beta(c) subunit and constitutively induces its tyrosine phosphorylation. *Cancer Res* 1996; **56:** 3426–30.
46. Hallek M, Danhauser-Riedl S, Herbst R et al, Interaction of the receptor tyrosine kinase p145c-kit with the p210bcr/abl kinase in myeloid cells. *Br J Haematol* 1996; **94:** 5–16.
47. Lord JD, McIntosh BC, Greenberg PD, Nelson BH, The IL-2 receptor promotes lymphocyte proliferation and induction of the c-myc, bcl-2, and bcl-x genes through the trans-activation domain of stat5. *J Immunol* 2000; **164:** 2533–41.
48. Ahmed NN, Grimes HL, Bellacosa A et al, Transduction of interleukin-2 antiapoptotic and proliferative signals via Akt protein kinase. *Proc Natl Acad Sci USA* 1997; **94:** 3627–32.
49. Miyazaki T, Liu ZJ, Kawahara A et al, Three distinct IL-2 signaling pathways mediated by bcl-2, c-myc, and lck cooperate in hematopoietic cell proliferation. *Cell* 1995; **81:** 223–31.
50. Askew DS, Ashmun RA, Simmons BC, Cleveland JL, Constitutive c-myc expression in an IL-3-dependent myeloid cell line suppresses

cell cycle arrest and accelerates apoptosis. *Oncogene* 1991; **6:** 1915–22.
51. Nunez G, London L, Hockenbery D et al, Deregulated Bcl-2 gene expression selectively prolongs survival of growth factor-deprived hemopoietic cell lines. *J Immunol* 1990; **144:** 3602–10.
52. Fairbairn LJ, Cowling GJ, Reipert BM, Dexter TM, Suppression of apoptosis allows differentiation and development of a multipotent hemopoietic cell line in the absence of added growth factors. *Cell* 1993; **74:** 823–32.
53. Otani H, Erdos M, Leonard WJ, Tyrosine kinase(s) regulate apoptosis and bcl-2 expression in a growth factor-dependent cell line. *J Biol Chem* 1993; **268:** 22733–6.
54. McKenna SL, Cotter TG, Functional aspects of apoptosis in hematopoiesis and consequences of failure. *Adv Cancer Res* 1997; **71:** 121–64.
55. Muller AJ, Young JC, Pendergast AM et al, BCR first exon sequences specifically activate the BCR/ABL tyrosine kinase oncogene of Philadelphia chromosome-positive human leukemias. *Mol Cell Biol* 1991; **11:** 1785–92.
56. Van Etten RA, Jackson P, Baltimore D, The mouse type IV c-abl gene product is a nuclear protein, and activation of transforming ability is associated with cytoplasmic localization. *Cell* 1989; **58:** 669–78.
57. McWhirter JR, Wang JY, An actin-binding function contributes to transformation by the Bcr–Abl oncoprotein of Philadelphia chromosome-positive human leukemias. *EMBO J* 1993; **12:** 1533–46.
58. Satoh T, Nakafuku M, Miyajima A, Kaziro Y, Involvement of ras p21 protein in signal-transduction pathways from interleukin 2, interleukin 3, and granulocyte/macrophage colony-stimulating factor, but not from interleukin 4. *Proc Natl Acad Sci USA* 1991; **88:** 3314–18.
59. Lewis TS, Shapiro PS, Ahn NG, Signal transduction through MAP kinase cascades. *Adv Cancer Res* 1998; **74:** 49–139.
60. Robinson MJ, Cobb MH, Mitogen-activated protein kinase pathways. *Curr Opin Cell Biol* 1997; **9:** 180–6.
61. Goga A, McLaughlin J, Afar DE et al, Alternative signals to RAS for hematopoietic transformation by the BCR–ABL oncogene. *Cell* 1995; **82:** 981–8.
62. Druker B, Okuda K, Matulonis U et al, Tyrosine phosphorylation of rasGAP and associated proteins in chronic myelogenous leukemia cell lines. *Blood* 1992; **79:** 2215–20.
63. Sawyers CL, McLaughlin J, Witte ON, Genetic requirement for Ras in the transformation of fibroblasts and hematopoietic cells by the Bcr–Abl oncogene. *J Exp Med* 1995; **181:** 307–13.
64. Tauchi T, Boswell HS, Leibowitz D, Broxmeyer HE, Coupling between p210bcr–abl and Shc and Grb2 adaptor proteins in hematopoietic cells permits growth factor receptor-independent link to ras activation pathway. *J Exp Med* 1994; **179:** 167–75.
65. Mandanas RA, Leibowitz DS, Gharehbaghi K et al, Role of p21 RAS in p210 bcr–abl transformation of murine myeloid cells. *Blood* 1993; **82:** 1838–47.
66. Koh EY, Chen T, Daley GQ, Complementation of cytokine signaling using a retroviral expression cloning strategy. Manuscript in preparation.
67. McCubrey JA, Steelman LS, Hoyle PE et al, Differential abilities of activated Raf oncoproteins to abrogate cytokine dependency, prevent apoptosis and induce autocrine growth factor synthesis in human hematopoietic cells. *Leukemia* 1998; **12:** 1903–29.
68. Neshat MS, Raitano AB, Wang HG et al, The survival function of the Bcr–Abl oncogene is mediated by Bad-dependent and -independent pathways: roles for phosphatidylinositol 3-kinase and Raf. *Mol Cell Biol* 2000; **20:** 1179–86.
69. Lanfrancone L, Pelicci G, Brizzi MF et al, Overexpression of Shc proteins potentiates the proliferative response to the granulocyte–macrophage colony-stimulating factor and recruitment of Grb2/SoS and Grb2/p140 complexes to the beta receptor subunit. *Oncogene* 1995; **10:** 907–17 [Erratum 1995; **11:** 607].
70. Bollag G, Clapp DW, Shih S et al, Loss of NF1 results in activation of the Ras signaling pathway and leads to aberrant growth in haematopoietic cells. *Nature Genet* 1996; **12:** 144–8.
71. Emanuel PD, Bates LJ, Castleberry RP et al, Selective hypersensitivity to granulocyte–macrophage colony-stimulating factor by juvenile chronic myeloid leukemia hematopoietic progenitors. *Blood* 1991; **77:** 925–9.
72. Largaespada DA, Brannan CI, Jenkins NA, Copeland NG, Nf1 deficiency causes Ras-mediated granulocyte/macrophage colony stimulating factor hypersensitivity and chronic myeloid leukaemia. *Nature Genet* 1996; **12:** 137–43.

73. Cogswell PC, Morgan R, Dunn M et al, Mutations of the ras protooncogenes in chronic myelogenous leukemia: a high frequency of ras mutations in bcr/abl rearrangement-negative chronic myelogenous leukemia. *Blood* 1989; **74:** 2629–33.
74. Janssen JW, Steenvoorden AC, Lyons J et al, RAS gene mutations in acute and chronic myelocytic leukemias, chronic myeloproliferative disorders, and myelodysplastic syndromes. *Proc Natl Acad Sci USA* 1987; **84:** 9228–32.
75. Urbano-Ispizua A, Gill R, Matutes E et al, Low frequency of ras oncogene mutations in Philadelphia-positive acute leukemia and report of a novel mutation H61 Leu in a single case. *Leukemia* 1992; **6:** 342–6.
76. Berns K, Hijmans EM, Koh EY et al, A genetic screen to identify genes that rescue the slow growth phenotype of *c-myc* null fibroblasts. *Oncogene* 2000; **19:** 3330–4.
77. Isfort RJ, Ihle JN, Multiple hematopoietic growth factors signal through tyrosine phosphorylation. *Growth Factors* 1990; **2:** 213–20.
78. Nieborowska-Skorska M, Wasik MA, Slupianek A et al, Signal transducer and activator of transcription (STAT) 5 activation by BCR/ABL is dependent on intact Src homology (SH) 3 and SH2 domains of BCR/ABL and is required for leukemogenesis. *J Exp Med* 1999; **189:** 1229–42.
79. Afar DE, Goga A, McLaughlin J et al, Differential complementation of Bcr–Abl point mutants with c-Myc. *Science* 1994; **264:** 424–6.
80. Afar DE, McLaughlin J, Sherr CJ et al, Signaling by ABL oncogenes through cyclin D1. *Proc Natl Acad Sci USA* 1995; **92:** 9540–4.
81. Afar DE, Goga A, Cohen L et al, Genetic approaches to defining signaling by the CML-associated tyrosine kinase BCR–ABL. *Cold Spring Harb Symp Quant Biol* 1994; **59:** 589–94.
82. Jena N, Deng M, Whoriskey W et al, Cyclin D2 is a critical mediator of hematopoietic cell transformation by BCR/ABL. Submitted 2000.
83. Gold MR, Duronio V, Saxena SP et al, Multiple cytokines activate phosphatidylinositol 3-kinase in hemopoietic cells. Association of the enzyme with various tyrosine-phosphorylated proteins. *J Biol Chem* 1994; **269:** 5403–12.
84. Sattler M, Salgia R, Shrikhande G et al, Steel factor induces tyrosine phosphorylation of CRKL and binding of CRKL to a complex containing c-kit, phosphatidylinositol 3-kinase, and p120(CBL). *J Biol Chem* 1997; **272:** 10248–53.
85. Rinaudo MS, Su K, Falk LA et al, Human interleukin-3 receptor modulates bcl-2 mRNA and protein levels through protein kinase C in TF-1 cells. *Blood* 1995; **86:** 80–8.
86. Kennedy SG, Wagner AJ, Conzen SD et al, The PI 3-kinase/Akt signaling pathway delivers an anti-apoptotic signal. *Genes Dev* 1997; **11:** 701–13.
87. Sattler M, Salgia R, Okuda K et al, The proto-oncogene product p120CBL and the adaptor proteins CRKL and c-CRK link c-ABL, p190BCR/ABL and p210BCR/ABL to the phosphatidylinositol-3′ kinase pathway. *Oncogene* 1996; **12:** 839–46.
88. Harrison-Findik D, Susa M, Varticovski L, Association of phosphatidylinositol 3-kinase with SHC in chronic myelogeneous leukemia cells. *Oncogene* 1995; **10:** 1385–91.
89. Varticovski L, Daley GQ, Jackson P et al, Activation of phosphatidylinositol 3-kinase in cells expressing abl oncogene variants. *Mol Cell Biol* 1991; **11:** 1107–13.
90. Rodriguez-Viciana P, Warne PH, Dhand R et al, Phosphatidylinositol-3-OH kinase as a direct target of Ras. *Nature* 1994; **370:** 527–32.
91. Ihle JN, Kerr IM, Jaks and Stats in signaling by the cytokine receptor superfamily. *Trends Genet* 1995; **11:** 69–74.
92. Watowich SS, Wu H, Socolovsky M et al, Cytokine receptor signal transduction and the control of hematopoietic cell development. *Annu Rev Cell Dev Biol* 1996; **12:** 91–128.
93. Ihle JN, Signaling by the cytokine receptor superfamily in normal and transformed hematopoietic cells. *Adv Cancer Res* 1996; **68:** 23–65.
94. Carlesso N, Frank DA, Griffin JD, Tyrosyl phosphorylation and DNA binding activity of signal transducers and activators of transcription (STAT) proteins in hematopoietic cell lines transformed by Bcr/Abl. *J Exp Med* 1996; **183:** 811–20.
95. Ilaria RL Jr, Van Etten RA, P210 and P190(BCR/ABL) induce the tyrosine phosphorylation and DNA binding activity of multiple specific STAT family members. *J Biol Chem* 1996; **271:** 31704–10.
96. Shuai K, Halpern J, ten Hoeve J et al, Constitutive activation of STAT5 by the BCR–ABL oncogene in chronic myelogenous leukemia. *Oncogene* 1996; **13:** 247–54.
97. Socolovsky M, Fallon AE, Wang S et al, Fetal anemia and apoptosis of red cell progenitors in

Stat5a−/−5b−/− mice: a direct role for Stat5 in Bcl-X(L) induction. *Cell* 1999; **98:** 181–91.
98. Mui AL, Wakao H, Kinoshita T et al, Suppression of interleukin-3-induced gene expression by a C-terminal truncated Stat5: role of Stat5 in proliferation. *EMBO J* 1996; **15:** 2425–33.
99. Matsumura I, Kitamura T, Wakao H et al, Transcriptional regulation of the cyclin D1 promoter by STAT5: its involvement in cytokine-dependent growth of hematopoietic cells. *EMBO J* 1999; **18:** 1367–77.
100. Grigorieva I, Grigoriev VG, Rowney MK, Hoover RG, Regulation of c-myc transcription by interleukin-2 (IL-2). Identification of a novel IL-2 response element interaction with stat-4. *J Biol Chem* 2000; **275:** 7343–50.
101. Hoover RR, Gerlach MJ, Koh EY, Daley GQ, Multiple signaling pathways contribute to cell survival, proliferation, and resistance to radiation-induced apoptosis in BCR/ABL-transformed BaF3 cells. Submitted 2000.
102. Sokol L, Luhovy M, Guan Y et al, Primary familial polycythemia: a frameshift mutation in the erythropoietin receptor gene and increased sensitivity of erythroid progenitors to erythropoietin. *Blood* 1995; **86:** 15–22.
103. Kralovics R, Indrak K, Stopka T et al, Two new EPO receptor mutations: truncated EPO receptors are most frequently associated with primary familial and congenital polycythemias. *Blood* 1997; **90:** 2057–61.
104. Kralovics R, Sokol L, Broxson EH Jr, Prchal JT, The erythropoietin receptor gene is not linked with the polycythemia phenotype in a family with autosomal dominant primary polycythemia. *Proc Assoc Am Physicians* 1997; **109:** 580–5.
105. Percy MJ, McMullin MF, Roques AW et al, Erythrocytosis due to a mutation in the erythropoietin receptor gene. *Br J Haematol* 1998; **100:** 407–10.
106. Kondo T, Okabe M, Sanada M et al, Familial essential thrombocythemia associated with one-base deletion in the 5′-untranslated region of the thrombopoietin gene. *Blood* 1998; **92:** 1091–6.
107. Alexander WS, Nicola NA, Hemopoietic growth factor receptor abnormalities in leukemia. *Leuk Res* 1998; **22:** 1097–111.
108. McMullin MF, Percy MJ, Erythropoietin receptor and hematological disease. *Am J Hematol* 1999; **60:** 55–60.
109. Gonda TJ, D'Andrea RJ, Activating mutations in cytokine receptors: implications for receptor function and role in disease. *Blood* 1997; **89:** 355–69.
110. D'Andrea AD, Cytokine receptors in congenital hematopoietic disease. *N Engl J Med* 1994; **330:** 839–46.
111. Hahn WC, Counter CM, Lundberg AS et al, Creation of human tumour cells with defined genetic elements. *Nature* 1999; **400:** 464–8.
112. Carroll M, Tomasson MH, Barker GF et al, The TEL/platelet-derived growth factor beta receptor (PDGF beta R) fusion in chronic myelomonocytic leukemia is a transforming protein that self-associates and activates PDGF beta R kinase-dependent signaling pathways. *Proc Natl Acad Sci USA* 1996; **93:** 14845–50.
113. Golub TR, Goga A, Barker GF et al, Oligomerization of the ABL tyrosine kinase by the Ets protein TEL in human leukemia. *Mol Cell Biol* 1996; **16:** 4107–16.
114. Ho JM, Beattie BK, Squire JA et al, Fusion of the ets transcription factor TEL to Jak2 results in constitutive Jak–Stat signaling. *Blood* 1999; **93:** 4354–64.
115. Schwaller J, Frantsve J, Aster J et al, Transformation of hematopoietic cell lines to growth-factor independence and induction of a fatal myelo- and lymphoproliferative disease in mice by retrovirally transduced TEL/JAK2 fusion genes. *EMBO J* 1998; **17:** 5321–33.
116. Lacronique V, Boureux A, Valle VD et al, A TEL–JAK2 fusion protein with constitutive kinase activity in human leukemia. *Science* 1997; **278:** 1309–12.
117. Peeters P, Raynaud SD, Cools J et al, Fusion of TEL, the ETS-variant gene 6 (ETV6), to the receptor-associated kinase JAK2 as a result of t(9;12) in a lymphoid and t(9;15;12) in a myeloid leukemia. *Blood* 1997; **90:** 2535–40.
118. Golub TR, Barker GF, Lovett M, Gilliland DG, Fusion of PDGF receptor beta to a novel ets-like gene, tel, in chronic myelomonocytic leukemia with t(5;12) chromosomal translocation. *Cell* 1994; **77:** 307–16.
119. Papadopoulos P, Ridge SA, Boucher CA et al, The novel activation of ABL by fusion to an ets-related gene, TEL. *Cancer Res* 1995; **55:** 34–8.
120. Okuda K, Golub TR, Gilliland DG, Griffin JD, p210BCR/ABL, p190BCR/ABL, and TEL/ABL activate similar signal transduction pathways in

hematopoietic cell lines. *Oncogene* 1996; **13:** 1147–52.

121. Holtschke T, Lohler J, Kanno Y et al, Immunodeficiency and chronic myelogenous leukemia-like syndrome in mice with a targeted mutation of the ICSBP gene. *Cell* 1996; **87:** 307–17.

5

Progenitor cell dynamics

Connie J Eaves, Allen C Eaves

CONTENTS • Introduction • Structure of the chronic-phase malignant clone and residual normal cells • Mechanisms of deregulated hematopoiesis in chronic phase • Progenitor changes associated with disease progression • Questions for the future

INTRODUCTION

This chapter will review what is currently known about the cellular composition of the hematopoietic system of patients with chronic myeloid leukemia (CML) under three major headings: (i) the quantitatively distorted structure of the chronic-phase malignant clone and residual normal cells; (ii) mechanisms responsible for the deregulated hematopoiesis characteristic of chronic-phase disease; (iii) disease progression. As has been the case for all other aspects of CML, significant advances have been made in the last few years in the characterization of the subpopulation of leukemic 'stem' cells in CML that initiate and maintain the disease in vivo. These observations have allowed many of the 'normal' as well as the 'abnormal' features of the leukemic stem cells and their immediate progeny to be identified. At the same time, they have revealed the importance of differentiation-stage-specific perturbations in the turnover and expansion of the leukemic cells in the chronic phase of the disease. This perspective has provided unique clues to the fascinating biology of CML, and offers a framework for explaining the highly variable pathogenesis of the disease in individual patients. Indeed, it seems likely that the eventual successful treatment of CML may well depend on approaches to patient evaluation and therapy that more fully exploit emerging information about normal and leukemic progenitor cells and their properties.

STRUCTURE OF THE CHRONIC-PHASE MALIGNANT CLONE AND RESIDUAL NORMAL CELLS

The leukemic clone in chronic-phase CML is hierarchically organized but the relative sizes of its different compartments are distorted by comparison to normal hematopoiesis (Figure 5.1).

The *BCR/ABL*-positive clone undergoes normal differentiation

CML results from an excessive production of granulocytes, sometimes accompanied by an increased output of platelets. At the cellular level, this is usually associated with complete replacement of normal hematopoiesis by a deregulated clone of cells of pluripotent hematopoietic stem cell origin (Figure 5.1). The presence of this clone is typically first indicated by symptoms related to the high concentrations of circulating granulocytes or the

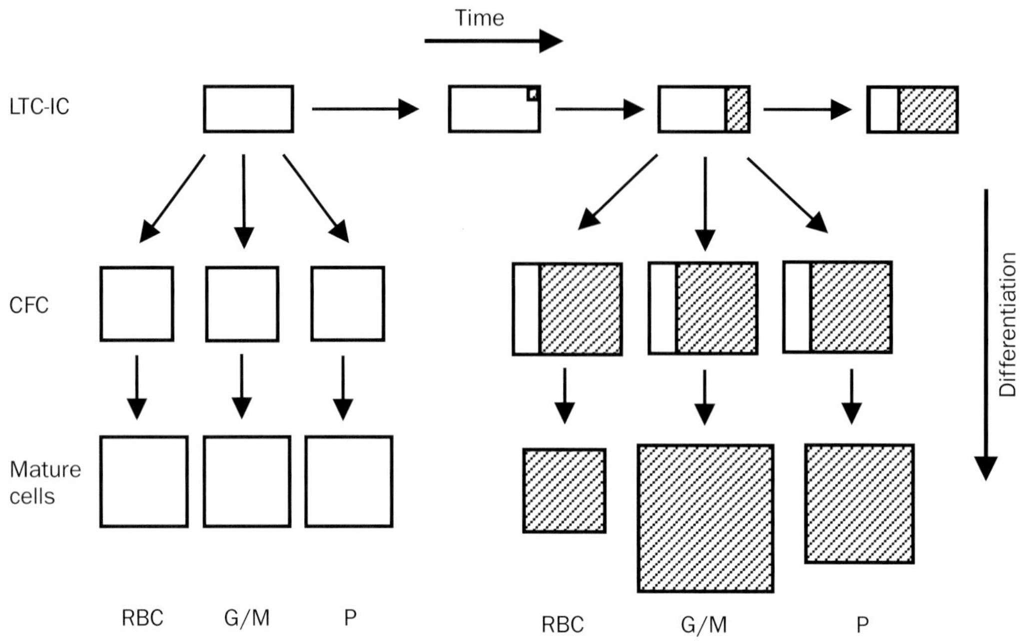

Figure 5.1
Schematic representation of the relative distributions of normal and leukemic cells in different compartments of hematopoietic cells in CML patients and the evolution of these compartments over time. The hatched areas refer to the leukemic component, and the open areas to the progeny of residual normal hematopoietic stem cells. Changes in compartment size are shown to indicate quantitative trends, but are not scaled according to actual numerical estimates. *Abbreviations:* LTC-IC, long-term culture-initiating cells; CFC, colony-forming cells; RBC, red blood cells; G/M, granulocytes/macrophages; P, platelets.

extramedullary hematopoiesis that is initiated (e.g. in the spleen) by leukemic progenitors that enter the circulation from the marrow in large numbers. The marrow is typically hypercellular owing to the presence of increased numbers of terminally differentiating myeloid cells. However, a definitive diagnosis of CML now relies on the demonstration in blood or marrow cells of the presence of the *BCR/ABL* fusion gene using either cytogenetic or molecular methods.

Whether or not the formation of the *BCR/ABL* oncogene is sufficient to cause CML is an entirely different question – and one for which a clear answer is not yet available. In gene transfer experiments using both primitive murine and human hematopoietic cell targets, an abnormal myeloproliferative 'disease' with many features of human CML can be induced.[1–9] However, these same vectors can also produce other hematopoietic disorders using the same or slightly modified transduction protocols, indicating that other factors (e.g. level of expression, initial target cell, and host genotype) may also be important determinants of the disease phenotype. Evidence of *BCR/ABL* transcripts in the blood cells of a large proportion of normal adults reinforces this notion.[10,11]

Although the granulopoietic lineage is the one that appears to be most affected, the presence in the marrow of increased numbers of recognizable precursors of all of the myeloid lineages was appreciated more than 50 years ago. Moreover, even at that time, this observation was correctly interpreted as evidence that the leukemic cells originate from a deregulated pluripotent precursor.[12] This concept was subsequently confirmed by the demonstration of the Philadelphia (Ph) chromosome in erythroid cells and megakaryocytes as well as granulopoietic cells,[13–15] and then later also in B-lineage cells[16,17] and early T-cell precursors.[18] Recently, evidence that some of the leukemic cells can also differentiate into endothelial cells has been reported.[19] The use of other clonal markers further established that, by the time of diagnosis, the leukemic clone in most chronic-phase patients produces over 95% of the red blood cells (RBC) and platelets, as well as the increased numbers of circulating granulocytes, even though the absolute number of RBC is often subnormal and the platelets are only variably increased.[20] In contrast, usually only a proportion of the B-cell compartment is Ph-positive, and mature Ph-positive T cells are absent.

The reasons for the lesser penetrance of the leukemic clone into the lymphoid lineages is not well understood. One possibility is that the BCR/ABL oncoprotein may be toxic in certain cell types (e.g. differentiating T-cell precursors), as has been suggested to be the case in fibroblasts.[21] However, regardless of the explanation for the poor output of mature Ph-positive/*BCR/ABL*-positive lymphoid cells in patients with chronic-phase disease, it is clear that the initial leukemogenic process in CML has little or no effect on the mechanisms of multilineage myeloid differentiation. Likewise, the average numbers of cell divisions required for the development of mature RBC, granulocytes, monocytes, and platelets from a pluripotent stem cell in the normal adult seem to be unaffected.

The colony-forming cell compartment in chronic-phase CML

Further evidence of the preservation of a normal myeloid differentiation program in CML was obtained when patients' cells were first examined in assays that detect different types of lineage-restricted and pluripotent colony-forming cell (CFC) progenitors from normal individuals. When suspensions of normal marrow are cultured in semisolid media containing all of the growth factors required to support the proliferation and complete maturation of cells of a particular lineage, various sizes of colonies are produced. These reflect the range of proliferative potentialities of progenitors that can divide under such conditions. Cells from chronic-phase CML patients produce the full spectrum of colony types and sizes seen in assays of normal cells. Moreover, upon cytogenetic analysis, the vast majority of these colonies, regardless of their lineage, are found to contain Ph-positive cells.[22] Taken together, these observations reinforce the view that the leukemic clone of chronic-phase patients retains the hierarchical structure characteristic of normal adult hematopoiesis (Figure 5.2). Later studies of the surface markers present on the different types of CML progenitors that make up this hierarchy indicated additional similarities with their normal counterparts, except for the more primitive subsets that have been found to display markers known to be altered by mitogenic stimulation.[23–26] Since one of the features of primitive CML progenitors is that their cycling activity is deregulated (see the discussion later in this chapter of deregulated hematopoiesis), such phenotypic changes are not surprising. Taken together, these findings indicate that clonal dominance in the terminal compartments is accompanied by clonal dominance of much earlier compartments (Figure 5.1).

Although the BCR/ABL oncoprotein does not appear to have significant direct effects on the in vitro detection of leukemic CFC, nor on their ability to execute normal differentiation programs in vivo, the total size of the CFC compartment in patients at diagnosis appears to be expanded several-fold owing to an excessive overproduction of leukemic CFC. This is inferred from the normal or slightly increased frequency of CFC (most of which are Ph-positive/*BCR/ABL*-positive) in marrow samples from CML patients, coupled with the increased cellularity of marrow biopsies. However, rigorous

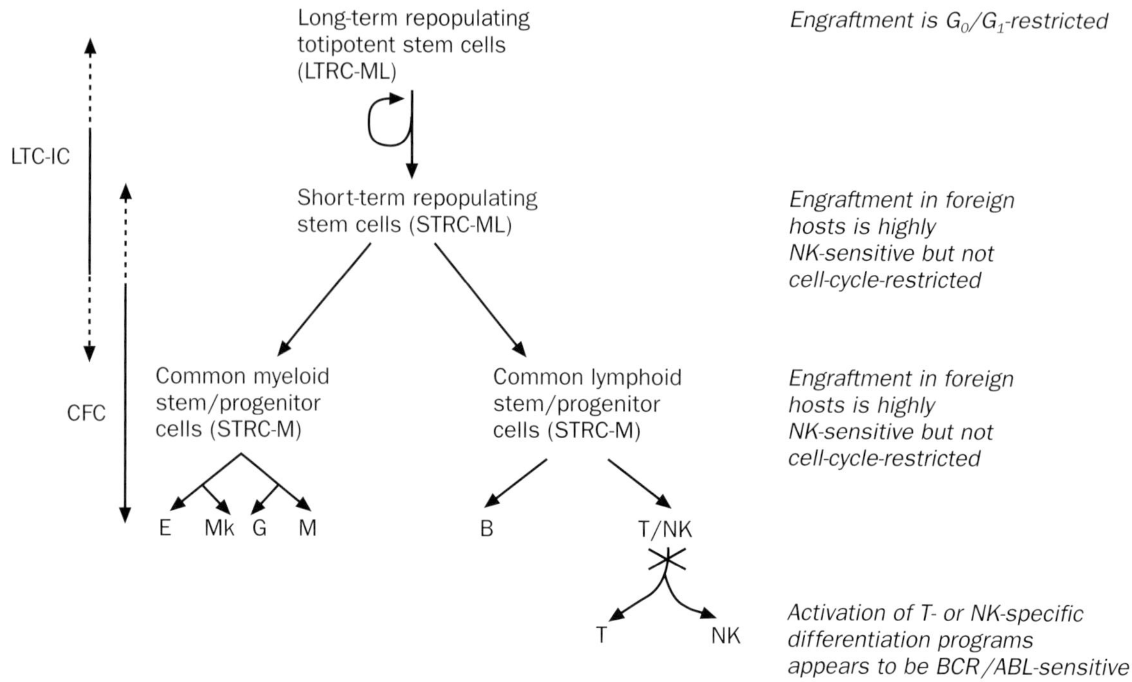

Figure 5.2
Schematic representation of sequential early steps defining the hierarchical structure of the hematopoietic system in the normal adult and the ability of various in vivo and in vitro assays to discriminate cells at each stage. (Note that this model assumes a unidirectional sequence of gene reprogramming events during differentiation – which may need to be reconsidered in the context of leukemia.) For simplicity, this model also excludes alternative (normally minor) possibilities in the mode and rate of lineage restriction. These should not, however, be ignored, since both have been documented in vitro,[141] where they may also be manipulated.[142,143] Normal long-term repopulating cells (LTRC) of the lympho-myeloid lineage (LTRC-ML) are responsible for the human lympho-myeloid repopulation seen after 6–8 weeks in transplanted non-obese diabetic/severe combined immunodeficient (NOD/SCID) mice.[41] These cells also self-renew themselves in these mice, as shown by their ability to engraft secondary NOD/SCID mice.[62] Short-term repopulating cells (STRC) of the lympho-myeloid lineage (STRC-ML) are responsible for most of the lympho-myeloid repopulation seen after 6–8 weeks in transplanted NOD/SCID–β_2-microglobulin double-negative ($\beta_2m^{-/-}$) mice, since they are usually more prevalent than LTRC-ML, although both engraft NOD/SCID–$\beta_2m^{-/-}$ mice.[58] STRC-ML do not undergo significant self-renewal. Myeloid-restricted STRC (STRC-M) produce a transient wave of trilineage myelopoiesis (peaking at 3 weeks) in NOD/SCID–$\beta_2m^{-/-}$ mice. STRC-M are believed to correspond to cells referred to as common myeloid progenitors in mice.[144] Human STRC of the lymphoid lineage (STRC-L) have not yet been identified, but are presumed to exist based on evidence of common lymphoid progenitors in mice[145] and the recent characterization of a type of human lymphoid-restricted long-term culture-initiating cells (LTC-IC).[146] *Other abbreviations:* CFC, colony-forming cells; E, erythroid; Mk, megakaryopoietic; G, granulopoietic; M, macrophage; B, B cell; T, T cell; NK, natural killer cell.

quantitation of the absolute numbers of leukemic CFC present in a given patient is difficult, because of inherent problems in sampling defined volumes of marrow.

Large numbers of almost exclusively Ph-positive/*BCR/ABL*-positive CFC are also found in the blood, where they increase rapidly with the white blood cell (WBC) count (Figure 5.3) to ultimately reach or exceed the numbers of CFC present in the marrow (reviewed in references 27 and 28). The mechanisms that cause these cells to be released from the marrow may be related, at least in part, to abnormalities in integrin expression and signaling, as discussed in Chapter 3. However, the release of these leukemic CFC into the blood may also be secondary to intrinsically activated production of interleukin-3 (IL-3) and granulocyte-colony-stimulating factor (G-CSF) production (described later in this chapter), since exogenous administration of both of these growth factors is known to cause the mobilization of normal CFC.

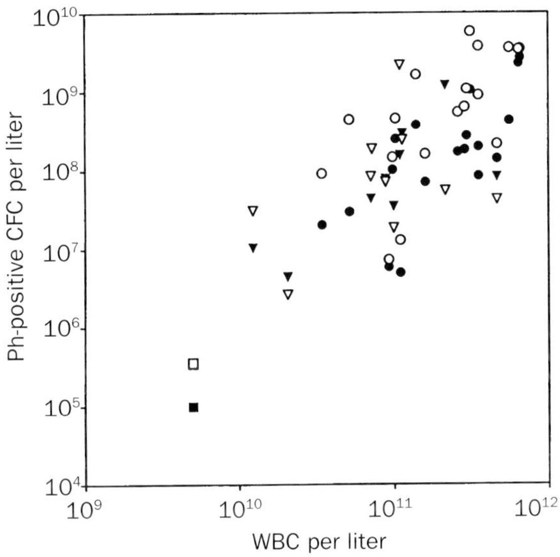

Figure 5.3
Circulating numbers of Ph-positive/*BCR-ABL*-positive CFC increase exponentially as a function of the WBC count. These increases are lineage-independent, as shown by equivalent effects on granulopoietic (solid symbols) and erythroid (open symbols) progenitors. They are also treatment-independent, as shown by equivalent increases of both types of progenitors in previously untreated patients (circles) or patients given hydroxyurea or interferon-α for varying periods (triangles). No patient is represented more than once after treatment. Squares indicate normal blood values. Reprinted from *Leuk Res* **22**, Defective regulation of leukemic hematopoiesis in chronic myeloid leukemia. Eaves C, Cashman J, Eaves A, pp 1085–96. Copyright © 1998, with permission from Elsevier.

Interestingly, the CFC for each of the different lineages, as well as pluripotent CFC, are all equivalently expanded in most patients (reviewed in reference 27). This observation suggests that a common mechanism may be responsible. It also suggests that the normal mechanisms of hematopoietic lineage restriction in pluripotent stem cells are not perturbed in human CML and that the enhanced granulopoiesis is *not* due to a preferential expansion of granulopoietic CFC. Recent studies to examine this issue in various models of *BCR/ABL*-induced disease have produced examples of both enhanced granulopoiesis[29] and enhanced erythropoiesis[30] in the progeny of primitive hematopoietic cells expressing *BCR/ABL* driven by a retroviral long terminal repeat (LTR). These findings underscore the likely importance of other factors in determining the ability of transduced *BCR/ABL* to generate populations of hematopoietic cells that faithfully recapitulate the biological features of human CML, and call for caution in interpreting data obtained from such models.

The lack of any selectivity in the amplification of granulopoietic CFC also means that both the overproduction of granulocytes and the inadequate production of RBC typical of newly diagnosed patients are not solely determined by the numbers of corresponding lineage-specific progenitors produced. The direct relationship of the circulating granulopoietic CFC numbers with the WBC (granulocyte) count would be consistent with the CFC compartment reflecting the potential clone size achievable in an individual patient. On the other hand, there must also be additional, as yet undefined, mechanisms that operate downstream of the erythroid CFC to limit their ability to terminally differentiate in vivo, but that are not effective in vitro and are reversed when the leukemic clone in vivo is reduced.

Long-term culture-initiating cells in chronic-phase CML

The introduction of stromal-cell-containing cultures to detect more primitive cells than the majority of those identified as CFC was rapidly followed by an analysis of CML cell behavior in this system. Initially the results of these studies were confusing, because the Ph-positive CFC were frequently found to disappear within the first 5 weeks in such cultures, often being replaced by normal (Ph-negative)[31] and non-clonal[32,33] CFC, even when normal CFC had not been detected in the original inoculum (Figure 5.4). Because of the known prevalence of leukemic elements in the CFC compartment of CML patients, it was assumed that the switching of CFC genotypes in these cultures reflected a reduced ability of primitive leukemic cells to be maintained under these conditions.

Later, when the kinetics of normal hematopoietic progenitor activation, turnover, and differentiation in such cultures were better defined, it became clear that the CFC present after 5 weeks represent the progeny of a more primitive type of cell (referred to as long-term culture-initiating cells: LTC-IC). Experimental strategies were then devised to allow LTC-IC numbers, their average CFC output (per LTC-IC) and their self-maintenance to be measured independently.[34] Application of these more specific endpoints to analyses of CML cells showed that Ph-positive/*BCR/ABL*-positive LTC-IC are present in highly variable numbers in different patients, but, when detectable, produce the same number and distribution of different types of CFC (granulopoietic versus erythroid versus mixed) as LTC-IC from normal adults.[35] However, in contrast to the CFC compartment, leukemic LTC-IC are frequently greatly outnumbered by normal LTC-IC. In addition, even the number of normal LTC-IC in patients with CML appears to be reduced (Figure 5.5).[24,28]

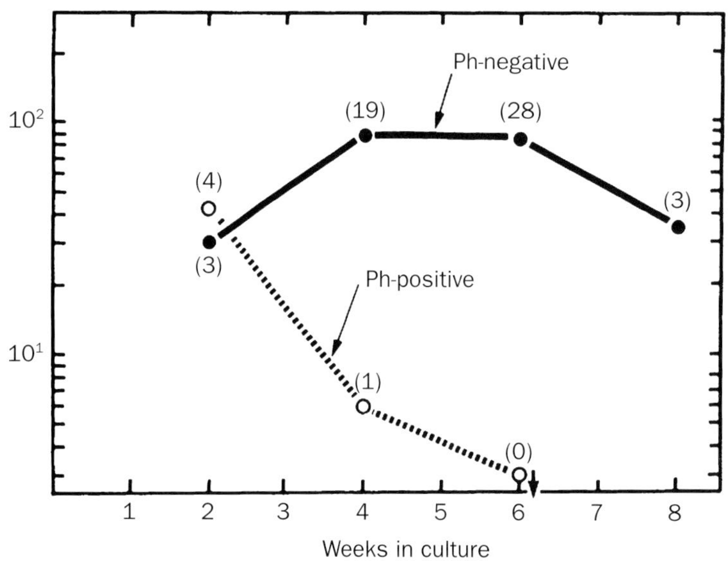

Figure 5.4
Different types of normal (Ph-negative, solid circles) and CML (Ph-positive, open circles) CFC (in this case shown for erythroid progenitors: burst-forming units erythroid, BFU-E) in long-term cultures of CML marrow. Results shown are from a single representative experiment. Reprinted with permission from Coulombel L, Kalousek DK, Eaves CJ et al, Long-term marrow culture reveals chromosomally normal hematopoietic progenitor cells in patients with Philadelphia chromosome-positive chronic myelogeneous leukemia. *N Engl J Med* 1983; **308:** 1493–8. Copyright © 1983 Massachusetts Medical Society. All rights reserved.

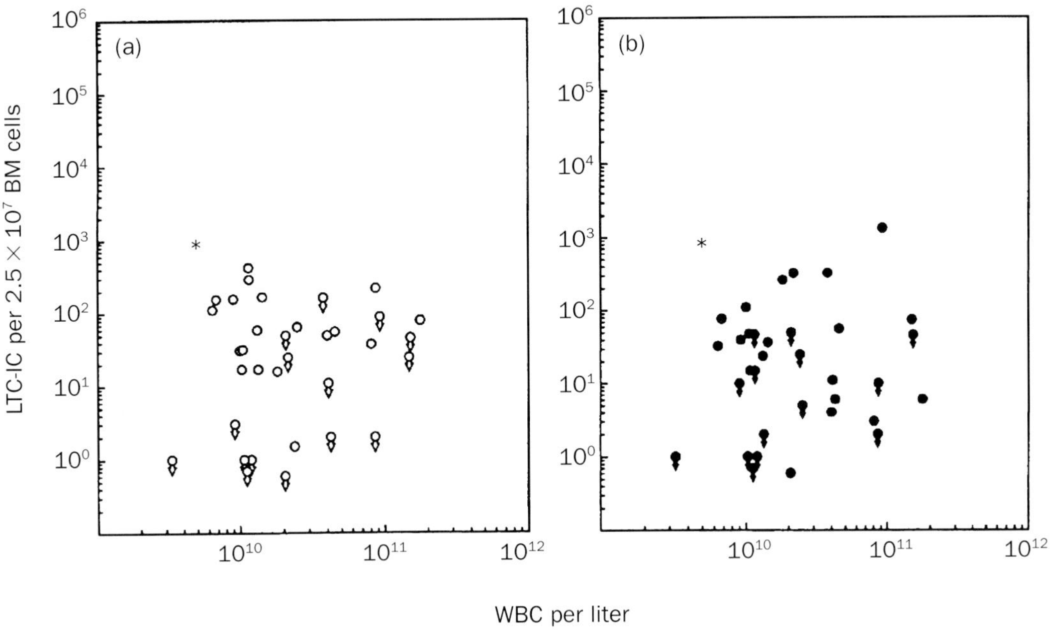

Figure 5.5
Frequencies of (a) normal (Ph-negative, open circles) and (b) Ph-positive (solid circles) LTC-IC in the bone marrow (BM) of 34 CML patients in chronic phase. Both are unrelated to the WBC count and, in general, reduced over tenfold below the frequency of LTC-IC in the marrow of normal individuals (asterisk). Reprinted with permission from Eaves CJ, Cashman JD, Zoumbos NC et al, Biological strategies for the selective manipulation of normal and leukemic stem cells. *Stem Cells* 1993; **11**(Suppl 3): 109–21. © AlphaMed Press 1993.

Thus, in most instances, long-term cultures initiated with CML cells will start off containing CFC that are predominantly Ph-positive, but these will rapidly disappear over the next 3–4 weeks as these progenitors differentiate into more mature (non-dividing) cells. If the majority of the LTC-IC in the input inoculum are normal (as is most commonly the case), then the type of switch in CFC genotypes frequently seen during the first 5 weeks would be expected. The actual extent of such a switch in any given experiment will, however, depend on both the absolute and the relative numbers of normal and leukemic LTC-IC present in the original population. Such differences likely explain the apparent discrepant results of CML CFC behavior in long-term cultures reported by different groups.[36,37]

Using selected patients' samples in which the LTC-IC were predominantly leukemic, the self-maintenance ability of these cells in vitro was then evaluated. Interestingly, the results of these latter studies demonstrated that this aspect of leukemic LTC-IC function is defective both in stromal-cell-containing[35] and in stroma-free cultures where support is assured by the provision of soluble growth factors.[38] Thus, the initial concept that primitive CML cells have a defective ability to maintain themselves in vitro proved to be correct, although the explanation for the switching of CFC genotypes typically seen is generally due to the different ratios of normal versus leukemic CFC and LTC-IC in the original samples. These observations provided a rationale for evaluating 'culture purging' as a strategy for removing Ph-positive/*BCR/ABL*-positive stem cells from autologous marrow transplants[39] (and discussed in detail in Chapter 27).

LTC-IC, like CFC, are found in the blood in elevated numbers, and a similar positive correlation with the WBC count has been demonstrated.[24] However, in contrast to the Ph-positive/*BCR/ABL*-positive genotype of most of the circulating CFC, the LTC-IC in the blood are often predominantly normal.[26,40] Initially, this observation was unexpected, since it indicated that the increase in the numbers of primitive hematopoietic cells in the blood of chronic-phase CML patients was due, at least in part, to an indirect mechanism, and hence was not an exclusive consequence of intrinsic changes in the adhesive properties of the leukemic cells. However, given that indirect mechanisms do play a role in stimulating primitive cells to enter the circulation, it is perhaps not surprising that the relative proportions of normal and leukemic progenitors mobilized (both CFC and LTC-IC) mirror those of the corresponding progenitor compartments in the marrow from which they come.

Are CML stem cells transplantable?

The ability of human hematopoietic cells to engraft the bone marrow of various types of highly immunodeficient mice was first recognized in the late 1980s, and has since formed the basis of powerful assays for primitive normal cells with in vivo engrafting properties (Figure 5.2). This xenotransplant system has also provided new opportunities to explore some of the mechanisms that regulate normal human stem cell self-renewal,[41–45] homing,[46] and turnover in vivo.[47] These advances have, of course, prompted efforts to address similar questions about the malignant cells present in various human hematopoietic malignancies, including CML. Several groups have now reported the engraftment of both severe combined immunodeficient (SCID) and non-obese diabetic (NOD)/SCID mice with human cells following intravenous injection of the mice with cells from chronic-phase patients.[48–52] In some instances, the presence of leukemic (Ph-positive/*BCR/ABL*-positive) B-lymphoid as well as myeloid cells in the marrow has also been demonstrated.[52] These findings have established that some CML cells can produce leukemic progeny upon their transplantation into sublethally irradiated immunodeficient mice, thus extending much older observations of low but persisting numbers of Ph-positive cells in occasional allogeneic (human) recipients of unirradiated granulocyte transfusions collected from CML patients.[53–55]

It should be noted, however, that the transplantation of very large inocula has been required to obtain positive animals in immunodeficient mice, and subsequent (unpublished) attempts to repeat these findings using the same models have met with variable success. In fact, even in the published studies, it was shown that cells from newly diagnosed CML patients frequently generate many normal progeny and predominantly normal CFC and LTC-IC.[49–52] Thus, these xenotransplant models have not lived up to initial hopes of being able to consistently transfer the human disease to animal hosts at frequencies or levels adequate for their further study. For the same reasons, it has also not yet been feasible to use these models to develop efficient assays for the detection and characterization of CML stem cells. Other lines of evidence suggest that CML stem cells may have intrinsically poor engraftment abilities in comparison with their normal counterparts. For example, gene transfer experiments have failed to show significant regrowth of retrovirally marked CML cells in autografted patients,[56] and *BCR/ABL*-transduced 'leukemic' mouse bone marrow cells have shown a relatively poor ability to engraft secondary mice.[8,57] Although there may be alternative explanations for these latter observations, they are all consistent with the possibility that CML stem cells in the circulation do not efficiently re-enter the bone marrow. More recently, specific subsets of normal human hematopoietic cells that can engraft immunodeficient mice have begun to be defined, some of the properties that can affect their seeding efficiency have been identified, and their turnover and differentiation post transplant have been partially characterized

(Figure 5.2).[58] This newer information has provided a number of insights that may help to explain the unexpectedly 'poor' results obtained with xenotransplanted CML cells from chronic-phase patients.

For several years, the NOD/SCID mouse has been the preferred host for assessing the frequency of (and effects of various ex vivo manipulations on) transplantable normal human hematopoietic cells. This is due to the higher levels of engraftment that can be achieved with smaller transplants by comparison with SCID mice.[59] In fact, even with NOD/SCID mouse hosts, most studies have used cord blood as the source of normal human cells to be transplanted because of the relatively high numbers of transplantable cells present compared with adult sources.[41,60–62] In normal adult human marrow, the frequency of lympho-myeloid repopulating cells able to engraft a sublethally irradiated NOD/SCID mouse has been determined from limiting-dilution assays to be only approximately 1 per 3×10^6 low-density cells or approximately 1 per 10^5 $CD34^+$ cells. In contrast, the corresponding frequencies for cord blood are 3- to 6-fold higher. Such transplantable human hematopoietic 'stem' cells are not present at detectable levels in normal adult human blood. They can be detected in mobilized peripheral blood, but at frequencies that are even lower than in adult marrow and that vary widely among samples from different individuals.[60,61] It should be noted that the true frequency of normal human hematopoietic cells with NOD/SCID-mouse engrafting potential is thought to be approximately 20 times higher than the frequencies measured by limiting-dilution assays. The need for a 'correction' is based on experiments indicating that only about 5% will successfully seed into the marrow of the injected NOD/SCID assay mice.[63] Such corrections are important when comparing the frequencies of cells detected by different assay procedures, particularly when these may be either in vitro (e.g. the LTC-IC assay) or in vivo.

Although significant differences in seeding efficiency between fetal and neonatal sources of human hematopoietic cells that engraft NOD/SCID mice have not been found,[63] marked changes in engraftment ability have been noted as transplantable adult human hematopoietic stem cells enter G_1 from G_0.[64] In experiments both with murine bone marrow[65,66] and with human cord blood,[67] an even more dramatic decrease has been noted as the stem cells transit $S/G_2/M$. This is particularly relevant to the poor NOD/SCID engrafting activity encountered with leukemic cells from CML patients in chronic phase. Based on the greatly increased proliferative activity characteristic of all primitive leukemic cell types (see below), it would be expected that a large proportion of the leukemic stem cells would share this behavior and thus be highly compromised in their ability to engraft NOD/SCID mice.

Other studies have now shown that different types of human hematopoietic stem cell subsets engraft different types of immunodeficient mice with different efficiencies (Figure 5.2).[58] Specifically, cells with short-term myelo-restricted repopulating activity produce a transient burst of trilineage myelopoiesis that peaks at 3 weeks post transplant when these cells are injected into sublethally irradiated NOD/SCID–β_2-microglobulin double-negative (NOD/SCID–$\beta_2m^{-/-}$) mice. In these same mice, another type of short-term repopulating human cell will produce large numbers of lymphoid and myeloid progeny for at least 3 months. Interestingly, both of these short-term repopulating cell types are unable to engraft NOD/SCID mice efficiently. In contrast, human repopulating cells with long-term lympho-myeloid regenerative activity appear to engraft both genotypes of murine recipients with equal efficiency, although their frequency is 5- to 10-fold lower. The substantially higher levels of human cell engraftment seen in NOD/SCID–$\beta_2m^{-/-}$ mice transplanted with primitive hematopoietic cells[58,68] can be simply explained by this differential engraftment ability of the three populations and the greater prevalence of the short-term repopulating cells in most human hematopoietic tissues. Importantly, the ability of the short-term lympho-myeloid repopulating cells to engraft NOD/SCID–$\beta_2m^{-/-}$ mice is not affected by cell cycle progression. It thus might be anticipated that CML cells would also engraft NOD/SCID–$\beta_2m^{-/-}$ mice more efficiently than NOD/SCID mice on the assumption that the point of rapid expansion of the Ph-positive/*BCR/ABL*-positive clone in patients occurs as the leukemic stem cells enter the short-term repopulating cell compartments. However, preliminary experiments have not borne out this prediction,[69] suggesting that this expansion occurs further downstream.

Summary

By the time of diagnosis, the single initially transformed Ph-positive/*BCR/ABL*-positive hematopoietic stem cell responsible for the disease has proliferated to generate a clone of at least 10^{12} cells comprising all of the known types of hematopoietic cells except those of the T-cell lineage. Follow-up of survivors of the atomic bomb explosions in Japan at the end of World War II indicates that the latency period required for the disease to become symptomatic is, on average, 6–7 years.[70] The cell types represented in the leukemic clone include all of the normal stages of differentiation, reflecting the same hierarchical structure typical of normal adult hematopoiesis. However, there is a dramatic change from a predominance of normal cells in the most primitive compartments (detectable in LTC-IC and NOD/SCID repopulation assays) to a predominance of leukemic elements at all later stages and in all of the myeloid lineages. The size of the most primitive cell population is not increased, but evidence of a deregulated lineage-non-specific expansion of the clone becomes apparent as the most primitive leukemic cells outcompete their normal counterparts in entering the CFC compartment. There is also a non-specific exodus of all types of primitive hematopoietic cells (irrespective of their genotype) from the marrow. The progenitors remaining in the marrow are responsible for the dramatic increase in granulocyte production, a modest and variable increase in platelet production, and usually a deficient output of RBC that are the hallmarks of this disease.

MECHANISMS OF DEREGULATED HEMATOPOIESIS IN CHRONIC PHASE

This section discusses the mechanisms underlying the deregulated proliferation and apoptosis of the leukemic progenitors in chronic-phase CML and their pattern of expansion in vivo.

The proliferative activity of all types of primitive leukemic cells is increased, but a quiescent subpopulation is also present

The hierarchical organization of normal hematopoietic cell differentiation offers enormous flexibility in the regulation of mature cell output. At each successive cell division, mechanisms that control cell viability, cell cycle progression, and the rate of molecular differentiation will together determine the extent of cell amplification that occurs between the stem cell compartment and the final end cells. Thus, where a given type of progenitor is increased above the norm, alterations in one or more of these parameters must exist.

Interest in elucidating such changes in CML is driven in part by a desire to define the mechanisms by which the clonal stem cells achieve a competitive advantage. However, the disease may also be viewed as a ‘naturally’ occurring perturbation of normal stem cell dynamics whose analysis can yield novel insights into how these cells and their immediate progeny are normally controlled. From either perspective, such investigations pose major challenges, both because the cells of interest are relatively rare ($<$0.1–1% of all the nucleated cells in a blood or marrow sample) and because they cannot be readily obtained in pure form or uniquely identified by direct methods. Thus standard labeling techniques to measure S-phase cells, or cells undergoing apoptosis, have not been useful for assessing the behavior of the most primitive hematopoietic cells in either normal adults or patients with CML.

Three approaches have allowed these problems to be circumvented. The first involves exposing the population to be evaluated (independent of its purity) to an agent that is specifically toxic to S-phase cells (e.g. high- specific-activity [^{3}H]thymidine or hydroxyurea) for a period of one cell cycle or less. As illustrated in Figure 5.6, a very brief exposure will kill only those cells in S phase at that moment. Because S phase occupies about 50% of the cell cycle, this will result in a maximum reduction in progenitor numbers (determined in subsequent quantitative functional assays) of approximately twofold when most of the progenitors are proliferating (asynchronously) and no reduction when most are quiescent. Prolonging the exposure to allow all cells in the G_1, G_2, or M phases of the cell cycle to enter S phase improves discrimination of proliferating populations (as percentage kill values can then exceed 90%), but this also reduces the resolution of quiescent populations (owing to some non-specific toxicity).[71]

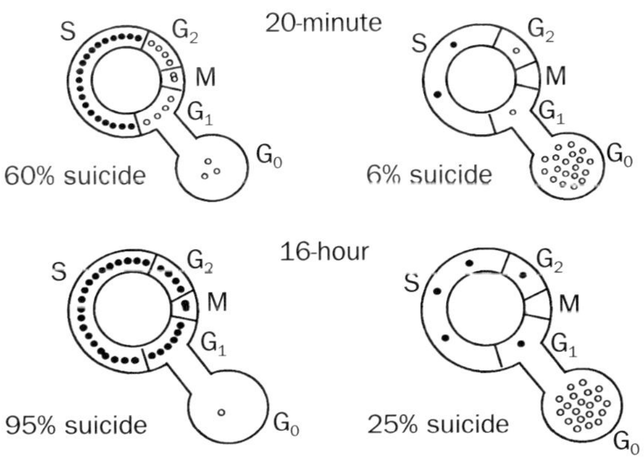

Figure 5.6
Schematic representation of the different distributions of largely cycling (left) and largely quiescent (right) populations in the different phases of the cell cycle. These predict the proportions of cells in each case expected to be killed (solid circles) or not (open circles) by a short (20-minute) or prolonged (16-hour) exposure to high-specific-activity [^{3}H]thymidine.

Such procedures were first used to demonstrate that the majority of CFC in normal adult marrow are proliferating, although the most primitive subsets of these, identified by their ability to produce very large and/or multilineage colonies, are mostly quiescent. In addition, only quiescent CFC (regardless of their proliferative or differentiation potential) are found in the blood of normal adults. In contrast, analogous measurements applied to CFC from CML patients showed that the majority of the leukemic CFC, regardless of their location or differentiation state, are cycling (reviewed in reference 27). Later, the prolonged [^{3}H]thymidine suicide procedure was used to show that most of the LTC-IC in normal adults are, like primitive CFC, quiescent,[71] whereas most of their leukemic counterparts are proliferating.[72] As discussed in the previous section, normal hematopoietic stem cells cannot engraft when they are in S phase at the time of transplantation. Thus, even if normal and leukemic sources of transplantable stem cells could be accessed in sufficient numbers and at sufficient purity to compare their cycling status, it is likely that [^{3}H]thymidine suicide assays would be uninformative.

A second approach to measuring the cell cycle status of primitive hematopoietic cells exploits FACS technology for isolating viable cells in G_0, G_1, and $S/G_2/M$ based on their DNA and RNA content after staining with Hoechst 33342 and Pyronin Y (Figure 5.7).[73,74] The isolated cells can then be assayed for particular progenitor activities and the numbers in each fraction calculated. Such experiments have confirmed the increased turnover of leukemic LTC-IC in chronic-phase CML patients.

At the same time, these studies provided the first direct evidence that there is a consistently detectable subpopulation of primitive *quiescent* leukemic cells present in chronic-phase CML patients. The G_0 leukemic cells include members of both the CFC and LTC-IC compartments.

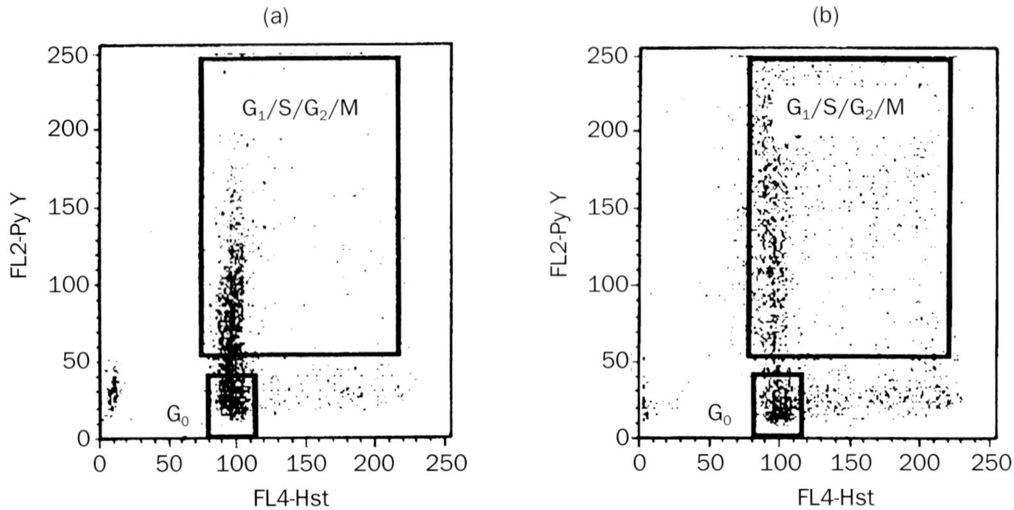

Figure 5.7
Use of Hoechst 33342 (Hst) and Pyronin Y (Py Y) staining to distinguish cells in different phases of the cell cycle. Results for fluorescence-activated cell sorting (FACS)-purified $CD34^+$ cells from a representative normal bone marrow (a) are shown in comparison with similarly purified $CD34^+$ cells from a chronic-phase CML patient in whom most of the LTC-IC were Ph-positive/*BCR/ABL*-positive (b). Reprinted with permission from Holyoake T, Jiang X, Eaves C, Eaves A, Isolation of a highly quiescent subpopulation of primitive leukemic cells in chronic myeloid leukemia. *Blood* 1999; **94:** 2056–64.

However, they are more prevalent within the leukemic LTC-IC population, where as many as 59% may be in G_0 phase.[74] More stringent evidence of their 'deeply' quiescent status has been provided by the demonstration that they can remain viable and functionally unaltered, but without dividing, when cultured for 5 days in the presence of a growth factor cocktail that is potently mitogenic for most primitive normal LTC-IC. Interestingly, the primitive quiescent leukemic cells contain *BCR/ABL* transcripts at levels readily detectable by single cell reverse transcriptase polymerase chain reaction (RT-PCR),[74] as shown previously for the majority of the cells in purified populations of leukemic cells exhibiting a 'primitive' phenotype (e.g. $CD34^+CD38^-$ cells).[75] This suggests that the actions of the BCR/ABL oncoprotein are not sufficient on their own to counteract all of the inhibitory cues emanating from the environment.

The existence of quiescent leukemic stem cells in CML patients has, in fact, been inferred from various clinical findings for many years. These include the failure of intensive chemotherapy regimens to eradicate the disease[76,77] and the observation of relapses many years post transplant.[78,79] However, both of these findings could have other explanations, and neither allows estimation of the frequency of such cells in individual patients. The introduction of methods for their routine isolation and further characterization should thus facilitate future investigations of the role of this subpopulation in disease progression and response to therapy.

A third approach to evaluating normal and leukemic stem cell dynamics has involved an assessment of telomere length in granulocytes from normal individuals and from CML patients. Telomere length in somatic cells decreases with each division (approximately 50–100 bp/year),[80,81] and can thus serve as an indicator of their mitotic history. In the hematopoietic system, the very short half-life of mature granulocytes makes these cells particularly useful for monitoring hematopoietic stem cell turnover rates. Telomere length measurements performed on granulocytes from normal individuals of different ages suggest that in the adult, all of the stem cells will divide, on average, only once every 1–2 years (Figure 5.8).[82] As also illustrated in Figure 5.8, such measurements show the telomere length of leukemic cells from patients with chronic-phase CML to be significantly shorter (over 1 kbp or so shorter) than in the granulocytes of age-matched controls, indicating a somewhat faster turnover of the leukemic stem cells.[83] Assuming no change in other kinetic parameters, this can be estimated to represent about 10 more self-renewal divisions than would be executed by normal stem cells prior to the time of diagnosis (i.e. about 1–2 extra divisions per year over an estimated average 6- to 7-year latency period[70]). Note that because of the wide variations in telomere length seen among different individuals,[82,84,85] assessment of either very large numbers of people or of matched non-clonal (e.g. T cells) and leukemic cells (blood or marrow) from the same individuals is necessary for meaningful comparisons.

Altered responses of primitive leukemic progenitors to proliferation inhibitors

Over the last 15 years, experimental systems for analyzing the mitogenic responses of primitive hematopoietic progenitors to external treatments both in vitro and in vivo have been devised. A multiplicity of growth factors that can stimulate normal quiescent CFC to proliferate have been identified, some of which have also been shown to activate quiescent LTC-IC.[86] These latter factors include Flt3 ligand (FL), Steel factor (SF; also known as stem cell factor (SCF) and c-Kit ligand), and IL-3. Others, such as thrombopoietin (TPO), appear poorly mitogenic to very primitive cells, but can maintain their viability.[74,87,88] Thus, as primitive hematopoietic cells differentiate, they may continue to be responsive to the same factors, but the outcome of their stimulation by a given agent and the requirement for signals from different types of factors changes markedly. A similar picture has emerged for factors that inhibit primitive hematopoietic cell proliferation, as shown by their ability to cause the target cells to either stop proliferating (without disappearing) or to persist in G_0 in the presence of an activating stimulus. Transforming growth

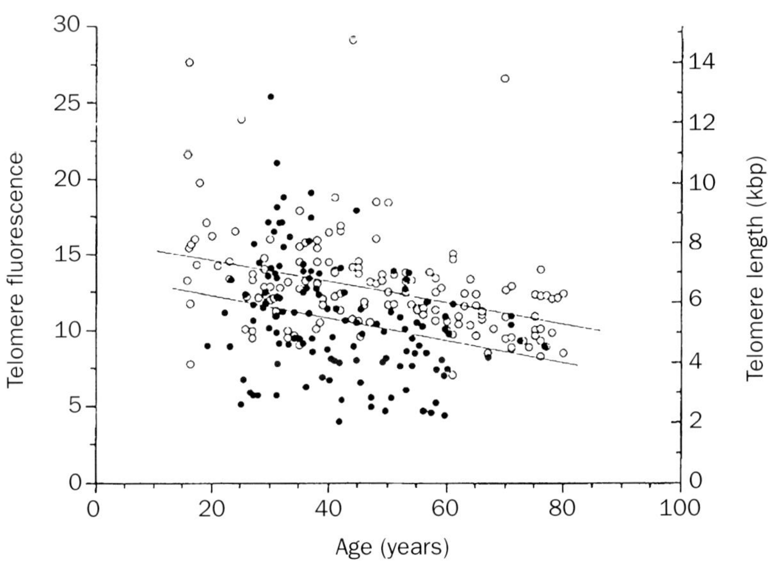

Figure 5.8
Telomere length in blood or marrow cells from CML patients (solid circles) is shorter than in blood cells from age-matched normal individuals (open circles). Telomere length was determined by flow fluorescence in situ hybridization (FISH). Reprinted with permission from Brummendorf TH, Holyoake TL, Rufer N et al, Prognostic implications of differences in telomere length between normal and malignant cells from patients with chronic myeloid leukemia measured by flow cytometry. *Blood* 2000; **95:** 1883–90.

Table 5.1 Cycling of normal human long-term culture-initiating cells (LTC-IC) and different types of colony-forming cells is responsive to different inhibitors in vivo[a]

Inhibitor[b]	Target progenitor[c]			
	LTC-IC	pCFU-GM	pBFU-E	mCFU-GM
MIP-1α	−	−	+	+
MCP-1	−	+	+	−
SDF-1	+	+	+	−
TGF-β	+	+	+	−

[a]Data from references 47 and 90.
[b]MIP-1α, macrophage inflammatory protein-1α; MCP-1, monocyte chemotactic protein-1; SDF-1, stromal-cell-derived factor-1; TFG-β, transferring growth factor-β.
[c]CFU-GM, colony-forming unit-granulocyte–macrophage; BFU-E, burst-forming unit-erythroid; p, primitive (high proliferative potential); m, mature (low proliferative potential); −, no effect on progenitor cycling (or numbers); +, inhibition of progenitor cycling (with no effect on progenitor numbers).

factor-β (TGF-β) is an example of an inhibitor that can block the cycling of a broad spectrum of hematopoietic progenitors, including transplantable human stem cells that repopulate NOD/SCID mice (lympho-myeloid long-term repopulating cells (LTRC-ML), Figure 5.2),[47,89] as well as LTC-IC and primitive CFC.[90] In addition, there are a number of chemokines that can block the cell cycle progression of primitive hematopoietic cells, but exhibit very specific ranges of target cell specificity (Table 5.1).[90–92]

Primitive CML cells appear normally sensitive to the inhibitory action of TGF-β, but do not respond to any of the chemokines that block the S-phase entry of primitive normal hematopoietic cells (see references 91–93 and unpublished data). These findings have two important implications. First, they indicate a mechanism by which some primitive CML cells could be forced to enter a quiescent state in vivo where there is likely to be considerable heterogeneity in the local concentrations of many cytokines, including TGF-β, throughout the marrow microenvironment. Secondly, they suggest that primitive CML cells utilize a common mechanism to override a shared intracellular signaling pathway that is activated by inhibitory chemokines to block the cell cycle progression of primitive normal hematopoietic cells. One possibility for such a mechanism would be an action of the BCR/ABL oncoprotein, itself. However, another might be the antagonizing action of autocrine IL-3 and/or G-CSF, which is a unique mechanism operative in primitive CML cells,[94] discussed in the next subsection.

Autocrine mechanisms of deregulated viability, proliferation, and stem cell self-renewal in CML

The increased turnover of primitive CML cells has been well established for more than two decades. Nevertheless, a precise delineation of the molecular mechanisms responsible has remained elusive. Difficulties in obtaining large numbers of purified populations of leukemic progenitors have been a major impediment in the use of these cells for biochemical studies of perturbed intracellular signaling events. As a result, most of the information obtained to date on this subject has been derived from the more mature CML cells that are predominant in unpurified samples of blood and marrow cells from chronic-phase patients, or from *BCR/ABL*-transduced cells, or from various Ph-positive/*BCR/ABL*-positive cell lines established in vitro (from samples obtained from CML patients in blast crisis). One of the early findings from the studies of transduced factor-dependent cell lines was the activation of autocrine mechanisms that conferred partial or complete growth factor autonomy.[95–97] However, careful examination of primary samples of CML marrow and blood failed to replicate these observations in primary CML cells.[98,99] Moreover, the leukemic CFC from chronic-phase CML patients had not been found to have a decreased sensitivity to exogenously provided growth factors when assayed under standard assay conditions in vitro.[100,101] Thus, for many years, autocrine mechanisms were largely discounted as irrelevant to the pathogenesis of naturally occurring CML.

The acquired factor *independence* of many of the *BCR/ABL*-positive cell lines studied has also focused attention on the potential of the BCR/ABL oncoprotein to protect primary CML cells and progenitors from various apoptosis-inducing treatments. The results of experiments to examine this question have been conflicting.[102–104] However, five studies that have compared the effect specifically of growth factor withdrawal on normal and leukemic CFC survival have all shown a superior response by the leukemic cells.[94,105–108] In fact, in those from our own group, the numbers of all types of CFC were found not only to be maintained upon factor withdrawal, but had actually *increased* several-fold after 3 weeks of culture in serum-free medium (see e.g. Figure 5.9).

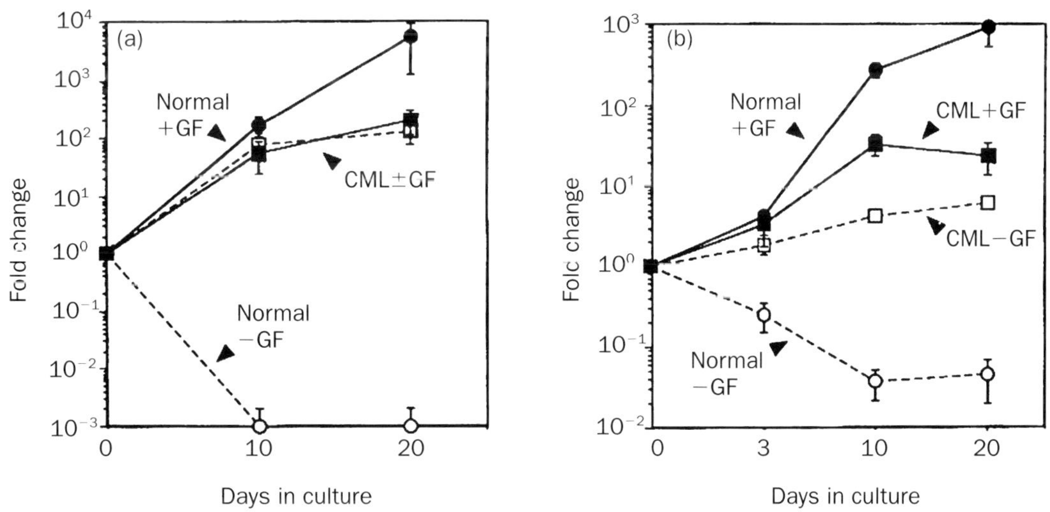

Figure 5.9
Factor-independent expansion of cells in serum-free cultures initiated with primitive CML cells. Increase in total cells (a) and CFC (b) in cultures initiated with CD34$^+$CD45RA$^-$CD71$^-$ cells from patients with predominantly Ph-positive LTC-IC is similar in the presence (solid squares) or absence (open squares) of growth factors (GF) that stimulate normal cells of the same primitive phenotype (solid circles). In the absence of growth factors, most normal cells die rapidly (open circles). Adapted from data published in reference 107.

Further investigation showed that this factor independence is a prominent but exclusive feature of the most primitive subpopulations of CML cells (e.g. as defined by a $CD34^{+}CD45RA^{-}CD71^{-}$ or $CD34^{+}CD38^{-}$ phenotype). These subpopulations contain most of the LTC-IC, varying proportions of which are normal and leukemic, depending on the patient. However, very few of the CFC (which are predominantly leukemic in most samples, as already noted) have either of these 'primitive' phenotypes. When samples with a high content of Ph-positive/*BCR/ABL*-positive LTC-IC are cultured under serum-free culture conditions in the absence of exogenous factors, the rapid generation of large numbers of leukemic CFC of all of the myeloid lineages can be quite dramatic, and, within 10 days, most of the cells present have already reached the terminal stages of differentiation.[108] Thus, by that time, morphologically recognizable maturing cells of all lineages, including the megakaryocyte lineage, are predominant (Figure 5.10). However, this burst of factor-independent growth and differentiation is short-lived because of the compromised self-renewal function of the primitive leukemic cells used to initiate the cultures (see the discussion of LTC-IC in chronic phase earlier in the chapter). Later subsets of $CD34^{+}$ cells that contain most of the CFC originally present show less pronounced factor-independent growth, as indicated by a smaller and even shorter net increase in cell number. By the time the leukemic cells have exited the $CD34^{+}$ (CFC) compartment, their requirement for exogenous factor provision to support their terminal growth and survival in vitro becomes almost indistinguishable from normal.[94]

These observations have now made it possible to reconcile many previous results that originally seemed contradictory, including the widely observed *factor dependence* of CML CFC in standard colony assays. These assays depend heavily on the ability of terminal $CD34^{-}$ cells to execute their final amplifying divisions. Thus, the majority of the cells that allow a leukemic CFC-derived colony to become detectable would be produced during the factor-depen-

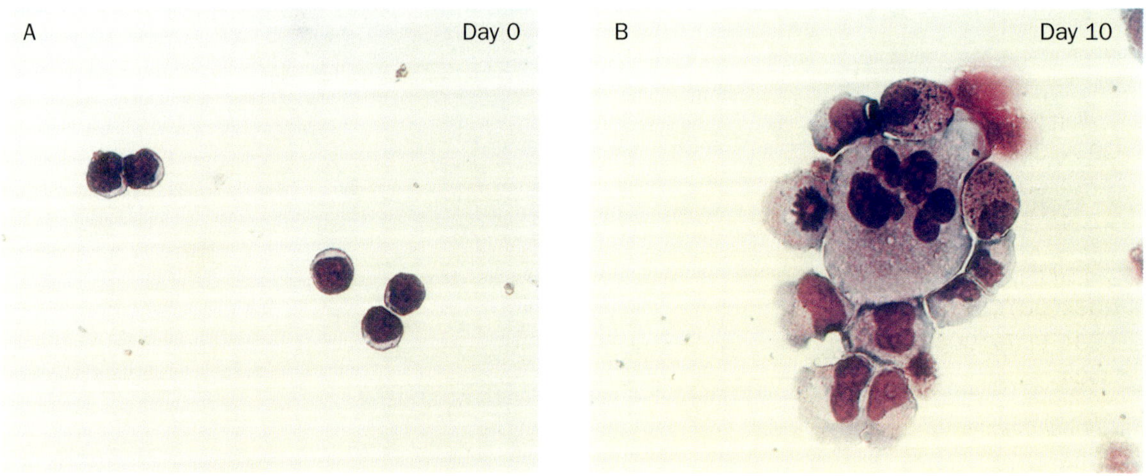

Figure 5.10
$CD34^{+}$ CML cells undergo rapid multilineage differentiation in vitro in the absence of exogenous growth factors. Panel A shows the initially isolated cells and panel B the differentiating granulopoietic cells and megakaryocytes present 10 days later. Reprinted by permission from Jiang X, Fujisaki T, Nicotini F et al, Autonomous multilineage differentiation in vitro of primitive $CD34^{+}$ cells from patients with chronic myeloid leukemia. *Leukemia* 2000; **14:** 1112–21. Copyright © 2000 Macmillan Magazines.

dent phase of CD34$^-$ leukemic cell proliferation, even though the initial CFCs might be CD34$^+$. In standard colony assays in which exogenous growth factors are not present, and in which the most 'mature' CFC types are the most numerous, abortive colony starts would be the expected outcome, as was originally observed by Strife et al.[105] Only when highly purified populations of very primitive and predominantly leukemic CML cells are evaluated does a convincing picture of factor independence emerge.

These findings prompted a renewed search for evidence of an autocrine mechanism operating in primitive CML cells. Using sensitive RT-PCR procedures, the presence of IL-3 and G-CSF transcripts were immediately demonstrated in the CD34$^+$ cells from all of a large number of chronic-phase patients evaluated, and single-cell RT-PCR analyses showed this to be a consistent feature of over 80% of the CD34$^+$ *BCR/ABL*-positive cells.[94] Moreover, the activation of IL-3 and G-CSF expression was found to mirror the stage-specific decline of factor independence as the cells become increasingly differentiated. It also appeared to be quite specific (Table 5.2). Bioactivity and antibody neutralization experiments confirmed the ability of primitive CML cells to release IL-3 and G-CSF into the medium, and demonstrated a partial dependence of their growth on this mechanism of autostimulation. Presumably, an additional autocrine effect not accessible to inhibition by exogenous antibodies would be initiated by intracellular binding of these two growth factors to receptors expressed on the endoplasmic reticulum.[96,109,110] In addition, it is possible that primitive CML progenitors produce other autocrine growth factors that have not yet been identified.

The constitutive production of IL-3 and G-CSF by primitive CML cells fits remarkably with the known differentiation stage-specific responses of normal cells to high levels of both

Table 5.2 Growth factor mRNAs in CD34$^+$ and CD34$^-$ subpopulations[a]

Cells	IL-3	G-CSF	SF	GM-GSF	IL-6	TPO
CML (Ph-positive LTC-IC)						
CD34$^+$CD71$^-$CD45RA$^-$	15/15	15/15	2/8	0/8	0/8	0/6
CD34$^+$CD71$^+$CD45RA$^+$	15/15	15/15	2/8	0/8	0/8	0/6
CD34$^+$	2/10	2/10	0/8	0/8	0/8	0/6
CML (Ph-negative LTC-IC)						
CD34$^+$CD71$^-$CD45RA$^-$	0/2	0/2	0/2	0/2	0/2	ND
CD34$^+$CD71$^+$CD45RA$^+$	2/2	2/2	0/2	0/2	0/2	ND
CD34$^+$	0/2	0/2	0/2	0/2	0/2	ND
Normal marrow						
CD34$^+$CD71$^-$CD45RA$^-$	0/4	0/4	0/4	0/4	0/4	0/4
CD34$^+$CD71$^+$CD45RA$^+$	0/4	0/4	0/4	0/4	0/4	0/4
CD34$^-$	0/3	0/3	0/3	0/3	0/3	0/3

[a]Data from reference 94.
Abbreviations: IL, interleukin; G-CSF, granulocyte-colony-stimulating factor; SF, Steel factor (stem cell factor, c-Kit ligand); GM-CSF, granulocyte–macrophage-colony-stimulating factor; TPO, thrombopoietin.

of these factors or either alone. (Such levels can be assumed because of the autocrine source of the ligand.) For example, IL-3 as a single factor has been shown to support the survival of normal $CD34^{+}CD38^{-}$ bone marrow cells[87] and to activate the proliferation of quiescent LTC-IC and CFC.[111] However, in the absence of adequate co-stimulation by FL and SF, excess IL-3 delivers a potent differentiation-inducing stimulus to LTC-IC, and helps to maximize the amplification of CFC,[112] which is further amplified when the cells are also stimulated by G-CSF.[113] Interestingly, IL-3 is also associated with an enhanced production of basophils and mast cells,[114,115] which are frequently elevated in CML patients. Likewise, G-CSF is a major stimulator in vivo of terminal granulopoiesis.[115,116] These parallelisms between the progenitor dynamics characteristic of the leukemic clone and the known effects of IL-3 and G-CSF on different subpopulations of normal progenitors are illustrated in Figure 5.11.

Further support that IL-3, in particular, plays a significant role in contributing to the 'CML disease phenotype' comes from the demonstration of a CML-like myeloproliferative disease in mice transplanted with syngeneic marrow cells transduced to overexpress IL-3.[117–119] The spectrum of signaling events characteristic of *BCR/ABL*-expressing cells also shows many similarities with those induced by IL-3 stimulation (reviewed in reference 120). Indeed, some of these, such as the increased phosphorylation of STAT5, whose activation in *BCR/ABL*-expressing cells has been thought to be a function of the BCR/ABL oncoprotein, now appear,

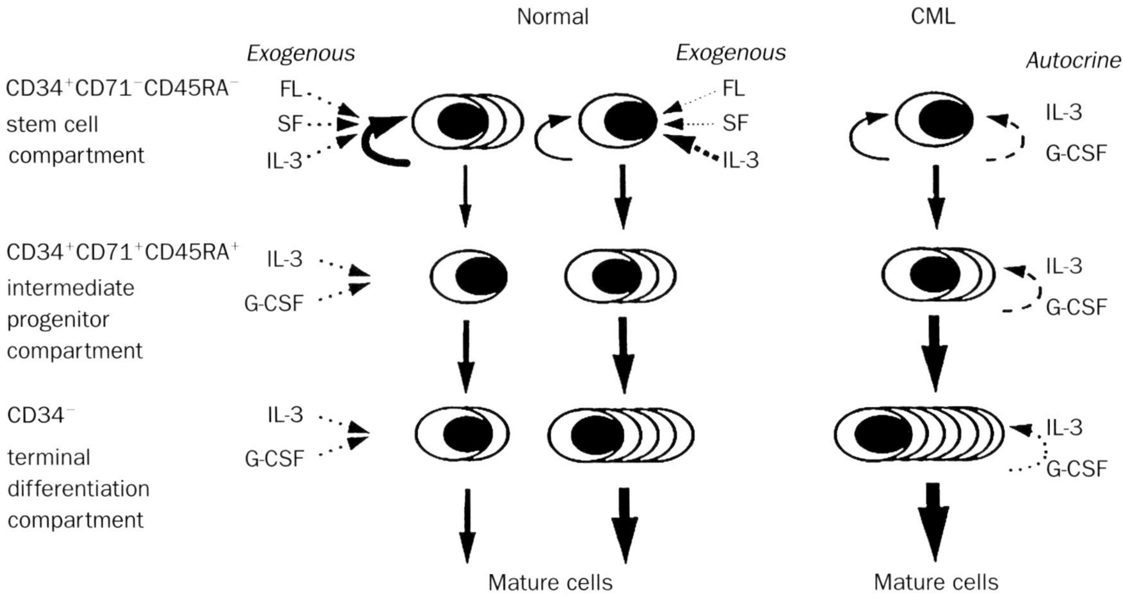

Figure 5.11
Schematic representation of the differential effects of different levels of interleukin-3 (IL-3) and granulocyte-colony-stimulating factor (G-CSF) stimulation on primitive normal cells in comparison with the observed alterations in CML patients where an autocrine IL-3/G-CSF loop in the earliest leukemic compartments has been demonstrated. (FL, Flt3 ligand; SF, Steel factor.) Reprinted with permission from Jiang X, Lopez A, Holyoake T et al, Autocrine production and action of IL-3 and granulocyte colony-stimulating factor in chronic myeloid leukemia. *Proc Natl Acad Sci USA* 1999; **96:** 12804–9. Copyright © 1999 The National Academy of Sciences of the United States of America.

at least in part, to be secondary to IL-3-induced signaling in primary CML progenitors.[94]

Although it is clear that the vast majority of CD34$^+$ leukemic cells produce both IL-3 and G-CSF, the recent discovery of a subset of quiescent cells among the most primitive elements of this leukemic progenitor compartment has raised the interesting question of their factor-independent status. It turns out that, in the absence of growth factors, many of these initially quiescent progenitors can survive for several days in vitro, and then they may spontaneously begin to proliferate, albeit quite inefficiently.[74,121] Interestingly, upon initial isolation, IL-3 and G-CSF expression is seen to be markedly downregulated in these quiescent but *BCR/ABL*-expressing leukemic cells. Then, within a few days (at about the same time as the cells begin to divide), transcripts for IL-3 reappear. The correlation between the production of IL-3 and G-CSF by primitive *BCR/ABL*-positive cells and their factor independence provides strong evidence that these two phenomena are causally linked. These findings also show, however, that the expression of *BCR/ABL* in primitive cells is not sufficient to ensure the activation of IL-3 and G-CSF production. Subsequent studies have demonstrated that the production of both IL-3 and G-CSF is consistently activated in murine bone marrow cells transduced with a *BCR/ABL* retrovirus.[7,8] We have confirmed these findings, and have also shown that this occurs in very primitive cells. Furthermore, activation of expression of both IL-3 and G-CSF in this model occurs a few days after transduction but *following* the onset of *BCR/ABL* expression. These experimental data are thus consistent with a causal linkage of factor-independent growth and an autocrine IL-3/G-CSF mechanism that is secondary to *BCR/ABL* expression.[122] At present, very little else is known about the mechanism by which the BCR/ABL oncoprotein elicits this autocrine activity, except that its SH2 domain appears to be important for this to occur.[97]

The fact that quiescent leukemic cells can remain viable in the absence of IL-3 and G-CSF expression strongly suggests that a primary function of the BCR/ABL oncoprotein in very primitive cell types may be to protect these cells against apoptosis when exogenous ligands with this potential are limiting. Although the results of studies to address this question have appeared conflicting (as discussed above), perhaps this may be explained by the use of different starting populations, culture conditions, and progenitor assays. It is well known that very primitive quiescent normal cells (including LTC-IC) can survive for several days in the absence of exogenous growth factors or other cells.[74,87,123] Hence, more extensive comparisons may be required to determine the extent to which *BCR/ABL* may (or may not) enhance this property in different early compartments of CML patients' cells. There are certainly a number of signaling pathways that BCR/ABL is known to activate and that may be candidates for promoting primitive CML cell viability. These may also contribute to the leukemic potential of *BCR/ABL*-transduced myeloid cells in various models, independent of autocrine IL-3 or G-CSF.[124–126]

Summary

Primitive CML cells show an increased proliferative activity and compartment turnover in comparison with their normal counterparts, both in the same patients and in normal individuals. Although sensitive to the cytostatic activity of TGF-β, these cells show a generic lack of responsiveness to chemokines that can arrest or block the activation of primitive normal hematopoietic cells both in vitro and in vivo. Both of these features may be explained, at least in part, by the activation within primitive Ph-positive/*BCR/ABL*-positive cells of an autocrine IL-3/G-CSF mechanism. This mechanism may also be responsible for the defective self-renewal of CML stem cells, which mimics the response of normal stem cells to excess IL-3. A close correlation between *BCR/ABL* expression and the activation of IL-3 and G-CSF production both in naturally occurring CML and following *BCR/ABL* transduction of various hematopoietic targets indicates a close linkage between these two processes, with one important exception. This relates to the observation that CML patients also harbor a small but readily detectable subpopulation of primitive quiescent *BCR/ABL*-expressing cells whose cell cycle progression can be reactivated spontaneously in vitro, even in the absence of stimulation by exogenous growth factors. Interestingly, when these cells become quiescent, their expression of IL-3 and G-CSF is turned off, but then reappears as the cells begin to cycle.

PROGENITOR CHANGES ASSOCIATED WITH DISEASE PROGRESSION

The emergence of a subclone of leukemic cells that no longer differentiate normally and accumulate rapidly marks the terminal phase of CML referred to as blast crisis. These subclones arise as a result of the acquisition of additional mutations within the chronic-phase clone, and create a clinical condition resembling other forms of acute leukemia that are very refractory to conventional treatments and have an abysmal prognosis. At the time of blast crisis, the blastic-phase subclone usually already overshadows the presence of the underlying chronic-phase clone. Since the secondary mutations responsible for the outgrowth of the blastic-phase subclone may arise in any of the amplified progenitor compartments, blastic-phase disease is typically classified as 'myeloid' or 'lymphoid'. In the first case, this may include examples where the subclone actually arises from within the stem cell compartment; in the second, some evidence of lymphoid restriction, usually to the B-cell lineage, is used to make the assignment.

In both cases, the perturbation of normal differentiation mechanisms makes detection and analysis of progenitors within the blastic-phase clone a difficult problem. These cells often proliferate poorly in conventional in vitro assays for normal progenitors (CFC and LTC-IC), and, even when they do proliferate, they may or may not differentiate normally. It is therefore impossible to quantitate those progenitors that are part of the blastic-phase subclone as distinct from those that are part of the underlying chronic-phase clone (or even residual normal cells) in a rigorous fashion. In addition, the use of cytogenetics or fluorescence in situ hybridization (FISH) is crucial to a definitive identification of the origin of any colonies obtained.

The mechanism by which secondary mutations capable of generating blastic-phase disease are generated within the chronic-phase clone is unknown, although this appears to have a stochastic component, which has made anticipating the timing of this event in individual CML patients very difficult. Occasionally, blast crisis may occur even without the clinical recognition of a prior period of chronic-phase disease. Alternatively, at the opposite extreme, blast crisis may not appear for more than two decades. In the former case, the chronic-phase clone may not yet have reached a size to be clinically obvious, and would thus escape notice unless looked for using more sensitive procedures (such as the detection of CFC that are Ph-positive/*BCR/ABL*-positive). Under these circumstances, the patient may appear to be presenting with Ph-positive/*BCR/ABL*-positive acute myeloid leukemia (AML) or acute lymphoblastic leukemia (ALL). Because of the preferential association of the p190 BCR/ABL oncoprotein with ALL in both adults and children, there has been much controversy concerning the frequency with which this disease actually originates de novo in a B-lineage precursor. Many examples of patients with Ph-positive/*BCR/ABL*-positive ALL have now been found to also have some clonal myeloid cells, clearly establishing that the disease arose in a pluripotent stem cell in these cases.[127–131] Although this has also not been a universal finding, the resolution of current methods for undertaking such analyses is low, and populations comprising less than 10% of the total would be unlikely to be detected. On the other hand, whether the identification of an underlying chronic-phase clone of myeloid precursors is of clinical significance when these are not sufficiently numerous to be detectable is also not known.

Although the onset of blast crisis in relation to the time of diagnosis can certainly vary over many years, it seems likely that the size of the chronic-phase clone would influence the probability of such an event occurring. Thus, part of the variability in the timing of this event might reflect variations in the size of the chronic-phase clone at the time of diagnosis. If it is assumed that this, in turn, is a direct function of the 'age' of the chronic-phase clone and/or the extent of prior clonal stem cell turnover, then surrogate measures of these parameters should offer some prognostic predictive power. As discussed earlier, two potential endpoints would be the presence of an LTC-IC compartment that was predominantly Ph-positive/*BCR/ABL*-positive (relative to the normal LTC-IC) and a severe reduction in the telomere length in the mature leukemic cells. Measurements of these parameters have suggested that they may both have predictive value.[83,132,133] Specifically, patients who developed blast crisis within the following 2 years were found to have predominantly leukemic LTC-IC and shorter telomeres in their leukemic cells more frequently than patients who took longer to develop blastic-phase disease.

Although cells responsible for contributing to blastic-phase disease have been generally refractory to propagation in vitro, they have been found to engraft sublethally irradiated immunodeficient mice more readily than chronic-phase CML cells.[48,52] The explanation for this is not yet clear, although it is known that many types of AML and B-lineage ALL, including diseases classified as Ph-positive/BCR/ABL^{p190}-ALL, engraft immunodeficient mice relatively efficiently.[134–136]

QUESTIONS FOR THE FUTURE

Our understanding of the biology of chronic-phase CML is now well advanced, and includes the identification of a number of mechanisms that can account for the perturbed dynamics of the expanding leukemic clone. Central to these is the differentiation-stage-specific activation of autocrine IL-3 and G-CSF production within the most primitive leukemic cells. These factors and the critical downstream signaling intermediates they activate would therefore be potential targets for new therapies. For example, if the autocrine IL-3 produced by leukemic stem cells limits their ability to expand by increasing their probability of differentiation, then an enhancement of this effect might promote their complete extinction, whereas a blockade might be ultimately deleterious. One in vitro study has provided some evidence of a selective 'therapeutic effect' of exposing CML progenitors to increasing concentrations of IL-3.[137] However, without more information, it is difficult to predict what the actual outcome might be in vivo. Working out these possibilities using gene transfer strategies and various growth factor knockout mice should be helpful in this regard.

Of even more immediate and practical importance may be questions pertaining to the effects of STI571 on different types of CML progenitors. This potent inhibitor of the kinase function of BCR/ABL oncoproteins[138] has shown dramatic effects in patients with chronic-phase disease while demonstrating minimal toxicity.[139,140] However, the extent to which STI571 actually kills the leukemic *stem* cells in these individuals, and how this may vary according to the number of leukemic stem cells that are present and their quiescent or proliferative status, are questions currently under investigation. The answers to these are important, because they may help to predict the length of treatments required to achieve durable effects. Such studies might also help to distinguish patients that will be more or less responsive to this agent. See also Chapters 33 and 34 for further discussion of STI571.

Finally, the continued development of xenotransplant models should offer new opportunities for understanding the transition from chronic phase to blast crisis, and eventually for evaluating new treatment strategies for CML patients who are refractory to or ineligible for currently available modalities. It is noteworthy that the first benefits of a rational approach to curing leukemia have been a product of basic research in CML. The challenge now is to extend this philosophy to encompass all patients who present with this diagnosis.

ACKNOWLEDGEMENTS

The authors are deeply indebted to a large team of co-workers, trainees, and support staff, who have, over the years, made possible many of the observations described in this chapter, and to the National Cancer Institute of Canada, who have provided continuous support of this work with funds from the Terry Fox Foundation and the Canadian Cancer Society. Particular thanks are extended to Drs Xiaoyan Jiang and Yves Chalandon for critically reading the manuscript and making helpful suggestions, and to Amy Ahamed for expert secretarial assistance.

REFERENCES

1. Daley GQ, Van Etten RA, Baltimore D, Induction of chronic myelogenous leukemia in mice by the $P210^{bcr/abl}$ gene of the Philadelphia chromosome. *Science* 1990; **247:** 824–30.
2. Kelliher MA, McLaughlin J, Witte ON, Rosenberg N, Induction of a chronic myelogenous leukemia-like syndrome in mice with v-abl and BCR/ABL. *Proc Natl Acad Sci USA* 1990; **87:** 6649–53.
3. Elefanty AG, Hariharan IK, Cory S, bcr–abl, the hallmark of chronic myeloid leukaemia in man, induces multiple haemopoietic neoplasms in mice. *EMBO J* 1990; **9:** 1069–78.
4. Gishizky ML, Johnson-White J, Witte ON, Efficient transplantation of *BCR–ABL*-induced chronic myelogenous leukemia-like syndrome in mice. *Proc Natl Acad Sci USA* 1993; **90:** 3755–9.
5. Honda H, Oda H, Suzuki T et al, Development of acute lymphoblastic leukemia and myeloproliferative disorder in transgenic mice expressing $p210^{bcr/abl}$: a novel transgenic model for human Ph^1-positive leukemias. *Blood* 1998; **91:** 2067–75.
6. Pear WS, Miller JP, Xu L et al, Efficient and rapid induction of a chronic myelogenous leukemia-like myeloproliferative disease in mice receiving P210 bcr/abl-transduced bone marrow. *Blood* 1998; **92:** 3780–92.
7. Zhang X, Ren R, BCR–ABL efficiently induces a myeloproliferative disease and production of excess interleukin-3 and granulocyte–macrophage colony-stimulating factor in mice: a novel model for chronic myelogenous leukemia. *Blood* 1998; **92:** 3829–40.
8. Li S, Ilaria RL, Million RP et al, The p190, p210, and p230 forms of the BCR/ABL oncogene induce a similar chronic myeloid leukemia-like syndrome in mice but have different lymphoid leukemogenic activity. *J Exp Med* 1999; **189:** 1399–412.
9. Zhao RC, Jiang Y, Verfaillie CM, A model of human $p210^{bcr/ABL}$ mediated CML by transduction of primary normal human $CD34^+$ cells with a BCR/ABL containing retroviral vector. *Blood* 2001; **97:** 2406–12.
10. Biernaux C, Loos M, Sels A et al, Detection of major bcr–abl gene expression at a very low level in blood cells of some healthy individuals. *Blood* 1995; **86:** 3118–22.
11. Bose S, Deininger M, Gora-Tybor J et al, The presence of typical and atypical BCR–ABL fusion genes in leukocytes of normal individuals: biologic significance and implications for the assessment of minimal residual disease. *Blood* 1998; **92:** 3362–7.
12. Dameshek W, Some speculations on the myeloproliferative syndromes. *Blood* 1951; **6:** 372–5.
13. Whang J, Frei III E, Tjio JH et al, The distribution of the Philadelphia chromosome in patients with chronic myelogenous leukemia. *Blood* 1963; **22:** 664–73.
14. Rastrick JM, Fitzgerald PH, Gunz FW, Direct evidence for presence of Ph^1 chromosome in erythroid cells. *BMJ* 1968; **i:** 96–8.
15. Tough IM, Jacobs PA, Court Brown WM et al, Cytogenetic studies on bone-marrow in chronic myeloid leukaemia. *Lancet* 1963; **i:** 844–6.
16. Martin PJ, Najfeld V, Hansen JA et al, Involvement of the B-lymphoid system in chronic myelogenous leukaemia. *Nature* 1980; **287:** 49–50.
17. Bernheim A, Berger R, Preud'Homme JL et al, Philadelphia chromosome positive blood B lymphocytes in chronic myelocytic leukemia. *Leuk Res* 1981; **5:** 331–9.
18. Takahashi N, Miura I, Saitoh K, Miura AB, Lineage involvement of stem cells bearing the Philadelphia chromosome in chronic myeloid leukemia in the chronic phase as shown by a

combination of fluorescence-activated cell sorting and fluorescence in situ hybridization. *Blood* 1998; **92:** 4758–63.
19. Gunsilius E, Duba H-C, Petzer AL et al, Evidence from a leukaemia model for maintenance of vascular endothelium by bone-marrow-derived endothelial cells. *Lancet* 2000; **355:** 1688–91.
20. Raskind WH, Fialkow PJ, The use of cell markers in the study of human hematopoietic neoplasia. *Adv Cancer Res* 1987; **49:** 127–67.
21. Lugo TG, Witte ON, The BCR–ABL oncogene transforms rat-1 cells and cooperates with v-*myc*. *Mol Cell Biol* 1989; **9:** 1263–70.
22. Dube ID, Gupta CM, Kalousek DK et al, Cytogenetic studies of early myeloid progenitor compartments in Ph1-positive chronic myeloid leukaemia (CML). I. Persistence of Ph1-negative committed progenitors that are suppressed from differentiating in vivo. *Br J Haematol* 1984; **56:** 633–44.
23. Verfaillie CM, Miller WJ, Boylan K, McGlave PB, Selection of benign primitive hematopoietic progenitors in chronic myelogenous leukemia on the basis of HLA-DR antigen expression. *Blood* 1992; **79:** 1003–10.
24. Eaves CJ, Cashman JD, Zoumbos NC et al, Biological strategies for the selective manipulation of normal and leukemic stem cells. *Stem Cells* 1993; **11**(Suppl 3): 109–21.
25. Ghaffari S, Dougherty GJ, Lansdorp PM et al, Differentiation-associated changes in CD44 isoform expression during normal hematopoiesis and their alteration in chronic myeloid leukemia. *Blood* 1995; **86:** 2976–85.
26. Petzer AL, Eaves CJ, Lansdorp PM et al, Characterization of primitive subpopulations of normal and leukemic cells present in the blood of patients with newly diagnosed as well as established chronic myeloid leukemia. *Blood* 1996; **88:** 2162–71.
27. Eaves CJ, Eaves AC, Cell culture studies in CML. *Baillière's Clin Haematol* 1987; **1:** 931–61.
28. Eaves C, Cashman J, Eaves A, Defective regulation of leukemic hematopoiesis in chronic myeloid leukemia. *Leuk Res* 1998; **22:** 1085–96.
29. Era T, Witte ON, Regulated expression of P210 Bcr–Abl during embryonic stem cell differentiation stimulates multipotential progenitor expansion and myeloid cell fate. *Proc Natl Acad Sci USA* 2000; **97:** 1737–42.
30. Chalandon Y, Jiang X, Conneally E et al, BCR–ABL transduction of multiple $CD34^+$ subsets of human cord blood cells leads to an excessive generation of erythroid progeny. *Blood* 2000; **96**(Suppl 1): 94a.
31. Coulombel L, Kalousek DK, Eaves CJ et al, Long-term marrow culture reveals chromosomally normal hematopoietic progenitor cells in patients with Philadelphia chromosome-positive chronic myelogenous leukemia. *N Engl J Med* 1983; **308:** 1493–8.
32. Dube ID, Arlin ZA, Kalousek DK et al, Nonclonal hemopoietic progenitor cells detected in long-term marrow cultures from a Turner syndrome mosaic with chronic myeloid leukemia. *Blood* 1984; **64:** 1284–7.
33. Hogge DE, Coulombel L, Kalousek DK et al, Nonclonal hemopoietic progenitors in a G6PD heterozygote with chronic myelogenous leukemia revealed after long-term marrow culture. *Am J Hematol* 1987; **24:** 389–94.
34. Sutherland HJ, Lansdorp PM, Henkelman DH et al, Functional characterization of individual human hematopoietic stem cells cultured at limiting dilution on supportive marrow stromal layers. *Proc Natl Acad Sci USA* 1990; **87:** 3584–8.
35. Udomsakdi C, Eaves CJ, Swolin B et al, Rapid decline of chronic myeloid leukemic cells in long-term culture due to a defect at the leukemic stem cell level. *Proc Natl Acad Sci USA* 1992; **89:** 6192–6.
36. Bernstein ID, Singer JW, Smith FO et al, Differences in the frequency of normal and clonal precursors of colony-forming cells in chronic myelogenous leukemia and acute myelogenous leukemia. *Blood* 1992; **79:** 1811–16.
37. Cornelissen JJ, Wognum AW, Ploemacher RE et al, Efficient long term maintenance of chronic myeloid leukemic cobblestone area forming cells on a murine stromal cell line. *Leukemia* 1997; **11:** 126–33.
38. Petzer AL, Eaves CJ, Barnett MJ, Eaves AC, Selective expansion of primitive normal hematopoietic cells in cytokine-supplemented cultures of purified cells from patients with chronic myeloid leukemia. *Blood* 1997; **90:** 64–9.
39. Barnett MJ, Eaves CJ, Phillips GL et al, Autografting with cultured marrow in chronic myeloid leukemia: results of a pilot study. *Blood* 1994; **84:** 724–32.
40. Lewis ID, Haylock DN, Moore S et al, Peripheral blood is a source of BCR–ABL-negative pre-progenitors in early chronic phase

chronic myeloid leukemia. *Leukemia* 1997; **11:** 581–7.
41. Conneally E, Cashman J, Petzer A, Eaves C, Expansion in vitro of transplantable human cord blood stem cells demonstrated using a quantitative assay of their lympho-myeloid repopulating activity in nonobese diabetic–*scid/scid* mice. *Proc Natl Acad Sci USA* 1997; **94:** 9836–41.
42. Bhatia M, Bonnet D, Kapp U et al, Quantitative analysis reveals expansion of human hematopoietic repopulating cells after short-term ex vivo culture. *J Exp Med* 1997; **186:** 619–24.
43. Kollet O, Aviram R, Chebath J et al, The soluble interleukin-6 (IL-6) receptor/IL-6 fusion protein enhances in vitro maintenance and proliferation of human $CD34^{+}CD38^{-/low}$ cells capable of repopulating severe combined immunodeficiency mice. *Blood* 1999; **94:** 923–31.
44. Ueda T, Tsuji K, Yoshino H et al, Expansion of human NOD/SCID-repopulating cells by stem cell factor, Flk2/Flt3 ligand, thrombopoietin, IL-6, and soluble IL-6 receptor. *J Clin Invest* 2001; **105:** 1013–21.
45. Lewis ID, Almeida-Porada G, Du J et al, Umbilical cord blood cells capable of engrafting in primary, secondary and tertiary xenogeneic hosts are preserved after ex-vivo culture in a non-contact system. *Blood* 2001; (in press).
46. Peled A, Petit I, Kollet O et al, Dependence of human stem cell engraftment and repopulation of NOD/SCID mice on CXCR4. *Science* 1999; **283:** 845–8.
47. Cashman J, Clark-Lewis I, Eaves C, SDF-1 and TGF-β enhance the detection of transplantable human stem cells regenerating in NOD/SCID mice. *Exp Hematol* 2000; **28**(Suppl 1): 85.
48. Sirard C, Lapidot T, Vormoor J et al, Normal and leukemic SCID-repopulating cells (SRC) co-exist in the bone marrow and peripheral blood from CML patients in chronic phase while leukemic SRC are detected in blast crisis. *Blood* 1996; **87:** 1539–48.
49. Lewis ID, McDiarmid LA, Samels LM et al, Establishment of a reproducible model of chronic-phase chronic myeloid leukemia in NOD/SCID mice using blood-derived mononuclear or $CD34^{+}$ cells. *Blood* 1998; **91:** 630–40.
50. Wang JCY, Lapidot T, Cashman JD et al, High level engraftment of NOD/SCID mice by primitive normal and leukemic hematopoietic cells from patients with chronic myeloid leukemia in chronic phase. *Blood* 1998; **91:** 2406–14.
51. Dazzi F, Capelli D, Hasserjian R et al, The kinetics and extent of engraftment of chronic myelogenous leukemia cells in non-obese diabetic/severe combined immunodeficiency mice reflect the phase of the donor's disease: an in vivo model of chronic myelogenous leukemia biology. *Blood* 1998; **92:** 1390–6.
52. Verstegen MMA, Cornelissen JJ, Terpstra W et al, Multilineage outgrowth of both malignant and normal hemopoietic progenitor cells from individual chronic myeloid leukemia patients in immunodeficient mice. *Leukemia* 1999; **13:** 618–28.
53. Levin RH, Whang J, Tjio JH et al, Persistent mitosis of transfused homologous leukocytes in children receiving antileukemic therapy. *Science* 1963; **142:** 1305–11.
54. Bronson WR, McGinniss MH, Morse EE, Hematopoietic graft detected by a change in ABO group. *Blood* 1964; **23:** 239–49.
55. Graw RGJ, Buckner CD, Whang-Peng J et al, Complication of bone-marrow transplantation. Graft-versus-host disease resulting from chronic-myelogenous-leukaemia leucocyte transfusions. *Lancet* 1970; **ii:** 338–41.
56. Deisseroth AB, Zu Z, Claxton D et al, Genetic marking shows that Ph^{+} cells present in autologous transplants of chronic myelogenous leukemia (CML) contribute to relapse after autologous bone marrow in CML. *Blood* 1994; **83:** 3068–76.
57. Daley GQ, Van Etten RA, Baltimore D, Blast crisis in a murine model of chronic myelogenous leukemia. *Proc Natl Acad Sci USA* 1991; **88:** 11335–8.
58. Glimm H, Eisterer W, Lee K et al, Previously undetected human hematopoietic cell populations with short term repopulating activity selectively engraft NOD/SCID-β_2 microglobulin null mice. *J Clin Invest* 2001; **107:** 199–206.
59. Cashman JD, Lapidot T, Wang JCY et al, Kinetic evidence of the regeneration of multilineage hematopoiesis from primitive cells in normal human bone marrow transplanted into immunodeficient mice. *Blood* 1997; **89:** 4307–16.
60. Wang JCY, Doedens M, Dick JE, Primitive human hematopoietic cells are enriched in cord blood compared with adult bone marrow or mobilized peripheral blood as measured by the quantitative in vivo SCID-repopulating cell

assay. *Blood* 1997; **89:** 3919–24.

61. Van der Loo JCM, Hanenberg H, Cooper RJ et al, Nonobese diabetic/severe combined immunodeficiency (NOD/SCID) mouse as a model system to study the engraftment and mobilization of human peripheral blood stem cells. *Blood* 1998; **92:** 2556–70.
62. Holyoake TL, Nicolini FE, Eaves CJ, Functional differences between transplantable human hematopoietic stem cells from fetal liver, cord blood, and adult marrow. *Exp Hematol* 1999; **27:** 1418–27.
63. Cashman JD, Eaves CJ, High marrow seeding efficiency of human lymphomyeloid repopulating cells in irradiated NOD/SCID mice. *Blood* 2000; **96:** 3979–81.
64. Gothot A, Van der Loo JCM, Clapp W, Srour EF, Cell cycle-related changes in repopulating capacity of human mobilized peripheral blood $CD34^+$ cells in non-obese diabetic/severe combined immune-deficient mice. *Blood* 1998; **92:** 2641–9.
65. Orschell-Traycoff CM, Hiatt K, Dagher RN et al, Homing and engraftment potential of Sca-1^+lin^- cells fractionated on the basis of adhesion molecule expression and position in cell cycle. *Blood* 2000; **96:** 1380–7.
66. Habibian HK, Peters SO, Hsieh CC et al, The fluctuating phenotype of the lymphohematopoietic stem cell with cell cycle transit. *J Exp Med* 1998; **188:** 393–8.
67. Glimm H, Oh I, Eaves C, Human hematopoietic stem cells stimulated to proliferate in vitro lose engraftment potential during their $S/G_2/M$ transit and do not reenter G_0. *Blood* 2000; **96:** 4185–93.
68. Kollet O, Peled A, Byk T et al, β2 microglobulin-deficient ($B2m^{null}$) NOD/SCID mice are excellent recipients for studying human stem cell function. *Blood* 2000; **95:** 3102–5.
69. Eisterer W, Jiang X, Glimm H et al, Regeneration of $CD34^+$ $BCR–ABL^+$ $IL\text{-}3^+$ $G\text{-}CSF^+$ cells in NOD/SCID and NOD/SCID-β_2 microglobulin null ($\beta_2M^{-/-}$) mice transplanted with chronic myeloid leukemia (CML) cells. *Blood* 2000; **96**(Suppl 1): 349a.
70. Ichimaru M, Ishimaru T, Mikami M et al, Incidence of leukemia in a fixed cohort of atomic bomb survivors and controls, Hiroshima and Nagasaki October 1950–December 1978. Hiroshima: Radiation Effects Research Foundation, Technical Report RERF TR 13–81, 1981.
71. Ponchio L, Conneally E, Eaves C, Quantitation of the quiescent fraction of longterm culture-initiating cells (LTC-IC) in normal human blood and marrow and the kinetics of their growth factor-stimulated entry into S-phase in vitro. *Blood* 1995; **86:** 3314–21.
72. Ponchio L, Cashman J, Zoumbos N et al, Primitive CML cells show a deregulation of their cycling status both in vivo and in longterm cultures which is not normalized in the presence of interferon-α. *Blood* 1995; **86**(Suppl 1): 493a.
73. Shapiro HM, Flow cytometric estimation of DNA and RNA content in intact cells stained with Hoechst 33342 and Pyronin Y. *Cytometry* 1981; **2:** 143–50.
74. Holyoake T, Jiang X, Eaves C, Eaves A, Isolation of a highly quiescent subpopulation of primitive leukemic cells in chronic myeloid leukemia. *Blood* 1999; **94:** 2056–64.
75. Maguer-Satta V, Petzer AL, Eaves AC, Eaves CJ, BCR–ABL expression in different subpopulations of functionally characterized Ph^+ $CD34^+$ cells from patients with chronic myeloid leukemia. *Blood* 1996; **88:** 1796–804.
76. Goto T, Nishikori M, Arlin Z et al, Growth characteristics of leukemic and normal hematopoietic cells in Ph^1+ chronic myelogenous leukemia and effects of intensive treatment. *Blood* 1982; **59:** 793–808.
77. Kantarjian HM, Vellekoop L, McCredie KB et al, Intensive combination chemotherapy (ROAP 10) and splenectomy in the management of chronic myelogenous leukemia. *J Clin Oncol* 1985; **3:** 192–200.
78. Gratwohl A, Hermans J, Niederwieser D et al, Bone marrow transplantation for chronic myeloid leukemia: long-term results. *Bone Marrow Transplant* 1993; **12:** 509–16.
79. Yong ASM, Goldman JM, Relapse of chronic myeloid leukaemia 14 years after allogeneic bone marrow transplantation. *Bone Marrow Transplant* 1999; **23:** 827–8.
80. Allsopp R, Vaziri H, Patterson C et al, Telomere length predicts replicative capacity of human fibroblasts. *Proc Natl Acad Sci USA* 1992; **89:** 10114–18.
81. Vaziri H, Dragowska W, Allsopp RC et al, Evidence for a mitotic clock in human hematopoietic stem cells: Loss of telomeric DNA with age. *Proc Natl Acad Sci USA* 1994; **91:** 9857–60.

82. Rufer N, Brummendorf TH, Kolvraa S et al, Telomere fluorescence measurements in granulocytes and T lymphocyte subsets point to a high turnover of hematopoietic stem cells and memory T cells in early childhood. *J Exp Med* 1999; **190:** 157–67.
83. Brummendorf TH, Holyoake TL, Rufer N et al, Prognostic implications of differences in telomere length between normal and malignant cells from patients with chronic myeloid leukemia measured by flow cytometry. *Blood* 2000; **95:** 1883–90.
84. Slagboom PE, Droog S, Boomsma DI, Genetic determination of telomere size in humans: a twin study of three age groups. *Am J Hum Genet* 1994; **55:** 876–82.
85. Engelhardt M, Mackenzie K, Drullinsky P et al, Telomerase activity and telomere length in acute and chronic leukemia, pre and post-ex vivo culture. *Cancer Res* 2000; **60:** 610–17.
86. Ponchio L, Eaves CJ, Very primitive hematopoietic cells (LTC-IC) in normal adult human blood and marrow show differences in the regulation of their cycling state. *Blood* 1995; **86**(Suppl 1): 493a.
87. Borge OJ, Ramsfjell V, Cui L, Jacobsen SEW, Ability of early acting cytokines to directly promote survival and suppress apoptosis of human primitive $CD34^+CD38^-$ bone marrow cells with multilineage potential at the single-cell level: key role of thrombopoietin. *Blood* 1997; **90:** 2282–92.
88. Oh I-H, Lau A, Eaves CJ, During ontogeny primitive ($CD34^+CD38^-$) hematopoietic cells show altered expression of a subset of genes associated with early cytokine and differentiation responses of their adult counterparts. *Blood* 2000; **96:** 4160–8.
89. Glimm H, Tang P, von Kalle C, Eaves C, Increased transplantability of in vitro expanded human cord blood stem cells after a two day incubation with inhibitors of stem cell cycling. *Mol Ther* 2001; (in press).
90. Cashman JD, Clark-Lewis I, Eaves AC, Eaves CJ, Differentiation stage-specific regulation of primitive human hematopoietic progenitor cycling by exogenous and endogenous inhibitors in an in vivo model. *Blood* 1999; **94:** 3722–9.
91. Eaves CJ, Cashman JD, Wolpe SD, Eaves AC, Unresponsiveness of primitive chronic myeloid leukemia cells to macrophage inflammatory protein 1α, an inhibitor of primitive normal hematopoietic cells. *Proc Natl Acad Sci USA* 1993; **90:** 12015–19.
92. Cashman JD, Eaves CJ, Sarris AH, Eaves AC, MCP-1, not MIP-1α is the endogenous chemokine that cooperates with TGF-β to inhibit the cycling of primitive normal but not leukemic (CML) progenitors in long-term human marrow cultures. *Blood* 1998; **92:** 2338–44.
93. Cashman JD, Eaves AC, Eaves CJ, Granulocyte–macrophage colony-stimulating factor modulation of the inhibitory effect of transforming growth factor-β on normal and leukemic human hematopoietic progenitor cells. *Leukemia* 1992; **6:** 886–92.
94. Jiang X, Lopez A, Holyoake T et al, Autocrine production and action of IL-3 and granulocyte colony-stimulating factor in chronic myeloid leukemia. *Proc Natl Acad Sci USA* 1999; **96:** 12804–9.
95. Hariharan IK, Adams JM, Cory S, BCR–ABL oncogene renders myeloid cell line factor independent: potential autocrine mechanism in chronic myeloid leukemia. *Oncogene Res* 1988; **3:** 387–99.
96. Sirard C, Laneuville P, Dick J, Expression of *bcr–abl* abrogates factor-dependent growth of human hematopoietic M07E cells by an autocrine mechanism. *Blood* 1994; **83:** 1575–85.
97. Anderson SM, Mladenovic J, The BCR–ABL oncogene requires both kinase activity and src-homology 2 domain to induce cytokine secretion. *Blood* 1996; **87:** 238–44.
98. Specchia G, Liso V, Capalbo S et al, Constitutive expression of IL-1β, M-CSF and c-fms during the myeloid blastic phase of chronic myelogenous leukaemia. *Br J Haematol* 1992; **80:** 310–16.
99. Otsuka T, Eaves CJ, Humphries RK et al, Lack of evidence for abnormal autocrine or paracrine mechanisms underlying the uncontrolled proliferation of primitive chronic myeloid leukemia progenitor cells. *Leukemia* 1991; **5:** 861–8.
100. Moore MAS, Williams N, Metcalf D, In vitro colony formation by normal and leukemic human hematopoietic cells: characterization of the colony-forming cells. *J Natl Cancer Inst* 1973; **50:** 603–23.
101. Metcalf D, *Hemopoietic Colonies. In Vitro Cloning of Normal and Leukemic Cells.* Berlin: Springer-Verlag, 1977.

102. Amos TAS, Lewis JL, Grand FH et al, Apoptosis in chronic myeloid leukaemia: normal responses by progenitor cells to growth factor deprivation, X-irradiation and glucocorticoids. *Br J Haematol* 1995; **91:** 387–93.

103. Santucci MA, Anklesaria P, Laneuville P et al, Expression of p210 bcr/abl increases hematopoietic progenitor cell radiosensitivity. *Int J Radiat Oncol Biol Phys* 1993; **26:** 831–6.

104. Bedi A, Barber J, Bedi G et al, BCR–ABL-mediated inhibition of apoptosis with delay of G2/M transition after DNA damage: a mechanism of resistance to multiple anticancer agents. *Blood* 1995; **86:** 1148–58.

105. Strife A, Lambek C, Wisniewski D et al, Discordant maturation as the primary biological defect in chronic myelogenous leukemia. *Cancer Res* 1988; **48:** 1035–41.

106. Bedi A, Zehnbauer BA, Barber J et al, Inhibition of apoptosis by BCR–ABL in chronic myeloid leukemia. *Blood* 1994; **83:** 2038–44.

107. Maguer-Satta V, Burl S, Liu L et al, BCR–ABL accelerates C2-ceramide-induced apoptosis. *Oncogene* 1998; **16:** 237–48.

108. Jiang X, Fujisaki T, Nicolini F et al, Autonomous multi-lineage differentiation in vitro of primitive $CD34^+$ cells from patients with chronic myeloid leukemia. *Leukemia* 2000; **14:** 1112–21.

109. Keating MT, Williams LT, Autocrine stimulation of intracellular PDGF receptors in v-*sis*-transformed cells. *Science* 1988; **239:** 914–16.

110. Dunbar CE, Browder TM, Abrams JS, Nienhuis AW, COOH-terminal-modified interleukin-3 is retained intracellularly and stimulates autocrine growth. *Science* 1989; **245:** 1493–6.

111. Ponchio L, Eaves C, Steel factor and Flk-2/Flt-3 ligand alone trigger quiescent human LTC-IC into S-phase more effectively than primitive quiescent clonogenic progenitor cells. *J Hematother* 1995; **4**(Suppl 3): 217.

112. Zandstra PW, Conneally E, Petzer AL et al, Cytokine manipulation of primitive human hematopoietic cell self-renewal. *Proc Natl Acad Sci USA* 1997; **94:** 4698–703.

113. Petzer AL, Zandstra PW, Piret JM, Eaves CJ, Differential cytokine effects on primitive ($CD34^+CD38^-$) human hematopoietic cells: novel responses to flt3-ligand and thrombopoietin. *J Exp Med* 1996; **183:** 2551–8.

114. Saito H, Hatake K, Dvorak AM et al, Selective differentiation and proliferation of hematopoietic cells induced by recombinant human interleukins. *Proc Natl Acad Sci USA* 1988; **85:** 2288–92.

115. Metcalf D, Control of granulocytes and macrophages: molecular, cellular, and clinical aspects. *Science* 1991; **254:** 529–33.

116. Souza LM, Boone TC, Gabrilove J et al, Recombinant human granulocyte colony-stimulating factor: effects on normal and leukemic myeloid cells. *Science* 1986; **232:** 61–5.

117. Chang JM, Metcalf D, Lang RA et al, Nonneoplastic hematopoietic myeloproliferative syndrome induced by dysregulated multi-CSF (IL-3) expression. *Blood* 1989; **73:** 1487–97.

118. Wong PMC, Chung S, Dunbar CE et al, Retrovirus-mediated transfer and expression of the interleukin-3 gene in mouse hematopoietic cells result in a myeloproliferative disorder. *Mol Cell Biol* 1989; **9:** 798–808.

119. Just U, Katsuno M, Stocking C et al, Targeted in vivo infection with a retroviral vector carrying the interleukin-3 (multi-CSF) gene leads to immortalization and leukemic transformation of primitive hematopoietic progenitor cells. *Growth Factors* 1993; **9:** 41–55.

120. Sattler M, Salgia R, Activation of hematopoietic growth factor signal transduction pathways by the human oncogene BCR/ABL. *Cytokine Growth Factor Rev* 1997; **8:** 63–79.

121. Holyoake TL, Jiang X, Jorgensen HG et al, Primitive quiescent leukemic cells from patients with chronic myeloid leukemia spontaneously initiate factor-independent growth in vitro in association with up-regulation of expression of interleukin-3. *Blood* 2001; **97:** 720–8.

122. Jiang X, Yip C, Eisterer W et al, Reduced tyrosine phosphorylation of $p210^{BCR-ABL}$ and lack of STAT5 activation in BCR–ABL-transduced $IL-3^{-/-}$ primitive hematopoietic cells. *Blood* 2000; **96**(Suppl 1): 92a.

123. Sutherland HJ, Hogge DE, Cook D, Eaves CJ, Alternative mechanisms with and without Steel factor support primitive human hematopoiesis. *Blood* 1993; **81:** 1465–70.

124. Gesbert F, Griffin JD, Bcr/Abl activates transcription of the *Bcl-X* gene through STAT5. *Blood* 2000; **96:** 2269–76.

125. Horita M, Andreau EJ, Benito A et al, Blockade of the Bcr–Abl kinase activity induces apoptosis of chronic myelogenous leukemia cells by suppressing signal transducer and activator of transcription 5-dependent expression of $Bcr-x_L$. *J Exp Med* 2000; **191:** 977–84.

126. Sexl V, Piekorz R, Moriggl R et al, Stat5a/b contribute to interleukin 7-induced B-cell precursor expansion, but *abl*- and *bcr/abl*-induced transformation are independent of Stat5. *Blood* 2000; **96:** 2277–83.
127. Tachibana N, Raimondi SC, Lauer SJ et al, Evidence for a multipotential stem cell disease in some childhood Philadelphia chromosome-positive acute lymphoblastic leukemia. *Blood* 1987; **70:** 1458–61.
128. Kalousek DK, Dube ID, Eaves CJ, Eaves AC, Cytogenetic studies of haemopoietic colonies from patients with an initial diagnosis of acute lymphoblastic leukaemia. *Br J Haematol* 1988; **70:** 5–11.
129. Anatasi J, Feng J, Dickstein JL et al, Lineage involvement by BCR/ABL in Ph^+ lymphoblastic leukemias: chronic myelogenous leukemia presenting in lymphoid blast phase vs Ph^+ acute lymphoblastic leukemia. *Leukemia* 1996; **10:** 795–802.
130. Schenk TM, Keyhani A, Bottcher S et al, Multilineage involvement of Philadelphia chromosome positive acute lymphoblastic leukemia. *Leukemia* 1998; **12:** 666–74.
131. Kasprzyk A, Harrison CJ, Secker-Walker LM, Investigation of clonal involvement of myeloid cells in Philadelphia-positive and high hyperdiploid acute lymphoblastic leukemia. *Leukemia* 1999; **13:** 2000–6.
132. Iwama H, Ohyashiki K, Ohyashiki JH et al, The relationship between telomere length and therapy-associated cytogenetic responses in patients with chronic myeloid leukemia. *Cancer* 1997; **79:** 1552–60.
133. Boultwood J, Fidler C, Shepherd P et al, Telomere length shortening is associated with disease evolution in chronic myelogenous leukemia. *Am J Hematol* 1999; **61:** 5–9.
134. Dick JE, Normal and leukemic human stem cells assayed in SCID mice. *Semin Immunol* 1996; **8:** 197–206.
135. Bonnet D, Dick JE, Human acute myeloid leukemia is organized as a hierarchy that originates from a primitive hematopoietic cell. *Nature Med* 1997; **3:** 730–6.
136. Cobaleda C, Gutierrez-Cianca N, Perez-Losada J et al, A primitive hematopoietic cell is the target for the leukemic transformation in human Philadelphia-positive acute lymphoblastic leukemia. *Blood* 2000; **95:** 1007–13.
137. Bedi A, Griffin CA, Barber JP et al, Growth factor-mediated terminal differentiation of chronic myeloid leukemia. *Cancer Res* 1994; **54:** 5535–8.
138. Druker BJ, Tamura S, Buchdunger E et al, Effects of a selective inhibitor of the Abl tyrosine kinase on the growth of Bcr–Abl positive cells. *Nature Med* 1996; **2:** 561–6.
139. Druker BJ, Lydon NB, Lessons learned from the development of an Abl tyrosine kinase inhibitor for chronic myelogenous leukemia. *J Clin Invest* 2000; **105:** 3–7.
140. Kantarjian H, Sawyers C, Hochhaus A et al, Phase II study of STI571, a tyrosine kinase inhibitor, in patients (pts) with resistant or refractory Philadelphia chromosome-positive chronic myeloid leukemia. *Blood* 2000; **96**(Suppl 1): 470a.
141. Ogawa M, Differentiation and proliferation of hematopoietic stem cells. *Blood* 1993; **81:** 2844–53.
142. Borzillo GV, Ashmun RA, Sherr CJ, Macrophage lineage switching of murine early pre-B lymphoid cells expressing transduced fms genes. *Mol Cell Biol* 1990; **10:** 2703–14.
143. Krystal G, Lam V, Dragowska W et al, Transforming growth factor β1 is an inducer of erythroid differentiation. *J Exp Med* 1994; **180:** 851–60.
144. Akashi K, Traver D, Miyamoto T, Weissman IL, A clonogenic common myeloid progenitor that gives rise to all myeloid lineages. *Nature* 2000; **404:** 193–7.
145. Kondo M, Weissman IL, Akashi K, Identification of clonogenic common lymphoid progenitors in mouse bone marrow. *Cell* 1997; **91:** 661–72.
146. Hao Q-L, Zhu J, Price MA et al, CD7 expression defines a $CD34^+CD38^-$ subpopulation with differentiation potential restricted to lymphoid lineages. *Blood* 2000; **96**(Suppl 1): 662a.

6

Animal models of Philadelphia-positive leukemia

Richard A Van Etten

CONTENTS • Why use animal models of Ph-positive leukemia? • Xenotransplantation of human CML cells into immunodeficient mice • Propagation of *BCR/ABL*-transformed hematopoietic cell lines in mice • *BCR/ABL* transgenic mice • Retroviral bone marrow transduction/transplantation models of *BCR/ABL*-induced leukemia • Conclusions

WHY USE ANIMAL MODELS OF Ph-POSITIVE LEUKEMIA?

The *BCR/ABL* oncogene was first isolated in 1984[1] and found to be a fusion of *BCR* and c-*ABL*. Shortly thereafter, the product of this chimeric gene, BCR/ABL, was shown to be a dysregulated tyrosine kinase[2] capable of transformation of primary bone-marrow-derived B-lymphoid cells in vitro.[3] Subsequent studies demonstrated that BCR/ABL could weakly transform Rat-1[4] and NIH 3T3[5] fibroblasts to anchorage independence. Finally, BCR/ABL was shown to transform cytokine-dependent lymphoid[6] and myeloid[7] hematopoietic cell lines to become independent of cytokine for survival and proliferation. These semiquantitative assays demonstrated that *BCR/ABL* is a classical oncogene, allowed a comparison of the transforming activity of different isoforms of BCR/ABL,[8,9] and permitted mutagenic analysis of the requirements for different structural domains of BCR/ABL for transformation.[10,11] Studies in cell lines and primary cells in vitro demonstrated that BCR/ABL constitutively activated many cell signaling pathways,[12] several of which were demonstrated to be required for transformation. Given the ready availability of these different in vitro assays for *BCR/ABL* function and the wealth of information gleaned from them, the question might naturally arise why animal models of *BCR/ABL*-induced leukemia are needed?

First and most obviously, if one wishes to understand the pathophysiology of leukemia, this process must be studied in the context of the hematopoietic system of a living organism. *BCR/ABL* is associated with two very different human leukemias: B-cell acute lymphoblastic leukemia (B-ALL) and chronic myeloid leukemia (CML). The former is characterized by a profound differentiation arrest in B-lymphoid development and overgrowth of marrow and hematopoietic organs with proliferating immature blasts. In contrast, in CML, there is greatly increased production of neutrophils, with preservation of differentiation, and gradual evolution to acute leukemia in blast crisis. While transformation of primary B-lymphoid cells in culture[3] is a reasonable in vitro correlate of B-ALL, there is no corresponding in vitro assay that realistically models CML. Attempts to transform primary bone-marrow-derived myeloid cells with *BCR/ABL* in vitro have been unsuccessful.[13] Hematopoietic cell lines exist that undergo differentiation in vitro to a limited extent, but the response of such cell lines to *BCR/ABL* is often paradoxical. For example, *BCR/ABL* blocks the G-CSF-induced differentiation of 32D cells to neutrophils.[14] Embryonic stem (ES) cells differentiate in culture into multiple myeloid and B-lymphoid lineages, but cannot be propagated after differentiation, making longitudinal studies of the effects of *BCR/ABL* expression difficult. The lack of an accurate in vitro model of *BCR/ABL*-induced CML likely reflects the difficulty in establishing myelopoiesis in vitro; significantly, no cell lines have ever been derived from chronic-phase CML patients. In the absence of an accurate model for induction of CML-like leukemia, whether *BCR/ABL* was indeed the principal cause of this disease was in some doubt.[15]

As a corollary, in vivo models of Ph-positive leukemia are required to understand the essential mechanisms and pathways through which *BCR/ABL* induces leukemia. The pathophysiologies of Ph-positive B-ALL and CML are likely to be very different, and it is plausible that entirely distinct mechanisms of leukemogenesis are involved in these diseases. A great deal about the pathophysiology of CML has been learned by study of primary cells from CML patients (see Chapter 3 and Chapter 5). However, such studies are largely descriptive and comparative in nature, and experimental manipulation of these systems is difficult. Knowledge of critical leukemogenesis pathways is essential to selecting targets for rational therapy of Ph-positive leukemia. In this regard, studies in cultured cells have often yielded conflicting results. For example, BCR/ABL contains a direct binding site for the Src homology 2 (SH2) domain of the adapter protein Grb2 at tyrosine 177 in BCR[16] (see Chapter 2), that links BCR/ABL to activation of the Ras pathway. A tyrosine-to-phenylalanine mutation at this site (Y177F) in BCR/ABL renders the protein unable to transform fibroblasts,[16] but capable of transforming cytokine-dependent hematopoietic cell lines[17,18] and primary marrow B-lymphoid cells in vitro.[18] These results leave the importance of direct binding of Grb2 by BCR/ABL in lymphoid and myeloid leukemogenesis unclear. Similarly, the SH2 domain of ABL is required for transformation of fibroblasts by activated ABL,[19,20] but dispensable for transformation of cytokine-dependent hematopoietic cells[21,22] and primary B-lymphoid cells.[20] Recently, the use of mouse model systems of *BCR/ABL*-induced leukemia has provided definitive answers about the relevance of both these pathways to lymphoid and myeloid leukemogenesis by *BCR/ABL* (see below).

Finally, animal models of Ph-positive leukemia would have great utility as platforms for the testing of new therapies for these diseases. They could be useful as secondary assays for compounds identified via high-throughput biochemical or cell-line-based screens, and for testing of structure–activity relationships in promising compounds. Such models would be valuable for investigating synergistic interactions between different drugs in vivo, and for studying the acquisition and mechanisms of drug resistance. Lastly, animal models are a requirement for the development and preclinical testing of immune-based therapies of Ph-positive leukemia. Relevant examples of the use of animal models of *BCR/ABL*-associated leukemia in preclinical therapeutics will be highlighted below.

This chapter will describe four distinct approaches to the modeling of Ph-positive leukemia in the laboratory mouse, *Mus musculus*. These model systems include

(i) xenotransplantation of primary human CML cells in immunodeficient mice;
(ii) the propagation of *BCR/ABL*-transformed hematopoietic cell lines in mice;
(iii) *BCR/ABL* transgenic mice;
(iv) retroviral transduction of *BCR/ABL* into murine bone marrow followed by transplantation.

With each method, emphasis will be placed on what has been learned from the approach, as well as the strengths and weaknesses of the system. The intent is to allow investigators considering the use of an animal model of Ph-positive leukemia to select the system that best fits their particular experimental requirements.

XENOTRANSPLANTATION OF HUMAN CML CELLS INTO IMMUNODEFICIENT MICE

Immunodeficient mice as tools for studying normal and malignant human hematopoiesis in vivo

The classic severe combined immunodeficiency (SCID) mouse strain[23] lacks functional B and T cells owing to a mutation in the catalytic subunit of DNA-dependent protein kinase and the accompanying defect in V(D)J recombination. Both normal and malignant human hematopoietic cells can engraft SCID mice.[24] Interestingly, while human umbilical cord blood cells engraft SCID recipients without cytokine support,[25] progenitors from adult bone marrow efficiently engraft only with concomitant administration of exogenous human cytokines[26] or in the presence of human marrow stroma.[27,28] Similarly, exogenous cytokines are required for engraftment of human acute myeloid leukemia cells in SCID mice,[29–31] but not for acute lymphoblastic leukemia cells.[32–34] The relative difficulty in establishing human myelopoiesis in SCID mice may be due in part to persistent natural killer (NK) cell immunity in these hosts, and has motivated the use of strains lacking NK activity, such as *bg/nu/xid* mice[35,36] and non-obese diabetic/LtSz *scid/scid* (NOD/SCID) mice. The latter strain is profoundly immunodeficient, with impairment of macrophage and NK function,[37] and is superior to SCID mice for engraftment of human myeloid cells.[38,39] Human myeloid engraftment of NOD/SCID recipients is cytokine-independent with large cell doses, but exogenous cytokines or co-transplantation of accessory cells are required with limiting cell numbers.[40] Cell fractionation and limiting-dilution studies have defined the SCID-repopulating cell (SRC) as a $CD34^+CD38^-$ human hematopoietic progenitor that is more primitive than most long-term culture-initiating cells (LTC-IC) and colony-forming cells (CFC),[39,41] although a distinct subset of SRC may be $CD34^-$.[42]

Engraftment of CML blast-crisis cells and cell lines in SCID mice

Early experiments demonstrated that, like many other established cell lines, cell lines derived from CML blast-crisis patients efficiently engraft and disseminate in SCID mice.[43–45] Malignant cells are detectable first in lung and liver, then in marrow, and finally in metastatic sites such as peritoneum and the central nervous system. Engrafted mice provide a useful model for testing therapy with antisense oligodeoxynucleotides and/or chemotherapy,[46,47] but obviously do not offer a representative model of chronic-phase CML. Attempts to propagate primary cells from CML patients were generally successful when the patients were in blast crisis,[29,43,48,49] but stable engraftment of primary chronic-phase cells was not achieved in early attempts,[43,49] although transient focal growth of maturing human myeloid cells was often observed at the site of inoculation.

Engraftment of chronic-phase CML cells in SCID mice

These difficulties were subsequently overcome by using very large cell inocula ($(8\text{–}14) \times 10^7$ cells) from chronic-phase CML patients into SCID mice.[50] Intravenous injection of primary CML patient cells from either peripheral blood or bone marrow resulted in engraftment of recipient bone marrow with human hematopoietic cells at levels from 1% to 10% within 30–60 days after injection, as judged by flow-cytometric analysis of human-specific CD45 cell surface antigen expression or analysis of genomic DNA with a human-specific probe. Human myeloid ($CD13^+$), B-lymphoid ($CD19^+$), and progenitor

($CD34^+$) cells, as well as multilineage CFC, were detected in recipient bone marrow, but there was no apparent dissemination to peripheral blood, spleen, or other organs, and nor did recipients develop any clinical illness. Surprisingly, treatment of recipients with exogenous human cytokines was not required for efficient engraftment, which may reflect aberrant production of cytokines by primitive CML progenitors,[51] with autocrine and paracrine effects after transplantation. Surprisingly, only about one-third of CFC were derived from Ph-positive progenitors, even when peripheral blood was used as the graft, demonstrating that primitive normal cells are mobilized in chronic-phase CML along with their malignant counterparts, and may engraft SCID mice more efficiently. The degree of engraftment was cell-dose-dependent, with very low engraftment observed at lower inocula ($(1–4) \times 10^7$ cells). In agreement with the earlier studies, primary cells from CML lymphoid and myeloid blast-crisis patients engrafted very efficiently at low cell doses,[50] with the morphology and phenotype of the engrafted cells being similar to those of the original blast population.

Superiority of NOD/SCID mice as recipients

Three different groups have reported that NOD/SCID mice are superior to SCID mice for engraftment of primary cells from chronic-phase CML patients.[52–54] When injected with similar numbers of cells from chronic-phase patients, NOD/SCID recipients reproducibly had higher levels of human hematopoietic engraftment than SCID recipients;[53] when assessed by human- and *BCR/ABL*-specific interphase fluorescence in situ hybridization (FISH), 84% of mice receiving more than 4×10^7 cells showed evidence of engraftment, with half of these demonstrating greater than 10% human cells in their BM.[52] As was observed in SCID recipients, exogenous cytokines were not required for engraftment,[52,53] and both normal and Ph-positive engraftment was observed (although cytokines are also not required for engraftment of cells from normal controls in this strain[40]). In one study, the percentage of *BCR/ABL*-positive cells as assessed by FISH was between 23% and 64% in three highly engrafted mice,[52] while another study found an average of 66% of total human bone marrow cells and 71% of bone marrow-derived human CFC were Ph-positive by Southern blot or karyotype analysis, respectively.[53] This contrasts with SCID recipients, in which an average of 70% of human CFC were Ph-negative.[50] Interestingly, some NOD/SCID recipients demonstrated human cells in the spleen;[52,53] in one study, about two-thirds of recipients with bone marrow engraftment also had detectable human cells in the spleen at variable (average 16%) levels, with moderate splenomegaly in some cases.[52] Cell fractionation studies demonstrated that the bone-marrow-engrafting cell was $CD34^+$.[52,53] Comparison of engraftment of NOD/SCID recipients with cells derived from CML patients in chronic, accelerated, and blastic phases demonstrated that the extent of engraftment increased and the time to engraftment decreased between chronic phase and blast crisis.[54] Interestingly, the NOD/SCID leukemia-initiating cell in Ph-positive ($p190^+$) acute B-lymphoblastic leukemia is also $CD34^+$ $CD38^-$,[55] but the relationship of this target cell to the engrafting cell in CML requires further study.

Advantages and drawbacks of xenotransplant model systems

The NOD/SCID assay system holds great promise for elucidating the characteristics of the clonogenic leukemia cell in CML,[30,56] for understanding the cellular biology of CML,[57] and for testing new therapies for CML, such as gene therapy approaches. Given the quantitative differences in engraftment of chronic-, accelerated-, and blastic-phase cells,[54] it is conceivable that xenotransplantation might yield useful prognostic information when performed serially with samples from the same CML patient. However, the current system has several apparent problems that may limit its usefulness. First, engraftment appears to be quite variable, so that the degree of engraftment of individual mice transplanted with cells derived from the same patient may vary over three orders of magnitude.[53] In addition, the average overall engraftment observed among recipients of cells from clinically similar patients varied greatly from patient to patient,[52] although it is plausible that some of this variability may represent more advanced disease in some patients.[54] Although engraftment of normal human hematopoietic progenitors in NOD/SCID recipients is also somewhat inconsistent, it is reproducible enough to allow statistically significant limiting-dilution analysis, enabling estimation of the frequency of the repopulating cells.[41] It is unclear whether similar quantitative analysis of engraftment will be possible with CML cells. Second, it remains to be seen whether NOD/SCID recipients engrafted with chronic-phase CML cells accurately recapitulate the pathophysiology of human CML. Recipients do not appear to have circulating human myeloid cells or dissemination of human cells to liver or other extramedullary sites. Although NOD/SCID recipients do often exhibit human hematopoietic cells in the spleen, with concomitant splenomegaly, most of these cells appear to be of T-cell origin,[52] the majority of which are Ph-negative.[52,53] Most significantly, recipients of CML chronic-phase cells do not appear to develop progressive clinical myeloproliferative disease or to evolve to acute leukemia, although long-term studies of such recipients have not been reported. In part, these difficulties may reflect the same fundamental problem, namely that NOD/SCID mice may not be able to efficiently support long-term human normal[58] or CML-derived myelopoiesis. It seems likely that factors other than host immune responses, such as the marrow microenvironment, may account for this. In addition, Ph-positive cells appear to engraft even the highly immunodeficient NOD/SCID recipients less efficiently than normal cells. This could explain the poor engraftment with bone marrow, where the most primitive progenitors are largely Ph-negative in most chronic-phase CML patients,[59] but does not account for similar results with peripheral blood, where the vast majority of LTC-IC are Ph-positive. Alternatively, poor engraftment of Ph-positive stem/progenitors may be a consequence of abnormalities in SDF-1/CXCR4-mediated bone marrow homing and adhesion, which is required for efficient engraftment of NOD/SCID mice by human cells,[60] and inhibited by the action of BCR/ABL.[61] Lastly, the xenotransplant system is difficult to manipulate experimentally, for example to directly analyze the role of BCR/ABL and downstream pathways in the leukemic process. Although this can be attempted through use of chemical inhibitors and antisense treatments, it is not possible to express different forms of BCR/ABL or introduce other modulatory genes or proteins into the system. Despite these limitations, there is certain to be great interest in this model system, and many of these issues should be addressed in the near future.

PROPAGATION OF *BCR/ABL*-TRANSFORMED HEMATOPOIETIC CELL LINES IN MICE

Transformation of cytokine-dependent hematopoietic cell lines by *BCR/ABL*

Hematopoietic cytokine-dependent cell lines are derived from long-term in vitro culture of mouse bone marrow, and are absolutely dependent on particular cytokines for survival and proliferation. The most commonly used myeloid lines include 32D[62] and FDCP-1[63], that require interleukin-3 (IL-3) and IL-3 or granulocyte–macrophage colony-stimulating factor (GM-CSF), respectively. The prototypic B-lymphoid cell line is the widely used IL-3-dependent Ba/F3 cell line.[64] Upon cytokine deprivation, these cells undergo rapid death by apoptosis. When introduced into immunodeficient or syngeneic immunocompetent mice by subcutaneous or intravenous injection, the cells are unable to form tumors or induce leukemia, probably because the ambient levels of cytokine in vivo are insufficient to allow cell survival.

These cell lines can be transformed by almost any oncogene that encodes a dysregulated tyrosine kinase, including v-*abl* and *BCR/ABL*,[6,7,14,65,66] to become independent of exogenous cytokine for survival and growth. Although expression of *BCR/ABL* induces autocrine production of cytokines, including IL-3, in some cell types,[7] the mechanism of transformation of such cells to cytokine independence by *BCR/ABL* does not require autocrine stimulation.[6,7]

In vivo models using *BCR/ABL*-transformed cell lines

Intravenous injection of *BCR/ABL*-transformed cytokine-independent cells into syngeneic recipient mice (e.g. Balb/c mice for Ba/F3 cells[21] and C3H mice for 32D cells[67]) results in cell proliferation and a rapidly fatal leukemia-like disease. At autopsy, mice exhibit extensive infiltration of marrow, spleen, liver, and often other organs with cells that phenotypically resemble the input cells and express BCR/ABL protein, with the cause of death likely due to bone marrow failure and severe anemia.[21,67] The use of immunodeficient nude or SCID mice as recipients results in a similar disease process.[67–69] Syngeneic or immunodeficient mice probably serve merely as 'living incubators' for the autonomous growth of these *BCR/ABL*-transformed cells, and the disease process therefore does not represent a bona fide acute leukemia. However, several aspects of the biology of the *BCR/ABL*-transformed cells that are not apparent in vitro, such as disease latency and patterns of organ homing and involvement, can be assessed in this model system. In addition, the system has the advantage that the cells employed are permanent cell lines that can be manipulated and extensively characterized in vitro, and then tested for leukemogenicity in vivo. Because the parental cytokine-dependent cells and their *BCR/ABL*-transformed derivatives are identical except for the presence or absence of the *BCR/ABL* gene, differences in biological behavior can be directly attributed to the action of *BCR/ABL*. For example, while the SH2 or SH3 domains of BCR/ABL are not required for transformation of cytokine-dependent hematopoietic cells to cytokine independence in vitro, adoptive transfer of cells transformed by these mutants into recipient mice is associated with prolonged survival and evidence of altered cell homing in vivo.[21,68] Conditional expression of *BCR/ABL* in Ba/F3 cells has recently been used to demonstrate that tumorigenicity requires high levels of BCR/ABL protein expression, and tumorigenic variants that lack *BCR/ABL* expression but exhibit constitutive activation of STAT5 can be selected in vivo.[70]

Cell-line-based models of immune therapy

Because syngeneic recipient mice have an intact immune system, this adoptive transplant system is useful for investigating cellular immune responses to *BCR/ABL*-transformed cells. Expression of the T-cell co-stimulatory molecule B7–1 in *BCR/ABL*-transformed 32D cells renders the cells immunogenic, and syngeneic C3H mice receiving intermediate doses of this cell line eradicate the leukemia by a mechanism that requires $CD8^+$ cells.[67] Immunized animals are protected against rechallenge with the fully leukemogenic parental 32D–*BCR/ABL* line, and hyperimmunization can also eradicate previously established 32D–*BCR/ABL* leukemia if initiated early. B7–1 is superior to the related B7–2 co-stimulatory molecule in this cellular vaccination strategy.[71] Similar immunogenic effects are observed upon co-expression of the interferon consensus sequence binding protein (ICSBP) in *BCR/ABL*-transformed Ba/F3 cells.[72] The mechanism and antigen(s) responsible for these antitumor immune effects are not known, but it is possible that the BCR/ABL protein sequence itself plays a role, since peptides from the junction between BCR and ABL sequences can elicit T-cell responses in mice[73] and humans.[74] Alternatively, the immune response could be to a non-*BCR/ABL*-specific antigen present on the parental cells or induced by oncogene expression; this could be determined in principle by testing whether immunized mice are cross-resistant to the same cells when transformed by other oncogenes.

Cell-line-based models in drug testing

This type of model system also has utility for in vivo testing of new compounds for treatment of *BCR/ABL*-induced leukemias. Promising compounds can be tested for cytostatic and cytotoxic effects on *BCR/ABL*-expressing cells in vitro, and in vivo activity then rapidly assessed by determining whether administration of the compound can prolong survival of syngeneic mice inoculated with the same cells. A novel 2-phenylaminopyrimidine compound that is a potent and relatively selective inhibitor of the ABL tyrosine kinase activity was shown to specifically inhibit the leukemogenicity of 32D–*BCR/ABL* cells in C3H mice,[75] and to allow in vivo eradication of Ph-positive cell lines from nude mice.[76] Similarly, *BCR/ABL*-transformed Ba/F3 cells have been used as a secondary screen for several compounds identified in a large screening cell panel.[77]

Limitations of cell-line-based model systems

The central limitation of these cell-line-based models is that the cytokine-dependent parental cells are aneuploid, immortalized cell lines that are likely to have abnormalities in the ARF–p53 pathway, as well as other mutations. Therefore, any conclusions about leukemogenic mechanisms drawn from this model system must necessarily be limited. The system does not allow expression of *BCR/ABL* in primary cells in vivo, and nor does it provide a accurate model of chronic-phase CML. For these reasons, much effort has been devoted to expression of *BCR/ABL* in primary hematopoietic cells in mice. There are two principal methods to accomplish this: generation of transgenic strains of mice carrying the *BCR/ABL* oncogene, and retroviral transduction of the *BCR/ABL* gene into murine bone marrow ex vivo, followed by transplantation into syngeneic or immunodeficient recipient mice. These efforts will be described in detail in the next two sections.

BCR/ABL TRANSGENIC MICE

Use of transgenic mice to study oncogenesis in vivo

Transgenic mice are generated by injection of the pronucleus of a fertilized mouse egg with purified DNA, followed by implantation of injected eggs into pseudopregnant female mice. The transgene DNA construct contains the gene to be expressed, usually containing an intron and polyadenylation sequence, with a promoter and/or enhancer sequence placed 5' to the coding sequence. Following birth, pups are screened for the presence of the transgene in somatic tissues by Southern blot or PCR. The transgene usually integrates at a single chromosomal location, is present in one to several copies in a tandem repeat, and is found in all cells of the animal, including the germline. The expression of the transgene in the mice is predominantly controlled by the particular promoter/enhancer element utilized in the DNA construct. Usually, the transgene can be passed from a founder mouse to offspring, inherited in a Mendelian fashion. Transgenic mice expressing oncogenes such as activated *ras* genes have been invaluable tools for studying mechanisms of malignant transformation in vivo.[78] They have the advantage of allowing the generation of additional identical mice for study by simple breeding. The effects of genetic background, mutations in other endogenous genes, or interactions with additional transgenes can all be assessed by appropriate crosses. However, transgenic mice have some disadvantages for the expression of oncogenes. The most significant limitation is that traditional transgenic mice contain the transgene in all tissues, and expression of some oncogenes (including those encoding dysregulated tyrosine kinases such as

BCR/ABL) may have deleterious effects during embryogenesis. The consequence may be decreased efficiency in generating transgenic founders, or poor or absent expression of the transgene in those founders that are obtained. This has been a particular problem with *BCR/ABL* transgenes (see below). In contrast with human disease, where the Ph translocation occurs in a single stem or progenitor cell, *BCR/ABL* transgenic mice carry the oncogene in all hematopoietic cells, which may alter the pathophysiology of a resultant leukemia or its response to therapy. On a more practical note, transgenic mice also have the drawback that the study of different isoforms or mutants of a given oncogene requires the generation, characterization, and maintenance of additional transgenic lines – a time-consuming and costly effort. The different *BCR/ABL* transgenic mice that have been generated to date are summarized in Table 6.1.

A *BCR*/v-*abl* transgene induces lymphoid malignancies

The first attempt to generate *BCR/ABL* transgenic mice came before the *BCR/ABL* cDNA was widely available,[79] and utilized a facsimile where the human *BCR* gene was fused to the mouse v-*abl* gene, the transforming gene of Abelson murine leukemia virus. This transgene was similar to the p210 *BCR/ABL* fusion gene but lacked some sequences from *BCR* and *ABL* near the junction of the two genes. Two different promoter/enhancer constructs were employed to direct expression of *BCR*/v-*abl*, the murine immunoglobulin heavy-chain enhancer and variable promoter (EμV_H) that expresses predominantly in pre-B- and pre-T-lymphoid cells,[80] and the promoter/enhancer from the long terminal repeat (LTR) of the murine myeloproliferative sarcoma virus (MPSV),[81] known to express in a wide variety of somatic cells and particularly in undifferentiated and stem cell types. There appeared to be a decreased efficiency of generation of transgenic offspring from eggs injected with either transgene DNA, most prominently with the more widely expressed MPSV-LTR/*BCR*/v-*abl* construct, suggesting embryonic toxicity. A small number of transgenic founders of both types and some progeny developed fatal lymphomas, predominantly T-cell but some of B-cell phenotype. The tumors were clonal by analysis of T-cell receptor or immunoglobulin gene rearrangement status, and expressed high levels of the *BCR*/v-*abl* transgene. However, healthy *BCR*/v-*abl* transgenic founders and littermates exhibited no hematologic abnormalities and did not express the transgene by Northern blot analysis, even in pre-B and pre-T cells.[79] This contrasts with EμV_H/c-*myc* transgenic mice generated by the same group, which constitutively express c-*myc* in pre-B cells, leading to a premalignant expansion of this population and subsequent development of clonal B-cell lymphomas.[82] This suggests that expression of the *BCR*/v-*abl* transgene was silenced during embryonic development owing to toxicity, and activated in lymphoid cells as a somatic event. These studies demonstrated that *BCR/ABL* could induce lymphoid malignancies in vivo, but did not provide a suitable model of CML.

Lethal effect of *BCR/ABL* on embryogenesis

A subsequent study confirmed that some *BCR/ABL* transgenes can indeed have a lethal effect during embryonic development. When the *BCR* promoter, which is widely expressed in somatic cells and during fetal development,[83,84] was used to express p210 *BCR/ABL*, there was a greatly decreased yield of pups from injected eggs, and no transgenic founders were obtained.[85] Analysis of preterm reimplanted foster mothers demonstrated loss of transgenic embryos from embryonic day 9.5 to day 18.5, with later-stage transgenic embryos lacking any apparent vascular system. Reverse-transcriptase (RT)-PCR and Northern analysis detected expression of the *BCR/ABL* transgene in most transgenic embryos, but no morphologic evidence of leukemia was apparent. The precise mechanism of toxicity was not identi-

Table 6.1 *BCR/ABL* transgenic mice

Transgene	Promoter	Disease	Comments	Ref[a]
BCR/v-*abl* hybrid (p210-like)	$E\mu V_H$, MPSV-LTR	B-, T-ALL	Transgene silenced but expressed in tumors	79
p190 *BCR/ABL*	Metallothionein (δMT-1)	B-ALL	Transgene expressed widely at low levels	88, 89
p210 *BCR/ABL*	*BCR*	Embryonic lethal	Lack of vasculature in more mature transgenic embryos	85
p210 *BCR/ABL*	Metallothionein (δMT-1)	B-, T-ALL	Longer latency and reduced penetrance than δMT-1/p190	98
p210 *BCR/ABL*	Metallothionein	T-ALL	Transgene expression in thymus but not bone marrow	97
p190 *BCR/ABL*	*BCR* (knock-in)	B-ALL	Leukemias induced in chimeras via blastocyst injection	108
p210 *BCR/ABL*	*tec*	T-ALL, MPD[b]	Long-latency MPD with thrombocytosis and anemia; accelerated T-ALL in *p53*$^{+/-}$ background	103, 104
p210 *BCR/ABL*	MMTV-LTR/tTA TRE/CMV/p210	B-ALL	Conditional induction and maintenance of leukemia	95

[a] Transgenic mice are listed chronologically by publication date, but discussed in the text in slightly different order.
[b] MPD, myeloproliferative disease with moderate leukocytosis (WBC (15–20) $\times 10^3/\mu l$) and excess neutrophils.

fied, but the lack of leukemia suggests that the lethality was due to the effect of *BCR/ABL* expression on non-hematopoietic tissues.

B-lymphoid leukemia in p190 *BCR/ABL* transgenic mice

After considerable effort, success in generating transgenic mice that reproducibly developed *BCR/ABL*-induced leukemia came when the p190 form of *BCR/ABL* was expressed under the control of a segment of the mouse metallothionein (δMT-1) promoter, which is inducible with heavy metals[86] but constitutively and widely expressed in transgenic mice.[87] In initial experiments, 10 transgenic founder mice were obtained (a frequency of 17%), of which eight rapidly developed fatal leukemia within 58 days of birth in the absence of treatment with heavy metals.[88] Three mice died within two weeks of birth, suggesting that the leukemia had likely initiated in utero. Two mice demonstrated some degree of differentiation towards mature neutrophils in their marrow, suggestive of myeloid leukemia. The other six mice succumbed to B-lymphoblastic leukemia, while the two transgenic progeny that remained healthy were chimeric and did not contain the transgene in bone marrow. Owing to the rapidity of the disease, none of the leukemic founders was successfully bred.

Subsequent efforts by this group led to the generation of 14 additional δMT-1/p190 *BCR/ABL* founders.[89] Nine of these founders died prematurely, one of unknown causes, and the remaining eight of B-lymphoid leukemia/lymphoma between 28 and 79 days of age, with one founder (No. 623) surviving 198 days. The leukemic cells were positive for B220 (CD45R) and 6C3/BP1 antigens, suggestive of an immature B-lymphoid cell phenotype.[90] Five founders did not develop disease. Transgenic progeny were obtained from seven founders, including the five healthy founders, and offspring of six out of seven (including four of the healthy founders) also developed B-lymphoid malignancies, with an overall incidence of 67%. Founder 623 was used to establish a permanent transgenic line from which over 90% of mice die of B-cell leukemia/lymphoma within 40–150 days of age (mean survival 68 days).[91] The *BCR/ABL* transgene was found by RT-PCR to be expressed in the bone marrow of leukemic founders and progeny, but not in the healthy founders. Studies in the 623 line demonstrated widespread transgene expression by RT-PCR in marrow, brain, liver, kidney, and muscle in day 14–16 embryos, at birth, and at 1–2 weeks of age, but expression in peripheral blood was not detected until 20–30 days of age, probably coincident with the appearance of circulating leukemia cells. With a more quantitative RNase protection assay, the expression of the transgene was higher in brain than liver, kidney, or muscle, but the average expression in leukemic cells was 50- to 500-fold higher than in brain.[89] These observations demonstrate that the oncogenic effects of *BCR/ABL* are restricted to the hematopoietic system, but also suggest that either the expression of the *BCR/ABL* transgene is upregulated in lymphoid cells, or a small subpopulation of cells with high expression is selected for during the development of leukemia. A follow-up study showed that lymphoid leukemogenesis by p190 *BCR/ABL* does not require the endogenous murine *bcr* gene product.[92]

Is *BCR/ABL* sufficient to induce leukemia in transgenic mice?

These seminal studies established that *BCR/ABL* was a leukemia-specific oncogene, but raised the question of whether *BCR/ABL* alone was sufficient to induce B-lymphoid leukemia or whether additional events were required. In transgenic models of cancer, the issue of sufficiency is classically addressed by determining if transgene expression can be detected in cells that are not fully malignant (as assessed by secondary transplantation, for example), and by whether the malignant tumors or leukemias that develop are polyclonal as opposed to oligo- or monoclonal.[82] However, detailed studies of the δMT-1/p190 transgenic mice have not yielded a clear answer to this question. Secondary transplantation studies have been reported only from animals with established leukemia, not from young mice.[91,93] The issue of clonality of the leukemia is also unclear. The bone marrow karyotype of line 623 animals sacrificed at day 19, after detectable expression of *BCR/ABL* in peripheral blood but prior to development of overt leukemia, is normal. Karyotype analysis of advanced primary leukemias in line 623 and secondary transplants from this line,[91] and in clonal cell lines derived from peripheral blood leukemia cells,[93] demonstrated that multiple non-random cytogenetic abnormalities tend to arise in the leukemic cells, with preference for trisomy involving chromosomes 10, 12, 14, and 17. However, a few mice with advanced leukemia retained normal karyotypes, and normal metaphases were found in some leukemic cells from the majority of animals with chromosomal abnormalities.[91] While these findings are consistent with the expansion of a pool of early leukemic cells that have *BCR/ABL* as a sole abnormality, the lack of clonal karyotypic abnormalities does not necessarily imply that these leukemias are polyclonal. Analysis of IgH gene rearrangements in the leukemic cells demonstrated a complex pattern, with some tumors having largely germline IgH configuration and others with oligoclonal rearrangements.[89] An oligoclonal IgH rearrangement pattern is prima facie evidence of clonality, but because *BCR/ABL* transgene expression appears to be increased in tumors, one cannot exclude the possibility that the observed clonality results from this event rather than a distinct secondary mutation. Conversely, it was suggested that tumors with germline IgH bands might actually represent polyclonal rearrangements of a single IgH allele, but such a polyclonal pattern is typically quite distinct by Southern blot, and could be verified by a PCR-based assay for IgH gene rearrangement.[94] It seems more likely that these tumors represent cells arrested at the pro-B stage of development with germline IgH alleles, in which case the clonality status of these leukemias is unknown. While it is clear that these *BCR/ABL*-induced leukemias undergo clonal evolution in primary and secondary animals, further studies of these transgenic mice are necessary to determine whether expression of *BCR/ABL* alone is sufficient to induce B-lymphoid leukemia. Significantly, studies in a conditional transgenic model of *BCR/ABL*-induced B-lymphoid leukemia[95] and in retroviral transduction models[8,96] (see below) support the hypothesis that expression of *BCR/ABL* alone is insufficient for lymphoid leukemogenesis.

p210 *BCR/ABL* has distinct leukemogenic activity in transgenic mice

Recently, the MT-1 promoter has also been used to generate p210 *BCR/ABL* transgenic mice. In one study, six transgenic founders were obtained, two of which developed fatal lymphoma, with one of these founders generating a transgenic line that developed similar disease with a penetrance of about 30%.[97] The lymphomas were exclusively of T-cell origin and had rearrangements of T-cell receptor (TCR) β and γ gene loci, although it is not clear whether the rearrangements were clonal. The expression of the *BCR/ABL* transgene was easily detected by Western blotting in the tumor cells, but was undetectable by Western or Northern blotting in any tissues before development of leukemia. Expression was observed by RT-PCR in the leukemia-prone line in kidney, liver, heart, brain, spleen, and particularly highly in thymus, but interestingly not in bone marrow. In three transgenic lines that never developed leukemia, low-level expression in kidney alone was observed in two lines and no detectable expression in any tissue in the other line. In a second study, using the same δMT-1 promoter segment employed in the p190 transgenic mice, several δMT-1/p210 *BCR/ABL* transgenic founders and lines were generated,[98] and these animals developed predominantly T- and B-cell leukemia/lymphoma, with a penetrance of about 60% by 44 weeks of age. One offspring developed a myeloblastic leukemia with Gr-1$^+$ cells. The clonality of the lymphoid tumors was not assessed. This disease pattern was significantly different from the δMT-1/p190 mice, which exhibit greater than 90% incidence of leukemia by 24 weeks of age and never develop T-cell disease.[89,91] By RT-PCR, the p210 *BCR/ABL* transgene was expressed at low levels (50- to >100-fold lower than in leukemic cells) in testis, brain, bone marrow, and spleen of transgenic mice, both in utero and after birth, without induction with heavy metals. As with the p190 transgenics, peripheral blood p210 transgene expression was a prerequisite for development of disease, but overt leukemia did not immediately follow in all cases, since some mice with expression of p210 *BCR/ABL* in circulating leukocytes remained free of disease for months. Collectively, these studies suggest that p210 *BCR/ABL* has less potent and distinct lymphoid leukemogenic activity in transgenic mice when compared with p190.

Why don't *BCR/ABL* transgenic mice develop myeloid leukemia?

The obvious question that arises is why these mice do not develop myeloid leukemias or CML. Initially, there was some doubt whether the p190 form of *BCR/ABL*, found nearly exclusively in Ph-positive ALL in humans,[99] could induce CML at all. However, recent studies with retroviral transduction of *BCR/ABL* have shown definitively that p190 can induce CML-like disease in mice (see below),[96] and in any case this would not explain the nearly complete absence of myeloid disease in the p210 transgenic mice. The most direct explanation may be lack of sufficient expression of the *BCR/ABL* transgene in myeloid and early progenitor/stem cells. Although expression of the p190 and p210 *BCR/ABL* transgenes can be detected in the bone marrow of these mice, it is possible that the expression is heterogeneous and restricted to lymphoid progenitors. There is no reason that the δMT-1 promoter should not express in myeloid progenitors, but it is possible that expression of this promoter is downregulated in these transgenic mice because of transgene toxicity, and the resulting low levels of *BCR/ABL* expression are below a threshold required for oncogenic transformation by tyrosine kinases.[70,100] This might explain the very low levels of bone marrow expression in young δMT-1/*BCR/ABL* transgenic mice, but much greater expression in the lymphoid leukemia cells. In support of this hypothesis, when efforts were made to direct p210 *BCR/ABL* expression to myeloid cells by use of the CD11b[101] or cathepsin G[102] promoters, which are known to direct high-level position-independent expression of reporter transgenes to myeloid cells, the p210 transgenic founders that were obtained did not express detectable levels of *BCR/ABL* in their myeloid cells nor develop disease (S Dziennis, RA Van Etten, and DG Tenen, unpublished work; PP Pandolfi, personal communication).

A novel transgenic model of p210-induced myeloproliferative disease

Recently, the p210 *BCR/ABL* gene has been expressed under control of the promoter of the *tec* gene, which encodes a cytoplasmic kinase preferentially expressed in the hematopoietic system.[103] Five founders were obtained, and two died of T-cell lymphoblastic leukemia between 3 and 4 months of age. One of these leukemic founders gave rise to a permanent line that showed no evidence of T-ALL but instead developed a slow myeloproliferative-like syndrome with 100% penetrance by 8 months of age. This syndrome was characterized by modestly increased peripheral blood leukocyte counts ($(9\text{–}15) \times 10^3/\mu l$) composed predominantly of mature neutrophils, moderate thrombocytosis ($(80\text{–}200) \times 10^4/\mu l$), and mild anemia (hemoglobin 8.0–14.5 g/dl). Some mice became moribund at around 1 year of age, and showed infiltration of spleen and mesenteric lymph nodes with neutrophils, marked thrombocytosis, and severe anemia. *BCR/ABL* transgene expression was detected in circulating neutrophils by RT-PCR. This novel transgenic model is intriguing, but further studies are necessary to determine whether it represents an accurate model of CML. In particular, it is not clear whether the disease process is progressive or fatal in all offspring or whether the illness is transplantable, and the cause of death in some mice appeared to be severe anemia, which is not a prominent feature of chronic-phase CML in human patients. Crossing the *tec*/p210 transgene into a $p53^{+/-}$ heterozygous background results in development of T-lymphomas from 2 to 11 months of age,[104] often accompanied by loss of the wild-type *p53* allele, but it is unclear whether this is a model of CML disease progression or merely oncogene cooperativity.

Embryonic stem-cell-based approaches to *BCR/ABL* expression in mice

A distinct approach to expression of *BCR/ABL* in mice is through the use of embryonic stem (ES) cells. ES cells are totipotent undifferentiated cells that can be propagated in culture, genetically modified and selected, then introduced into mice by injection into 3.5-day-old blastocysts, followed by implantation into the uterus of pseudopregnant foster mothers. Chimeric offspring with ES cell contribution to somatic tissues (including the hematopoietic system) and often the germline can be identified by scoring coat color alleles or by molecular analysis of polymorphic markers. The ES cell system has principally been used to inactivate genes by homologous recombination ('knockout'), but the potential also exists to introduce oncogenes, either as simple transgenes or by homologous recombination into the corresponding endogenous murine gene ('knock-in').[105,106] ES cells can also be differentiated into multiple hematopoietic lineages in culture,[107] allowing the opportunity to determine if oncogene expression might perturb hematopoietic development in vitro. However, the differentiation conditions do not allow continued growth of the cells, and it has not been possible to demonstrate consistent contributions of undifferentiated or differentiated ES cells to hematopoiesis upon direct transfer into mice.

Utilizing the knock-in approach, a p190 *BCR/ABL* transgene was created by homologous recombination in ES cells using a construct with fusion of mouse *bcr* exon 1 sequence with human *BCR* exon 1/*ABL* cDNA, with the resulting chimeric DNA expressed from the endogenous mouse *bcr* promoter.[108] Expression of the knock-in gene in the ES cell clone was documented by RT-PCR. Of 40 chimeric mice generated by blastocyst injection with the targeted ES cell clone, 38 developed B-lymphoid leukemia of the pre-B type by 4 months of age, with the majority of leukemias exhibiting clonal IgH gene rearrangements. The *bcr/ABL* gene was presumably expressed in all ES-derived tissues in the chimeras (although this was not directly demonstrated) yet only leukemia developed, again suggesting that the oncogenic action of *BCR/ABL* is specific to the hematopoietic system. Using a second round of targeting, the remaining normal *bcr* allele was inactivated in the *bcr/ABL* ES clone, and these cells induced identical leukemia in chimeras, again demonstrating that *BCR/ABL* does not require the *bcr* gene product for leukemogenesis. It was not determined if expression of the transgene was increased in leukemic cells, as was observed in the δMT-1/p190 transgenic mice.[89] It was also not reported whether any of the chimeras were bred and successfully passed the *BCR/ABL* gene to offspring. Because of the toxicity of p210 *BCR/ABL* when expressed from a *bcr* promoter,[85] one might anticipate similar toxicity with the knock-in oncogene, resulting in failure of germline transmission of *BCR/ABL*. Although this model system was suggested to be a superior model of Ph-positive B-ALL, it is not apparent that there are significant advantages over the δMT-1/p190 transgenic mice. It was claimed that the histopathology of the disease in these chimeras more closely resembled human Ph-positive ALL because of a predominant leukemia rather than lymphoma, but the importance of this is not clear, because the δMT-1/p190 mice all have circulating malignant cells and are therefore leukemic, and human Ph-positive ALL patients can certainly present with lymphadenopathy. The ES cell system as employed in this model is clearly more cumbersome and labor-intensive than transgenic mice, because blastocyst harvesting, injection, and reimplantation is necessary to obtain diseased animals, and genetic manipulation of the leukemic clone requires modification of the original *bcr/ABL* ES cell clone, as opposed to simply breeding transgenic mice with other strains.

Other groups have pursued the approach of expression of *BCR/ABL* in ES cells by retroviral transduction or electroporation, with the goal of obtaining *BCR/ABL*-expressing ES cells or hematopoietic derivatives of ES cells that might induce hematologic disease upon direct inoculation of adult mice. Stable *BCR/ABL* expression in ES cells decreased the efficiency of embryoid body (EB) formation but increased the generation of myeloid hematopoietic progenitors in vitro,[109] while conditional expression of BCR/ABL stimulated multipotential progenitor expansion and myeloid lineage commitment.[173] Others have isolated a primitive EB-derived hematopoietic-like cell line expressing *BCR/ABL* that generates a myeloproliferative-like disorder upon transfer into irradiated syngeneic recipient mice.[110] More work is necessary to determine if these novel approaches will yield useful models of *BCR/ABL*-induced leukemia.

Conditional transgenic systems

Despite over a decade of effort in generation of *BCR/ABL* transgenic mice by conventional techniques, there is no transgenic mouse model of CML (with the possible exception of the *tec*/p210 *BCR/ABL* mice, which require further validation). Recently, attention has turned to the use of conditional transgenic systems as an approach to developing a model of CML. There are several types of conditional transgenic system available, and the utility of any of these for generating a CML model depends in large part on what the fundamental problem is with traditional transgenic mice. The obvious goal is to develop mice that reproducibly express *BCR/ABL* at high levels in myeloid and progenitor/stem cells. This has not been achieved in any of the published *BCR/ABL* transgenic mice, despite the use of promoters that should express at high levels in these cells. The most likely explanation is transgene toxicity, as discussed above. In theory, the toxicity of *BCR/ABL* during embryogenesis could be due to expression within the developing blood system or to non-hematopoietic expression. A non-hematopoietic mechanism of toxicity is supported by the observation that toxicity is more severe with widely expressed promoters,[79] and by the lack of vasculature in more mature *bcr* promoter/*BCR/ABL* transgenic embryos[85] (although it should be noted that the hematopoietic system and vasculature have a common embryonic origin). In theory, the use of promoters to express *BCR/ABL* that are more specific for myeloid/stem cells might alleviate this toxicity. Unfortunately, toxicity was still observed when the myeloid-specific CD11b and cathepsin G promoters were used to express p210 *BCR/ABL* (see above). Perhaps this was due to expression of these promoters at low to intermediate levels outside the hematopoietic system. If this is the case, then the problem may be helped by the use of binary systems, where the product of one transgene controls the expression of another. There are two principal types of these systems, distinguished by whether the controlling transgene encodes a transcription factor or a recombinase. In the first system, a transgenic strain expressing the yeast Gal4p transcriptional activator under a hematopoietic-specific promoter is mated with a strain containing a *BCR/ABL* transgene under control of *GAL4* upstream activating sequences.[111] In the second system, a strain expressing a DNA recombinase from bacteriophage P1 (Cre[112]) or yeast (FLP[113]) from a hematopoietic-specific promoter is mated with a strain containing a *BCR/ABL* gene in inverted orientation from a strong promoter or with a transcriptional terminator inserted between promoter and transgene, in either case flanked by the appropriate recombination signal sequences (*lox* or *FRT*, respectively). In double transgenic mice from either system, the controlling transgene product induces expression of *BCR/ABL* specifically in hematopoietic cells by transcriptional activation or recombination. Because fairly high levels of expression of Gal4p or recombinase are necessary for efficient induction of the target transgene, the binary system tends to eliminate non-specific expression of the target transgene outside the tissue of interest. To date, the application of either of these binary systems for expression of *BCR/ABL* in mice has not been reported.

Recently, the retroviral transduction/transplantation model system (see the next section) has been used to rapidly and efficiently induce CML-like myeloproliferative illness in mice. This disease process is fatal and extremely rapid, despite transduction of limiting numbers of stem/progenitor target cells. These observations suggest that high-level expression of *BCR/ABL* in stem/progenitor cells in transgenic mice, if achieved, would result in prenatal demise from myeloproliferative disease, or at best, very brief survival after birth. If this scenario is correct, then the only feasible way to develop a transgenic model of CML would be to suppress expression of *BCR/ABL* until after birth. This is possible with the use of a binary transgene system that utilizes the tetracycline-regulated transcriptional activator tTA[114] (Figure 6.1). tTA is a fusion of the *E. coli* tetracycline operon repressor and the herpes virus transactivator VP16, which binds to tet operator DNA sequences and activates transcription in the absence of tetracycline, but not in its presence. In a recent study,[95] four lines of transgenic mice with p210 *BCR/ABL* under control of the tet-response element (TRE) fused to a minimal cytomegalovirus (CMV) promoter ('transresponders') were generated, and transgenic offspring were born with the expected Mendelian frequency and developed normally, indicating that the TRE/CMV/p210 transgene was not toxic. Transresponder mice were then mated to 'transactivator' mice with tTA under control of the mouse mammary tumor virus long terminal repeat (MMTV-LTR) promoter/enhancer,[115] known to express tTA in epithelial cells and bone marrow. Females were maintained on tetracycline beginning five days prior to mating to suppress expression of the *BCR/ABL* transgene. Double transgenic mice were obtained at the predicted Mendelian frequency, and remained healthy as long as tetracycline administration was continued. Withdrawal of tetracycline resulted in development of fatal B-lymphoid leukemia with 100% incidence in all four lines. Leukemia induction was fairly rapid (50% death by 16–28 days) in three of the lines, but delayed (50% death by 45 days) in the other. Kinetic studies demonstrated that immature lymphoid cells expressing B220 and 6C3/BP1 antigens appeared in peripheral blood within 10 days of cessation of tetracycline treatment in the three lines with more acute disease, but was somewhat delayed in the fourth line. The disease was transplantable at death, and analysis of IgH gene rearrangements demonstrated oligoclonal rearrangements, suggesting that additional events were necessary for complete malignant transformation. Bone marrow fractionation demonstrated that the MMTV-LTR/tTA transgene was expressed in $B220^+$ cells but not $CD11b^+$ or $Thy1^+$ cells, which could explain the induction of B-lymphoid leukemia rather than myeloid leukemia in the double transgenic mice. Surprisingly, re-administration of tetracycline resulted in rapid disappearance of leukemic cells from blood and involved lymph nodes, with the majority of malignant lymphoblasts undergoing apoptosis.[95] These studies demonstrate that *BCR/ABL*-induced lymphoid leukemia is absolutely dependent on continued expression of the *BCR/ABL* oncogene, even at advanced stages of disease.

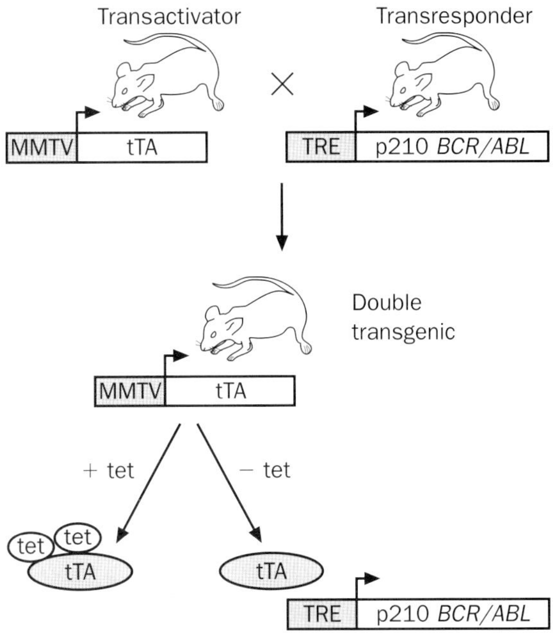

Figure 6.1 Schematic representation of binary transgene system employing the tetracycline-regulated transactivator (tTA) to control expression of a *BCR/ABL* transgene. The transactivator strain (upper left) expresses the tTA protein from the mouse mammary tumor virus (MMTV) LTR, while the transresponder strain (upper right) contains a p210 *BCR/ABL* transgene under control of the tetracycline-responsive promoter element (TRE). Double transgenic mice express tTA constitutively, but the p210 transgene is only expressed in the absence of tetracycline (lower right).

Future prospects

A great deal has been learned from *BCR/ABL* transgenic mice. These studies have shown that *BCR/ABL* is a leukemia-specific oncogene, and the available strains provide novel reagents for dissecting the different signaling pathways required for *BCR/ABL*-induced leukemogenesis, and for testing new treatments and therapies. In particular, the tetracycline-regulated transgene system holds great promise for studying *BCR/ABL* biology. The existing MMTV-LTR/tTA/p210 *BCR/ABL* double transgenic mice provide an ideal model system for investigating the earliest events during *BCR/ABL*-induced lymphoid leukemogenesis, and for elucidating the mechanism of anti-apoptotic action of *BCR/ABL* in primary lymphoid cells. In addition, the use of myeloid- or stem-cell-specific promoters such as MRP8,[116] human CD34,[117] or Sca1[118] to express the tTA transactivator offer the possibility of generating the long-sought transgenic model of CML.

RETROVIRAL BONE MARROW TRANSDUCTION/TRANSPLANTATION MODELS OF *BCR/ABL*-INDUCED LEUKEMIA

Background and early studies

Currently, the most accurate and informative animal model of CML involves transfer of the *BCR/ABL* gene into primary murine bone marrow cells ex vivo, followed by transplantation of the genetically modified cells into syngeneic or immunodeficient recipient mice (Figure 6.2). The preferred method of gene transfer has been to use replication-defective ecotropic retroviral vectors, because of their unparalleled efficiency at stable transduction of hematopoietic progenitor and stem cells, and because the retroviral DNA integrates into the cell chromosomal DNA and serves as a unique clonal marker of that cell and its progeny. In initial experiments, *BCR/ABL*-transduced primary bone marrow was propagated in liquid culture under conditions favoring expansion and development of B-lymphoid cells (Whitlock–Witte cultures[119]). Under these conditions, untransduced marrow will undergo expansion to cell densities of $(2–4) \times 10^5$ cells/ml over a 6-week period and the resulting population, a mixture of immature and differentiated B-lymphoid cells, is non-malignant and capable of reconstitution of B-cell function upon adoptive transfer into SCID mice. In contrast, marrow transduced with p210 *BCR/ABL* retrovirus expands to higher densities ($(4–10) \times 10^5$ cells/ml) over the same time

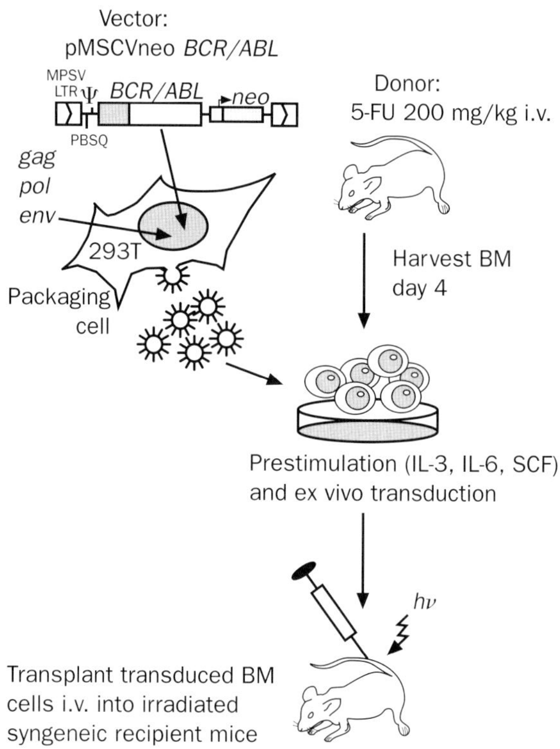

Figure 6.2 Schematic diagram of the retroviral bone marrow (BM) transduction/transplantation model system for *BCR/ABL* leukemogenesis. A retroviral vector containing the *BCR/ABL* cDNA is introduced into a packaging cell (upper left) to produce replication-defective retrovirus stock; bone marrow is harvested from donor mice pretreated with 5-fluorouracil (5-FU, upper right) and transduced with virus stock ex vivo (middle) in the presence of cytokines, followed by transplantation into irradiated (*hν*) syngeneic recipient mice (bottom).

period owing to oligoclonal outgrowth of *BCR/ABL*-transduced pre-B cells.[3] Unlike v-*abl*-transduced cultures, which become independent of stroma by 4 weeks and are highly malignant upon transfer to syngeneic mice,[120] p210-transduced cultures remained stromal-dependent for up to 15 weeks and were only weakly leukemogenic in vivo. Substitution of a cloned stromal cell line for the bone-marrow-derived adherent layer in these cultures permitted the isolation of clonal p210-expressing B-progenitor lines that were non-leukemogenic and underwent Ig rearrangements in vitro and in vivo,[121] confirming the ability of p210 to stimulate growth without arresting differentiation. p190 *BCR/ABL* is more potent than p210 in this assay, with p190-transduced cultures reaching maximal density more often and becoming stromal-independent and leukemogenic sooner.[8] Subsequently, transduction of p210 *BCR/ABL* was shown to decrease the requirement of myeloid CFC for IL-3 or stem cell factor for clonogenic in vitro growth, allowing isolation of clonal mast, macrophage, granulocyte–macrophage, and B-lymphoid cell lines that eventually became cytokine-independent but remained non-leukemogenic.[122] Together, these studies provide strong support for the concept that the principal consequence of *BCR/ABL* expression in primary hematopoietic cells is a very subtle stimulation of growth without appreciable effects on differentiation.

p210 *BCR/ABL* induces multiple hematopoietic malignancies in vivo, including a CML-like myeloproliferative disease

To assess the in vivo leukemogenic potential of *BCR/ABL*-transduced bone marrow, it can be transplanted into syngeneic or immunodeficient recipient mice that have been conditioned with sublethal or lethal doses of ionizing radiation (Figure 6.2). Published studies utilizing the retroviral bone marrow transduction/transplantation model of *BCR/ABL* leukemogenesis are summarized in Table 6.2. The first experiments were modeled on earlier studies transplanting v-*fms*-transduced marrow, where recipients developed several hematopoietic diseases, including myeloproliferative-like syndromes.[123] After considerable effort, a major breakthrough was achieved in 1990 when several groups were able to induce CML-like myeloproliferative disease and other hematologic malignancies in recipients of p210 *BCR/ABL*-transduced bone marrow.[124–126] Key reasons for this success likely include the use of retroviral vectors derived from the myeloproliferative sarcoma virus (MPSV) variant[81] or its predecessor Moloney sarcoma virus (MSV)[127] to express *BCR/ABL*, rather than the traditional Moloney murine leukemia virus, and pretreatment of donor mice with 5-fluorouracil (5-FU), a thymidylate synthetase inhibitor with cell-cycle-specific cytotoxicity that increases the relative abundance and transduction efficiency of hematopoietic progenitor/stem cells.[128] The choice of mouse strain was probably also a factor, since Balb/c mice appear to be more sensitive to induction of leukemia by v-*abl* and *BCR/ABL* than other inbred strains.[126,129,130] The CML-like disease was a fatal illness arising 4–12 weeks post-transplant, characterized by dramatic increases in peripheral blood leukocyte counts (($50–500 \times 10^3/\mu l$), composed largely of neutrophils, metamyelocytes, and myelocytes, and hepatosplenomegaly with extensive infiltration with maturing myeloid cells. The cause of death in most animals appeared to be myeloid infiltration of the lung parenchyma, often with hemorrhage. Bone marrow of these mice exhibited myeloid hyperplasia with minimal fibrosis and less than 10% blasts. Myeloid cells were found to carry the *BCR/ABL* provirus, usually in a monoclonal pattern, and expressed p210 protein,[124,125] confirming that the disease was directly induced by *BCR/ABL*. In addition, provirus was present in the majority of day 12–14 spleen colonies ($CFU\text{-}S_{12}$) derived from a mouse with CML-like disease,[124] suggesting that the target cell that was transduced by *BCR/ABL* to induce the CML-like disease was an early multipotential progenitor that can generate $CFU\text{-}S_{12}$. Transplantation experiments

Table 6.2 *BCR/ABL* retroviral bone marrow transduction/transplantation studies

Authors (date)	Oncogene	Disease[a]	Comments
Daley et al[124] (1990)	p210	CML, B-ALL, Mϕ disease	Original demonstration that p210 induced CML-like disease in mice
Kelliher et al[125] (1990)	p210 v-*abl*	CML, B-ALL, Mϕ disease	Retroviral stocks contained helper virus; v-*abl* later found not to induce CML-like disease[162,164]
Elefanty et al[126] (1990)	p210	B-ALL, Mϕ disease, EL	Did not observe CML-like disease in C57Bl/6 and DBA mouse strains
Daley et al[131] (1991)	p210	CML, mast cell disease, B-, T-ALL	Secondary transplantation of CML-like disease and clonally related acute myeloid and lymphoid leukemias
Kelliher et al[172] (1991)	p210 p190	CML, B-ALL, Mϕ disease	p190 induced leukemias of shorter latency than p210
Elefanty and Cory[130] (1992)	p210	CML, B-ALL, Mϕ disease, EL	*BCR/ABL*-induced leukemias influenced by mouse strain and transduction conditions
Gishizky et al[132] (1993)	p210	CML, B-, T-ALL, Mϕ disease	Efficient secondary transplantation of CML-like disease; heterogeneity of target cells
Skorski et al[168] (1996)	p210	CML, AML	SCID mouse recipients; *p53*$^{+/+}$ donor marrow gave long latency MPD, while *p53*$^{-/-}$ donors gave AML-like disease
Skorski et al[154] (1997)	p210 ΔSH2	CML, AML	SCID recipients; p210 SH2 mutants induced less aggressive CML/AML-like disease
Pear et al[147] (1998)	p210	CML, T-ALL	Efficient induction and secondary transplantation of CML-like disease
Zhang and Ren[148] (1998)	p210	CML	Efficient induction/secondary transplantation of CML; elevated plasma IL-3/GM-CSF
Li et al[96] (1999)	p190 p210 p230	CML, B-ALL, Mϕ disease	Efficient/similar induction of CML by all three oncogenes; p190 more potent for induction of B-ALL
Gross et al[156] (1999)	p210 b3a3	CML	SH3-deleted p210 efficiently induces CML
Hao and Ren[167] (2000)	p210+ ICSBP	CML	Co-expression of ICSBP delays p210-induced CML-like disease
Million and Van Etten[164] (2000)	p210 Y177F	B-, T-ALL	Grb2 binding site required for induction of CML-like disease by p210

[a] Disease phenotypes are defined in the text. Mϕ, macrophage; EL, erythroleukemia.

demonstrated that the CML-like disease could be transferred from some but not all primary mice to secondary mice by injection of bone marrow and/or spleen cells;[131,132] surprisingly, other secondary transplant recipients developed clonally related acute leukemias of myeloid, B-lymphoid, and T-lymphoid origin, strongly suggesting that the CML-like disease involved a pluripotent hematopoietic stem cell, and mimicking the blast-crisis phase of human CML. These observations demonstrated that p210 *BCR/ABL* induces a disease in mice that is a very close pathophysiologic match to human CML.

In addition to the CML-like disease, which was observed in about 25% of recipients of p210 *BCR/ABL*-transduced marrow, other recipients developed distinct hematopoietic malignancies, including B-lymphoid leukemia, tumors of monocyte–macrophage lineage, and occasionally erythroleukemia and T-lymphoid leukemia.[124–126] The B-lymphoid leukemia involved marrow and spleen, with less consistent involvement of peripheral blood and lymph nodes, appearing 8–30 weeks post transplant. The malignant cells expressed p210 protein and had a pre-B-cell phenotype, positive for B220 (CD45R), CD43, CD24, and 6C3/BP1 antigens,[90] with clonal rearrangements of one or both IgH gene loci. These leukemias were readily transplanted to secondary recipients, and were easily established as permanent cell lines in cultures supplemented with 2-mercaptoethanol but no other growth factors. This disease is very similar to that arising in δMT-1/p190 *BCR/ABL* transgenic mice[88] and induced in adult Balb/c mice by Abelson murine leukemia virus,[129] and is a reasonable model of human Ph-positive acute lymphoblastic leukemia. The macrophage disease was characterized by discrete tumors in liver, spleen, bone marrow, and mesentery, often with malignant ascites, appearing at prolonged intervals (up to 50 weeks) after transplant. The tumor cells had large nuclei and abundant vacuolated cytoplasm, and pathologically resembled reticulum cell sarcoma or malignant histiocytosis, neither of which is commonly associated with a Ph-chromosome translocation in humans.[133,134] The cells were $CD11b^{+}$ and esterase-positive, expressed p210 protein, and grew poorly in culture but could transfer the disease to secondary recipients after long latent periods. Interestingly, some animals with more extensive macrophage tumors were observed to have moderate expansion of mature neutrophils in peripheral blood, marrow, and sometimes the spleen, suggestive of myeloproliferative disease. However, when purified populations of neutrophils were analyzed, they were found to lack the p210 provirus,[124,126] and were therefore not part of the malignant clone, but represented a reactive process to excess GM-CSF and granulocyte colony-stimulating factor (G-CSF) produced by these tumors.[126]

Efficient induction of CML-like disease in mice by *BCR/ABL*

The above studies provided convincing evidence that *BCR/ABL* was the direct cause of human CML, but the inefficiency of induction of the CML-like disease, which likely reflected low levels of retroviral transduction of stem/progenitor cells, made it difficult to use the model to study the pathophysiology of CML in mice. The principal reason for inefficient transduction was the use of stable retroviral packaging cell lines,[135] because the toxic effect of BCR/ABL protein expression within the packaging cells caused a progressive decrease in the titer of *BCR/ABL* producer clones. A significant advance in the field came when several groups took advantage of the highly transfectable human embryonic kidney cell line 293[136,137] to develop transient retroviral packaging systems.[138–140] These transient packaging systems allowed the rapid and reproducible production of high-titer, replication-defective ecotropic *BCR/ABL* retrovirus stocks lacking detectable replication-competent virus. Improvements in retroviral vector design also led to improved titers[141] and stability of expression.[142,143] Lastly, alterations in transduction conditions, including cytokine prestimulation,[144] co-sedimentation of cells and virus,[145] and transduction on fibronectin[146] further improved transduction of primary hematopoietic cells.

Using these improvements, several groups recently reported efficient induction of CML-like disease in mice by p210 *BCR/ABL*,[96,147,148] where 100% of recipients of p210-transduced marrow succumbed to fatal CML-like disease, identical to that described earlier, within 4 weeks after transplantation. The CML-like disease in these mice was polyclonal by provirus integration rather than the monoclonal pattern observed previously, which confirmed increased transduction efficiency, and suggested that *BCR/ABL* transduction alone was sufficient to induce the CML-like disease. However, because the number of transduced target cells received by each animal was not known, this could not be definitively established by these studies. The CML-like disease was efficiently transplanted from most, but not all, primary mice by transfer of bone marrow or spleen cells. Interestingly, only a small subset of the clones present in the primary mice contributed to day-12 spleen colonies[96] and induced disease in secondary recipients,[96,148] suggesting there was heterogeneity between individual clones contributing to the expansion of myeloid cells in the primary animal, with only a minor subset capable of self-renewal as assessed by secondary transplantation. The same phenomenon may account for the heterogeneity in secondary transplantation observed in earlier studies.[131,132] Further evidence of improved retroviral transduction came from experiments where the donors were not pretreated with 5-FU.[96] Recipients of p210 *BCR/ABL*-transduced bone marrow derived from untreated donors developed a mixture of CML-like disease, B-lymphoid leukemia, and macrophage disease that was very similar to that observed in the earlier, less efficient model system.[124] The B-lymphoid leukemias and macrophage tumors were mono- or oligoclonal by provirus integration, suggesting that *BCR/ABL* transduction alone may be insufficient for full malignant transformation in these diseases, although this also cannot be proved by these data alone.

Distinct bone marrow target cells for *BCR/ABL*-induced leukemias

Why do different recipients of the same transduced marrow develop distinct hematologic malignancies? The most plausible explanation is that these diseases are the consequence of transduction of different target cells within the bone marrow. In mice with *BCR/ABL*-induced CML-like disease, the same spectrum of proviral clones is observed in neutrophils, macrophages, nucleated erythroid progenitors, B-lymphoid cells, and sometimes T-lymphoid cells, suggesting that the target cell for the CML-like disease has multilineage repopulating ability.[96] This finding supports the original hypothesis that the target cell for induction of CML-like disease is an early multipotential progenitor/stem cell.[124] In contrast, in mice with *BCR/ABL*-induced B-lymphoid leukemia or macrophage disease, the provirus is found in the malignant B-lymphoid and monocyte–macrophage cells, respectively, but not in normal myeloid cells or in CFU-S_{12} derived from these mice,[96] suggesting that the target cells for these diseases are distinct progenitors with lineage-restricted differentiation potential. The target cell for *BCR/ABL*-induced B-lymphoid leukemia is likely to be similar to the Abelson virus target cell, an early B-lymphoid progenitor,[149,150] while it is similarly plausible that the target cell for the macrophage disease is a monocytic progenitor. With the most efficient retroviral transduction, all recipients receive multiple *BCR/ABL*-transduced stem cells and rapidly develop CML-like disease.[96,147,148] However, under less efficient or altered[130] transduction conditions, some animals may receive no transduced stem cells and survive to develop B-lymphoid and monocyte– macrophage malignancies of longer latency that require multiple events in addition to *BCR/ABL*. Some mice develop several leukemias simultaneously,[96,124,126] and knowledge of the distinctive pathologic features of the different malignancies is required for accurate diagnosis. To complicate matters further, in occasional mice with monoclonal CML-like disease, it is possible to observe B-lymphoid leukemia that is derived from the same malignant clone, essentially representing blast crisis in a primary recipient (S Li and RA Van Etten, unpublished work). The existence of multiple *BCR/ABL*-induced leukemias arising from different target cells makes the system quite complex, and great care is required to avoid incorrect conclusions. Validation of this model of multitarget leukemogenesis by *BCR/ABL* will require isolation of these distinct target cells from bone marrow, and is an important goal of current work in this system.

Advantages and disadvantages of the retroviral transduction/transplantation model system

Expression of *BCR/ABL* in vivo by retroviral transduction has a number of distinct advantages over the use of transgenic mice. In this system, it is relatively easy to test different forms and mutants of *BCR/ABL*, simply by making new retroviral stocks. When comparing the leukemogenic activity of different stocks, it is, of course, imperative that the efficiency of marrow transduction between stocks be very similar. It is also easy, at least in principle, to test the leukemogenicity of *BCR/ABL* in different genetic backgrounds and in mice with targeted mutations in different genes by employing mutant mice as donors and/or recipients in the system. As a practical matter, results with mutant strains are most informative if the strain in question has normal baseline hematopoiesis and bone marrow donor and recipient function. The retroviral transduction system has been extended to the study of other leukemia oncogenes,[151,152] although not all putative oncogenes induce leukemia in this system. Using simultaneous transduction of bone marrow with two distinct retroviruses, it is possible to observe synergistic interactions between two genes in leukemogenesis,[153] but the relatively low incidence of co-transduction of stem cells with two viruses makes it implausible that dominant-negative effects can be detected in such experiments.[154] An alternative to efficiently co-express two genes is the use of retroviral vectors with the internal ribosome entry site (IRES) derived from encephalomyocarditis virus,[155] which allows expression of two cistrons from the same proviral mRNA transcript. Co-expression of *BCR/ABL* with enhanced green fluorescent protein (eGFP) facilitates rapid titering of retroviral stocks, and has been used to directly identify *BCR/ABL*-expressing cells in vivo.[147,148] However, there is significant discordance between expression of eGFP and *BCR/ABL* from IRES vectors in malignant cells in vivo[156] (S Li and Van RA Etten, unpublished work), and therefore eGFP expression cannot be reliably used as a surrogate marker for the presence of *BCR/ABL* provirus or BCR/ABL protein expression in this system.

The retroviral transduction/transplantation model has several disadvantages as well. The biggest drawback is that the generation of diseased mice for study requires the performance of a new transduction/transplantation procedure, which is somewhat laborious. Great care must be taken with each of the many steps involved (e.g. 5-FU priming, harvesting, virus production and titering, transduction, and injection of recipients) to obtain reproducible results, and control experiments are essential. It is possible that some of this repetitive effort may be circumvented by cryopreservation of transduced marrow, but this has not yet been tested. An additional concern is that *BCR/ABL* is expressed from the retroviral LTR in most of the vectors utilized, which obviously differs from the *BCR* promoter that expresses *BCR/ABL* in human CML. The LTR is probably a stronger promoter than *BCR*, and this may in part account for the short survival of mice with *BCR/ABL*-induced CML-like disease. As a consequence, the current system does not model the long latency period required for human CML patients to develop clinical symptoms following exposure to ionizing radiation.[157,158] However, the short latency of murine CML-like disease may also reflect the requirement for stem cells to be cycling in order to be transduced by retroviral vectors, and the use of different vectors or transduction conditions may allow models of CML latency to be developed in mice.[132]

Studying the pathophysiology of CML using the retroviral transduction/transplantation model system

The ability to induce CML-like disease in 100% of recipients of *BCR/ABL*-transduced marrow has allowed the system to be used as an actual assay for the first time, and several different types of experiments are now feasible. The first was a comparison of the leukemogenic activity of the three principal forms of *BCR/ABL*: p190, p210, and p230. These oncogenes arise from different breakpoints on chromosome 22, generating three distinct fusion proteins that contain the same portion of c-Abl with different amounts of Bcr polypeptide sequence at the N-terminus (see Chapter 1), and exhibit different intrinsic tyrosine kinase activity.[9,96] In humans, the three forms of *BCR/ABL* are predominantly associated with distinct forms of leukemia.[99] The p210 form is of course found in chronic-phase CML, while p190 is commonly observed in Ph-positive ALL but is very rarely detected in CML. Recently, several patients with p230 *BCR/ABL* and a mild form of CML were described, with less leukocytosis and requirement for myelosuppressive therapy, less splenomegaly, and delayed or absent transformation to blast crisis.[159] It was suggested that p230-positive CML represented a distinct and less aggressive variant, denoted neutrophilic CML. However, several subsequent reports described patients with p230 *BCR/ABL* and typical CML.[160,161] These observations raise the question of whether different forms of *BCR/ABL* have intrinsically different leukemogenic activity in hematopoietic cells. The retroviral transduction/transplantation model offers an ideal system to compare the in vivo leukemogenic activity of these different *BCR/ABL* oncogenes after transduction of an identical spectrum of hematopoietic cells. All three forms of *BCR/ABL* were equally potent in the induction of CML-like disease when marrow from 5-FU-treated donors was employed.[96] There were no significant differences in survival, peripheral blood leukocyte counts, or spleen weights at death, suggesting that all three *BCR/ABL* oncogenes induced a similar proliferative stimulus to myeloid cells under these conditions. These results do not support the hypothesis that p230 induces a distinct and less aggressive form of CML, and suggest that the rarity of p190 in chronic-phase CML may reflect infrequent *BCR* intron 1 breakpoints during the genesis of the Ph chromosome in stem cells, rather than intrinsic differences in myeloid leukemogenicity between p190 and p210.

A related question of considerable interest is whether the v-*abl* oncogene of Abelson murine leukemia virus can also induce CML-like disease. In an early version of the marrow transduction/transplantation model system that employed helper virus to increase transduction efficiency, it was reported that v-*abl* could induce CML-like disease,[125] with moderate elevations of neutrophils in peripheral blood and spleen. However, the neutrophils in such mice lack the v-*abl* provirus,[162] and probably represent a reactive process to cytokines produced by co-existing macrophage tumors, as discussed above. Others have described a chronic myeloproliferative disease induced by transduction of bone marrow with helper-free stocks of v-*abl*,[163] but careful analysis of the description and histopathology of the disease process suggests that these animals developed a mixture of B-lymphoid leukemia and tumors of macrophage and mast cell origin. When tested in the current efficient model system, none of the recipients of v-*abl*-transduced marrow developed CML-like disease, with recipients instead succumbing to B-lymphoid leukemias, mast cell tumors, and macrophage disease.[164] These results demonstrate conclusively that v-*abl* is unable to induce CML-like disease in this model system, presumably because the viral Gag/Abl fusion protein is unable to activate one or more critical signaling pathways necessary for stimulation of myelopoiesis in vivo.

Similar comparative studies can be carried

out with *BCR/ABL* genes containing mutations in distinct structural domains of the BCR/ABL fusion protein. Despite cell culture studies that suggested a role for the SH3 domain of BCR/ABL in leukemogenicity,[68] SH3 can be deleted from p210 BCR/ABL with no effect on induction of CML-like disease in vivo.[156] In contrast, the p210 BCR/ABL Y177F Grb2 binding site mutant is profoundly defective for induction of CML-like disease in mice, with recipients instead developing B-lymphoid leukemia or a novel T-cell lymphoma.[164,165] This result resolves the controversy over the importance of direct binding of Grb2 to BCR/ABL for leukemogenesis, and validates the Grb2 pathway as an important target for rational drug design in CML. The SH2 domain is not required for induction of B-lymphoid leukemia by *BCR/ABL*,[166] but contributes to efficient induction of CML-like disease in mice.[154,166] Although the SH2 domain of BCR/ABL was initially reported to be required for activation of the phosphatidylinositol 3-kinase (PI3-K) pathway in hematopoietic cells,[154] other studies have found no defect in PI3-K activation in cells transduced with *BCR/ABL* SH2 mutants,[166] and the mechanism of the modest defect in induction of CML-like disease by these mutants requires further study. The effect of co-expression of other genes with *BCR/ABL* can be tested using an IRES vector; for example, enforced expression of the ICSBP protein, normally downregulated in CML cells, delays the development of *BCR/ABL*-induced CML-like disease.[167]

A final type of experiment examines the influence of mutations in other genes on leukemogenesis by *BCR/ABL*. Transduction of bone marrow from *p53*$^{-/-}$ mice with p210 *BCR/ABL* is associated with rapidly fatal myeloblastic leukemia in SCID mouse recipients, as opposed to a more indolent myeloproliferative-like disease induced in *p53*$^{+/+}$ cells.[168] These results suggest that the p53 status of hematopoietic cells may influence the leukemogenic response to *BCR/ABL* transduction. Other experiments have examined the role of hematopoietic cytokines in the pathogenesis of CML. Recently, studies in primitive Ph-positive human CML progenitors have identified aberrant transcripts for IL-3 and G-CSF that may account in part for the autonomous in vitro growth of these cells[51] (see Chapter 5). Interestingly, increased plasma levels of IL-3[96,148] and GM-CSF[148] have been detected in plasma of mice with *BCR/ABL*-induced CML-like disease. Because the *il3*[169] and *gmcsf*[170] genes have been deleted in mice through homologous recombination, and the homozygous mutant mice have essentially normal hematopoiesis and marrow function, the role of these cytokine genes in the pathogenesis of the murine CML-like disease can be definitively established. Neither the *il3* nor the *gmcsf* gene is required in donor bone marrow for efficient induction of CML-like disease by p210 *BCR/ABL*,[171] but further studies are necessary to determine if other cytokines such as G-CSF are required for initiation or maintenance of the CML phenotype in vivo.

Future prospects

This improved retroviral transduction/transplantation model system should be very valuable for further investigation of the cellular and molecular pathophysiology of CML. We can anticipate that the structural requirements for induction of leukemia by BCR/ABL will be thoroughly defined in the near future, and experiments with chemical inhibitors, dominant-negative mutants, complementing genes, and genetically modified mouse strains will elucidate the critical signaling pathways for induction of myeloproliferative disease. Continued correlative studies between human CML and the murine CML-like disease are necessary, and conclusions reached in the mouse model system require validation, if possible, in human CML patients and cells.

CONCLUSIONS

It is apparent that we have learned an enormous amount about CML in the recent past, and one could argue fairly convincingly that it is the best understood of all human malignant disorders. In no small part, this is because of what has been learned from animal models of the disease. The power of animal model systems of Ph-positive leukemia derives from their ability to accurately recapitulate the complex physiology of CML and Ph-positive ALL in vivo. This suggests that the most productive future applications of these model systems will be in areas related to therapy of CML that are controversial today, as illustrated by the other chapters of this book. The mechanism of action of interferon-α in CML is unknown (see Chapter 7), and an assay that would predict responsiveness of CML patients to this drug is badly needed. While a specific chemical inhibitor of the ABL tyrosine kinase has demonstrated significant activity in interferon-unresponsive chronic-phase CML patients (see Chapter 32 and Chapter 33) it can be anticipated that resistance to this compound will develop, and novel methods to avoid and treat resistant disease will need to be identified. Autologous transplantation in CML has been shown to be feasible (see Chapter 28), but further improvements in disease-free survival after autografting will require a better understanding of the nature of the most primitive clonogenic CML cells. Finally, it is now apparent that most of the beneficial effect of allogeneic bone marrow transplantation is from the transplanted donor immune system (see Chapter 23), yet the mechanism of this effect is unknown. Critical advances in these areas will be facilitated by the careful and creative application of the animal model systems considered here.

ACKNOWLEDGEMENTS

The author would like to thank Drs John Dick, George Daley, and Mark Showers for critical reading of the manuscript. This work was supported by NIH Grant CA57593. The author is a Scholar of the Leukemia and Lymphoma Society of America and the Carl and Margaret Walter Scholar in Blood Research at Harvard Medical School.

REFERENCES

1. Groffen J, Stephenson JR, Heisterkamp N et al, Philadelphia chromosomal breakpoints are clustered within a limited region, *bcr*, on chromosome 22. *Cell* 1984; **36:** 93–9.
2. Konopka JB, Watanabe SM, Witte ON, An alteration of the human c-*abl* protein in K562 leukemia cells unmasks associated tyrosine kinase activity. *Cell* 1984; **37:** 1035–42.
3. McLaughlin J, Chianese E, Witte ON, In vitro transformation of immature hematopoietic cells by the P210 *bcr/abl* oncogene product of the Philadelphia chromosome. *Proc Natl Acad Sci USA* 1987; **84:** 6558–62.
4. Lugo TG, Witte ON, The *bcr–abl* oncogene transforms rat-1 cells and cooperates with v-*myc*. *Mol Cell Biol* 1989; **9:** 1263–70.
5. Renshaw MW, McWhirter JR, Wang JYJ, The human leukemia oncogene *bcr–abl* abrogates the anchorage requirement but not the growth factor requirement for proliferation. *Mol Cell Biol* 1995; **15:** 1286–93.
6. Daley G, Baltimore D, Transformation of an interleukin 3-dependent hematopoietic cell line by the chronic myelogenous leukemia-specific P210 *bcr/abl* protein. *Proc Natl Acad Sci USA* 1988; **85:** 9312–16.
7. Hariharan IK, Adams JM, Cory S, bcr–abl oncogene renders myeloid cell line factor independent: potential autocrine mechanism in chronic myeloid leukemia. *Oncogene Res* 1988; **3:** 387–99.
8. McLaughlin J, Chianese E, Witte ON, Alternative forms of the *bcr–abl* oncogene have quantitatively different potencies for stimulation of immature lymphoid cells. *Mol Cell Biol* 1989; **9:** 1866–74.
9. Lugo TG, Pendergast A, Muller AJ, Witte ON, Tyrosine kinase activity and transformation potency of bcr–abl oncogene products. *Science* 1990; **247:** 1079–82.
10. Muller AJ, Young JC, Pendergast A et al, BCR first exon sequences specifically activate the BCR/ABL tyrosine kinase oncogene of Philadelphia chromosome-positive leukemias. *Mol Cell Biol* 1991; **11:** 1785–92.
11. McWhirter JR, Wang JYJ, Activation of tyrosine kinase and microfilament-binding functions of c-*abl* by bcr sequences in *bcr/abl* fusion proteins. *Mol Cell Biol* 1991; **11:** 1785–92.
12. Sawyers CL, Signal transduction pathways involved in BCR-ABL transformation. *Baillière's*

Clin Haematol 1997; **10:** 223–31.

13. Young JC, Witte ON, Selective transformation of primitive lymphoid cells by the *bcr/abl* oncogene expressed in long-term lymphoid or myeloid cultures. *Mol Cell Biol* 1988; **8:** 4079–87.
14. Laneuville P, Heisterkamp N, Groffen J, Expression of the chronic myelogenous leukemia-associated p210 *bcr/abl* oncoprotein in a murine IL-3 dependent myeloid cell line. *Oncogene* 1991; **6:** 275–82.
15. Fialkow PJ, Martin PJ, Naifield V et al, Evidence for a multistep pathogenesis of chronic myelogenous leukemia. *Blood* 1981; **58:** 158–63.
16. Pendergast AM, Quilliam LA, Cripe LD et al, BCR–ABL-induced oncogenesis is mediated by direct interaction with the SH2 domain of the GRB-2 adaptor protein. *Cell* 1993; **75:** 175–85.
17. Cortez D, Kadlec L, Pendergast AM, Structural and signaling requirements for BCR–ABL-mediated transformation and inhibition of apoptosis. *Mol Cell Biol* 1995; **15:** 5531–41.
18. Goga A, McLaughlin J, Afar DE et al, Alternative signals to RAS for hematopoietic transformation by the BCR–ABL oncogene. *Cell* 1995; **82:** 981–8.
19. Mayer BJ, Jackson PK, Van Etten RA, Baltimore D, Point mutations in the *abl* SH2 domain coordinately impair phosphotyrosine binding in vitro and transforming activity in vivo. *Mol Cell Biol* 1992; **12:** 609–18.
20. Afar DEH, Goga A, McLaughlin J et al, Differential complementation of Bcr–Abl point mutants with c-myc. *Science* 1994; **264:** 424–6.
21. Ilaria RL, Van Etten RA, The SH2 domain of $P210^{BCR/ABL}$ is not required for transformation of hematopoietic factor-dependent cells. *Blood* 1995; **86:** 3897–904.
22. Anderson SM, Mladenovic J, The BCR/ABL oncogene requires both kinase activity and *src*-homology 2 domain to induce cytokine secretion. *Blood* 1996; **87:** 238–44.
23. Bosma GC, Custer RP, Bosma MJ, A severe combined immunodeficiency mutation in the mouse. *Nature* 1983; **301:** 527–30.
24. Dick JE, Normal and leukemic human stem cells assayed in SCID mice. *Semin Immunol* 1996; **8:** 197–206.
25. Vormoor J, Lapidot T, Pflumio F et al, Immature human cord blood progenitors engraft and proliferate to high levels in severe combined immunodeficient mice. *Blood* 1994; **83:** 2489–97.
26. Lapidot T, Pflumio F, Doedens M et al, Cytokine stimulation of multilineage hematopoiesis from immature human cells engrafted in SCID mice. *Science* 1992; **255:** 1137–41.
27. Namikawa R, Weilbaecher KN, Kaneshima H et al, Long-term human hematopoiesis in the SCID-hu mouse. *J Exp Med* 1990; **172:** 1055–63.
28. Kyoizumi S, Baum CM, Kaneshima H et al, Implantation and maintenance of functional human bone marrow in SCID–hu mice. *Blood* 1992; **79:** 1704–11.
29. Cesano A, Hoxie JA, Lange B et al, The severe combined immunodeficient (SCID) mouse as a model for human myeloid leukemias. *Oncogene* 1992; **7:** 827–36.
30. Lapidot T, Sirard C, Vormoor J et al, A cell initiating human acute myeloid leukaemia after transplantation into SCID mice. *Nature* 1994; **367:** 645–8.
31. Chelstrom L, Gunther R, Simon J et al, Childhood acute myeloid leukemia in mice with severe combined immunodeficiency. *Blood* 1994; **84:** 20–6.
32. Kamel-Reid S, Letarte M, Sirard C et al, A model of human acute lymphoblastic leukemia in immune-deficient SCID mice. *Science* 1989; **246:** 1597–600.
33. DeLord C, Clutterbuck R, Titley J et al, Growth of primary human acute leukemia in severe combined immunodeficient mice. *Exp Hematol* 1991; **19:** 991.
34. Uckun FM, Sather H, Reaman G et al, Leukemic cell growth in SCID mice as a predictor of relapse in high-risk B-lineage acute lymphoblastic leukemia. *Blood* 1995; **85:** 873–8.
35. Kamel-Reid S, Dick JE, Engraftment of immune-deficient mice with human hematopoietic stem cells. *Science* 1998, **242:** 1706–9.
36. Nolta JA, Hanley MB, Kohn DB, Sustained human hematopoiesis in immunodeficient mice by cotransplantation of marrow stroma expressing human interleukin-3: analysis of gene transduction of long-lived progenitors. *Blood* 1994; **83:** 3041–51.
37. Shultz LD, Schweitzer PA, Christianson SW et al, Multiple defects in innate and adaptive immunologic function in NOD/LtSz-scid mice. *J Immunol* 1995; **154:** 180–91.
38. Bock TA, Orlic D, Dunbar CE et al, Improved engraftment of human hematopoietic cells in severe combined immunodeficient (SCID) mice

carrying human cytokine transgenes. *J Exp Med* 1995; **182:** 2037.

39. Larochelle A, Vormoor J, Hanenberg H et al, Identification of primitive human hematopoietic cells capable of repopulating NOD/SCID mouse bone marrow: implications for gene therapy. *Nature Med* 1996; **2:** 1329–37.
40. Bonnet D, Bhatia M, Wang JC et al, Cytokine treatment or accessory cells are required to initiate engraftment of purified primitive human hematopoietic cells transplanted at limiting doses into NOD/SCID mice. *Bone Marrow Transplant* 1999; **23:** 203–9.
41. Bhatia M, Wang JCY, Kapp U et al, Purification of primitive human hematopoietic cells capable of repopulating immune-deficient mice. *Proc Natl Acad Sci USA* 1997; **94:** 5320–5.
42. Bhatia M, Bonnet D, Murdoch B et al, A newly discovered class of human hematopoietic cells with SCID-repopulating activity. *Nature Med* 1998; **4:** 1038–45.
43. Sawyers CL, Gishizky ML, Quan S et al, Propagation of human blastic myeloid leukemias in the SCID mouse. *Blood* 1992; **79:** 2089–98.
44. Skorski T, Nieborowska-Skorska M, Calabretta B, A model of Ph′ positive chronic myeloid leukemia-blast crisis cell line growth in immunodeficient SCID mice. *Folia Histochem Cytobiol* 1992; **30:** 91–6.
45. Beran M, Pisa P, O'Brien S et al, Biological properties and growth in SCID mice of a new myelogenous leukemia cell line (KBM-5) derived from chronic myelogenous leukemia cells in the blastic phase. *Cancer Res* 1993; **53:** 3603–10.
46. Skorski T, Nieborowska-Skorska M, Wlodarski P et al, Antisense oligodeoxynucleotide combination therapy of primary chronic myelogenous leukemia blast crisis in SCID mice. *Blood* 1996; **88:** 1005–12.
47. Skorski T, Nieborowska-Skorska M, Wlodarski P et al, Treatment of Philadelphia leukemia in severe combined immunodeficient mice by combination of cyclophosphamide and bcr/abl antisense oligodeoxynucleotides. *J Natl Cancer Inst* 1997; **89:** 124–33.
48. Namikawa R, Ueda R, Kyoizumi S, Growth of human myeloid leukemias in the human marrow environment of SCID–hu mice. *Blood* 1993; **82:** 2526–36.
49. McGuirk J, Yan Y, Childs B et al, Differential growth patterns in SCID mice of patient-derived chronic myelogenous leukemias. *Bone Marrow Transplant* 1998; **22:** 367–74.
50. Sirard C, Lapidot T, Vormoor J et al, Normal and leukemic SCID-repopulating cells (SRC) coexist in the bone marrow and peripheral blood from CML patients in chronic phase, whereas leukemic SRC are detected in blast crisis. *Blood* 1996; **87:** 1539–48.
51. Jiang X, Lopez A, Holyoake T et al, Autocrine production and action of IL-3 and granulocyte colony-stimulating factor in chronic myeloid leukemia. *Proc Natl Acad Sci USA* 1999; **96:** 12804–9.
52. Lewis ID, McDiarmid LA, Samels LM et al, Establishment of a reproducible model of chronic-phase chronic myeloid leukemia in NOD/SCID mice using blood-derived mononuclear or CD34+ cells. *Blood* 1998; **91:** 630–40.
53. Wang JCY, Lapidot T, Cashman JD et al, High level engraftment of NOD/SCID mice by primitive normal and leukemic hematopoietic cells from patients with chronic myeloid leukemia in chronic phase. *Blood* 1998; **91:** 2406–14.
54. Dazzi F, Capelli D, Hasserjian R et al, The kinetics and extent of engraftment of chronic myelogenous leukemia cells in non-obese diabetic/severe combined immunodeficiency mice reflect the phase of the donor's disease: an in vivo model of chronic myelogenous leukemia biology. *Blood* 1998; **92:** 1390–6.
55. Cobaleda C, Gutiérrez-Cianca N, Pérez-Losada J et al, A primitive hematopoietic cell is the target for the leukemic transformation in human Philadelphia-positive acute lymphoblastic leukemia. *Blood* 2000; **95:** 1007–13.
56. Bonnet D, Dick JE, Human acute myeloid leukemia is organized as a hierarchy that originates from a primitive hematopoietic cell. *Nature Med* 1997; **3:** 730–7.
57. Holyoake T, Jiang X, Eaves C, Eaves A, Isolation of a highly quiescent subpopulation of primitive leukemic cells in chronic myeloid leukemia. *Blood* 1999; **94:** 2056–64.
58. Cashman JD, Lapidot T, Wang JC et al, Kinetic evidence of the regeneration of multilineage hematopoiesis from primitive cells in normal human bone marrow transplanted into immunodeficient mice. *Blood* 1997; **89:** 4307–16.
59. Eaves C, Udomsakdi C, Cashman J et al, The biology of normal and neoplastic stem cells in CML. *Leuk Lymphoma* 1993; **11**(Suppl 1): 245–53.

60. Peled A, Petit I, Kollet O et al, Dependence of human stem cell engraftment and repopulation of NOD/SCID mice on CXCR4. *Science* 1999; **283:** 845–8.
61. Salgia R, Quackenbush E, Lin J et al, The BCR/ABL oncogene alters the chemotactic response to stromal-derived factor-1α. *Blood* 1999; **94:** 4233–46.
62. Greenberger JS, Sakakeeny MA, Humphries RK et al, Demonstration of permanent factor-dependent multipotential (erthyroid/neutrophil/basophil) hematopoietic progenitor lines. *Proc Natl Acad Sci USA* 1983; **80:** 2931–5.
63. Dexter TM, Garland J, Scott D et al, Growth of factor-dependent hematopoietic precursor cell lines. *J Exp Med* 1980; **152:** 1036–47.
64. Palacios R, Steinmetz M, IL3-dependent mouse clones that express B-220 surface antigen, contain Ig genes in germ-line configuration, and generate B lymphocytes in vivo. *Cell* 1985; **41:** 727–34.
65. Cook WD, Metcalf D, Nicola NA et al, Malignant transformation of a growth factor-dependent myeloid cell line by Abelson virus without evidence of an autocrine mechanism. *Cell* 1985; **41:** 677–83.
66. Mathey-Prevot B, Nabel G, Palacios R, Baltimore D, Abelson virus abrogation of interleukin-3 dependence in a lymphoid cell line. *Mol Cell Biol* 1986; **6:** 4133–5.
67. Matulonis UA, Dosiou C, Lamont C et al, Role of B7–1 in mediating an immune response to myeloid leukemia cells. *Blood* 1995; **85:** 2507–15.
68. Skorski T, Nieborowska-Skorska M, Wlodarski P et al, The SH3 domain contributes to BCR/ABL-dependent leukemogenesis in vivo: role in adhesion, invasion, and homing. *Blood* 1998; **91:** 406–18.
69. Salomoni P, Wasik MA, Riedel RF et al, Expression of constitutively active Raf-1 in the mitochondria restores antiapoptotic and leukemogenic potential of a transformation-deficient BCR/ABL mutant. *J Exp Med* 1998; **187:** 1995–2007.
70. Klucher KM, Lopez DV, Daley GQ, Secondary mutation maintains the transformed state in BaF3 cells with inducible BCR/ABL expression. *Blood* 1998; **91:** 3927–34.
71. Matulonis U, Dosiou C, Freeman G et al, B7–1 is superior to B7–2 costimulation in the induction and maintenance of T cell-mediated antileukemia immunity. *J Immunol* 1996; **156:** 1126–31.
72. Deng M, Jena N, Tamura T et al, ICSBP expression abrogates BCR/ABL-induced leukemia in immunocompetent mice. *Blood* 1999; **94**(Suppl 1): 104a.
73. Chen W, Peace DJ, Rovira DK et al, T-cell immunity to the joining region of p210 BCR–ABL protein. *Proc Natl Acad Sci USA* 1992; **89:** 1468–72.
74. Bocchia M, Korontsvit T, Xu Q et al, Specific human cellular immunity to bcr–abl oncogene-derived peptides. *Blood* 1996; **87:** 3587–92.
75. Druker BJ, Tamura S, Buchdunger E et al, Effects of a selective inhibitor of the Abl tyrosine kinase on the growth of Bcr–Abl positive cells. *Nature Med* 1996; **2:** 561–6.
76. le Coutre P, Mologni L, Cleris L et al, In vivo eradication of human BCR/ABL-positive leukemia cells with an ABL kinase inhibitor. *J Natl Cancer Inst* 1999; **91:** 163–8.
77. Yang Q-E, Fong SE, Hagenau H et al, Establishment of a cell-line-based mouse model of Bcr/Abl-induced leukemia: detection of antileukemic activity of an amino-methyl cyclopentanone. *Cancer Res* 2001; submitted.
78. Pattengale PK, Stewart TA, Leder A et al, Animal models of human disease. Pathology and molecular biology of spontaneous neoplasms occurring in transgenic mice carrying and expressing activated cellular oncogenes. *Am J Pathol* 1989; **135:** 39–61.
79. Hariharan IK, Harris AW, Crawford M et al, A *bcr–v-abl* oncogene induces lymphomas in transgenic mice. *Mol Cell Biol* 1989; **9:** 2798–805.
80. Banerji J, Olson L, Schaffner W, A lymphocyte-specific cellular enhancer is located downstream of the joining region in immunoglobulin heavy chain genes. *Cell* 1983; **33:** 729–40.
81. Stocking C, Kollek R, Bergholz U, Ostertag W, Long terminal repeat sequences impart hematopoietic transformation properties to the myeloproliferative sarcoma virus. *Proc Natl Acad Sci USA* 1985; **82:** 5746–50.
82. Langdon WY, Harris AW, Cory S, Adams JM, The c-myc oncogene perturbs B lymphocyte development in E-mu-myc transgenic mice. *Cell* 1986; **47:** 11–18.
83. Lifshitz B, Fainstein E, Marcelle C et al, *bcr* genes and transcripts. *Oncogene* 1988; **2:** 113–17.
84. Shah NP, Witte ON, Denny CT, Characterization of the *BCR* promoter in Philadelphia chromosome-positive and -negative cell lines. *Mol Cell Biol* 1991; **11:** 1854–60.

85. Heisterkamp N, Jenster G, Kioussis D et al, Human *bcr–abl* gene has a lethal effect on embryogenesis. *Transgenic Res* 1991; **1:** 45–53.
86. Stuart GW, Searle PF, Chen HY et al, A 12 base-pair DNA motif that is repeated several times in metallothionein gene promoters confers metal regulation to a heterologous gene. *Proc Natl Acad Sci USA* 1984; **81:** 7318.
87. Palmiter RD, Norstedt G, Gelinas RE et al, Metallothionein–human GH fusion gene stimulates growth of mice. *Science* 1983; **222:** 809–14.
88. Heisterkamp N, Jenster G, ten Hoeve J et al, Acute leukemia in bcr/abl transgenic mice. *Nature* 1990; **344:** 251–3.
89. Voncken JW, Griffiths S, Greaves MF et al, Restricted oncogenicity of BCR/ABL p190 in transgenic mice. *Cancer Res* 1992; **52:** 4534–9.
90. Hardy RR, Carmack CE, Shinton SA et al, Resolution and characterization of pro-B and pre-pro-B cell stages in normal mouse bone marrow. *J Exp Med* 1991; **173:** 1213–25.
91. Voncken JW, Morris C, Pattengale P et al, Clonal development and karyotype evolution during leukemogenesis of BCR/ABL transgenic mice. *Blood* 1992; **79:** 1029–36.
92. Voncken JW, Kaartinen V, Groffen J, Heisterkamp N, Bcr/Abl associated leukemogenesis in *bcr* null mutant mice. *Oncogene* 1998; **16:** 2029–32.
93. Griffiths SD, Healy LE, Ford AM et al, Clonal characteristics of acute lymphoblastic cells derived from *BCR/ABL* p190 transgenic mice. *Oncogene* 1992; **7:** 1391–9.
94. Schlissel M, Baltimore D, Activation of immunoglobulin kappa gene rearrangement correlates with induction of germline kappa gene transcription. *Cell* 1989; **58:** 1001–7.
95. Huettner CS, Zhang P, Van Etten RA, Tenen DG, Reversibility of acute B-cell leukaemia induced by *BCR–ABL1*. *Nature Genet* 2000; **24:** 57–60.
96. Li S, Ilaria RL, Million RP et al, The P190, P210, and P230 forms of the *BCR/ABL* oncogene induce a similar chronic myeloid leukemia-like syndrome in mice but have different lymphoid leukemogenic activity. *J Exp Med* 1999; **189:** 1399–412.
97. Honda H, Fujii T, Takatoku M et al, Expression of $p210^{bcr/abl}$ by metallothionein promoter induced T-cell leukemia in transgenic mice. *Blood* 1995; **10:** 2853–61.
98. Voncken JW, Kaartinen V, Pattengale PK et al, *BCR/ABL* P210 and P190 cause distinct leukemia in transgenic mice. *Blood* 1995; **86:** 4603–11.
99. Melo JV, The diversity of BCR–ABL fusion proteins and their relationship to leukemia phenotype. *Blood* 1996; **88:** 2375–84.
100. Jakobovits EB, Majors JE, Varmus HE, Hormonal regulation of the rous sarcoma virus *src* gene via a heterologous promoter defines a threshold dose for cellular transformation. *Cell* 1984; **38:** 757–65.
101. Dziennis S, Van Etten RA, Pahl HL et al, The CD11b promoter directs high level expression of reporter genes in macrophages in transgenic mice. *Blood* 1995; **85:** 319–29.
102. Grisolano JL, Sclar GM, Ley TJ, Early myeloid cell-specific expression of the human cathepsin G gene in transgenic mice. *Proc Natl Acad Sci USA* 1994; **91:** 8989–93.
103. Honda H, Oda H, Suzuki T et al, Development of acute lymphoblastic leukemia and myeloproliferative disorder in transgenic mice expressing $p210^{bcr/abl}$: a novel transgenic model for human Ph[1]-positive leukemias. *Blood* 1998; **91:** 2067–75.
104. Honda H, Ushijima T, Wakazono K et al, Acquired loss of p53 induces blastic transformation in $p210^{bcr/abl}$-expressing hematopoietic cells: a transgenic study for blast crisis of human CML. *Blood* 2000; **95:** 1144–50.
105. Corral J, Lavenir I, Impey H et al, An *MLL–AF9* fusion gene made by homologous recombination causes acute leukemia in chimeric mice: a method to create fusion oncogenes. *Cell* 1996; **85:** 853–61.
106. Yergeau DA, Hetherington CJ, Wang Q et al, Embryonic lethality and impairment of haematopoiesis in mice heterozygous for an AML1–ETO fusion gene. *Nature Genet* 1997; **15:** 303–6.
107. Wiles MV, Keller G, Multiple hematopoietic lineages develop from embryonic stem (ES) cells in culture. *Development* 1991; **111:** 259–67.
108. Castellanos A, Pintado B, Weruaga E et al, A $BCR–ABL^{p190}$ fusion gene made by homologous recombination causes B-cell acute lymphoblastic leukemias in chimeric mice with independence of the endogenous *bcr* product. *Blood* 1997; **90:** 2168–74.
109. Turhan AG, Bonnet ML, Le Pesteur D et al, Generation of an embryonic stem (ES) cell model of chronic myelogenous leukemia (CML). *Blood* 1999; **94**(Suppl 1): 101a.

110. Peters DG, Perlingeiro RCR, Klucher KM et al, Generation of a hematopoietic stem cell line from ES cells using the oncogene BCR/ABL. *Blood* 1999; **94**(Suppl 1): 252a.
111. Ornitz DM, Moreadith RW, Leder P, Binary system for regulating transgene expression in mice: targeting *int-2* gene expression with yeast *GAL4/UAS* control elements. *Proc Natl Acad Sci USA* 1991; **88:** 698–702.
112. Kühn R, Schwenk F, Aguet M, Rajewsky K, Inducible gene targeting in mice. *Science* 1995; **269:** 1427–9.
113. O'Gorman S, Fox DT, Wahl GM, Recombinase-mediated gene activation and site-specific integration in mammalian cells. *Science* 1991; **251:** 1351–5.
114. Furth PA, St. Onge L, Boger H et al, Temporal control of gene expression in transgenic mice by a tetracycline-responsive promoter. *Proc Natl Acad Sci USA* 1994; **91:** 9302–6.
115. Hennighausen L, Wall RJ, Tillmann U et al, Conditional gene expression in secretory tissues and skin of transgenic mice using the MMTV-LTR and the tetracycline responsive system. *J Cell Biochem* 1995; **59:** 463–72.
116. Brown D, Kogan S, Lagasse E et al, A PML/RAR alpha transgene initiates murine acute promyelocytic leukemia. *Proc Natl Acad Sci USA* 1997; **94:** 2551–6.
117. Huettner CS, Radomska HS, Burn TC et al, Colocalization of human and murine CD34 in mice transgenic for the human CD34 locus. *Blood* 1997; **90**(Suppl 1): 160a.
118. Miles C, Sanchez MJ, Sinclair A, Dzierzak E, Expression of the Ly-6E.1 (Sca-1) transgene in adult hematopoietic stem cells and the developing mouse embryo. *Development* 1997; **124:** 537–47.
119. Whitlock CA, Witte ON, Long-term culture of B lymphocytes and their precursors from murine bone marrow. *Proc Natl Acad Sci USA* 1982; **79:** 3608–12.
120. Whitlock CA, Ziegler SF, Witte ON, Progression of the transformed phenotype in clonal lines of Abelson virus-infected lymphocytes. *Mol Cell Biol* 1983; **3:** 596–604.
121. Scherle PA, Dorshkind K, Witte ON, Clonal lymphoid progenitor cell lines expressing the *BCR/ABL* oncogene retain full differentiative function. *Proc Natl Acad Sci USA* 1990; **87:** 1908–12.
122. Gishizky ML, Witte ON, *BCR/ABL* enhances growth of multipotent progenitor cells but does not block their differentiation potential in vitro. *Curr Top Microbiol Immunol* 1992; **182:** 65–72.
123. Heard JM, Roussel MF, Rettenmier CW, Sherr CJ, Multilineage hematopoietic disorders induced by transplantation of bone marrow cells expressing the v-*fms* oncogene. *Cell* 1987; **51:** 663–73.
124. Daley GQ, Van Etten RA, Baltimore D, Induction of chronic myelogenous leukemia in mice by the P210$^{bcr/abl}$ gene of the Philadelphia chromosome. *Science* 1990; **247:** 824–30.
125. Kelliher MA, McLaughlin J, Witte ON, Rosenberg N, Induction of a chronic myelogenous leukemia-like syndrome in mice with v-abl and bcr/abl. *Proc Natl Acad Sci USA* 1990; **87:** 6649–53.
126. Elefanty AG, Hariharan IK, Cory S, *bcr–abl*, the hallmark of chronic myeloid leukemia in man, induces multiple hematopoietic neoplasms in mice. *EMBO J* 1990; **9:** 1069–78.
127. Prince VE, Rigby PW, Derivatives of Moloney murine sarcoma virus capable of being transcribed in embryonal carcinoma cells have gained a functional Sp1 site. *J Virol* 1991; **65:** 1803–11.
128. Wieder R, Cornetta K, Kessler SW, Anderson WF, Increased efficiency of retroviral-mediated gene transfer and expression in primate bone marrow progenitors after 5-fluorouracil-induced hematopoietic suppression and recovery. *Blood* 1991; **77:** 448–55.
129. Risser R, Potter M, Rowe WP, Abelson virus-induced lymphomagenesis in mice. *J Exp Med* 1978; **148:** 714–26.
130. Elefanty AG, Cory S, Hematologic disease induced in BALB/c mice by a bcr/abl retrovirus is influenced by infection conditions. *Mol Cell Biol* 1992; **12:** 1755–63.
131. Daley GQ, Van Etten RA, Baltimore D, Blast crisis in a murine model of chronic myelogenous leukemia. *Proc Natl Acad Sci USA* 1991; **88:** 11335–8.
132. Gishizky MI, Johnson-White J, Witte ON, Efficient transplantation of *BCR–ABL*-induced chronic myelogenous leukemia-like syndrome in mice. *Proc Natl Acad Sci USA* 1993; **90:** 3755–9.
133. Tamura K, Araki Y, Makino S et al, Ph1+ malignant histiocytosis – a case report. *Nippon Ketsueki Gakkai Zasshi* 1988; **51:** 1063–8.
134. Piccinini L, Bonacorsi G, Artusi T, Blast crisis of Ph1-CML, with the prevalent features of malig-

nant histiocytosis. *Haematologica* 1998; **83:** 187–8.
135. Danos O, Mulligan RC, Safe and efficient generation of recombinant retroviruses with amphotropic and ecotropic host ranges. *Proc Natl Acad Sci USA* 1988; **85:** 6460–4.
136. Graham FL, Smiley J, Russell WC, Narin R, Characteristics of a human cell line transformed by DNA from human adenovirus type 5. *J Gen Virol* 1977; **36:** 59–74.
137. DuBridge RB, Tang P, Hsia HC et al, Analysis of mutation in human cells by using an Epstein–Barr virus shuttle system. *Mol Cell Biol* 1987; **7:** 379–87.
138. Pear WS, Nolan GP, Scott ML, Baltimore D, Production of high-titer helper-free retroviruses by transient transfection. *Proc Natl Acad Sci USA* 1993; **90:** 8392–6.
139. Finer MH, Dull TJ, Qin L et al, *kat*: a high-efficiency retroviral transduction system for primary human T lymphocytes. *Blood* 1994; **83:** 43–50.
140. Soneoka Y, Cannon PM, Ramsdale EE et al, A transient three-plasmid expression system for the production of high titer retroviral vectors. *Nucleic Acids Res* 1995; **23:** 628–33.
141. Bender MA, Palmer TD, Gelinas RE, Miller AD, Evidence that the packaging signal of Moloney murine leukemia virus extends into the *gag* region. *J Virol* 1987; **61:** 1639–6.
142. Petersen R, Kempler G, Barklis E, A stem cell-specific silencer in the primer-binding site of a retrovirus. *Mol Cell Biol* 1991; **11:** 1214–21.
143. Hawley RG, Lieu FHL, Fong AZC, Hawley TS, Versatile retroviral vectors for potential use in gene therapy. *Gene Therapy* 1994; **1:** 136–8.
144. Luskey BD, Rosenblatt M, Zsebo K, Williams DA, Stem cell factor, interleukin-3, and interleukin-6 promote retroviral-mediated gene transfer into murine hematopoietic stem cells. *Blood* 1992; **80:** 396–402.
145. Kotani H, Newton PB, Zhang S et al, Improved methods of retroviral vector transduction and production for gene therapy. *Hum Gene Ther* 1994; **5:** 19–28.
146. Hannenberg H, Xiao XL, Dilloo D et al, Colocalization of retrovirus and target cells on specific fibronectin fragments increases genetic transduction of mammalian cells. *Nature Med* 1996; **2:** 876–82.
147. Pear WS, Miller JP, Xu L et al, Efficient and rapid induction of a chronic myelogenous leukemia-like myeloproliferative disease in mice receiving P210 bcr/abl-transduced bone marrow. *Blood* 1998; **92:** 3780–92.
148. Zhang X, Ren R, Bcr–Abl efficiently induces a myeloproliferative disease and production of excess interleukin-3 and granulocyte-macrophage colony-stimulating factor in mice: a novel model for chronic myelogenous leukemia. *Blood* 1998; **92:** 3829–40.
149. Tidmarsh GF, Heimfeld S, Whitlock CA et al, Identification of a novel bone marrow-derived B-cell progenitor population that coexpresses B220 and Thy-1 and is highly enriched for Abelson leukemia virus targets. *Mol Cell Biol* 1989; **9:** 2665–71.
150. Palumbo GJ, Ozanne BW, Kettman JR, Multistage progression of Abelson virus-infected murine pre-B cells to the tumorigenic state. *Cancer Res* 1990; **50:** 1917–23.
151. Pear WS, Aster JC, Scott ML et al, Exclusive development of T cell neoplasms in mice transplanted with bone marrow expressing activated notch alleles. *J Exp Med* 1996; **183:** 2283–91.
152. Schwaller J, Frantsve J, Aster J et al, Transformation of hematopoietic cell lines to growth-factor independence and induction of a fatal myeloid- and lymphoproliferative disease in mice by retrovirally transduced *TEL/JAK2* fusion gene. *EMBO J* 1998; **17:** 5321–33.
153. Kroon E, Krosl J, Thorsteindottir U et al, Hoxa9 transforms primary bone marrow cells through specific collaboration with Meis1a but not Pbx1b. *EMBO J* 1998; **17:** 3714–25.
154. Skorski T, Bellacosa A, Nieborowska-Skorska M et al, Transformation of hematopoietic cells by BCR/ABL requires activation of a PI-3K/Akt-dependent pathway. *EMBO J* 1997; **16:** 6151–61.
155. Mountford PS, Smith AS, Internal ribosome entry sites and dicistronic RNAs in mammalian transgenesis. *Trends Genet* 1995; **11:** 179–84.
156. Gross AW, Zhang X, Ren R, Bcr–Abl with an SH3 deletion retains the ability to induce a myeloproliferative disease in mice, yet c-Abl activated by an SH3 deletion induces only lymphoid malignancy. *Mol Cell Biol* 1999; **19:** 6918–28.
157. Lange RD, Moloney WC, Yamawaki T, Leukemia in atomic bomb survivors. I. General observations. *Blood* 1954; **9:** 574–85.
158. Berman E, Strife A, Wisniewski D et al, Duration of the preclinical phase of chronic myelogenous leukemia: a case report. *Blood* 1991; **78:** 2969–72.

159. Pane F, Frigeri F, Sindona M et al, Neutrophilic-chronic myeloid leukemia: a distinct disease with a specific molecular marker (*BCR/ABL* with C3/A2 junction). *Blood* 1996; **88:** 2410–14.
160. Emilia G, Luppi M, Marasca R, Torelli G, Relationship between BCR/ABL fusion proteins and leukemia phenotype. *Blood* 1997; **89:** 3889.
161. Mittre H, Leymarie P, Macro M, Leporrier M, A new case of chronic myeloid leukemia with c3/a2 BCR/ABL junction. Is it really a distinct disease? *Blood* 1997; **89:** 4239–41.
162. Scott ML, Van Etten RA, Daley GQ, Baltimore D, v-*abl* causes hematopoietic disease distinct from that caused by *bcr–abl*. *Proc Natl Acad Sci USA* 1991; **88:** 6506–10.
163. Han X, Wong PMC, Chung S-W, Chronic myeloproliferative disease induced by site-specific integration of Abelson murine leukemia virus-infected hemopoietic stem cells. *Proc Natl Acad Sci USA* 1991; **88:** 10129–33.
164. Million RP, Van Etten RA, The Grb2 binding site is required for induction of chronic myeloid leukemia-like disease in mice by the Bcr/Abl tyrosine kinase. *Blood* 2000; **96:** 664–70.
165. Pear WS, Miller J, Xu LW et al, Murine models for studying the pathogenesis of chronic myelogenous leukemia. *Blood* 1997; **90**(Suppl 1): 393a.
166. Roumiantsev S, de Aos IE, Varticovski L et al, The Src homology 2 domain of Bcr/Abl is required for efficient induction of chronic myeloid leukemia-like disease in mice but not for lymphoid leukemogenesis or activation of phosphatidylinositol 3 kinase. *Blood* 2001; **97:** 4–13.
167. Hao SX, Ren R, Expression of interferon consensus sequence binding protein (ICSBP) is downregulated in Bcr–Abl-induced murine chronic myelogenous leukemia-like disease, and forced coexpression of ICSBP inhibits Bcr–Abl-induced myeloproliferative disorder. *Mol Cell Biol* 2000; **20:** 1149–61.
168. Skorski T, Nieborowska-Skorska M, Wlodarski P et al, Blastic transformation of p53-deficient bone marrow cells by p210$^{bcr/abl}$ tyrosine kinase. *Proc Natl Acad Sci USA* 1996; **93:** 13137–42.
169. Mach N, Lantz CS, Galli SJ et al, Involvement of interleukin-3 in delayed-type hypersensitivity. *Blood* 1998; **91:** 778–83.
170. Dranoff G, Crawford AD, Sadelain M et al, Involvement of granulocyte–macrophage colony-stimulating factor in pulmonary homeostasis. *Science* 1994; **264:** 713–16.
171. Li S, Gillessen S, Thomasson MH et al, Interleukin-3 and granulocyte-macrophage colony-stimulating factor are not required for induction of chronic myeloid leukemia-like myeloproliferative disease in mice by BCR/ABl. *Blood* 2001; **97:** 1442–500.
172. Kelliher M, Knott A, McLaughlin J et al, Differences in oncogenic potency but not target cell specificity distinguish the two forms of the *BCR/ABL* oncogene. *Mol Cell Biol* 1991; **11:** 4710–16.
173. Eva T, Witte ON, regulated expression of P210 Bcr-Abl during embryonic stem cell differentiation stimulates multipotential progenitor expansion and myeloid cell fate. *Proc Natl Acad Sci USA* 2000; **97:** 1737–42.

Part 2

Conventional treatment for chronic myeloid leukaemia

7

Biology of interferon

Thomas Fischer, Moshe Talpaz

CONTENTS • Introduction • Interferon genes and proteins • The IFN-α receptor • IFN-α signal transduction • Direct effects of IFN-α involved in control of cell growth • Indirect mechanisms involved in growth control of malignant hematopoiesis by IFN-α • Molecular mechanisms of clinical resistance to IFN-α • Perspectives

INTRODUCTION

Interferons (IFNs) were first described as potent antiviral agents in 1957 by Isaacs and Lindenmann.[1] They were later shown to have pleiotropic functions not only in antiviral control but also in control of cell proliferation and in modulation of the immune system. The discovery that IFNs inhibit the growth of normal and malignant hematopoietic cells in vitro and in vivo led to pivotal phase I clinical studies using recombinant IFN-α in 1982.[2] IFNs were the first cytokines made available for clinical trials in cancer patients. Since then, the antitumor activity of IFN-α has been well documented in a variety of solid and hematologic malignancies. Today, recombinant IFN-α is approved worldwide in over 40 countries for the therapy of a variety of malignant and viral diseases, including condyloma acuminata, hepatitis B and C, non-Hodgkin's lymphoma, and chronic myeloid leukemia (CML).[3] However, the precise mechanism by which IFN-α works in the therapy of malignancies is still unknown. The same holds for our knowledge of the molecular mechanism of clinical resistance to IFN-α. This chapter will highlighten signal transduction of IFN-α and some of the direct and indirect effects that are believed to play an important role in control of cell growth and in the clinical response to IFN-α.

INTERFERON GENES AND PROTEINS

There are two major classes of human IFNs: type I and type II (Table 7.1). By virtue of binding to a common type I receptor, type I IFNs are represented by IFN-α, IFN-β, and IFN-ω. Type II IFN, IFN-γ, binds to a distinct type II receptor.[4] There are 21 distinct IFN-α genes and 4 IFN-α pseudo-genes. IFN-β, IFN-ω, and IFN-γ are represented by a single gene.[4] IFN-α proteins consist of approximately 170 amino acids and are partially homologous in their amino acid sequences (about 75–80%). They show a high level of species specificity in binding to the type I IFN receptor.[4]

Biosynthesis of IFN-α is induced by viruses, some bacteria, mycoplasma, and protozoa.[5] In addition, double-stranded (ds) RNA generated during viral replication is a classical stimulus of IFN-α biosynthesis.[5] Some cytokines and growth factors, such as interleukin-1 (IL-1), IL-2, tumor necrosis factor α (TNF-α), and macrophage colony-stimulating factor (M-CSF, CSF-1), are also able to induce IFN-α. There is a

Table 7.1 Interferons

	Type I	Type II
Subtypes	α1–22 β ω	γ
Genes	27	1
Amino acids	165–166	143
pH-stability	Stable	Labile
Source	Leukocytes, fibroblasts	T cells, NK cells
Receptors	IFN-αR1 IFN-αR2c	IFN-γR1 IFN-γR2

stringent transcriptional control of IFN-α synthesis, which is mediated via activation of so-called PRDI elements located in the promoters of IFN-α genes.[5]

THE IFN-α RECEPTOR

IFN-α, IFN-β and IFN-ω bind to a common type I IFN receptor.[3,6] Two subunits of the human IFN-α receptor have been identified to date: IFN-αR1 and IFN-αR2. IFN-αR1 is a 110 kDa protein consisting of 557 amino acids with a 21-amino-acid transmembrane segment and a 100-amino-acid cytoplasmic domain.[3,6] The encoding sequence of IFN-αR1 was identified by Uze et al[7] in 1990. It has subsequently been shown that a null mutation in the IFN-αR1 gene eliminates antiproliferative and antiviral responses to IFN-α and IFN-β.[8,9] The major ligand-binding component of the IFN-α receptor is IFN-αR2. IFN-αR2 exists in three distinct forms, which represent differentially spliced isoforms of the same IFN-αR2 gene. The largest form, IFN-αR2c, is composed of 515 amino acids and is the functional receptor in IFN-α signaling. The short form of the receptor is IFN-αR2a, whereas IFN-αR2b represents a soluble form.[3]

IFN-α SIGNAL TRANSDUCTION

In recent years significant progress has been made in elucidating the molecular mechanisms of IFN signaling (for reviews, see references 3 and 10–18).

The first step in the sequence of molecular events elicited by binding of IFN-α to the IFN-αR2 chain is oligomerization of receptor chains. IFN-αR1 and IFN-αR2 are constitutively associated with the Janus kinases (Jaks) Tyk2 and Jak1, respectively. Oligomerization of IFN-α receptor chains results in activation of these kinases, which become cross-phosphorylated on tyrosine residues. In addition, Jak1 and Tyk2 phosphorylate tyrosine residues on the cytoplasmic domains of the IFN-α receptor chains, activating specific docking sites for cytoplasmic STAT (signal transducer and activator of transcription) proteins. STAT2 then docks to the Tyk2-phosphorylated tyrosine 466 of IFN-αR1 and itself becomes phosphorylated by Tyk2 at tyrosine 690. Next, STAT1 binds to receptor-associated phosphorylated STAT2 and is phosphorylated at tyrosine 701. As a consequence of these events, STAT1–STAT1 homodimers and STAT1–STAT2 heterodimers are formed and translocate to the nucleus. Here, STAT1–STAT2 heterodimers associate with the p48 protein, a member of the IRF (IFN regulatory factors) family. This trimeric complex is called ISGF3 (IFN-stimulated gene factor 3), and binds to its specific recognition site within the promoter of

ISGs (IFN-stimulated genes) (Figure 7.1). The recognition sites specific for ISGF3 are termed the ISRE (IFN-stimulated response element) and are characterized by the consensus sequence GAAAN(N)GAAA. This consensus sequence is necessary and sufficient to mediate IFN-α activation of transcription. Cytoplasmic phospholipase A2 has also been show to be involved in activation of ISRE-containing genes. Some IFN-α-induced genes such as *IRF1* do not contain the ISRE sequence but rather the palindromic GAS (gamma-IFN activation site) sequence TTNNNNNAA. This sequence is recognized by STAT1 homodimers, thereby controlling transcription of GAS-dependent genes (Figure 7.1).

In addition to the Jak–STAT pathway, other Jak–dependent signaling elements are also activated by IFN-α (for a review, see reference 15). It has been described that IFN-α activates the phosphatidylinositol 3′-kinase (PI3-K) kinase pathway by inducing rapid and transient tyrosine phosphorylation of IRS1, a member of the insulin receptor substrate (IRS) signaling system.[19,20] IFN-α tyrosine-phosphorylated IRS1 would then associate with the p85 regulatory subunit of PI3-K, resulting in activation of its catalytic subunit.[19,20] Interestingly, all members of the IRS family have multiple tyrosine phosphorylation sites on binding motifs for the SH2 domains of various signaling molecules such as

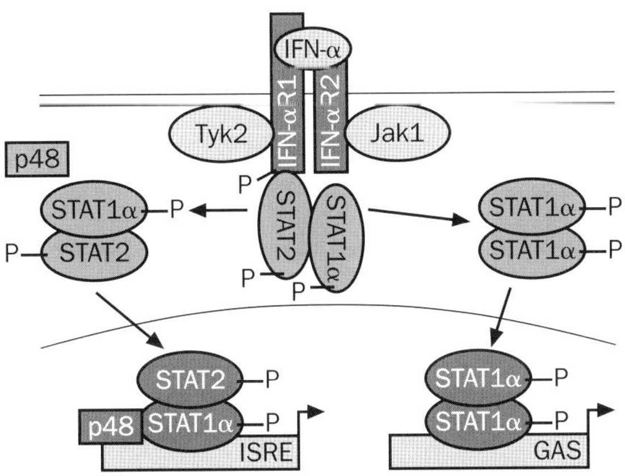

Figure 7.1 IFN-α signaling.

Grb2 and SHPTP2 phosphatase or for the above-described p85 subunit of PI3-K. Cbl ($p120^{Cbl}$) appears to be another signaling element that functions as an adapter protein in IFN-α signaling. Cbl associates with Tyk2 and undergoes phosphorylation in a type I IFN-dependent manner.[21] It then serves as a docking site for the Src family kinase Fyn and the Crkl adapter. As a result, Crkl becomes tyrosine-phosphorylated by IFN-α – an event that has been implicated in generation of the antiproliferative effects of IFNs.

In this context, it is interesting to note that Crkl has been identified recently as a nuclear adapter protein for STAT5.[22] According to this report, STAT5 constitutively associates with type I IFN-receptor-associated Tyk2 kinase and becomes tyrosine-phosphorylated upon IFN stimulation. Crkl then binds to STAT5 via its SH2 domain, and the resulting complex has been shown to regulate gene transcription of certain IFN-stimulated genes.

Another intriguing observation regarding non-Jak–STAT signaling molecules involved in type I IFN signal transduction is that Vav undergoes rapid tyrosine phosphorylation in response to type I IFN stimulation.[23] This phosphorylation appears to be mediated by Tyk2, with which Vav is constitutively associated.

While the mechanisms of generation of IFN-induced signals are well understood, little is known about the mechanisms of signal attenuation. Potential mechanisms include inhibition of phosphorylation or dephosphorylation of Jak kinases, IFN receptor chains and STAT proteins. SH2-domain-containing protein–tyrosine phosphatases (SHPTPs) are attractive candidates for such regulatory functions. Two members of this phosphatase family, SHPTP1 and SHPTP2, have been identified in mammalian cells and have been implicated in modulation of signals induced by type I IFNs.[24,25] SHPTP1 (PTP1C, HCP, SHP-1) is expressed primarily in hematopoietic cells. Lack of SHPTP1 as in *me/me* (motheaten) mice[26] leads to uncontrolled proliferation of hematopoetic cells, suggesting that its phosphatase activity is regulating signaling of cytokines that promote cell growth.[27,28]

Subsequent studies showed that SHPTP1 selectively regulates distinct components of Jak–STAT signaling pathways.[29] SHPTP1 reversibly associates with the type I IFN receptor complex upon IFN stimulation. In comparison with controls, *me/me* cells show hyperphosphorylation of Jak1 and STAT1 tyrosine residues, whereas Tyk2 and STAT2 activation remains largely unchanged.[29] Thus, SHPTP1 appears to play a role in regulating type I IFN responses.

SHPTP2 (Syp, PTP1D, PTP2C, SHP-2) is tyrosine-phosphorylated upon stimulation with a number of cytokines, including IL-6, granulocyte–macrophage colony-stimulating factor (GM-CSF), IL-3,[30] erythropoietin (EPO),[31] and IFN-α. A recent study showed that SHPTP2 functions as a negative regulator of the IFN-stimulated Jak–STAT pathway, although its precise role in cytokine signaling has not yet been defined.[32]

DIRECT EFFECTS OF IFN-α INVOLVED IN CONTROL OF CELL GROWTH

In the following, we shall discuss direct antiproliferative effects of IFN-α that may play a role in the successful treatment of CML. The molecular targets and mechanisms crucially involved in the control of malignant cell growth by IFN-α in CML are unknown. IFN-α can exhibit direct antiproliferative effects on a variety of cell types. The mechanisms involved include control of cell cycle transition, modulation of apoptosis, and induction of IFN-dependent genes directly involved in growth control. In addition, in hematopoietic progenitor cells, IFN-α has been show to exert inhibitory effects on clonogenic growth, and is profoundly involved in the regulation of adhesion molecules.

Effects on cell cycle transition and function of cell cycle regulatory elements

Cell cycle transition and DNA replication is a tightly controlled process regulated by a large number of cell cycle regulatory proteins (reviewed in references 33–37). In mammalian cells, G_1 cyclins, cyclin-dependent kinases (Cdks), and their regulatory kinases and phosphatases are involved in regulation of G_1–S phase transition. This regulation is controlled by signals deriving from growth factors, thereby driving the cell cycle. The final common pathway in G_1 phase is phosphorylation of Rb, the product of the retinoblastoma gene *Rb*.

Since the original discoveries of Tiefenbrun et al[38] and Zhang and Kumar[39] on the effects of IFN-α on cell cycle regulatory elements, it has been well documented that IFN-α profoundly affects G_1–S phase transition. The general theme in molecular events can be summarized by upregulation of Cdk inhibitors (such as p21 or p15) at a transcriptional level, followed by subsequent inhibition of Cdks such as Cdk2 or Cdk4.[40,41] This inhibition is due to increased association of Cdk inhibitors to their cognate Cdk binding partner. As a result, G_1 cyclin/Cdk-associated kinase activities are suppressed by IFN-α (Figure 7.2). In parallel, IFN-α suppresses G_1 cyclin levels at an mRNA level, and downregulates Cdc25A phosphatase.[38] As a consequence, IFN-α treatment results in increased expression of underphosphorylated Rb[39,42,43] and in alterations of expression and phosphorylation of other pocket proteins, such as p130 and p107.[43] This then leads to formation of E2F4–Rb and E2F4–p130 complexes, which

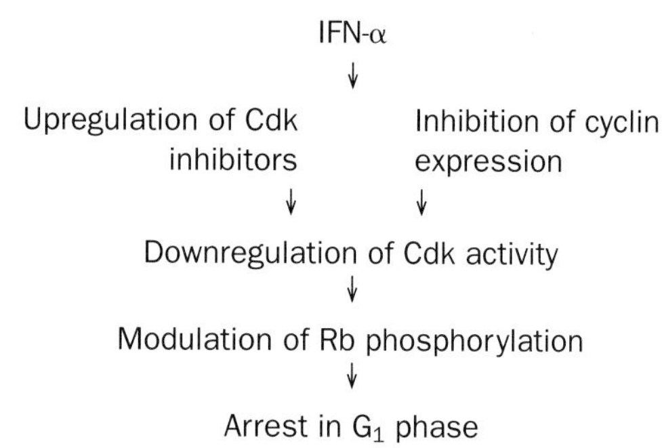

Figure 7.2 Effects of IFN-α on cell cycle transition and function of cell cycle regulatory elements.

transcriptionally repress the *E2F1* gene.[42] In addition, effects of IFN-α on p53[44] and c-Myc[38] have been described. Examples of these actions of IFN-α have been described in many cell lines and molecular scenarios, strengthening the view that IFN-α leads to a reversible G_0-like arrest.

Modulation of apoptosis

IFNs are crucially involved in the development of immunologic responses to viruses and other microbial pathogens. Negative and positive selection of immune effector cells often involves apoptosis. Depending on the cellular context, IFNs may either stimulate or inhibit apoptotic processes. Stimulation of apoptosis appears to be involved in the growth-inhibitory effects of IFN-α.[11] IFN-α has been shown to increase CD95 ligand (Fas ligand)-induced apoptosis via activation of caspase 3.[45] Another mechanism involved in stimulation of CD95 (Fas)-induced apoptosis is upregulation of caspase protein levels.[46] Interestingly, IFN-α also upregulates phospholipid scramblase I (PLSCR-I) at a transcriptional level.[47] This effect by itself is not accompanied by increased cell surface exposure of phosphatidylserine. Thus, IFN-α may also have a modulatory function in apoptosis via regulation of PLSCR-I protein levels.

Induction of PKR and RNaseL

The double-stranded RNA (dsRNA)-dependent IFN-induced protein kinase (PKR) is involved in mediating antiproliferative activities of IFN-α (for reviews, see references 11 and 48). Activated PKR phosphorylates eIF-2, thereby inhibiting protein synthesis. Inducible expression of wild-type but not kinase-inactive PKR results in inhibition of growth in a yeast model. Mutant PKR proteins have been shown to induce tumor formation. In addition, PKR plays an important role as a signal transducer. It is activated by extracellular signals such as dsRNA, lipopolysaccharide (LPS), and different cytokines, and it phosphorylates intracellular targets.

I-κB, the inhibitor of the transcription factor NF-κB, has been identified as a prominent target of PKR. PKR is also involved in mediating apoptosis and induction of cell adhesion molecules. The IFN-inducible RNaseL[49] and the 2-5A system[49] have also been implicated as playing a role in apoptosis, since expression of a dominant-negative RNaseL mutant inhibited apoptosis.[11]. Induction of PKR, RNaseL, and 2-5 OA synthetase[11] has been shown to be induced by IFN-α in CML cells both in vitro and in vivo.[50]

Direct effects of IFN-α on hematopoietic progenitors

Recently, it has been shown that in co-cultures of CML progenitors with endothelial cells, IFN-α inhibited the generation of clonogenic cells. In contrast, in co-cultures of normal progenitors with endothelial cells, IFN-α increased the generation of clonogenic cells via upregulation of Flt3 ligand by endothelial cells.[51]

IFN-α also inhibits the clonogenic output in flask long-term cultures. After 8 weeks of long-term culture, the percentage of Philadelphia chromosome (Ph)-positive nucleated cells produced was significantly more inhibited by IFN-α in responding patients than in non-responders.[52] In addition, a recent study showed that IFN-α inhibits amplification of CML, but not normal, granulocyte–macrophage colony-forming units (CFU-GM) in vitro.[53] Direct inhibition of megakaryopoiesis by IFN-α was shown to be mediated via inhibition of thrombopoietin (TPO)-induced megakaryocyte growth. In a TPO-dependent hematopoietic cell line, IFN-α suppressed TPO-induced phosphorylation of c-Mpl and STAT5.[54] Interestingly, the molecular mechanism involved was induction of SOCS-I.[54]

Another mechanism possibly involved in restoration of normal hematopoesis in CML is regulation of cell adhesion.[55] In normal hematopoiesis, adhesive interactions between progenitor cells and stroma or extracellular matrix components are involved in the growth control of progenitors. In fact, at the level of progenitor cells, growth control appears to be the result of concerted action of cytokine and adhesive interactions.

Extracellular matrix is produced by stromal cells, which include endothelial cells, fibroblasts, osteoblasts, and macrophages, and consists of fibronectin, hyaluronic acid, integrins, and other components. Integrins are cell surface glycoproteins responsible for cell–cell and cell–matrix interactions. Stromal cells also express cell surface adhesive ligands, such as vascular cell adhesion molecule 1 (VCAM-1).[56]

CML progenitor cells have been found to exhibit several defects in adhesion functions. *BCR/ABL*-positive cytotoxic T lymphocytes (CTL) and long-term culture-initiating cells (LTC-IC) adhere significantly less to stromal cells and to fibronectin than normal progenitors.[55,57,58] In addition, a number of studies have indicated that growth of *BCR/ABL*-positive progenitors is not inhibited by contact with stromal cells.[59,60] Together, these data suggest that CML cells have a defective interaction with the bone marrow microenvironment. IFN-α has been shown to restore the fibronectin- and integrin-dependent adhesion functions of CML progenitors.[59] IFN-α treatment also results in restoration of adhesion-mediated inhibition of progenitor proliferation.[59]

INDIRECT MECHANISMS INVOLVED IN GROWTH CONTROL OF MALIGNANT HEMATOPOIESIS BY IFN-α

Indirect mechanisms potentially involved in the suppression of *BCR/ABL*-positive hematopoiesis by IFN-α include regulation of effector mechanisms exerted by the immune system and modulation of cytokine synthesis. Regarding the latter, it has been postulated that a finely tuned balance of positive and negative regulatory cytokines is involved in growth control of normal and malignant hematopoiesis.[61] This control is of particular importance for stem cell renewal, sustained hematopoiesis, and regulation of differentiation, and takes place at the level of interaction of hematopoietic cells with bone marrow stromal cells.

Bone marrow stromal cells have been found to produce a variety of cytokines and hematopoietic growth factors, such as IL-7, IL-11, stem cell factor (SCF, Steel factor),[62–64] and GM-CSF.[65,66] These factors are produced in small but biologically relevant amounts, and have a stimulatory effect on hematopoiesis. In addition, bone marrow stromal cells are able to secrete negative regulators, such as transforming growth factor β (TGF-β) and TNF-α.[67] IFN-α substantially inhibits the production of cytokines with stimulatory effect on hematopoiesis, such as GM-CSF, IL-1β, and granulocyte colony-stimulating factor (G-CSF).[61] On the other hand, it plays a role in the control of IL-1-mediated stimulatory effects by upregulating the production of IL-1 receptor antagonist (IL-1RA) by stromal cells.[61] Thus, these results indicate that the myelosuppressive effects of IFN-α are in part mediated by regulating humoral factors in the bone marrow microenvironment.

In comparison with type II IFN (IFN-γ), the immune-modulatory functions of type I IFNs are generally believed to be more restricted. However, genetic approaches using gene knockouts have clearly demonstrated that, in addition to IFN-γ, IFN-α profoundly affects the development of innate and adaptive immune responses. IFN-α exerts these functions basically by two mechanisms: it modulates the growth, differentiation, and function of various immunological effector cells (Table 7.2), and it regulates the ability of these effector cells to interact with infected or malignant cells.[3] Regarding the former mechanism, IFN-α has been described to exert either positive or negative influence on the activation of T cells.[68–70] A recent report describes that IFN-α reduces IL-2 production and IL-2 receptor function on primary $CD4^+$ T cells.[69] The mechanism involved is downregulation of CD3 and CD28 surface expression, which results in diminished phosphorylation of the mitogen-activated extracellu-

Table 7.2 Pleiotropic effects of IFN-α on the immune system*

- Increases in membrane antigens, especially class I MHC antigens and cellular adhesion molecules, on tumor cells and effector cells
- Promotion of differentiation of various lymphoid cells
- Activation of effector cells:
  - Augmentation of NK cell activity
  - Activation of macrophages
  - Stimulation of generation of immune T cells (weak relative to IFN-γ)
- Effects on multiple functions of lymphoid cells:
  - Cytotoxicity
  - Cytokine production
  - Possible alteration of homing patterns in vivo
- Effects on proliferation of lymphoid cells
  - Inhibition of proliferation of activated lymphocytes in vitro
  - Increase in number of NK cells in vivo

*Adapted with permission from Pfeffer LM, Dinarello CA, Herberman RB et al, *Cancer Research* 1998; **58:** 2489–99.[3]

lar signal-regulated activating kinase. In another study, IFN-α was found to inhibit proliferation of human T cells by abrogation of IL-2-induced changes in cell cycle regulatory proteins.[70] IFN-α prevented upregulation of G_1 cyclins and Cdks, as well as abrogating mitogen-induced reduction of $p27^{Kip1}$ levels. This latter effect was due to stabilization of p27 protein in IFN-α-treated cells. IFN-α has been shown to upregulate IL-2Rα, c-Myc and Pim-1 in anti-CD3-activated human T lymphocytes, and it sensitizes T cells to IL-2-induced proliferation and enhances tyrosine phosphorylation of STAT1, -3, -4, -5a, and 5b.[68] This is in line with results of a recent report describing that IFN-α may act in synergy with signals from the T-cell antigen receptor. The common pathway involved is induction of STAT1 transcriptional activity.[71] In this context, it is interesting to note that CML patients and normal controls reveal significant differences in the cytokine patterns of T-cell subsets.[72] A recent study investigated the cytokine pattern of phorbol-ester-activated $CD4^+$ and $CD8^+$ T-cell subsets of 81 CML patients and 21 normal controls using intracellular staining and flow-cytometric analysis. The percentages of $CD4^+$ and $CD8^+$ T cells from CML patients synthesizing the Th1 cytokines IL-2, IFN-γ, and TNF-α were significantly lower than those of patients in remission and of normal controls.[72]

The main mechanism enhancing interaction between immune effector cells and their target cells is IFN-α-induced upregulation of MHC class I antigen and adhesion molecule expression. IRF1, a pleiotropic immediate IFN-α response gene, is the main transcription factor in the control of MHC class I antigen expression. IFN-α-induced expression of MHC class I can be inhibited by other cytokines through suppression of IFN-α-stimulated IRF1 synthesis.[73] The role of MHC regulation as a potential mechanism in clearing malignant cells by T-cell immunity was stressed in a recent study.[74] Interestingly, a strong correlation between the presence of T cells specifically recognizing a peptide (PR1) from proteinase 3 and clinical responses after IFN-α therapy has been described. Proteinase 3 is a myeloid-tissue-restricted serine protease that is overexpressed by two- to fivefold in CML cells. It has been shown that the appearance of PR1-specific CTL correlates with a cytogenetic response to IFN-α. It has been suggested[74] that IFN-α may induce

Table 7.3 Effects of IFN-α on the activity of NK cells*

• Effector phase:
Increase in binders (seen with only some targets)
Non-lytic binders activated to lytic activity
Accelerated kinetics
Recycling (lysis of multiple targets)
• Effects on target cells:
Decreased susceptibility to NK cells (seen with only some targets)
IL-2-dependent growth:
Increased response to IL-2
Introduction of T-cell-dependent growth inhibition

*Adapted with permission from Pfeffer LM, Dinarello CA, Herberman RB et al, *Cancer Research* 1998; **58:** 2489–99.[3]

remissions by facilitating the expansion of autologous leukemia-reactive CTL. This may occur by upregulation of MHC class I or tumor antigens in the leukemic cells, thereby precipitating an immune response.[74]

In addition to the effects described above, IFN-α has been shown to enhance the cytotoxic activity of natural killer (NK) cells. Table 7.3 lists the main pathways suggested to contribute to this immunological effector mechanism.[3]

MOLECULAR MECHANISMS OF CLINICAL RESISTANCE TO IFN-α

It has been well established in cell lines that resistance to IFN-α can be linked to defects in signal transduction elements and to defective modulation of G_1 cell cycle regulatory elements. For example in IFN-resistant Daudi cells, IFN-induced STAT1 and Jak phosphorylation was partially reduced.[75] In parallel, these cells overexpress JAB, an inhibitor of the Janus kinases Jak1, Jak2, and Tyk2. This is in line with a recent observation that mutant cell lines resistant to IFN-α/β are defective in tyrosine phosphorylation of ISGF3 components.[76]

In lymphoid cell lines, IFN-α upregulates p21, p15, and p27, thereby suppressing G_1 Cdk activity.[43] As a result, phosphorylation of Rb and of other pocket proteins, such as p130 and p107, is inhibited.[43] Lymphoid cell lines featuring homozygous deletions of *p15* and *p16* genes and lacking p21 protein are resistant to IFN-α and show no effect of IFN-α on p27 expression or on pocket proteins. Lack of significant regulation of $p27^{Kip1}$ mRNA levels was also described in an IFN-α resistant small cell lung cancer cell line.[77] In this context, it is interesting to note that selection against the IFN-α/β system may also play a role in development of the malignant phenotype. Leukemic cell lines with alterations of IFN-α/β genes are also frequently resistant to the antiproliferative effects of IFN-α.[78]

In primary tumor cells, resistance to the antiproliferative actions of IFN-α may also be partly due to defects in signaling. In melanoma cells resistant to growth inhibition by IFN-α, defective Jak–STAT signal transduction has been described. This includes deficiencies in ISGF3 compounds such as STAT1, STAT2, and p48–ISGF3γ.[79] In hairy cell leukemia, defective IFN-α receptor internalization could be connected to IFN-α resistance.[80] However, it is not clear from the literature whether the above-described defects in signaling and cell cycle regulatory elements account for the vast majority of IFN-α-resistant cases in the treatment of lymphoma and melanoma patients.

In CML, a more thorough investigation of molecular mechanisms involved in primary or secondary resistance to IFN-α has been performed by several groups.[50,81,82] It is clear from these investigations that the vast majority of CML patients resistant clinically to IFN-α show no major defects in IFN-α induced activation of IFN-α signal transduction. Both IFN-α signaling pathways – ISGF3-dependent and STAT1-homodimer-dependent – were shown to be functional in primary *BCR/ABL* positive cells from these patients.[50] IFN-α-stimulated induction of IRF1, IRF2, PKR, RNaseL, 2-5 OAS, and other ISGs could be documented, ruling out

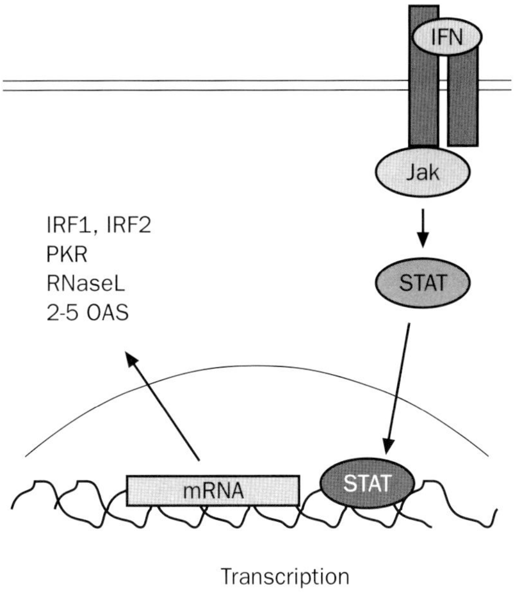

Figure 7.3 IFN-stimulated genes are inducible by IFN-α in clinically resistant CML patients.

major structural and functional deficiencies in signal transduction elements, such as lack of STATs or ISGF3 (Figure 7.3).[50]

This was independent of the state of differentiation and clonal evolution. However, these studies do not rule out that inhibition of IFN-α signaling at the level of hematopoietic progenitor cells may be a cause of the development of clinical resistance to IFN-α. It has recently been shown that growth factors such as GM-CSF suppress IFN-α signaling by a block in the activation of STAT1 DNA binding.[73] In this context, it is interesting to note that the phosphorylation and DNA-binding capacity of STAT1 has been described as representing a critical variable in malignant cell responsiveness to IFN-α therapy.[83]

Since GM-CSF is part of an autocrine loop in *BCR/ABL*-positive disease, it is intriguing to speculate that the above-described mechanism points to a potential molecular effect interfering with IFN-α-induced actions at the level of hematopoietic progenitors. In this scenario, insufficient activation of IFN signaling pathways would be at least partly involved in clinical resistance to IFN-α. Potential mediators include cytokines such as GM-CSF or IL-10. The latter has been described as being predominantly expressed in T-cell populations from CML patients.[72]

Development of autoantibodies to IFN-α has also been implicated in clinical resistance. However, detection of these antibodies and their quantification has been flawed by nonstandardized assay methodology.[3] Current concepts do not provide indications that autoantibodies to IFN-α may generally be of major relevance for the induction of clinically resistant disease.

PERSPECTIVES

IFN-α has been shown to directly exert inhibitory effects on malignant cell growth and to participate in elimination of malignant cells by stimulating specific T-cell immunity. In CML, IFN-α has been demonstrated to induce inhibition of the *BCR/ABL*-positive clone, resulting in hematologic and cytogenetic remissions. However, in many CML patients, therapy with IFN-α does not control the malignant clone sufficiently or is associated with intolerable side-effects. Combination of IFN-α with chemotherapeutic agents such as cytosine arabinoside has shown superior results in comparison with IFN-α therapy alone. However, this approach resulted in increased toxicity, and subsequent studies could not reproduce superior results. STI571 (Glivec), a specific tyrosine kinase inhibitor, suppresses malignant hematopoiesis in CML very efficiently by inducing apoptosis of *BCR/ABL*-positive cells (see Chapters 33 and 34). It is tempting to speculate that combination therapy with STI571 and IFN-α may be a curative approach in some patients by bringing together the effects of T-cell immunity with a direct apoptotic effect on Ph-positive cells.

REFERENCES

1. Isaacs A, Lindenmann J, Virus interference. I. The interferon. *Proc R Soc Lond, Ser B* 1957; **147:** 258.
2. Balkwill F, The interferons. In: *Cytokines in Cancer Therapy*, Oxford: Oxford University Press 1989: 8.
3. Pfeffer LM, Dinarello CA, Herberman RB et al, Biological properties of recombinant α-interferons: 40th anniversary of the discovery of interferons. *Cancer Res* 1998; **58:** 2489–99.
4. Pestka S, Lander JA, Zoon KC, Samuel CE, Interferons and their actions. *Annu Rev Biochem* 1987; **56:** 727.
5. Sen, GC, Lengyel P, The interferon system. *J Biol Chem* 1997; **267:** 5017–20.
6. Pestka S, The interferon receptors. *Semin Oncol* 1997; **24:** 9.
7. Uzé G, Lutfalla G, Gresser I, Genetic transfer of a functional human interferon α receptor into mouse cells; cloning and expression of its cDNA. *Cell* 1990; **60:** 225–34.
8. Müller U, Steinhoff U, Reis LF et al, Functional role of type I and type II interferons in antiviral defense. *Science* 1994; **264:** 1918–21.
9. Hwang SY, Hertzog PJ, Holland KA et al, A null mutation in the gene encoding a type I interferon receptor component eliminates antiproliferative and antiviral responses to interferon α and β and alters macrophage responses. *Proc Natl Acad Sci USA* 1995; **92:** 11284–8.
10. Borden EC, Waalen J, Schreiber R, Williams B, Response and resistance to interferons and interacting cytokines. *J Natl Cancer Inst* 1995; **87:** 257–64.
11. Stark GR, Kerr IM, Williams BRG, Silverman RH, Schreiber RD, How cells respond to interferons. *Annu Rev Biochem* 1998; **67:** 227–64.
12. Haque SJ, Williams BRG, Signal transduction in the interferon system. *Semin Oncol* 1998; **25**(1, Suppl 1): 14–22.
13. Williams BRG, Transcriptional regulation of interferon-stimulated genes. *Eur J Biochem* 1991; **200:** 1–11.
14. Williams BRG, Signal transduction and transcriptional regulation of interferon-α-stimulated genes. *J Interferon Res* 1991; **11:** 207–13.
15. Platanias LC, Fish EN, Signaling pathways activated by interferons. *Exp Hematol* 1999; **27:** 1583–92.
16. Ransohoff RM, Cellular responses to interferons and other cytokines: the JAK–STAT paradigm. *N Engl J Med* 1998; **338:** 616.
17. Ihle JN, Witthuhn BA, Quelle FW et al, Signaling by the cytokine receptor superfamily: JAKs and STATs. *Trends Biochem Sci* 1994; **19:** 222–7.
18. Darnell JE Jr, Kerr IM, Stark GR, JAK–STAT pathways and transcriptional activation in response to IFNs and other extracellular signaling proteins. *Science* 1993; **264:** 1415.
19. Uddin S, Yenush L, Sun X-J et al, Interferon α engages the insulin receptor substance-1 to associate with the phosphatidylinositol 3'-kinase. *J Biol Chem* 1995; **270:** 15938.
20. Uddin S, Fish EN, Sher DA et al, Activation of the phosphatidylinositol 3'- kinase serine kinase by IFNα. *J Immunol* 1997; **158:** 2390.
21. Uddin S, Gardziola C, Dangat A et al, Interaction of the c-cbl proto-oncogene product with the Tyk-2 protein tyrosine kinase. *Biochem Biophys Res Commun* 1996; **225:** 833.
22. Fish EN, Uddin S, Korkmaz M et al, Activation of a CrkL–Stat5 signaling complex by type I interferons. *J Biol Chem* 1999; **274:** 571.
23. Platanias LC, Sweet ME, Interferon α induces rapid tyrosine phosphorylation of the vav proto-oncogene product in hematopoietic cells. *J Biol Chem* 1994; **269:** 3143.
24. Feng GS, Pawson T, Phosphotyrosine phosphatases with Sh2 domains: regulators of signal transduction. *Trends Genet* 1994; **10:** 54–8.
25. Neel BG, Structure and function of SH2-domain containing tyrosine phosphatase. *Cell Biol* 1993; **4:** 419–43.
26. Tsui HW, Siminovitch KA, DeSouza L, Tsui FW, Motheaten and viable motheaten mice have mutations in the hematopoietic cell phosphatase gene. *Nature Genet* 1993; **4:** 124–9.
27. Kingmuller U, Lorenz U, Cantley LC et al, Specific recruitment of SH-PTP1 to the erythropoietin receptor causes inactivation of JAK2 and termination of proliferative signals. *Cell* 1995; **80:** 729–38.
28. Yi T, Mui ALF, Krystal G, Ihle J, Hematopoietic cell phosphatase associates with the interleukin-3 (IL-3) receptor β chain and down-regulates IL-3-induced tyrosine phosphorylation and mitogenesis. *Mol Cell Biol* 1993; **13:** 7577–86.
29. David M, Chen HE, Goelz S, Differential regulation of the alpha/beta interferon-stimulated Jak/Stat pathway by the SH2 domain-containing tyrosine phosphatase SHPTP1. *Mol Cell Biol* 1995; **15:** 7050–8.

30. Welham MJ, Dechert U, Leslie KB et al, Interleukin (IL)-3 and granulocyte/macrophage colony-stimulating factor, but not IL-4, induced tyrosine phosphorylation activation and association of SHPTP2 with Grb2 and phosphatidylinositol 3'- kinase. *J Biol Chem* 1994; **269:** 23764–8.
31. Tauchi T, Feng GS, Shen R et al, Involvement of SH2-containing phosphotyrosine phosphatase Syp in erythropoietin receptor signal transduction pathways. *J Biol Chem* 1995; **270:** 5631–5.
32. You M, Yu DH, Feng GS, Shp-2 tyrosine phosphatase functions as a negative regulator of the interferon-stimulated JAK/STAT pathway. *Mol Cell Biol* 1999; **19:** 2416.
33. Sherr CH, Mammalian G_1 cyclins. *Cell* 1993; **73:** 1059–65
34. Weinberg RA, The retinoblastoma protein and cell cycle control. *Cell* 1995; **81:** 323–30
35. Lewin B, Driving the cell cycle: M phase kinase, its partners, and substrates. *Cell* 1990; **61:** 743–52.
36. Sherr CJ, G1 phase progression: cycling on cue. *Cell* 1994; **79:** 551–5.
37. Nurse P, Ordering S phase and M phase on the cell cycle. *Cell* 1994; **79:** 547–50
38. Tiefenbrun N, Melamed D, Levy N et al, Alpha interferon suppresses the cyclin D3 and cdc25A genes, leading to a reversible G_0-like arrest. *Mol Cell Biol* 1996; **16:** 3934–44.
39. Zhang K, Kumar R, Interferon-α inhibits cyclin E- and cyclin D1-dependent CDK-2 kinase activity associated with RB protein and E2F in daudi cells. *Biochem Biophys Res Commun* 1994; **200:** 522–8.
40. Sangfelt O, Erickson S, Einhorn S, Grandér D, Induction of Cip/Kip and Ink4 cyclin dependent kinase inhibitors by interferon-α in hematopoietic cell lines *Oncogene* 1997; **14:** 415–23.
41. Mandal M, Bandyopadhyay D, Goepfert TM, Kumar R, Interferon-induces expression of cyclin-dependent kinase-inhibitors p21WAF1 and p27Kip1 that prevent activation of cyclin-dependent kinase by CDK-activating kinase (CAK). *Oncogene* 1998; **16:** 217–25.
42. Furukawa Y, Iwase S, Kikuchi J et al, Transcriptional repression of the E2F-1 gene by interferon-alpha is mediated through induction of E2F-4/pRB and E2F-4/p130 complexes. *Oncogene* 1999; **18:** 2003–14.
43. Sangfelt O, Erickson S, Castro J et al, Molecular mechanisms underlying interferon-alpha-induced G0/G1 arrest: CKI-mediated regulation of G1 Cdk-complexes and activation of pocket proteins. *Oncogene* 1999; **18:** 2798–810.
44. Ben Dori R, Resnitzki D, Kimchi A, Reduction in p53 synthesis during differentiation of Friend-erythroleukemia cells. Correlation with the commitment to terminal cell division. *FEBS Lett* 1983; **162:** 384.
45. Roth W, Wagenknecht B, Dichgans J, Weller M, Interferon-alpha enhances CD95L-induced apoptosis of human malignant glioma cells. *J Neuroimmunol* 1998; **87:** 121–9.
46. Kindler T, Panitzek S, Stevens T et al, Possible mechanisms of IFN-α triggered apoptosis: upregulation of proapoptotic proteins ICE, CASPASE 3 and BAK. *Onkologie* 2000; **23:** 21.
47. Zhou Q, Zhao J, Al-Zoghaibi F et al, Transcription control of the human plasma membrane phospholipid scramblase 1 gene is mediated by interferon-alpha. *Blood* 2000; **95:** 2593–9.
48. Williams BEG, The role of the dsRNA-activated kinase, PKR, in signal transduction. *Semin Virol* 1995; **6:** 191–202.
49. Zhou A, Hassel BA, Silverman RH, Expression cloning of 2-5A-dependent Rnase, a uniquely regulated mediator of interferon action. *Cell* 1993; **72:** 753–65.
50. Fischer F, Aman J, Van Der Kuip H et al, Induction of interferon regulatory factors, 2'-5' oligoadenylate synthetase, p68 kinase and Rnase L in chronic myelogenous leukaemia cells and its relationship to clinical responsiveness. *Br J Haematol* 1996; **92:** 595–603.
51. Solanilla A, El Andaloussi A, Grosset C et al, Differential effect of interferon alpha on chronic myelogenous leukaemia and normal haematopoietic progenitors in a stromal cell co-culture context: role of the flt3 ligand. *Br J Haematol* 2000; **109:** 382–7.
52. Cornelissen JJ, Ploemacher RE, Wognum BW et al, An in vitro model for cytogenetic conversion in CML. Interferon-alpha preferentially inhibits the outgrowth of malignant stem cells preserved in long-term culture. *J Clin Invest* 1998; **102:** 976–83.
53. Gordon MY, Marley SB, Lewis JL et al, Treatment with interferon-alpha preferentially reduces the capacity for amplification of granulocyte–macrophage progenitors (CFU-GM) from patients with chronic myeloid leukemia but spares normal CFU-GM. *J Clin Invest* 1998; **102:** 710–15.

54. Wang Q, Miyakawa Y, Fox N, Kaushansky K, Interferon-alpha directly represses megakaryopoiesis by inhibiting thrombopoietin-induced signaling through induction of SOCS-1. *Blood* 2000; **96:** 2093–9.
55. Verfaillie CM, McCarthy JB, McGlave PB, Mechanisms underlying abnormal trafficking of malignant progenitors in chronic myelogenous leukemia. Decreased adhesion to stroma and fibronectin but increased adhesion to the basement menbrane components laminin and collagen type IV. *J Clin Invest* 1992; **90:** 1232.
56. Simons PJ, Masinovsky B, Longenecker BM et al, Vascular cell adhesion molecule-1 expressed by bone marrow stromal cells mediates the binding of hematopoietic progenitor cells. *Blood* 1992; **80:** 388.
57. Bhatia R, Wayner E, Verfaillie CM, Interferon-α restores adhesion of malignant progenitors in CML by restoring β1 integrin function. *J Clin Invest* 1994; **94:** 384.
58. Gordon MY, Dowdling CR, Riley GP et al, Altered adhesive interactions with marrow stroma of hematopoietic progenitor cells in chronic myeloid leukaemia. *Nature* 1984; **328:** 342.
59. Bhatia R, McCarthy JB, Verfaillie CM, Interferon-α restores normal β1-integrin mediated negative regulation of chronic myelogenous leukemia progenitor proliferation. *Blood* 1996; **87:** 3883.
60. Eaves AC, Cashman JD, Gaboury LA et al, Unregulated proliferation of primitive chronic myeloid leukemia progenitors in the presence of normal marrow adherent cells. *Proc Natl Acad Sci USA* 1986; **83:** 5306.
61. Aman J, Keller U, Derigs G et al, Regulation of cytokine expression by interferon-α in human bone marrow stromal cells: inhibition of hematopoietic growth factors and induction of interleukin-1 receptor anatagonist. *Blood* 1994; **84:** 4142–50.
62. Namen AE, Schmierer AE, March CJ et al, B cell precursor growth-promoting activity. Purification and characterization of a growth factor active on lymphocyte precursors. *J Exp Med* 1988; **167:** 988.
63. Paul SR, Bennett F, Calvette JA et al, Molecular cloning or a cDNA encoding interleukin 11, a stromal cell-derived lymphopoietic and hematopoietic cytokine. *Proc Natl Acad Sci USA* 1990; **87:** 7512.
64. Heinrich MC, Dooley DC, Freed AC et al, Constitutive expression of Steel factor gene by human stromal cells. *Blood* 1993; **82:** 771.
65. Charbord P, Tamayo E, Sealand S et al, Granulocyte–macrophage colony-stimulating factor (GM-CSF) in human long-term bone marrow cultures: endogenous production in the adherent layer and effect of exogenous GM-CSF in granulomonopoiesis. *Blood* 1991; **78:** 1230.
66. Kittler ELW, McGrath H, Temeles D et al, Biologic significance of constitutive and subliminal growth factor production by bone marrow stroma. *Blood* 1992; **79:** 3168.
67. Khoury E, Lemoine FM, Baillou C et al, Tumor necrosis factor alpha in human long-term bone marrow cultures: distinct effects on nonadherent and adherent progenitors. *Exp Hematol* 1992; **20:** 991.
68. Matikainen S, Sareneva T, Ronni T et al, Interferon-alpha activities multiple STAT proteins and upregulates proliferation-associated IL-2Ralpha, c-myc, and pim-1 genes in human T cells. *Blood* 1999; **93:** 1980–91.
69. Zella D, Romerio F, Curreli S et al, IFN-alpha 2b reduces IL-2 production and IL-2 receptor function in primary CD4+ T cells. *J Immunol* 2000; **164:** 2296–302.
70. Erickson S, Sangfelt O, Castro J et al, Interferon-alpha inhibits proliferation in human T lymphocytes by abrogation of interleukin 2-induced changes in cell cycle-regulatory proteins. *Cell Growth Differ* 1999; **10:** 575–82.
71. Gamero AM, Larner AC, Signaling via the T cell antigen receptor induces phosphorylation of Stat1 on serine 727. *J Biol Chem* 2000; **275:** 16574–8.
72. Reuben JM, Lee BN, Johnson H et al, Restoration of Th1 cytokine synthesis by T cells of patients with chronic myelogenous leukemia in cytogenetic and hematologic remission with interferon-alpha. *Clin Cancer Res* 2000; **6:** 1671–7.
73. Kindler T, Panitzek S, Haque SJ et al, GM-CSF inhibits IFN-induced signals by a block in STAT1 activation. Submitted for publication.
74. Molldrem J, Lee P, Wang C et al, Evidence that specific T lymphocytes may participate in the elimination of chronic myelogenous leukemia. *Nature Med* 2000; **6:** 1018–23.
75. Sakamoto H, Yasukawa H, Masuhara M et al, A Janus kinase inhibitor, JAB, is an interferon-gamma-inducible gene and confers resistance to interferons. *Blood* 1998; **92:** 1668–76.

76. Loh JE, Schindler C, Ziemiecki A et al, Mutant cell lines unresponsive to alpha/beta and gamma interferon are defective in tyrosine phosphorylation of ISGF-3α components. *Mol Cell Biol* 1994; **14:** 2170–9.
77. Moro A, Calixto A, Suarez E et al, Differential expression of the p27Kip1 mRNA in IFN-sensitive and resistant cell lines. *Biochem Biophys Res Commun* 1998; **245:** 752–6.
78. Colamonici OR, Domanski P, Platanias C, Diaz MO, Correlation between interferon (IFN) α resistance and deletion of the IFN α/β genes in acute leukemia cell lines suggests selection against the IFN system. *Blood* 1992; **80:** 744–9.
79. Wong LH, Krauer KG, Hatzinisiriou I et al, Interferon-resistant human melanoma cells are deficient in ISGF3 components, STAT1, STAT2, and p-48–ISGF3gamma. *J Biol Chem* 1997; **272:** 28779–85.
80. Platanias LC, Expression of the IFN-alpha receptor in hairy cell leukemia. *Br J Haematol* 1992; **82:** 541.
81. Clauss IM, Vandenplas B, Wathelet MG et al, Analysis of interferon-inducible genes in cells of chronic myeloid leukemia patients responsive or resistant to an interferon-alpha treatment. *Blood* 1990; **76:** 2337–42.
82. Talpaz M, Chernajovsky Y, Troutman-Worden K et al, Interferon-stimulated genes in interferon-sensitive and -resistant chronic myelogenous leukemia patients. *Cancer Res* 1992; **52:** 1087–90.
83. Grimely PM, Fang H, Rui H et al, Prolonged STAT1 activation related to the growth arrest of malignant lymphoma cells by interferon-alpha. *Blood* 1998; **91:** 3017–27.

8

Interferon-α dosage regimens

Patricia CA Shepherd

CONTENTS • Introduction • Variables affecting response to IFN-α therapy • Initial studies on the use of IFN-α • Subsequent studies of IFN-α • Randomized trials of IFN-α versus chemotherapy in chronic-phase CML • IFN-α toxicities • Prospective randomized trials comparing low- and high-dose IFN-α • Studies using IFN-α and Ara-C • Conclusions

INTRODUCTION

Based on in vitro data showing that interferon-α (IFN-α) suppressed stem cell proliferation in both normal and chronic myeloid leukaemia (CML) bone marrow[1,2] and on its effect on other tumours, the first clinical studies on the effect of IFN-α in CML patients were published in 1983.[3] Initially with purified leukocyte IFN-α and later with recombinant IFN-α, the doses used ranged from 3 to 9 MU/day.[4,5]

The effect of IFN-α was to induce haematologic control of the disease, and in addition suppression of the Philadelphia chromosome (Ph)-positive clone was achieved in a proportion of these patients. Based on these data, and a comparison of complete haematologic response and karyotypic response from other single-agent studies using lower doses of IFN-α, over time a standard dose and schedule of IFN-α was established of 5 MU/m^2 given on a daily basis, with dose reduction permitted in the case of significant toxicity.[6–8]

A single randomized trial initially addressed the optimal dose of IFN-α, and supported the hypothesis that a higher dose given on a daily basis gives a higher rate of haematologic remission.[9–11]

Over the last decade, a number of large randomized trials comparing IFN-α with chemotherapy have been published, with most results showing that the use of IFN-α improved survival compared with standard chemotherapy, using either hydroxyurea or busulphan.[12–16] Two trials did not show a survival advantage for IFN-α over chemotherapy.[17,18] However, a meta-analysis of the data has confirmed the survival benefit, with no significant heterogeneity of treatment effect between the trials.[19]

Some of these randomized trials and a few other non-controlled studies have used lower doses of IFN-α, and have shown efficacy in terms of cytogenetic response[14,18,20] and in some cases survival.[14] This has again raised the issue of the dose of IFN-α and whether it is important as a variable in outcome. The early studies used IFN-α as a single agent in assessing control of the disease – in later studies IFN-α was often combined with other agents such as hydroxyurea, which maintained better immediate control of the white blood cell (WBC) count and allowed longer periods of time on IFN-α in which it could exert its effect. It is still not clear how IFN-α works in CML, but its maximum effect takes many months to occur, as assessed by continuing cytogenetic response, which can continue for a number of years.

It is also recognized that while high doses may be tolerable for a period of time, in many cases dose modification has to be applied because of significant non-haematologic toxicity. In addition, those patients who respond best to IFN-α tend to maintain low WBC and platelet counts while on this agent, which is an indication of the sensitivity of the cells to IFN-α, and may also require dose reduction to maintain a reasonable neutrophil and platelet count.

In addition to dose, a number of other factors have to be taken into account when assessing the effect of IFN-α on the course of the disease. Initial studies showed that patients in low Sokal risk groups had higher levels of complete haematologic remission and cytogenetic responses than those in higher-risk groups.[4,5] Also, those patients treated earlier in the disease with IFN-α tend to do better than those treated later in the disease.[9,21] The duration of IFN-α therapy is also important, since cytogenetic responses take time to develop, necessitating usually at least 12 months' therapy to achieve a major cytogenetic response. A substantial proportion may take significantly longer – up to a number of years – to achieve maximum benefit.

IFN-α therapy is toxic, with the majority of patients suffering at least mild flu-like symptoms and a significant minority being intolerant to the side-effects, particularly severe fatigue, weight loss, neuropsychiatric effects, and autoimmune phenomena. The toxicity appears to be related to the dose and schedule, being higher with higher doses and daily administration. Quality of life is an important issue, and will affect patient compliance with medication. Furthermore, in the case of a very expensive drug such as IFN-α, the issue of health care costs cannot be ignored. A number of papers on the cost-effectiveness of IFN-α therapy show marginal benefit.[22–24] If reducing the dose of IFN-α was efficacious (or the cost of the drug were to be lowered), this would have major effects on health care resources.

This chapter will review the studies in the published literature in relation to the dosage administration of IFN-α.

VARIABLES AFFECTING RESPONSE TO IFN-α THERAPY

In analysing the effects of IFN-α in the many reported studies of its use in CML, we have to look at a number of factors (Table 8.1). These include the prognostic risk profile of the patient studied, the time from diagnosis before IFN-α is started, the dose of IFN-α scheduled and actually given, the duration of IFN-α therapy, and the use of additional therapies in addition to IFN-α to control the disease.

The major outcomes reported are haematologic response, cytogenetic response, and survival. However, haematologic response and cytogenetic response are also subject to certain variables that affect interpretation of the reported studies (Table 8.2).

Ideally, one would like to see results reported in standardized ways for each of the major outcomes in each of the prognostic risk groups in order to be able to define more clearly the effects of other variables, such as IFN-α dose, in this disease. Problems arise, however, with the numbers of patients required in each of the subgroups to allow sufficient statistical power to enable confident prediction of a significant effect to occur. In practice, comparison of the various studies – even in the randomized trials comparing IFN-α with chemotherapy – is difficult to interpret because

Table 8.1 Possible variables affecting outcome of IFN-α therapy

- Prognostic risk group
- Time from diagnosis to starting IFN-α (early untreated versus late pretreated)
- Dose of IFN-α scheduled and delivered
- Duration of IFN-α therapy
- Use of additional therapy in conjunction with IFN-α

Table 8.2 Major outcomes in assessing response to IFN-α therapy

Outcomes	Variables in assessment
Haematologic response	• Prognostic risk group • Timing: 3 months, 6 months, best at any time • Criteria not standardized (no mature WBC, <5% immature WBC) • On IFN-α alone, or combined with other chemotherapy
Cytogenetic response	• Prognostic risk group • Timing: 6 months, 12 months, 24 months, best at any time • Degree of response – definition of minor, major, complete responders on evaluation of minimum number of metaphases • Durability of response • Frequency and timing of analyses
Survival	• Prognostic risk group • Median follow-up • Frequency of events • Statistical power of study

of these variables, and in addition there are differences in the entry criteria and exclusions and the protocol design of the trials.

A great deal of experience has now been gained from these studies, however, into expected outcomes from the use of IFN-α in CML.

- Response rates, both haematologic and cytogenetic, are higher in patients treated early in the course of their disease.
- Response rates, both haematologic and cytogenetic, are higher in those with a good prognostic risk profile than in those with poor prognostic risk factors. The commonest prognostic risk model reported is that of the Sokal index, but other prognostic systems may be equally valid.
- The attainment of a complete haematologic response is a prerequisite for the attainment of a major cytogenetic response.
- The complete haematologic response rate to IFN-α alone is probably inferior to the reported complete haematologic response rates when a combination of IFN-α and chemotherapies such as hydroxurea is allowed.
- Myelosuppression with a WBC of count of less than $4 \times 10^9/l$ is usually seen in those patients who obtain a cytogenetic response to IFN-α.
- Cytogenetic responses, particularly major cytogenetic ones, take a significant time to develop – usually at least 12 months and sometimes a number of years.
- Major cytogenetic responders (<35% Ph-positive cells) have significantly better survival than minor or non-responders when studied by analyses that take into account the time taken for the cytogenetic response to occur. Attainment of a major cytogenetic response is therefore a major goal of therapy, and should impact on survival outcomes if it occurs in a significant proportion

of patients. Minor cytogenetic responses are frequently not durable, and the outcome for such patients is probably not significantly different from that of non-responders to IFN-α.

- Major cytogenetic responses should be shown to be durable for more than 6–12 months before being accepted as indicating a very good prognosis.
- The assessment of minimal residual disease by quantitative polymerase chain reaction (PCR) techniques in complete cytogenetic responders may delineate those in whom relapse is likely to occur.[25]
- Patients who achieve less than a complete haematologic response on optimal therapy have a particularly poor prognosis, and there is probably little to gain from continuing IFN-α.

INITIAL STUDIES ON THE USE OF IFN-α

The initial clinical studies at the MD Anderson Cancer Center, Houston used leukocyte IFN-α at doses of 3–9 MU daily until haematologic remission. Maintenance doses after this ranged from 3 MU on alternate days to 9 MU daily to maintain haematologic remission.[1] Subsequently, recombinant IFN-α became available, and was given as a starting dose of 5 MU/m^2 daily, with dose modifications for significant toxicity and provision for dose escalation if there was resistance to therapy.[5] For 96 patients treated with IFN-α alone, either leukocyte-derived or recombinant, the complete haematologic response rate was 73% and the major cytogenetic response rate (<35% Ph-positive) was 26%. The median survival was 62 months.[26]

Randomized trials of different doses of IFN-α

Only one randomized trial has been published comparing different doses of IFN-α in early-stage CML. This has been published in a series of three papers studying a total of 71 patients from a single centre with early-stage chronic-phase CML (<12 months from diagnosis).[9–11] In this trial 63 patients were randomized to either 2 or 5 MU/m^2 three times a week. If after 4 weeks the white cell count was rising or if after 8 weeks the WBC count had shown no reduction, the patients were crossed over to the higher dose. The last 8 patients admitted to the study were given daily IFN-α, initially at 2 MU/m^2 and increased to 5 MU/m^2 if after 4 weeks the white count was increasing or if after 8 weeks the WBC count had not fallen. For those in the intermittent dose schedule, patients who showed a partial haematologic response after 6 months or those in whom complete haematologic response was unstable were permitted crossover to daily IFN-α administration at doses of 2–5 MU/m^2. The results are shown in Table 8.3. The authors of this study concluded that a higher complete haematologic response rate was seen with escalation of dose and with a daily rather than an intermittent dosage schedule. No other randomized trials comparing doses of IFN-α therapy in CML have been published.

A number of points should be noted in this study. The number of patients is small. The primary endpoint was haematologic response evaluated a short time after IFN-α alone was given. The complete haematologic response rate was related significantly to the Sokal risk group at diagnosis – however, no information was given as to the distribution of the risk groups in the randomized dose allocations. Haematologic and cytogenetic responses were seen in a substantial proportion of patients even at relatively low doses and on an intermittent treatment schedule. The duration of time to crossover to a higher dose or to daily administration was short (4–8 weeks). It is known that IFN-α takes time to induce haematologic and cytogenetic responses, and it could be that longer-term control would have occurred anyway if the dose had been unchanged. The trial studied monotherapy with IFN-α alone, and no additional chemotherapy was permitted. From the results in those patients who were treated in late chronic phase (>12 months) or in accelerated phase, when hydroxyurea was also per-

Table 8.3 Studies in 71 patients in early-stage, chronic-phase CML (<12 months' duration)[9–11]

Dose	Number of patients	Complete haematologic response
2 MU/m^2 t.i.w.	33	8 (24%)
5 MU/m^2 t.i.w.	30	13 (43%)
Crossover		
2 → 5 MU/m^2 t.i.w.	21	7 (33%)
2 MU/m^2 daily	8	3 (38%)
Crossover		
2 → 5 MU/m^2 daily	4	4 (100%)

mitted, it was suggested that the combination with hydroxyurea may be more efficacious than the use of IFN-α alone.

Other low-dose studies

In a further study, Freund et al[6] treated 27 patients at a dose of 5 MU/m^2 three times a week, and obtained a complete haematologic response in 37% of cases. No major cytogenetic responses were seen. However, only 10 of these patients had no pretreatment, with the remainder being a median of 26 months from diagnosis. On the basis that these results were inferior to those reported previously by investigators using a higher-dose schedule, Freund et al concluded that this was because of dose. Since responses, both haematologic and cytogenetic, are significantly less frequent in patients at a later stage of their disease, this may have had a significant bearing on the results.

In a study by the Cancer and Leukaemia Group B,[7] 16 patients were treated at a dose of 2 MU/m^2 five times a week. The authors of this study state that this was later considered to be ineffective, and future patients were treated at a dose of 5 MU/m^2 daily.

On the basis of an assessment of the results using a daily IFN-α schedule at a dose of 5 MU/m^2, predominantly from the MD Anderson Cancer Center and from the randomized trial by Alimena et al, most subsequent investigators have used daily IFN-α at a higher dose level in subsequent studies.

SUBSEQUENT STUDIES OF IFN-α

The MD Anderson Cancer Center later utilized IFN-α in combination with IFN-γ or with hydroxyurea. A total of 274 patients were reported, all of whom were less than 12 months from diagnosis and 50% of whom were within 1 month of diagnosis.[27] The dose was 5 MU/m^2 but no indication has been given as to the dose actually received or the duration of therapy, although dose modification for toxicity was permitted. The complete haematologic response was 80%, the major cytogenetic response rate was 38%, the median survival was 89 months, and the 5-year survival rate was 63%. The highest rate of major cytogenetic response was seen in the good-prognosis group, and the times to major response and complete response were 12 months (range 3–75 months) and 16 months (3–70 months) respectively. Other observational studies using doses of 4–5 MU/m^2 daily have reported major cytogenetic response rates of 25–43% and 5-year survival rates of 55–68%.[7,28,29]

A few studies have reported the use of lower doses of IFN-α than those described above. Thaler et al[8] used a dose of 3.5 MU/day, escalating to 7 MU/day after three months if no haematologic response was noted. They showed a lower rate of major cytogenetic response of 11%, but no details were given of the Sokal risk groups of the patients studied. They also noted that where dose escalation was performed according to protocol, 4 out of 11 patients succeeded in obtaining a better haematologic response. Eight patients were withdrawn from the study because of disease progression or severe side-effects, and in 15 patients the protocol dose was not increased because of side-effects. These patients remained on the low dose, and subsequently achieved a better haematologic response (although not complete at the time).

In a small study of 41 patients, Schofield et al[20] treated chronic-phase CML patients with 2 MU/m^2 daily for 4 weeks, then 2 MU/m^2 t.i.w. with hydroxyurea if necessary to control the blood counts. Again no information was given on prognostic risk groups in these patients. The major cytogenetic response rate was 20%, with a 5-year survival rate of 54%. This group contained a number of patients who were in the later stage of their disease (>1 year, 14 patients). When the early-stage patients were considered, the major cytogenetic response rate was 22% and the 5-year survival rate was 73%.

With small numbers of patients it is difficult to generalize, but the results of these two studies show that lower-dose IFN-α therapy can be effective in obtaining cytogenetic response, and the survival rate in the Schofield study was similar to that seen with higher-dose regimens.

RANDOMIZED TRIALS OF IFN-α VERSUS CHEMOTHERAPY IN CHRONIC-PHASE CML

Subsequent to the above studies, a number of large randomized trials have now been published comparing IFN-α with chemotherapy, either busulfan or hydroxyurea, in chronic-phase CML.[12–18] Not all of these trials have shown a survival advantage for IFN-α over conventional chemotherapy.[17,18] However, a meta-analysis of these trials has confirmed the survival advantage of patients treated with IFN-α compared with those treated with either busulfan or hydroxyurea.[19] The results seen in the different trials are not significantly different from each other. None of these studies are directly comparable – they vary in the numbers enrolled, the statistical power of the study, the entry/exclusion criteria, the characteristics of the populations studied as assessed by Sokal risk group, the dose of IFN-α to be used, the use of additional chemotherapy, and the criteria for establishing complete haematologic response. Major cytogenetic response has been almost uniformly taken across all these studies as suppression of the Ph clone to <35% metaphases present. Discussion in the literature has attempted to explain some of the discrepancies in the individual trials that are related to the above factors.[30–34]

The Italian and German groups attempted an analysis to correct for the differing criteria for entry to the two trials, and still found that no significant difference was noted in the German trial between the IFN-α and hydroxyurea arms, although the results obtained for the IFN-α group in the Italian and German studies were not significantly different.[33] Other major issues highlighted in the literature were the strict use of monotherapy alone in the German group, which led to many patients abandoning IFN-α early in the trial and so being unable to obtain a possible benefit from additional IFN-α if it had been combined with additional disease control with the use of hydroxyurea. The low level of major cytogenetic response in the German trial has been linked to the use of monotherapy and the infrequency of cytogenetic analysis. In the study by the Benelux group, the use of IFN-α in low doses resulted in a major cytogenetic response rate of 16%, yet no survival advantage was seen over hydroxyurea-treated patients. It was noted, however, that the median survival of hydroxyurea-treated patients in this study was longer at 68 months than was seen in the Italian trial (52 months), German trial (56 months), or British trial (52 months). It is not clear why the results of the hydroxyurea-treated arm were so much better in the Benelux trial – possible reasons are the strict control of the WBC count and, probably more importantly, individual heterogeneity of the disease process.

The attainment of a major cytogenetic response in most, but not all,[7,17] studies has been shown to be a major prognostic indicator, and should impact on improved survival if it occurs in a significant proportion of patients. Comparing the results of IFN-α therapy between studies on the basis of complete haematologic response and cytogenetic response without reference to Sokal risk groups and the major endpoint, survival, may be misleading. In addition, Hehlmann et al[35] showed that the Sokal risk group contributes more to differences in survival than the effect of IFN-α within each of these risk groups, although IFN-α therapy is of benefit within each of the risk groups – an effect confirmed by the recent meta-analysis of randomized trials of IFN-α in CML. The greater effect of prognostic risk groups compared with therapy effects has also been noted in the patients studied at the MD Cancer Center.[36]

Attainment of a major cytogenetic response has been linked to IFN-α dosage; however, it is difficult to compare cytogenetic response rates between trials, because these rates are influenced by the proportion of the population studied in each Sokal risk group. Indeed, complete haematologic response is also influenced by the proportion of each Sokal risk group.

The proportion of cytogenetic responders is also related to the number and frequency of cytogenetic analyses, in addition to the dose and duration of IFN-α given. The low proportion of major cytogenetic responders in the German trial has been attributed to the use of monotherapy alone whereby IFN-α was stopped if control of the WBC count was not achieved, to infrequency of cytogenetic analysis, and to a high proportion of Sokal high-risk patients.

In recent guidelines published by the American Society for Hematology, the criteria by which trials should be compared is by survival outcome and not solely by surrogate markers of response such as complete haematologic and cytogenetic response rates.[37]

A comparison of the randomized trials of IFN-α in CML and of some observational studies on newly diagnosed CML patients given high- and low-dose IFN-α is given in Table 8.4. This shows the distribution of the Sokal risk groups, the major cytogenetic response rates, the median survival, and the 5-year survival rates.

The highest rates of cytogenetic response are seen in the single-centre high-dose studies, but these are also the studies with the lowest percentage of Sokal high-risk groups. The randomized trials show lower major cytogenetic response rates. In addition, major cytogenetic response rates between the lower-dose trials (British and Benelux) and higher-dose trials (Italian, German, and Japanese) do not differ significantly, particularly if one takes account of the differing risk groups. The German trial has a lower cytogenetic response rate, which may be explained by the reasons previously discussed. The median survivals and 5-year survival rates, however, do not differ substantially among the randomized trials using higher or lower doses of IFN-α or, with the exception of the Mahon trial,[28] within any of the studies: 54–63%. The median survivals within the Sokal risk groups, where given, also seem quite similar, and this includes the British low-dose study.

Figure 8.1 shows the major cytogenetic response rates for these trials, including the high-dose IFN-α arm of the French randomized trial comparing IFN-α alone versus IFN-α plus Ara-C (cytosine arabinoside, cytarabine),[38] according to the proportion of patients in the Sokal low- or intermediate-risk group where the great majority of major cytogenetic responders will be found. There is very good correlation between cytogenetic response rates found in the respective trials and the Sokal risk profile. The low response rate in the German trial, as discussed, is probably related to the

Table 8.4 Summary of reported outcomes for various studies of IFN in CML

Study[a]	Target dose of IFN-α	Percentage in Sokal risk group			Cytogenetic response rate (%) (<35% Ph⁺ cells)				Median survival (months)				5-year survival rate (%)			
		L	I	H	Overall	L	I	H	Overall	L	I	H	Overall	L	I	H
Randomized trials																
Italian[12,13] (218)	5 MU/m² daily	43	33	24	19				72	>72 (L and I)			54	62[b]		
					21				76	64% 6-yr	72	54				
German[17,33] (133)	5 MU/m² daily	27	35	38	8 evaluable 5 total				66	80% 6-yr	65	47	59			
British[14,15] (293)	3 MU daily, escalating if WBC not controlled Aim: WBC <5 × 10⁹/l	24	35	41	11	18	15	4	63	97	73	48	54	66	63	34
Japan[16] (80)	9 MU daily, escalating if poor control Aim: WBC <5 × 10⁹/l Platelets >50 × 10⁹/l	37	33	29	16								54			
Benelux[18] (100)	3 MU 5 days per week	29	43	28	16				64				55			

High-dose studies																
Kantarjian[27] (274)	5 MU/m^2	52	25	23	38	52	32	24	89	104	90	62	63	78	62	46
Ozer[7] (107)	5 MU/m^2				29 (<50% Ph^+)				66				58			
Kloke[29] (71)	4 MU/m^2	49	32	20	25				NR				55			
Mahon[28] (116)	5 MU/m^2	50	36	14	43				NR				68			
Low-dose studies																
Thaler[8] (80)	3.5 MU daily, escalating if no response to 7 MU daily				11				NR				NR			
Schofield[20] (41)	2 MU/m^2 for 4 weeks then 2 MU/m^2 t. .w.				20				84				54			

[a] Reference; number of patients in parentheses.
[b] Estimated from survival curve. NR, not recorded.

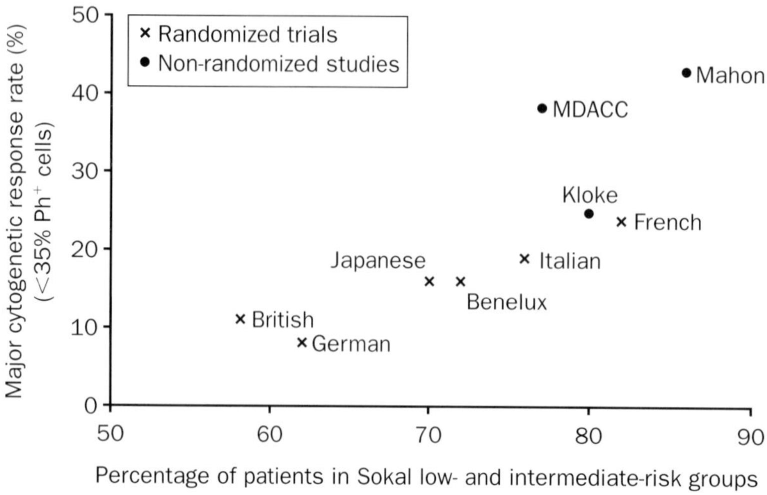

Figure 8.1 Correlation of major cytogenetic response rate with percentage of patients in Sokal low- and intermediate-risk groups.

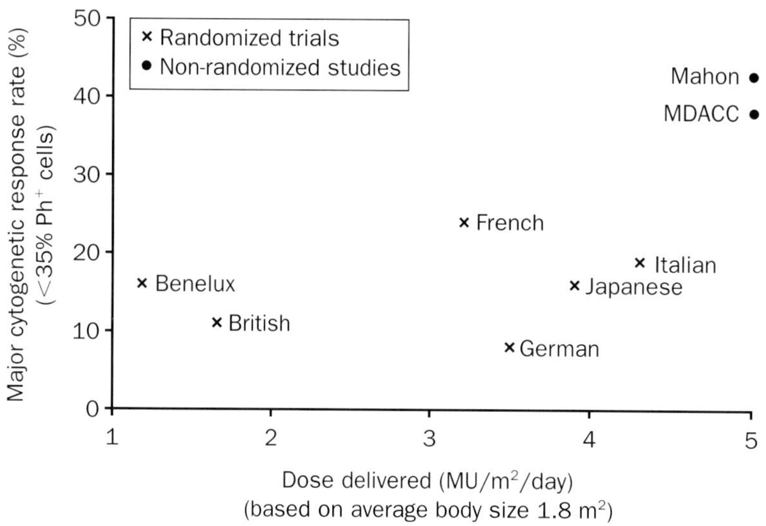

Figure 8.2 Correlation of major cytogenetic response rate with active dose of IFN-α delivered in first year.

infrequency of cytogenetic analysis and to the use of strictly IFN-α monotherapy, with early IFN-α discontinuation in non-responders. Figure 8.2 shows the major cytogenetic response rate attained according to the dose of IFN-α delivered in the first year of therapy, and this exhibits significantly poorer correlation.

These randomized trials all come from multi-centre studies. Non-randomized studies from single centres, particularly the MD Anderson group and the Bordeaux group, have shown higher major cytogenetic response rates and better survival, which may be a reflection of selection bias from referring centres, a low proportion of high-risk patients, and a strict adherence to the target dose of 5 MU/m^2, in addition to a consistent approach to modifying therapy at a single centre.

IFN-α TOXICITIES

IFN-α has significant toxicities, which appear to be dose-dependent. In all the randomized trials, some modification to dose is made because of toxicity. Table 8.5 summarizes these. In the Italian trial, a median dose of 4.3 MU/m^2 daily was maintained for the first 14 months, and thereafter the dose in cytogenetic responders, declined over time to 21 MU/week at 5 years. For the non-cytogenetic responders, after 14 months the protocol stated that the dose was reduced to 9 MU/week, but in fact significantly higher doses were given (15 MU/week in year 2, 11 MU/week in year 3). Additional chemotherapy to IFN-α was given in 21% of IFN-α-treated patients. Eighteen per cent of patients abandoned therapy because of side-effects.

In the Benelux study, although low doses were used and the dose was maintained, 25% stopped therapy at a median of 17.6 months from starting IFN-α because of side-effects. The median duration of IFN-α therapy was 25 months.

In the German study, the doses given were 3.5 MU/m^2 at 1 year, 3 MU/m^2 at 2 years, and 2 MU/m^2 thereafter. However, a substantial proportion of patients (20%) stopped IFN-α within 3 months because of non-response, and the median duration of therapy was 22 months. IFN-α was abandoned because of side-effects in 18% of patients.

In the Japanese study, a dose of 7 MU daily was achieved. The median duration of therapy was 40 months for complete cytogenetic response, 46 months for partial cytogenetic response, 16 months for minor cytogenetic response, and only 4.5 months for non-responders. These investigators noted that there was no difference in the dose given to cytogenetic responders and non-responders, but the duration of therapy was not optimal. Twenty-nine per cent of patients abandoned IFN-α because of side effects, 16% within 4 weeks.

In the British study, 90 patients (31%) abandoned IFN-α because of side-effects, 11% by 1 year, 20% by 2 years, and 26% by 3 years. In only a third of these cases was the WBC count well controlled ($<10 \times 10^9$/l) on IFN-α alone when it was abandoned. In a quarter of the cases, there was poor disease control (WBC $> 30 \times 10^9$/l) when the IFN-α was abandoned, and this probably contributed to the decision to stop IFN-α (unpublished data, P Shepherd).

Thus toxicity is a major problem in delivering IFN-α dose, and contributes to patients abandoning IFN-α over time. It should be noted, however, that toxicities were still significant even when low doses were used in the Benelux and UK MRC studies, although the lower doses may have enabled some patients to stay on IFN-α for longer. Overall, 18–31% of patients abandoned IFN-α because of adverse effects, many of them within the first year of IFN-α therapy. The degree of toxicity that patients will tolerate reflects patient/clinician interaction and motivation, and to an extent is possibly age-dependent.

Since the dose of IFN-α does not seem to have a clear-cut impact on the published results, there is a need for a randomized trial comparing lower and higher doses of IFN-α, with particular focus on actual compliance with therapy over time, adverse effects over time, and quality of life, in addition to measurements of efficacy – major cytogenetic response rates and survival.

PROSPECTIVE RANDOMIZED TRIALS COMPARING LOW- AND HIGH-DOSE IFN-α

In 1993, the Netherlands Hovon 20 Group opened a trial comparing a fixed low-dose IFN-α schedule of 3 MU 5 days/week with hydroxyurea, compared with 5 MU/m^2 daily with hydroxyurea. Control of the WBC count should be kept at less than 5×10^9/l. In 1995, the MRC CML Working Group recommended adopting a similar approach to see whether the dose as a single variable has any effect on outcomes.

Table 8.5 Summary of drug modifications in randomized trials of IFN in CML

Study[a]	Target dose and criteria for increasing or decreasing dose	Dose delivered	Comments	Percentage abandoning IFN-α because of side-effects	Median duration of IFN-α therapy	Additional chemotherapy permitted?
Italian[12,13] (218)	5 MU/m^2 daily to 8 months ↑ by 25% if < complete cytogenetic response at 8 months ↑ by 50% if no cytogenetic response at 8 months At 14 months, if no cytogenetic response, dose reduced to 3 MU t.i.w.	Median 4.3 MU/m^2 daily in first 14 months, thereafter progressive decrease to 21 MU/week at 5 years for cytogenetic response and 10 MU/week for no cytogenetic response	In first 14 months, percentage of scheduled dose: 76–100% in 53% 50–75% in 29% <50% in 18%	18	Not given	Yes for no haematologic response at 3 months, for < complete haematologic response, platelets $>750 \times 10^9$/l palpable spleen at 8 months: 21% hydroxyurea added to IFN-α
German[17,33] (133)	5 MU/m^2 daily to achieve WBC $<5 \times 10^9$/l with no intolerable adverse effects. IFN-α discontinued if <partial haematologic response within 4 months or intolerable adverse effects	3 MU/m^2 daily at 2 years 2 MU/m^2 daily thereafter	3.5 MU/m^2 daily at 1 year within first 3 months for non-response	20% stopped IFN-α	18	22 months No
Japanese[16] (80)	9 MU daily to achieve WBC of $<5 \times 10^9$/l, platelets $>50 \times 10^9$/l or more if required	7 MU daily	16% stopped IFN-α within 4 weeks	29	40 months, complete cytogenetic response 47 months, partial cytogenetic response 16 months, minor cytogenetic response 5 months, no cytogenetic response	No
Benelux[18] (100)	3 MU 5 days/week Hydroxyurea allowed in addition to keep WBC $<10 \times 10^9$/l	3 MU 5 days/week	No dose reduction	25 after median 18 months	25 months	Yes to keep WBC $<10 \times 10^9$/l if required
MRC[14,15] (293)	3 MU daily, escalating to 6, 9, or 12 MU daily to keep WBC $<5 \times 10^9$/l	3 MU daily	Cytogenetic responders: 21 MU/week Non cytogenetic responders 24 MU/week in 1st year	31 (11 in 1st year) (20 by 2 years) (26 by 3 years)	23 months (17 months for non cytogenetic responders)	Yes if WBC $>30 \times 10^9$/l on IFN-α alone

[a] Numbers of patients in parentheses.

Inclusion/exclusion criteria are similar. Endpoints are haematologic response, cytogenetic response, survival, toxicity, and quality of life. An economic costing analysis should also be produced.

These studies are still ongoing, and to date about 360 patients have been randomized. No information is yet available on outcomes; however, overall analyses show that haematologic and cytogenetic response rates are encouraging (P Shepherd and H Kluin-Nelemans, unpublished data).

The Spanish Group on CML and IFN-α has recently reported in abstract form a comparison of intermediate-dose IFN-α (maximum 4.5 MU daily) and standard-dose IFN-α (maximum 9 MU daily).[39] They studied 95 patients, and found no difference between the two dose levels in haematologic response or cytogenetic response after 1 year. Toxicity was also similar in the two groups. At 2 years, no difference in survival was noted. The numbers of patients here are small and the survival data are not mature, but in the short term there appeared to be no significant differences between the two dose levels, with significant cost-saving.

STUDIES USING IFN-α AND Ara-C

More recently, attempts have been made to improve on the results seen with IFN-α in CML by combining it with other agents such as Ara-C. The recently published French CML 91 multicentre randomized trial compared IFN-α with IFN-α plus Ara-C, and showed a survival benefit for the combination arm: 79% versus 86% at 3 years, $p = 0.02$.[38] Major cytogenetic response rates were also improved after 12 months of therapy in the IFN-α plus Ara-C arm (41% versus 24%). The dose of IFN-α in this study was also 5 MU/m^2 and the mean delivered dose was 5.6 MU daily (3.2 MU/m^2/day based on average surface area of 1.75 m^2). Only 14% of cases in the IFN-α plus Ara-C arm and 18% in the IFN-α arm were in the Sokal high-risk group.

A beneficial result in a similar trial by the Italian Cooperative Study Group has also been published in abstract form.[40,41] The MD Anderson Cancer Center group have also used IFN-α in combination with low-dose Ara-C, and have observed an improvement in their major cytogenetic response rate but not in survival compared with historical controls.[42] Of interest, they found that a lower-dose schedule of IFN-α was given (3.7 MU/m^2) predominantly because of significant regimen-related myelosuppression.

Thaler et al[43] used IFN-α at a dose of 3.5 MU daily with Ara-C 10 mg/m^2 for 10 days every month in 84 patients, and found higher major cytogenetic response rates (25%) than previously reported by their group with IFN-α alone.

It appears from the data so far that the combination of IFN-α with Ara-C is better (level I evidence, two randomized trials) and that the dose of IFN-α given in combination is lower and may be less critical for achieving significant responses than has previously been thought. Further studies using homoharringtonine either sequentially or in combination with IFN-α have suggested that lower doses of IFN-α in combination with this agent are efficacious in achieving cytogenetic responses, and are associated with less toxicity.[44,45]

CONCLUSIONS

The use of IFN-α in CML has evolved over the past 17 years of its use in clinical practice. The initial studies used IFN-α alone at a dose of 5 MU/m^2, which is a significantly lower dose than was used in the treatment of solid tumours. A dose–response relationship favoured higher doses of 5 MU/m^2 over lower doses, based primarily on a series of papers from one institution that showed that dose escalation of IFN-α alone over a short period of time improved haematologic control. The initial studies from the MD Anderson Cancer Center used IFN-α alone, and later combined with IFN-γ or hydroxyurea. The overall results from this group showed a major cytogenetic response rate of 38%, with a median survival of 89 months. The subsequent reporting of randomized trials comparing IFN-α with chemotherapy confirmed a survival benefit for IFN-α, but the major cytogenetic response rates and the median survivals were not so good.

Various reasons have been discussed in relation to the differences in outcome that are seen. One of these is dosage, but others include the comparison of single-centre studies against multicentre randomized trials, the population studied as assessed by Sokal risk groups, and the combination with IFN-α of other agents that could give better control of the disease and permit longer use of IFN-α to allow it to take effect in this disease.

Whether more is better, or less is just as good, or worse, is not clear when evaluating major cytogenetic rates and survival. Certainly major and complete cytogenetic responses are seen with lower-dose regimens, and the quality of that response as assessed by very low levels of *BCR/ABL* transcripts can be excellent, as shown in some of the patients treated in the British study and reported by Hochhaus et al.[25] This suggests that the sensitivity of the Ph-positive cells to IFN-α is a critical factor, which may not be overcome by dose escalation. In practice, dose modification for toxicity is seen in the majority of patients and its degree can be affected by patient motivation and patient/physician interaction, in addition to defined criteria. The standard dose of 5 MU/m^2 is modified to the maximal tolerated dose, which can vary considerably. Definite answers to the question of optimal dosage await the outcome of the currently running randomized trial in which dose is the only variable.

If efficacy is not reduced, the toxicities of IFN-α may be reduced, and patient compliance, duration of IFN-α therapy, and quality of life could be improved with increased cost-effectiveness of what is a very expensive drug. However, in relation to toxicities, even low doses can be intolerable for a significant number of patients.

The most recent studies of the combination of IFN-α and Ara-C show improved survival over IFN-α alone, and some studies have utilized lower doses of IFN-α than were previously given. The use of homoharringtonine with IFN-α also permits lower doses to be used to maintain response without apparent loss of efficacy in the patients studied. The use of these combinations may thus lessen the debate over the best dose of IFN-α.

The coming use of tyrosine kinase inhibitors opens up exciting opportunities for the treatment of CML patients. The benefit of these agents awaits comparison in randomized studies with IFN-α and Ara-C, but their combination with IFN-α, Ara-C, or other agents may hopefully improve on the benefits that have been seen to date with IFN-α alone.

REFERENCES

1. Verma DS, Spitzer G, Gutterman JU et al, Human leukocyte interferon preparation blocks granulopoietic differentiation. *Blood* 1979; **54:** 1423–7.
2. Williams CK, Svet-Moldavskaya I, Vilcek J et al, Inhibitory effects of human leukocyte and fibroblast interferons on normal and chronic myelogenous leukemic granulocytic progenitor cells. *Oncology* 1981; **38:** 356–60.
3. Talpaz M, McCredie KB, Mavligit GM, Gutterman JU, Leukocyte interferon-induced myeloid cytoreduction in chronic myelogenous leukemia. *Blood* 1983; **62:** 689–92.
4. Talpaz M, Kantarjian HM, McCredie KB et al, Clinical investigation of human alpha interferon in chronic myelogenous leukemia. *Blood* 1987; **69:** 1280–8.
5. Talpaz M, Kantarjian HM, McCredie K et al, Hematologic remission and cytogenetic improvement induced by recombinant human interferon alpha A in chronic myelogenous leukemia. *N Engl J Med* 1986; **314:** 1065–9.
6. Freund M, von Wussow P, Diedrich H et al, Recombinant human interferon (IFN) alpha-2b in chronic myelogenous leukaemia: dose dependency of response and frequency of neutralizing anti-interferon antibodies. *Br J Haematol* 1989; **72:** 350–6.
7. Ozer H, George SL, Schiffer CA et al, Prolonged subcutaneous administration of recombinant alpha 2b interferon in patients with previously untreated Philadelphia chromosome-positive

chronic-phase chronic myelogenous leukemia: effect on remission duration and survival: Cancer and Leukemia Group B Study 8583. *Blood* 1993; **82:** 2975–84.

8. Thaler J, Gastl G, Fluckinger T et al, Treatment of chronic myelogenous leukemia with interferon alfa-2c: response rate and toxicity in a phase II multicenter study. The Austrian Biological Response Modifier (BRM) Study Group. *Semin Hematol* 1993; **30**(3 Suppl 3): 17–19.
9. Alimena G, Morra E, Lazzarino M et al, Treatment of Ph′-positive chronic myelogenous leukemia (CML) with recombinant interferon alfa-2b (Intron A). *Cancer Treat Rev* 1988; **15**(Suppl A): 21–6.
10. Alimena G, Morra E, Lazzarino M et al, Interferon alpha-2b as therapy for Ph′-positive chronic myelogenous leukemia: a study of 82 patients treated with intermittent or daily administration. *Blood* 1988; **72:** 642–7.
11. Morra E, Alimena G, Lazzarino M et al, Evolving modalities of treatment with interferon alfa-2b for Ph1-positive chronic myelogenous leukaemia. *Eur J Cancer* 1991; **27**(Suppl 4): S14–17.
12. The Italian Cooperative Study Group on Chronic Myeloid Leukemia, Interferon alfa-2a as compared with conventional chemotherapy for the treatment of chronic myeloid leukemia. *N Engl J Med* 1994; **330:** 820–5.
13. The Italian Cooperative Study Group on Chronic Myeloid Leukaemia, Long term follow-up of the Italian trial of interferon-α versus conventional chemotherapy in chronic myeloid leukaemia. *Blood* 1998; **92:** 1541–8.
14. Allan NC, Richards SM, Shepherd PC, UK Medical Research Council randomised, multicentre trial of interferon-alpha n1 for chronic myeloid leukaemia: improved survival irrespective of cytogenetic response. The UK Medical Research Council's Working Parties for Therapeutic Trials in Adult Leukaemia. *Lancet* 1995; **345:** 1392–7.
15. Shepherd PC, Richards SM, Allan NC, Progress with interferon in CML – results of the MRC UK CML III Study. *Bone Marrow Transplant* 1996; **17**(Suppl 3): S15–18.
16. Ohnishi K, Ohno R, Tomonaga M et al, A randomized trial comparing interferon-alpha with busulfan for newly diagnosed chronic myelogenous leukemia in chronic phase. *Blood* 1995; **86:** 906–16.
17. Hehlmann R, Heimpel H, Hasford J et al, Randomized comparison of interferon-alpha with busulfan and hydroxyurea in chronic myelogenous leukemia. The German CML Study Group. *Blood* 1994; **84:** 4064–77.
18. The Benelux CML Study Group, Randomized study on hydroxyurea alone versus hydroxyurea combined with low-dose interferon-alpha 2b for chronic myeloid leukemia. *Blood* 1998; **91:** 2713–21.
19. Chronic Myeloid Leukemia Trialists' Collaborative Group, Interferon alfa versus chemotherapy for chronic myeloid leukemia: a meta-analysis of seven randomized trials. *J Natl Cancer Inst* 1997; **89:** 1616–20.
20. Schofield JR, Robinson WA, Murphy JR, Rovira DK, Low doses of interferon-alpha are as effective as higher doses in inducing remissions and prolonging survival in chronic myeloid leukemia. *Ann Intern Med* 1994; **121:** 736–44.
21. Niederle N, Moritz T, Kloke O et al, Interferon alfa-2b in acute- and chronic-phase chronic myelogenous leukaemia: initial response and long-term results in 54 patients. *Eur J Cancer* 1991; **27**(Suppl 4): S7–14.
22. Kattan MW, Inoue Y, Giles FJ et al, Cost-effectiveness of interferon-alpha and conventional chemotherapy in chronic myelogenous leukemia. *Ann Intern Med* 1996; **125:** 541–8.
23. Liberato NL, Quaglini S, Barosi G, Cost-effectiveness of interferon alfa in chronic myelogenous leukemia. *J Clin Oncol* 1997; **15:** 2673–82.
24. Messori A, Cost-effectiveness of interferon in chronic myeloid leukaemia: analysis of four clinical studies. *Ann Oncol* 1998; **9:** 389–96.
25. Hochhaus A, Reiter A, Saussele S et al, Molecular heterogeneity in complete cytogenetic responders after interferon-alpha therapy for chronic myelogenous leukemia: low levels of minimal residual disease are associated with continuing remission. German CML Study Group and the UK MRC CML Study Group. *Blood* 2000; **95:** 62–6.
26. Talpaz M, Kantarjian H, Kurzrock R et al, Interferon-alpha produces sustained cytogenetic responses in chronic myelogenous leukemia. Philadelphia chromosome-positive patients. *Ann Intern Med* 1991; **114:** 532–8.
27. Kantarjian HM, Smith TL, O'Brien S et al, Prolonged survival in chronic myelogenous leukaemia after cytogenetic response to interferon-alpha therapy. *Ann Intern Med* 1995; **122:** 254–61.

28. Mahon FX, Faberes C, Pueyo S et al, Response at three months is a good predictive factor for newly diagnosed chronic myeloid leukemia patients treated by recombinant interferon-alpha. *Blood* 1998; **92:** 4059–65.
29. Kloke O, Niederle N, Qiu JY et al, Impact of interferon alpha-induced cytogenetic improvement on survival in chronic myelogenous leukaemia. *Br J Haematol* 1993; **83:** 399–403.
30. Kantarjian HM, Talpaz M, Interferon-α therapy in chronic myelogenous leukemia: questions related to the German randomized trial. *Blood* 1995; **85:** 2998–9.
31. Tura S, Baccarani M, for The Italian Cooperative Study Group on Chronic Myeloid Leukemia, α-interferon in the treatment of chronic myeloid leukemia. *Blood* 1995; **85:** 2999–3000.
32. Hehlmann R, Heimpel H, Hasford J, Randomised comparison of interferon-α, hydroxyurea, and busulphan in chronic myeloid leukemia: response to Kantarjian and Talpaz and to Tura and Baccarani. *Blood* 1995; **85:** 3000–2.
33. Hasford J, Baccarani M, Hehlmann R et al, Interferon-alpha and hydroxyurea in early chronic myeloid leukemia: a comparative analysis of the Italian and German chronic myeloid leukemia trials with interferon-alpha. *Blood* 1996; **87:** 5384–91.
34. Kantarjian H, Talpaz M, Questions raised by the Benelux CML Study Group: results from the randomized study with hydroxyurea alone versus hydroxyurea combined with low-dose interferon-alpha2b for chronic myeloid leukemia. *Blood* 1998; **92:** 2984–7.
35. Hehlmann R, Ansari H, Hasford J et al, Comparative analysis of the impact of risk profile and of drug therapy on survival in CML using Sokal's index and a new score. German Chronic Myeloid Leukaemia (CML)-Study Group. *Br J Haematol* 1997; **97:** 76–85.
36. Giralt S, Kantarjian H, Talpaz M, Treatment of chronic myelogenous leukemia. *Semin Oncol* 1995; **22:** 396–404.
37. Silver RT, Woolf SH, Hehlmann R et al, An evidence-based analysis of the effect of busulfan, hydroxyurea, interferon, and allogeneic bone marrow transplantation in treating the chronic phase of chronic myeloid leukemia: developed for the American Society of Hematology. *Blood* 1999; **94:** 1517–36.
38. Guilhot F, Chastang C, Michallet M et al, Interferon alfa-2b combined with cytarabine versus interferon alone in chronic myelogenous leukemia. French Chronic Myeloid Leukemia Study Group. *N Engl J Med* 1997; **337:** 223–9.
39. Steegmann J, Pennarubia M, Odriozola J et al, Intermediate versus standard doses of interferon-alpha in chronic myelogenous leukemia Ph+. *Blood* 1999; **94**(10 Suppl 1 Part 1): 530a.
40. Tura S, On behalf of the Italian Cooperative Study Group on CML (ICSG on CML). Cytarabine increases karyotypic response in alpha-IFN treated chronic myeloid leukemia patients: results of a national prospective randomised trial. *Blood* 1998; **92**(10 Suppl 1 Part 1): 317a.
41. Rosti G, Bonifazi F, De Vivo A et al, Cytarabine increases karyotypic response and survival in αIFN treated chronic myelogenous leukemia patients: results of a national prospective randomised trial of the Italian Cooperative Study Group on CML. *Blood* 1999; **94**(10 Suppl 1 Part 1): 600a.
42. Kantarjian H, O'Brien S, Smith T et al, Treatment of Philadelphia chromosome-positive early chronic phase chronic myelogenous leukemia with daily doses of interferon alpha and low dose cytarabine. *J Clin Oncol* 1999; **17:** 284–92.
43. Thaler J, Hilbe W, Apfelbeck U et al, Interferon-alpha-2C and LD ara-C for the treatment of patients with CML: results of the Austrian multicenter phase II study. *Leuk Res* 1997; **21:** 75–80.
44. O'Brien S, Kantarjian H, Koller C et al, Sequential homoharringtonine and interferon-alpha in the treatment of early chronic phase chronic myelogenous leukemia. *Blood* 1999; **93:** 4149–53.
45. O'Brien S, Talpaz M, Giles FJ et al, Simultaneous interferon alpha (IFN-α) and homoharringtonine (HHT) is an effective regimen in Philadelphia chromosome (Ph) positive chronic myelogenous leukemia. *Blood* 1999; **94**(10 Suppl 1 Part 2): 278b.

9

Chemotherapy versus interferon: Long-term effects

Andreas Hochhaus, Rüdiger Hehlmann

CONTENTS • Introduction • Non-randomized trials • Randomized trial of IFN-α versus chemotherapy • Dose–response relationship • Combination of IFN-α with chemotherapy • Adverse effects • Effect of IFN-α and chemotherapy on bone marrow morphology • Impact of prognostic risk groups and stage of disease on response to IFN-α • Complete cytogenetic response after IFN-α therapy • IFN-α pretreatment prior to allogeneic BMT • Prediction of response • Pegylated interferons • Combination of signal transduction inhibitors and IFN-α • Conclusions

INTRODUCTION

Interferons are a family of multifunctional cytokines that play important roles in the induction of antiviral activities, inhibition of cell growth, induction of cell differentiation, and immunomodulation (for a review, see Pfeffer et al[1]). Interferon-α (IFN-α) in vitro also restores normal adhesion of chronic myeloid leukaemia (CML) progenitors to bone marrow stroma.[2] Interferons function by inducing a group of transcriptional factors called interferon regulatory factors (IRFs) (for a review see Harada et al[3]). IRFs regulate the expression of interferon-stimulated genes by binding to specific DNA sequences, i.e. interferon-stimulated response elements, in promoters of the genes regulated by interferons.

It is generally accepted that IFN-α and, to a lesser extent, also hydroxyurea prolong survival in CML patients. Initial studies used human leukocyte IFN-α,[4] but most subsequent clinical trials focused on the use of recombinant IFN-α 2a, 2b, and 2c. The first report on the efficacy of IFN-α was published in 1983 by Talpaz et al,[4] who demonstrated myeloid cytoreduction with haematological remission in five of seven untreated or minimally pretreated chronic-phase CML patients and control of severe, therapy-resistant thrombocytosis in nine patients with advanced CML.

NON-RANDOMIZED TRIALS

In 1986, Talpaz et al[5] reported not only good cytoreduction by recombinant IFN-α2a in 14 out of 17 patients but also the induction of complete cytogenetic remission in 6 out of 13 patients with haematological remission. The good cytoreductive property of IFN-α in CML was confirmed by other groups. Niederle et al[6] observed normalization of leukocyte counts in 13 out of 16 evaluable CML patients and a cytogenetic response of up to 50% Philadelphia chromosome (Ph) negativity in four patients at an IFN-α dosage of 4 MU/day.

Kantarjian et al[7] reported, from long-term

observations of 274 patients treated with IFN-α in early chronic phase, that 80% achieved complete haematological and 26% complete cytogenetic remissions. Cytogenetic remissions were durable and long-lasting in the majority of patients. Ozer and the CALGB[8] treated 107 Ph-positive CML patients in chronic phase with IFN-α at 5 MU/m^2 daily, and found haematological remissions in 63 patients (59%; 24 complete, 39 partial); 31 patients (40% of evaluable) achieved a cytogenetic response (14 complete, 17 partial). No survival advantage of cytogenetic responders over non-responders was found. Mahon et al[9] observed a major cytogenetic remission rate in 51 mostly good-risk patients according to Sokal on IFN-α at a dose level of 5 MU/day IFN-α. Thaler et al[10] treated 80 patients with a favourable risk profile with IFN-α2c at an absolute dose of 3.5 MU/day, and achieved haematological responses in 74% and cytogenetic responses in 28% (13% major) of patients. The estimated median survival is only 51 months, probably because of the low IFN-α dosage.

RANDOMIZED TRIALS OF IFN-α VERSUS CHEMOTHERAPY

Busulfan, introduced in the 1950s,[11] controls haematological variables and is inexpensive. Side-effects include severe, prolonged myelosuppression in 10% of patients and pulmonary fibrosis. Busulfan is given orally at 0.1 mg/kg daily until the leukocyte count decreases by 50%; at that point, the dose is reduced by 50%. In most patients receiving busulfan, disease cannot be controlled safely at the low leukocyte levels needed to induce a complete haematological response. In individual cases, therapy with busulfan is effective even in patients with disease refractory to hydroxyurea.[12]

In 1972, hydroxyurea, a cell-cycle-specific inhibitor of DNA synthesis, became available for CML therapy.[13] It allows rapid but transient haematological control, is well tolerated, and has few side-effects (megaloblastic anaemia, mucosal ulcers, and skin manifestations).[14–17] Hydroxyurea is given orally at 40 mg/kg daily, and doses are adjusted to maintain a leukocyte count of (2–4) × 10^9/l. Cytogenetic remissions are rare. The survival advantage of hydroxyurea over busulfan has been demonstrated by the German CML Study Group (Figure 9.1).[12]

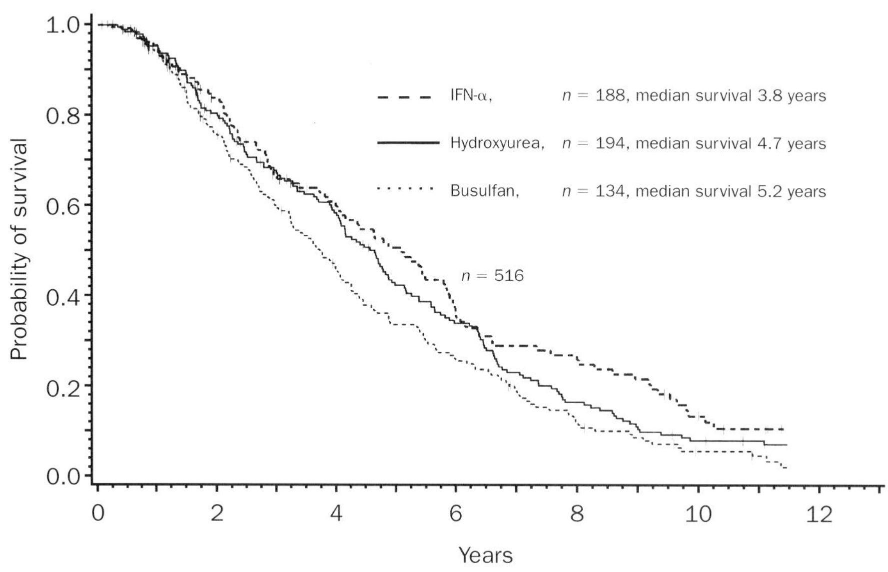

Figure 9.1 German CML study I: busulfan versus hydroxyurea versus IFN-α.[18]

Table 9.1 Randomized studies of IFN-α in CML

Study	Comparisons[a]	No. of patients	Outcome
Hehlmann et al (1994)[18]	IFN-α vs HU vs Bu	516	IFN-α superior to Bu; as effective as HU
Italian Cooperative Group (1994)[20]	IFN-α (±HU) vs CT	322	IFN-α superior
Allan et al (1995)[19]	IFN-α (±CHT) vs HU vs Bu	587	IFN-α superior
Ohnishi et al (1995)[21]	IFN-α (±CHT) vs Bu	159	IFN-α superior
Benelux Study Group (1998)[23]	Low-dose IFN-α + HU vs HU	195	IFN-α as effective as HU
German CML Study II (1999)[24]	IFN-α + HU vs HU	340	Not yet evaluable
Guilhot et al (1997)[25]	IFN-α (±HU) + Ara-C vs IFN-α (±HU)	721	IFN-α + Ara-C superior
Italian Cooperative Group (2000)	IFN-α (±HU) + Ara-C vs IFN-α (±HU)	584	Efficacy equal

[a] Bu, busulfan; HU, hydroxyurea; CT, chemotherapy.

Four randomized studies[18–21] and a meta-analysis[22] have shown that IFN-α prolongs survival by approximately 20 months compared with busulfan in the German study (Figure 9.1) and hydroxyurea in other studies (Table 9.1), depending on the risk profile at diagnosis.[18–21,23–26] Differences among the four studies are mainly due to variations in patient risk profiles (Figure 9.2). If patient populations are adjusted to uniform prognostic criteria, the survival curves are almost identical, as shown in a meta-analysis of the German and Italian randomized studies.[27] Evolving evidence suggests that outcome is better if treatment is started early (within 6 months of diagnosis) and in patients with less than 10% blasts in the peripheral blood and no other signs of acceleration.[28] IFN-α treatment is particularly advantageous in low-risk patients (Figure 9.3). A recent meta-analysis of seven randomized trials comparing IFN-α treatment with chemotherapy confirmed better survival with IFN-α treatment than with either hydroxyurea therapy ($p = 0.001$) or busulfan therapy ($p < 0.001$).[22] The 5-year survival rates were 57% with IFN-α therapy and 42% with chemotherapy (Figure 9.4).

DOSE–RESPONSE RELATIONSHIP

There is evidence for a dose–response relationship with IFN-α treatment.[28] The higher and daily IFN-α dosage was found to be more effective. Freund et al[29] also confirmed the dose dependence of response using IFN-α2b. In most studies showing that IFN-α improves survival, it has been combined with other drugs, mostly hydroxyurea. The single trial in which IFN-α was used as a monotherapy did not show a survival benefit compared with the use of hydroxyurea.[18] Although prolongation of survival is the most important benefit of IFN-α therapy, the available evidence suggests that prolonged survival is primarily achieved when IFN-α treatment is started during the early chronic phase and complete haematological and major cytogenetic remission (<35% Ph positivity) are induced. Complete haematological remission is accomplished after a median of 6 months;[18] complete cytogenetic remission (0% Ph positivity) occurs after a median of 12–17 months.[30]

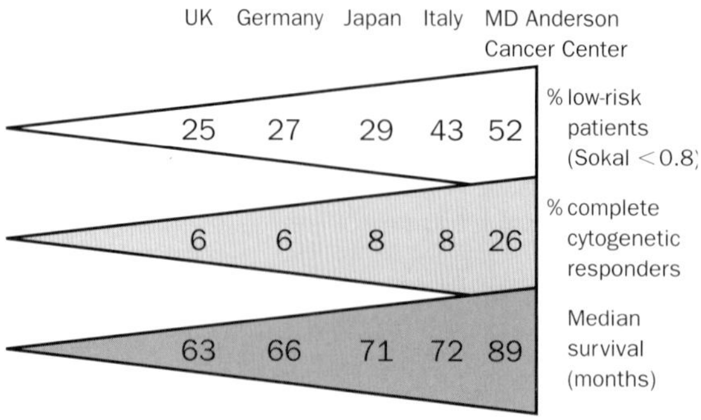

Figure 9.2 Risk profile, cytogenetic response, and median survival in IFN-α-treated CML patients. Comparison of the randomized multicentre trials from the UK,[19] Germany (CML study I),[18] Japan,[21] and Italy,[20] and the monocentric non-randomized experience of the MD Anderson Cancer Center, Houston.[7]

COMBINATION OF IFN-α WITH CHEMOTHERAPY

Several lines of evidence suggest that survival in CML patients correlates with tumour burden.[12,25,26,31–38] This evidence emerged from early studies using intensive chemotherapy, which demonstrated cytogenetic remission rates up to 70%,[39,40] and from survival analyses of 148 patients who relapsed after allogeneic bone marrow transplantations and had a significant survival advantage over 470 matched controls with conventional therapy ($p = 0.0002$). Intensification of treatment by the addition of low doses of Ara-C (cytosine arabinoside, cytarabine) further increases cytogenetic remission rate and survival, as shown by a recent randomized study.[25] Several ongoing studies apply this concept either by adding moderate doses of Ara-C and idarubicine to an induction treatment consisting of IFN-α and hydroxyurea or by using high-dose chemotherapy followed by autografting. Examples are Studies III and IIIA of the German CML Study Group and the autografting study recently launched by the European Group for Blood and Marrow Transplantation (EBMT).

ADVERSE EFFECTS

Virtually all patients receiving IFN-α experience some side-effects. Discontinuation of treatment due to toxicity is necessary for 4–18% of

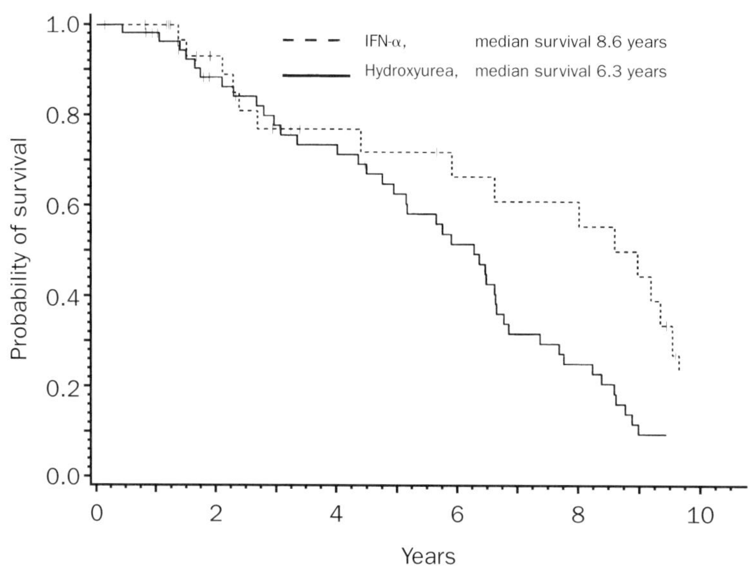

Figure 9.3 German CML study I: survival of low-risk patients according to Sokal.

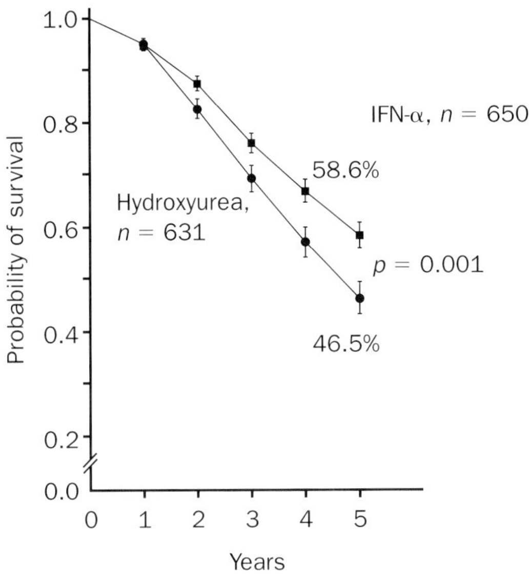

Figure 9.4 CML Trialists' Collaborative Group: IFN-α versus chemotherapy. Meta-analysis of seven randomized CML trials.[22]

patients, compared with 1% of those receiving hydroxyurea. Ozer et al[8] reported that in their study, patients received only 60% of the target dose owing to side-effects. Acute side-effects are generally mild to moderate, and include flu-like symptoms such as fever, chills, and malaise. Subacute side-effects include hair loss and exacerbation of autoimmune disorders. The most important chronic adverse events belong to the group of neurological and psychiatric problems, such as depression.[41,42] In contrast to busulfan, however, no life-threatening adverse effects have been described, and virtually all side-effects are reversible after discontinuation of the drug.

EFFECT OF IFN-α AND CHEMOTHERAPY ON BONE MARROW MORPHOLOGY

Following IFN-α administration, a decrease in neutrophil granulopoiesis accompanied by a significant expansion of erythroid precursors and an increased number of haemosiderin-laden macrophages has been observed. These changes corresponded to haematological response in most patients. Numbers of megakaryocytes and reticulin/collagen fibre density increased during treatment. In responding patients, atypical micromegakaryocytes were partially replaced by normal-sized megakaryocytes.[43,44]

IMPACT OF PROGNOSTIC RISK GROUPS AND STAGE OF DISEASE ON RESPONSE TO IFN-α

The widely used Sokal score[45] works well as a prognostic discriminator for survival of three different strata of patients treated with busulfan or hydroxyurea, but it has been repeatedly observed to be a poorer discriminator for survival of patients treated with IFN-α.[46] Since survival outcome is dependent on the risk profile at diagnosis, the establishment of reliable prognostic scores is important. Therefore the Sokal score has been improved and adapted to IFN-α treatment. An improved prognostic scoring system for estimating survival of chronic-phase CML patients treated with IFN-α has been developed and validated on the basis of 1377 IFN-α-treated patients by Hasford et al[46] for the collaborative CML Prognostic Factors Project (CPFP: www.pharmacoepi.de).[46] Low-risk patients according to Hasford show a 10-year survival of about 40% (Figure 9.5, see also Chapter 12, Figure 12.4). Long-term follow-up of the Italian trial of IFN-α versus conventional chemotherapy in CML showed a median survival and a 10-year survival rate for low-risk patients according to Sokal of 104 months and 47% in the IFN-α arm, and of 64 months and 30% in the chemotherapy arm ($p = 0.03$). Non-low-risk patients had a median survival and a 10-year survival rate of 69 months and 16% in the IFN-α arm, and of 46 months and 5% in the chemotherapy arm ($p = 0.006$).[26]

Therapy with IFN-α alone in the late chronic (>12 months after diagnosis) and accelerated phases of CML yields modest results. Complete haematological response has been achieved

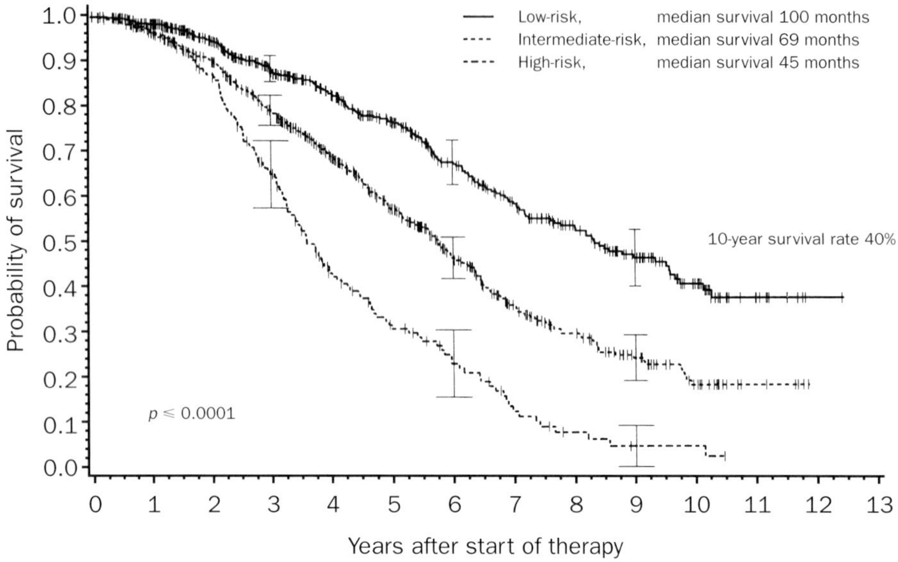

Figure 9.5 New IFN-α score applied to 1400 patients with early chronic-phase CML treated with IFN-α. About 40% of low-risk patients survive for more than 10 years.[46]

in 57% of patients, and major cytogenetic responses in only 10 out of 123 patients (8%).[47] However, even patients with clonal cytogenetic evolution (i.e. trisomy 8, double Ph, chromosome 17 abnormality) may respond to IFN-α, and this response is associated with longer survival.[48]

The prognostic risk for older patients (over 60 years of age) is worse than that for younger age groups, as would be expected. However, in elderly patients, acceptable rates of haematological and cytogenetic responses have been observed.[49] One publication reports that elderly patients tolerate IFN-α less well. Cortes et al[50] observed severe, dose-limiting toxicities in 26% of patients aged over 60 years, compared with 10–20% in the overall population.[51] Another study observed that the median ages of groups that discontinued IFN-α because of side-effects and of groups on continued IFN-α were identical.[18] Therefore, in older patients, a trial of IFN-α should be given.

COMPLETE CYTOGENETIC RESPONSE AFTER IFN-α THERAPY

A substantial minority of IFN-α-treated patients achieve a complete response, defined as the disappearance from the bone marrow of Ph-positive metaphases, which corresponds to a prolongation of the chronic phase and survival.[52] Currently, it is unclear for how long treatment with IFN-α should be continued for such patients. Quantitative monitoring of minimal residual disease is of major interest in these patients. At presentation, patients usually have a total burden of more than 10^{12} malignant cells.[53] Cytogenetics, Southern blot analysis, Western blotting, and conventional fluorescence in situ hybridization (FISH) have sensitivities of no better than 1%. Therefore a patient with negative results may harbour up to 10^{10} residual leukaemic cells.[54]

There is controversy regarding whether patients in long-term cytogenetic remission might be considered cured.[55,56] Recent evidence from 54 patients in complete cytogenetic remission due to IFN-α treatment shows that all patients had molecular evidence of residual disease, although three patients were intermittently negative according to reverse-transcriptase polymerase chain reaction (RT-PCR). In general, *BCR/ABL* transcript numbers were inversely related to the duration of complete remission. The median ratio of *BCR/ABL* to *ABL* at the time of maximal response for each patient was 0.045% (range 0–3.6%). During the period of observation, 14 patients relapsed: 11 cytogenetically to chronic-phase disease and three directly to blastic phase. The median ratio of *BCR/ABL* to *ABL* at maximal response was significantly higher in patients who relapsed than in those who remained in complete remission: 0.49% versus 0.021%, $p < 0.0001$ (Figures 9.6 and 9.7).[57] These findings demonstrate that the level of residual disease decreases with time in patients who maintain their cytogenetic response to IFN-α, but molecular evidence of disease is rarely (if ever) eliminated. The actual level of minimal residual disease correlates with the probability of relapse (Figure 9.7). It has been suggested to continue IFN-α in patients who achieve a complete response at least until relatively low levels of residual leukaemia as measured by *BCR/ABL* transcript levels are achieved (Figure 9.8).

Experience with some patients in continued complete cytogenetic remission has shown that remission may be maintained even after discontinuation of IFN-α.[57] It remains to be seen whether these are anecdotal observations in a few cases or observations relevant for a larger group of patients in the future. If prolonged survival is observed – even in the presence of residual disease – this would be relevant for the respective patients as an 'operational cure'.

A long-term follow-up of 71 patients with

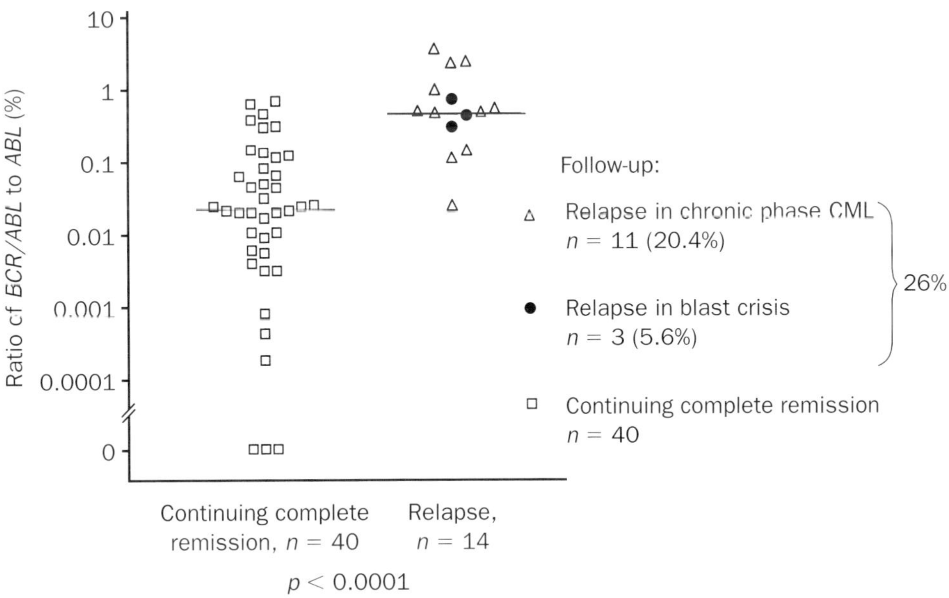

Figure 9.6 Maximum response on sequential analysis for the 54 CML patients in complete remission on IFN-α. For the 14 patients who relapsed, the minimum *BCR/ABL*-to-*ABL* ratio achieved was significantly higher ($p < 0.0001$, two-sided Mann–Whitney test) than that seen in patients who remained in complete remission.[57]

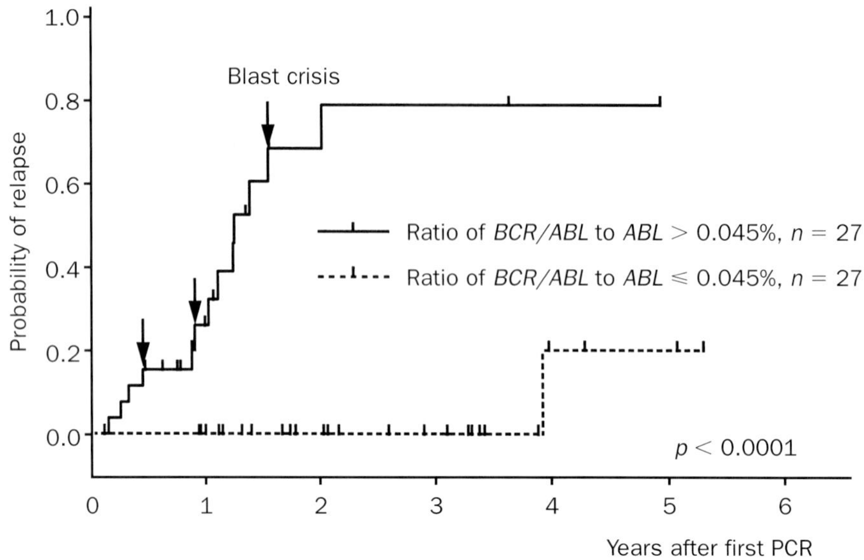

Figure 9.7 Relapse-free survival of patients in complete remission compared to the maximal response to IFN-α therapy. One of 27 patients with low levels of residual disease (*BCR/ABL*-to-*ABL* ratio ≤ 0.045%) relapsed, compared with 13 of 27 patients with relatively high levels (ratio > 0.045%; $p < 0.0001$, two-sided logrank test).[57]

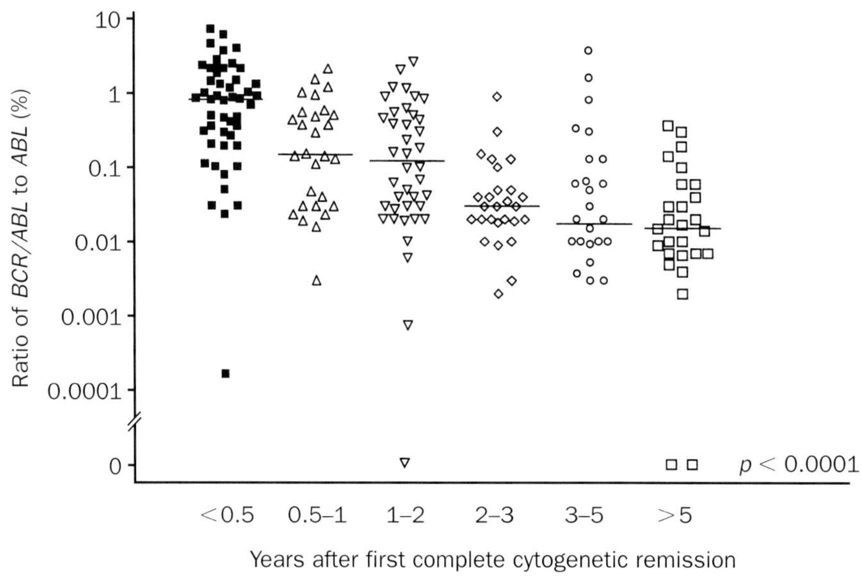

Figure 9.8 Residual disease measured as the ratio of *BCR/ABL* to *ABL* transcripts according to time in complete remission in 40 non-relapsing patients continuing IFN-α therapy.[57]

IFN-α as primary treatment for CML enrolled between 1984 and 1990 showed a significant survival advantage for patients with karyotypic response. Of 7 patients surviving more than 11 years, 6 were in continuous complete cytogenetic remission. All complete responders belonged to the low-risk group according to Sokal.[58]

IFN-α PRETREATMENT PRIOR TO ALLOGENEIC BMT

IFN-α pretreatment per se, in addition to the time aspect, may be harmful for subsequent transplantation because of increased transplantation-related early death rates due to graft rejection or graft-versus-host disease (GVHD). Such an IFN-α effect would appear plausible, since it is well known that IFN-α interferes with the cytokine network and its complex interactions. Dysregulation of cytokines by donor T cells has also been discussed as a mechanism underlying GVHD.

Five reports involving more than 300 patients did not confirm adverse effects of pretransplant IFN-α on subsequent allografting,[59–63] but two reports found a negative impact under some conditions, such as IFN-α pretreatment before transplantations with unrelated or mismatched donors, or duration of pretreatment with IFN-α of more than 5 or 12 months.[64,65] Since the reports with adverse outcome were not derived from controlled studies or predefined cohorts of patients and had no randomized pretreatments, they are subject to selection or referral bias. The referral aspect is critical, because IFN-α-treated patients who respond well to IFN-α are less likely to be referred to transplantation than patients who respond to IFN-α poorly or not at all. The issue was prospectively studied within two randomized studies of the German CML Study Group, which showed that IFN-α before transplantation does not affect outcome adversely (Figure 9.9), provided that it is discontinued at least 90 days before the procedure (Figure 9.10).[66]

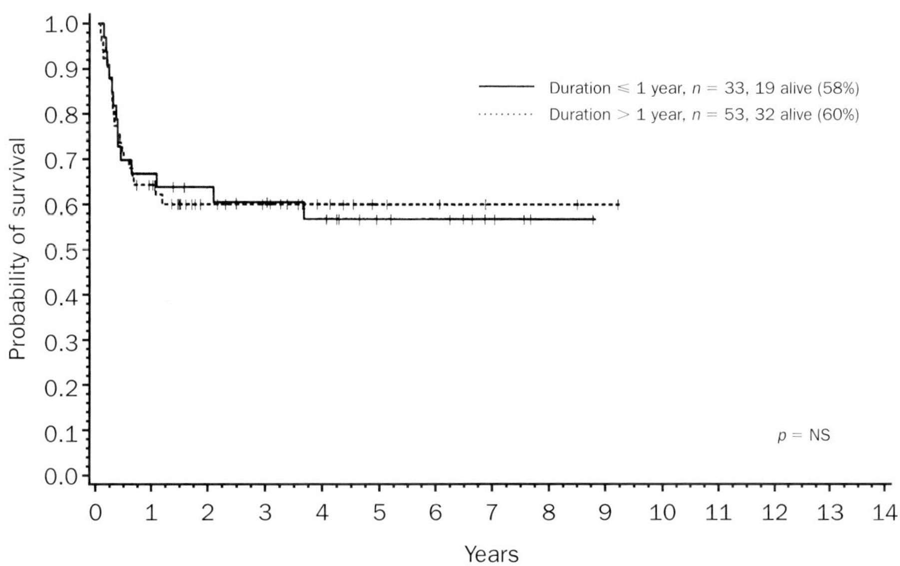

Figure 9.9 Survival of Ph/*BCR/ABL*-positive CML patients after bone marrow transplantation in chronic phase according to duration of pretransplant IFN-α treatment ($n = 86$).[66]

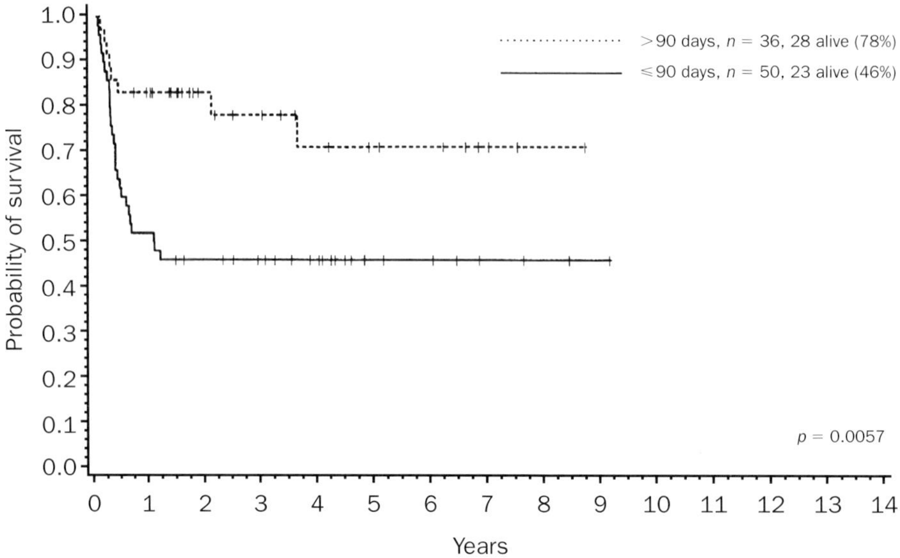

Figure 9.10 Survival of Ph/*BCR/ABL*-positive CML patients after bone marrow transplantation in chronic phase according to interval between discontinuation of IFN-α and transplantation ($n = 86$).[66]

In conclusion, there is no firm evidence in the literature against a trial procedure with IFN-α first, proceeding to transplantation only after an unsatisfactory response. There is suggestive evidence that IFN-α pretreatment may be beneficial for relapse-free or overall survival after transplantation, if IFN-α is given for a short period or if it is discontinued 3 months before transplantation.[66]

The evidence-based guidelines for the treatment of CML prepared by the American Society of Hematology state that there is no evidence of benefit of bone marrow transplantation from randomized controlled studies, and that it is uncertain to what extent results from uncontrolled observational studies are due to selection biases.[41] Therefore two retrospective studies comparatively analysed allografting versus IFN-α-based drug treatment. Both studies show that during the first 4–5 years, survival is better with drug treatment, but after 6 years, survival starts to be better with transplantation (Figure 9.11). The advantage of allografting is less clear in low-risk patients. In the study by the International Bone Marrow Transplant Registry (IBMTR) and the German CML Study Group, no significant advantage of allografting over drug treatment for low-risk patients is reached after 8 years,[67] and in the analysis by the Italian Cooperative Group, no survival advantage of allografting is reached after 10 years.[68]

Therefore, in 1995, the German CML Study Group decided to compare the two treatment strategies in a prospective randomized study and to quantify the differences. For the comparison, the instrument of genetic randomization was used, which requires the definition of a baseline sample by suitability for, and consent to, bone marrow transplantation and randomization by availability of a related donor. By spring 2000, 1010 patients were recruited, and 556 were allocated to the baseline sample as suitable for transplantation.[69]

PREDICTION OF RESPONSE

The most important factor predicting cytogenetic response to IFN-α is an early haematological

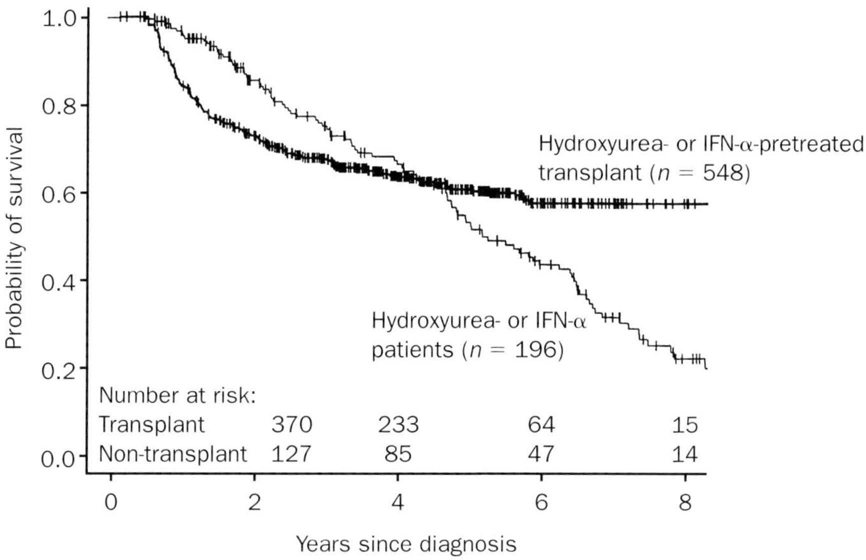

Figure 9.11 Adjusted probabilities (from Cox regression model) of survival after diagnosis of CML in persons receiving HLA-identical sibling bone marrow transplants within 1 year of diagnosis or non-transplant therapy with hydroxyurea or IFN-α (collaborative project of the German CML Study Group and the IBMTR).[67]

response. In patients achieving complete haematological remission within 3 months, the rate of major cytogenetic remission was over 80%.[9] The differential expression of IRF1 and IRF2 might influence cytogenetic responses. In major cytogenetic responders, the ratio of IRF1 to IRF2 mRNA transcripts is significantly higher than in non-responders[70], high expression of IRF4 is associated with a good response,[71] STAT1 expression was observed in complete responders, in contrast to STAT1 negativity in non-responders.[72] Pane et al[73] have demonstrated that in vitro downmodulation of *BCR/ABL* expression in bone marrow mononuclear cells within 24 hours corresponds to clinical response. *BCR/ABL* transcript levels in the course of IFN-α therapy may predict ultimate cytogenetic response.[74]

PEGYLATED INTERFERONS

It is expected that the pegylated forms of IFN-α may mitigate acute and chronic side-effects of recombinant IFN-α, such as flu-like effects, fatigue, weight loss, depression, and uncommon immunological events. PEG-interferons have a pharmacological profile that allows once-weekly dosing. A drug whose level in the circulation can be maintained (without the accentuated peaks and troughs) for a considerable length of time is much more advantageous than conventional IFN-α, with its typical undulating pharmacokinetic pattern.

Two phase I studies have been conducted with either PEG–IFN-α2a or PEG-IFN-α2b to determine the safety profile, and obtain some information on activity. Preliminary data from these trials suggest that PEG-interferons provide a significant advance over standard IFN-α.[75,76]

COMBINATION OF SIGNAL TRANSDUCTION INHIBITORS AND IFN-α

Recently, promising results have been reported in CML patients with the use of a novel inhibitor of the ABL protein tyrosine kinase,

STI571 (Glivec; Gleevec). Experience with IFN-α has demonstrated that sustained complete cytogenetic responses can be achieved, supporting the notion that Ph-negative haematopoiesis can be fully restored, as observed with immunostimulation by cytokine therapy. STI571 is the first compound that selectively inhibits activated forms of the ABL protein tyrosine kinase, in this case BCR/ABL.[77] These inhibitors may be successful as single agents, but it is likely that they will be more effective and/or will lead to more durable cytogenetic responses when given together with what is currently considered to be standard therapy for chronic-phase CML: hydroxyurea, IFN-α, and Ara-C.[78] It is believed that the ability of a signal transduction inhibitor to suppress the proliferation of the malignant clone together with the eradication of the clone by chemo- and immunotherapy may lead to a more permanent restitution of the haematopoietic system.

CONCLUSIONS

The evidence from randomized controlled trials suggest that, compared with busulfan and hydroxyurea, IFN-α improves survival in chronic-phase CML patients with a favourable risk profile: no or minimal prior treatment, normal platelet count, low blast counts in the bone marrow and peripheral blood, and treatment commencing soon after diagnosis.[41] IFN-α increases survival by a median of about 20 months. In low-risk patients, a 10-year survival rate of 40% can be achieved. Achievement of major cytogenetic remission is associated with prolonged survival. Combination with chemotherapy can increase the rate of cytogenetic remission and further prolong survival. The pegylation of the interferon molecule results in improved pharmacokinetic and pharmacodynamic profiles, with enhanced efficacy in patients refractory to conventional recombinant IFN-α. The role of STI571 for long-term control of CML remains to be determined.

REFERENCES

1. Pfeffer LM, Dinarello CA, Herberman RB et al, Biologic properties of recombinant alpha-interferon: 40th anniversary of the discovery of interferons. *Cancer Res* 1998; **58:** 2489–2499.
2. Bhatia R, Wayner EA, McGlave PB, Verfaillie CM, Interferon-alpha restores normal adhesion of chronic myelogenous leukemia hematopoietic progenitors to bone marrow stroma by correcting impaired beta 1 integrin receptor function. *J Clin Invest* 1994; **94:** 384–91.
3. Harada H, Taniguchi T, Tanaka N, The role of interferon regulatory factors in the interferon system and cell growth control. *Biochimie* 1998; **80:** 641–50.
4. Talpaz M, McCredie KB, Mavligit GM, Gutterman JU, Leukocyte interferon-induced myeloid cytoreduction in chronic myelogenous leukemia. *Blood* 1983; **62:** 689–92.
5. Talpaz M, Kantarjian HM, McCredie K et al, Hematologic remission and cytogenetic improvement induced by recombinant human interferon $alpha_{2a}$ in chronic myelogenous leukemia. *N Engl J Med* 1986; **314:** 1065–9.
6. Niederle N, Kloke O, Osieka R et al, Interferon alfa-2b in the treatment of chronic myelogenous leukemia. *Semin Oncol* 1987; **14:** 29–35.
7. Kantarjian HM, O'Brien S, Anderlini P, Talpaz M, Treatment of chronic myelogenous leukemia: current status and investigational options. *Blood* 1996; **87:** 3069–81.
8. Ozer H, George SL, Schiffer CA et al, Prolonged subcutaneous administration of recombinant alpha 2b interferon in patients with previously untreated Philadelphia chromosome-positive chronic-phase chronic myelogenous leukemia: effect on remission duration and survival: Cancer and Leukemia Group B Study 8583. *Blood* 1993; **82:** 2975–84.
9. Mahon FX, Montastruc M, Faberes C, Reiffers J, Predicting complete cytogenetic response in chronic myelogenous leukemia patients treated with recombinant interferon α. *Blood* 1994; **84:** 3592–4.
10. Thaler J, Gastl G, Fluckinger T et al, Austrian Biological Response Modifier (BRM) Study Group. Interferon alpha-2c therapy of patients with chronic myelogenous leukemia: long term results of a multicenter phase-II study. *Ann Hematol* 1996; **72:** 349–55.
11. Haut A, Abbott WS, Wintrobe MM, Cartwright

GE, Busulfan in the treatment of chronic myelocytic leukemia. The effect of long term intermittent therapy. *Blood* 1961; **17:** 1–19.
12. Hehlmann R, Heimpel H, Hasford J and the German CML Study Group, Randomized comparison of busulfan and hydroxyurea in chronic myelogenous leukemia: prolongation of survival by hydroxyurea. *Blood* 1993; **82:** 398–407.
13. Kennedy BJ, Hydroxyurea therapy in chronic myelogenous leukemia. *Cancer* 1972; **29:** 1052–6.
14. DeSimone C, Guerriero C, Guidi B et al, Multiple squamous cell carcinomas of the skin during long-term treatment with hydroxyurea. *Eur J Dermatol* 1998; **8:** 114–15.
15. Daoud MS, Gibson LE, Pittelkow MR, Hydroxyurea dermopathy: a unique lichenoid eruption complicating long-term therapy with hydroxyurea. *J Am Acad Dermatol* 1997; **36**(2 part 1): 178–82.
16. Weinlich G, Schuler G, Greil R et al, Leg ulcers associated with long-term hydroxyurea therapy. *J Am Acad Dermatol* 1998; **39:** 372–4.
17. Hehlmann R, Heimpel H, Hasford J, Randomized comparison of interferon-α, hydroxyurea, and busulfan in chronic myeloid leukemia: response to Kantarjian and Talpaz and to Tura and Baccarani. *Blood* 1995; **85:** 3000–2.
18. Hehlmann R, Heimpel H, Hasford J, and the German CML Study Group, Randomized comparison of interferon-alpha with busulfan and hydroxyurea in chronic myelogenous leukemia. The German CML Study Group. *Blood* 1994; **84:** 4064–77.
19. Allan NC, Richards SM, Shepherd PC, UK Medical Research Council randomized, multicentre trial of interferon-alpha n1 for chronic myeloid leukaemia: improved survival irrespective of cytogenetic response. The UK Medical Research Council's Working Parties for Therapeutic Trials in Adult Leukaemia. *Lancet* 1995; **345:** 1392–7.
20. The Italian Cooperative Study Group on Chronic Myeloid Leukemia, Interferon alfa-2a as compared with conventional chemotherapy for the treatment of chronic myeloid leukemia. *N Engl J Med* 1994; **330:** 820–5.
21. Ohnishi K, Ohno R, Tomonaga M and the Kouseisho Leukemia Study Group, A randomized trial comparing interferon-alpha with busulfan for newly diagnosed chronic myelogenous leukemia in chronic phase. *Blood* 1995; **86:** 906–16.
22. Chronic Myeloid Leukemia Trialists' Collaborative Group, Interferon alfa versus chemotherapy for chronic myeloid leukemia: a meta-analysis of seven randomized trials. *J Natl Cancer Inst* 1997; **89:** 1616–20.
23. The Benelux CML Study Group, Randomized study on hydroxyurea alone versus hydroxyurea combined with low-dose interferon-α2b for chronic myeloid leukemia. *Blood* 1998; **91:** 2713–21.
24. Hehlmann R, Heimpel H, Hossfeld DL and the German CML Study Group, Randomized study of the combination of hydroxyurea and interferon alpha versus hydroxyurea monotherapy during the chronic phase of chronic myelogenous leukemia (CML Study II). *Bone Marrow Transplant* 1996; **17**(Suppl 3): S21–4.
25. Guilhot F, Chastang C, Michallet M et al, for the French Chronic Myeloid Leukemia Study Group, Interferon alfa-2b combined with cytarabine versus interferon alone in chronic myelogenous leukemia. *N Engl J Med* 1997; **337:** 223–9.
26. The Italian Cooperative Study Group on Chronic Myeloid Leukemia, Long-term follow-up of the Italian trial of interferon-α versus conventional chemotherapy in chronic myeloid leukemia. *Blood* 1998; **92:** 1541–8.
27. Hasford J, Baccarani M, Hehlmann R et al, Interferon-α and hydroxyurea in early chronic myeloid leukemia: a comparative analysis of the Italian and German chronic myeloid leukemia trials with interferon-α. *Blood* 1996; **87:** 5384–91.
28. Alimena G, Morra E, Lazzarino M et al, Interferon alpha-2b as therapy for Ph′-positive chronic myelogenous leukemia: a study of 82 patients treated with intermittent or daily administration. *Blood* 1988; **72:** 642–7.
29. Freund M, von Wussow P, Diedrich H et al, Recombinant human interferon (IFN) alpha-2b in chronic myelogenous leukaemia: dose dependency of response and frequency of neutralizing anti-interferon antibodies. *Br J Haematol* 1989; **72:** 350–6.
30. Montastruc M, Mahon FX, Faberes C et al, Response to recombinant interferon alpha in patients with chronic myelogenous leukemia in a single center: results and analysis of predictive factors. *Leukemia* 1995; **9:** 1997–2002.
31. Hehlmann R, Heimpel H, Current aspects of drug therapy in Philadelphia-positive CML: correlation of tumor burden with survival. *Leuk Lymphoma* 1996; **22**(Suppl 1): 161–7.

32. Carella AM, Chimirri F, Podesta M et al, High-dose chemo-radiotherapy followed by autologous Philadelphia chromosome-negative blood progenitor cell transplantation in patients with chronic myelogenous leukemia. *Bone Marrow Transplant* 1996; **17:** 201–5.
33. Goldman JM, Autografting for CML – overview and perspectives. *Bone Marrow Transplant* 1996; **17**(Suppl 3): S71–4.
34. McGlave PB, De Fabritiis P, Deisseroth A et al, Autologous transplants for chronic myelogenous leukaemia: results from eight transplant groups. *Lancet* 1994; **343:** 1486–8.
35. Cunningham I, Gee T, Dowling M et al, Results of treatment of Ph'+ chronic myelogenous leukemia with an intensive treatment regimen (L-5 protocol). *Blood* 1979; **53:** 375–95.
36. Sharp JC, Joyner MV, Wayne AW et al, Karyotypic conversion in Ph^1-positive chronic myeloid leukaemia with combination chemotherapy. *Lancet* 1979; **i:** 1370–2.
37. Kolitz JE, Kempin SJ, Schulger A et al, A phase II pilot trial of high-dose hydroxyurea in chronic myelogenous leukemia. *Semin Oncol* 1992; **19:** 27–33.
38. Shepherd PCA, Richards SM, Allan NC, Progress with interferon in CML – Results of the MRC UK CML III study. *Bone Marrow Transplant* 1996; **17**(Suppl 3): S15–18.
39. Hehlmann R, Berger U, Hochhaus A and the German CML Study Group, Towards a cure by drug treatment? The German CML Study Group experience. In: *Autologous Blood and Marrow Transplantation. Proceedings of the Ninth International Symposium, Arlington, TX* (Dicke KA, Keating A, eds). Charlottesville, VA: Carden Jennings, 1999: 114–27.
40. Hehlmann R, Cytostatic therapy of chronic myelogenous leukemia: review and perspectives. In: *Chronic Myelocytic Leukemia and Interferon* (Huhn D, Hellriegel KP, Niederle N, eds). Berlin: Springer-Verlag, 1988: 102–12.
41. Silver RT, Woolf SH, Hehlmann R et al, An evidence-based analysis of the effect of busulfan, hydroxyurea, interferon, and allogeneic bone marrow transplantation in treating the chronic phase of chronic myeloid leukemia: developed for the American Society of Hematology. *Blood* 1999; **94:** 1517–36.
42. Trask PC, Esper P, Riba M, Redman B, Psychiatric side effects of interferon therapy: prevalence, proposed mechanisms, and future directions. *J Clin Oncol* 2000; **18:** 2316–26.
43. Thiele J, Zirbes TK, Kvasnicka HM et al, Effect of interferon therapy on bone marrow morphology in chronic myeloid leukemia: a cytochemical and immunohistochemical study of trephine biopsies. *J Interferon Cytokine Res* 1996; **16:** 217–24.
44. Thiele J, Kvasnicka HM, Schmitt-Graeff A et al, Effects of interferon and hydroxyurea on bone marrow fibrosis in chronic myelogenous leukemia: a comparative retrospective multicentre histological and clinical study. *Br J Haematol* 2000; **108:** 64–71.
45. Sokal JE, Cox EB, Baccarani M et al, Prognostic discrimination in 'good-risk' chronic granulocytic leukemia. *Blood* 1984; **63:** 789–99.
46. Hasford J, Pfirrmann M, Hehlmann R et al, A new prognostic score for survival of patients with chronic myeloid leukemia treated with interferon alfa. *J Natl Cancer Inst* 1998; **90:** 850–8.
47. Sacchi S, Kantarjian HM, O'Brien S et al, Long-term follow-up results of alpha-interferon-based regimens in patients with late chronic phase chronic myelogenous leukemia. *Leukemia* 1997; **11:** 1610–16.
48. Cortes J, Talpaz M, O'Brien S et al, Suppression of cytogenetic clonal evolution with interferon alfa therapy in patients with Philadelphia chromosome-positive chronic myelogenous leukemia. *J Clin Oncol* 1998; **16:** 3279–85.
49. Hilbe W, Apfelbeck U, Fridrik M et al, Interferon-α for the treatment of elderly patients with chronic myeloid leukaemia. *Leuk Res* 1998; **22:** 881–6.
50. Cortes J, Kantarjian H, O'Brien S et al, Results of interferon-alpha therapy in patients with chronic myelogenous leukemia 60 years of age and older. *Am J Med* 1996; **100:** 452–5.
51. Kantarjian HM, Deisseroth A, Kurzrock R et al, Chronic myelogeneous leukemia: a concise update. *Blood* 1993; **82:** 691–703.
52. Kantarjian HM, Smith TL, O'Brien S, and the Leukemia Service, Prolonged survival in chronic myelogenous leukemia after cytogenetic response to interferon-α therapy. *Ann Intern Med* 1995; **122:** 254–61.
53. Clarkson B, Strife A, Cytokinetic considerations relevant to development of a successful therapeutic strategy in chronic myelogenous leukemia (CML). *Leuk Lymphoma* 1993; **11**(Suppl 1): 101–7.
54. Morley A, Quantifying leukemia. *N Engl J Med* 1998; **339:** 627–9.

55. Kurzrock R, Estrov Z, Kantarjian H, Talpaz M, Conversion of interferon-induced, long-term cytogenetic remissions in chronic myelogenous leukemia to polymerase chain reaction negativity. *J Clin Oncol* 1998; **16:** 1526–31.
56. Hochhaus A, Lin F, Reiter A et al, Variable numbers of BCR–ABL transcripts persist in CML patients who achieve complete cytogenetic remission with interferon-α. *Br J Haematol* 1995; **91:** 126–31.
57. Hochhaus A, Reiter A, Saußele S et al, for the German CML Study Group and the U.K.MRC CML Study Group, Molecular heterogeneity in complete cytogenetic responders after interferon-α therapy for chronic myeloid leukaemia: low levels of minimal residual disease are associated with continuing remission. *Blood* 2000; **95:** 62–6.
58. Kloke O, Opalka B, Niederle N, Interferon alfa as primary treatment of chronic myeloid leukemia: long-term follow-up of 71 patients observed in a single center. *Leukemia* 2000; **14:** 389–92.
59. Tomás JF, López-Lorenzo JL, Requena MJ et al, Absence of influence of prior treatment with interferon on the outcome of allogeneic bone marrow transplantation for chronic myeloid leukemia. *Bone Marrow Transplant* 1998; **22:** 47–51.
60. Zuffa E, Bandini G, Bonini A et al, Prior treatment with alpha-interferon does not adversely affect the outcome of allogeneic BMT in chronic phase chronic myeloid leukemia. *Haematologica* 1998; **83:** 231–6.
61. Giralt SA, Kantarjian HM, Talpaz M et al, Effect of prior interferon alfa therapy on the outcome of allogeneic bone marrow transplantation for chronic myelogenous leukemia. *J Clin Oncol* 1993; **11:** 1055–61.
62. Giralt S, Szyldo R, Goldman JM et al, Effect of short-term interferon therapy on the outcome of subsequent HLA-identical sibling bone marrow transplantation for chronic myelogenous leukemia: an analysis from the International Bone Marrow Transplant Registry. *Blood* 2000; **95:** 410–15.
63. Shepherd P, Richards S, Allan N, Survival after allogeneic bone marrow transplantation (BMT) in patients randomised into a trial of IFN-α versus chemotherapy: no significant adverse effect of prolonged IFN-α administration. *Blood* 1996; **88:** 682a.
64. Morton JA, Gooley T, Hansen JA et al, Association between pretransplant interferon-α and outcome after unrelated donor marrow transplantation for chronic myelogenous leukemia in chronic phase. *Blood* 1998; **92:** 394–401.
65. Beelen DW, Elmaagacli AH, Schaefer UW, The adverse influence of pretransplant interferon-α (IFN-α) on transplant outcome after marrow transplantation for chronic phase chronic myelogenous leukemia increases with the duration of IFN-α exposure. *Blood* 1999; **93:** 1779–80.
66. Hehlmann R, Hochhaus A, Kolb HJ et al, for the German CML-Study Group and the SAKK, Interferon before allogeneic bone marrow transplantation in chronic myelogenous leukemia does not affect outcome adversely, provided it is discontinued at least 90 days before the procedure. *Blood* 1999; **94:** 3668–77.
67. Gale RP, Hehlmann R, Zhang MJ and the German CML Study Group, Survival with bone marrow transplantation versus hydroxyurea or interferon for chronic myelogenous leukemia (CML). *Blood* 1998; **91:** 1810–19.
68. The Italian Cooperative Study Group on Chronic Myeloid Leukemia and Italian Group for Bone Marrow Transplantation, Monitoring treatment and survival in chronic myeloid leukemia. *J Clin Oncol* 1999; **17:** 1858–68.
69. Hehlmann R, Berger U, Hochhaus A et al, Randomized comparison of allogeneic bone marrow transplantation and IFN based drug treatment in CML: early results. *Proc Am Soc Clin Oncol* 2000; **19:** 5a.
70. Hochhaus A, Yan XH, Willer A et al, Expression of interferon regulatory factor (IRF) genes and response to interferon-α in chronic myeloid leukaemia. *Leukemia* 1997; **11:** 933–9.
71. Schmidt M, Hochhaus A, König-Merediz SA et al, Expression of interferon regulatory factor 4 in chronic myeloid leukemia: correlation with response to interferon alfa therapy. *J Clin Oncol* 2000; **18:** 3331–8.
72. Landolfo S, Guarini A, Riera L et al, Chronic myeloid leukemia cells resistant to interferon-α lack STAT1 expression. *Hematol J* 2000; **1:** 7–14.
73. Pane F, Mostarda I, Selleri C et al, BCL/ABL mRNA and the $p210^{BCR/ABL}$ protein are down-modulated by interferon-α in chronic myeloid leukemia patients. *Blood* 1999; **94:** 2200–7.
74. Martinelli G, Testoni N, Amabile M et al, Quantification of BCR–ABL transcripts in CML patients in cytogenetic remission after interferon-α-based therapy. *Bone Marrow Transplant* 2000; **25:** 729–36.

75. Talpaz M, Cortes J, O'Brien S et al, Phase I study of polyethylene glycol (PEG) interferon alpha-2b (Intron-A) in CML patients. *Blood* 1998; **92**(Suppl 1): 251a.
76. Talpaz M, O'Brien S, Cortes J et al, Phase I study of pegylated-interferon α-2a (PEGASYS™) in patients with chronic myelogenous leukemia (CML). *Blood* 1999; **94**(Suppl 1): 530a.
77. Druker BJ, Tamura S, Buchdunger E et al, Effects of a selective inhibitor of the Abl tyrosine kinase on the growth of Bcr-Abl positive cells. *Nature Med* 1996; **2:** 561–6.
78. Thiesing JT, Ohno-Jones S, Kolibaba KS, Druker BJ, Efficacy of an ABL tyrosine kinase inhibitor in conjunction with other anti-neoplastic agents against BCR–ABL positive cells. *Blood* 1999; **94**(Suppl 1): 100a.

10

Chemotherapy

Bengt Simonsson

CONTENTS • Introduction • Mild chemotherapy to achieve palliation and symptom relief • Intensive chemotherapy to achieve Ph reduction or Ph negativity • Conclusions

INTRODUCTION

Patients with chronic myeloid leukaemia (CML) are often asymptomatic for a long time. They eventually develop symptoms such as tiredness, weight loss, sweats, bone pain, fever, and abdominal discomfort due to splenomegaly. All these symptoms can usually be handled with symptomatic therapy. The typical clinical culmination of CML is a fatal blast crisis. Only a small percentage of patients succumb to CML in the first and second years after diagnosis. Thereafter, however, the mortality rate is around 25% per year.

As far back as the 1950s, it was known that the symptoms of CML could be controlled with oral chemotherapy. For a long time, symptom relief was the only treatment option. Since the early 1980s, however, different treatment strategies have emerged, which now permit a choice between two major goals of treatment:

1. The first alternative is to relieve symptoms without attempting to cure the patient. The most common drugs used for symptomatic treatment of CML are hydroxyurea, interferon-α (IFN-α) in low dose, and busulfan.
2. The second alternative is to prolong the time to blast crisis, sometimes with the hope of curing the patient. The severe side-effects and increased initial mortality resulting from such therapy must be weighed against the reduced long-term survival associated with symptomatic treatment.

The best therapy for CML is allogeneic stem cell transplantation. It is a curative treatment, but owing to lack of bone marrow donors and to patient age, only a small percentage of CML patients benefit from this procedure. Intensive chemotherapy followed by autologous stem cell transplantation might also prolong survival, and quite a few patients also reach considerably long periods of Philadelphia chromosome (Ph) negativity.

IFN-α alone or combined with low-dose Ara-C also prolongs survival compared with single-dose chemotherapy. This drug fails, however, in most patients to induce long-term cytogenetic remissions.

This chapter discusses the effect of chemotherapy alone on CML. Chemotherapy alone does not cure CML, but can be used in two groups for two different purposes:

1. Mild chemotherapy to achieve palliation and symptom relief.
2. More intensive chemotherapy to achieve tumour regression to significant Ph reduction or Ph negativity.

MILD CHEMOTHERAPY TO ACHIEVE PALLIATION AND SYMPTOM RELIEF

If untreated and with poor supportive care, CML has from diagnosis a median survival of 31 months.[1] Nowadays patients seldom die in chronic-phase CML, because it is easy to control that phase of the disease. In up to 80% of patients, single-drug oral therapy can control symptoms caused by the disease, such as hyperproliferation, leukocytosis, and organomegaly. The drugs, however, have a marginal effect on the time to transformation to blastic phase or myelofibrosis with marrow failure.

In Table 10.1 are listed some drugs used for single-drug palliative and symptomatic treatment of CML. Patients treated with these drugs in palliative doses will die owing to transformation of their disease, with a median survival of 3–5 years. It should, however, be remembered that in interpreting the references cited in Table 10.1, the dosage of the drug is important, i.e. the dose used is for palliation alone. Besides low therapy intensity, patient risk groups (i.e. patient selection) also have to be considered.

Busulfan

In 1953, busulfan, an alkylating agent, was the first drug reported to be effective for haematological control in CML.[2] Fifteen years later, it was reported to control disease for longer periods than did radiotherapy.[7]

Busulfan is usually given daily at 0.1 mg/kg until the white blood cell (WBC) count is decreased by 50%, and then the dose is reduced to 0.05 mg/kg. Courses are repeated at 2–8 mg daily for 5–10 days. In most patients receiving busulfan, disease cannot be controlled safely at the low leukocyte levels needed to induce a complete haematological response. Generally the drug is discontinued when the leukocyte count declines to $(20–25) \times 10^9/l$, since this count will thereafter continue to fall for another 2–4 weeks.[8] Therefore, partial haematological response is the therapeutic aim (WBC $(20–50) \times 10^9/l$). Administration of large single doses (50–100 mg) at intervals of at least 4 weeks is seldom used, but is possible and effective.[9] Primary resistance to busulfan is uncommon. Side-effects of busulfan include severe prolonged myelosuppression (also after

Table 10.1 Drugs used for palliative and symptomatic chemotherapy

Drug	Refs
Busulfan	2–13
Hydroxyurea	3, 5, 14–20
Homoharringtonine	21–24
Ara-C (cytosine arabinoside, cytarabine)	25, 26
Etoposide (VP-16)	27
2-Chlorodeoxyadenosine (2-CdA, cladribine)	28
2'-Deoxycoformycin (DCF, pentostatin)	29
Fludarabine	29

standard doses). An uncommon side-effect is a severe idiosyncratic pulmonary reaction, a pronounced interstitial fibrosis, known as busulfan lung, which may be lethal.[10] Gonadal failure (usually irreversible?) may occur; males develop aspermia and females menopause after 3–6 months of therapy.[11,12] Other rare complications of busulfan treatment include cataract formation and Addison-disease-like clinical symptoms.[13]

Hydroxyurea

Introduced for use in CML in 1966,[14] hydroxyurea is now the drug of choice for disease control. The compound is a cycle-specific inhibitor of DNA synthesis. It has a better toxicity profile than busulfan. Hydroxyurea is less toxic to the bone marrow and does not produce prolonged or irreversible marrow aplasia. The WBC counts starts to increase within a few days after stopping (or reducing) treatment. It is usually given at a dose of 40 mg/kg daily, which is reduced by 50% when the WBC count drops below 20×10^9/l. The dose is then adjusted individually to keep the WBC count at $(2–5) \times 10^9$/l. The WBC count falls more rapidly than during treatment with busulfan. Treatment must be maintained indefinitely.

Hydroxyurea has a few side-effects, all of which are reversible on stopping treatment. Nausea and anorexia (more common at higher doses) are usually transient. Atrophy and scaling of the skin and partial alopecia may occur. Hydroxyurea may also cause red cell macrocytosis, megaloblastic changes in the bone marrow, and oral, genital or skin ulcers.[3,19] Hydroxyurea does not cause irreversible damage to the gonads. It may, however, be teratogenic, although normal births have been reported after hydroxyurea treatment.[20]

Busulfan and hydroxyurea produce haematological remissions in 50–80% of patients. Neither agent, however, as used routinely, achieves cytogenetic remission or significantly prevents progression to blastic transformation.

Hydroxyurea is, however, superior to busulfan. Thus Hehlman et al[5] showed in a prospective randomized study on 441 CML patients that treatment with hydroxyurea prolonged survival compared with treatment with busulfan (Figure 10.1). The median survivals

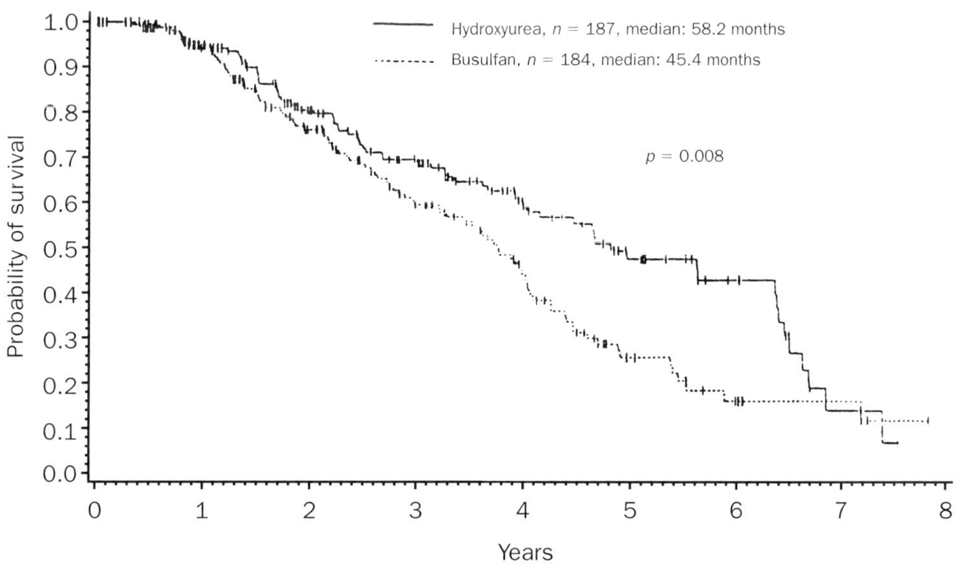

Figure 10.1 Survival of Ph-positive CML patients according to treatment group. Reproduced from reference 5 with permission from *Blood*.

were 58 months and 45 months respectively ($p = 0.008$). The survival advantage was recognized in all risk groups and as being due to a significant prolongation of the chronic phase. In other smaller studies, the superiority of hydroxyurea was not proven (see e.g. Allan et al[30]). In a meta-analysis of three national (Germany, UK, Sweden) randomized studies, however, Richards et al[18] confirmed that hydroxyurea is the drug of choice in CML and that patients on this drug survive around 10 months longer than those on busulfan.

Another advantage of hydroxyurea is that, in contrast to busulfan, exposure to hydroxyurea prior to stem cell transplantation has no adverse effects, and therefore is associated with a better outcome after allogeneic stem cell transplantation.[4,31]

Homoharringtonine

This drug is a cytotoxic alkaloid isolated from a Chinese tree (*Cephalotaxus fortuneii*). It blocks protein synthesis and thereby progression of cells from G_1 phase into S phase and from G_2 phase into M phase.[21] O'Brian et al[22] treated 71 patients with Ph-positive CML in late chronic phase with a continuous infusion of homoharringtonine at a daily dose of 2.5 mg/m^2 for 14 days for remission induction and then for 7 days every month for maintenance. Seventy-two per cent of the patients achieved complete and 16% partial haematological remission. Thirty-one per cent developed a cytogenetic response: major in 15% and complete in 7%. In early chronic disease, the haematological response was 92% and the cytogenetic response 68%.[23] The dose-limiting toxicities are hypotension and myelosuppression. The drug has relatively mild extramedullary toxicity and no cardiotoxicity.

These results suggest that homoharringtonine might have an effect on interferon-resistant patients. Combinations of homoharringtonine with IFN-α and Ara-C have shown promising preliminary results in the clinical setting.[24]

Low-dose Ara-C

Ara-C (cytosine arabinoside, cytarabine) has been given for extended periods in continuous infusion in patients with chronic-phase CML. The dose was 15–30 mg/m^2/day, usually for periods of 3–4 weeks. Haematological manifestations of the disease were controlled and a cytogenetic response was also achieved, including one complete cytogenetic remission.[25,26] The rationale for treatment with this drug is that prolonged exposure to low concentrations of Ara-C preferentially inhibit progenitor cells from CML patients compared with normal myeloid progenitors.

Other agents

Etoposide (VP-16),[27] 2-chlorodeoxyadenosine (2-CdA, cladribine),[28] 2'-deoxycoformycin (DCF, pentostatin), and fludarabine[29] have, in small studies with acceptable toxicity, also been shown to lead to a haematological response in chronic-phase CML.

INTENSIVE CHEMOTHERAPY TO ACHIEVE PH REDUCTION OR PH NEGATIVITY

Reports from the early 1970s showed that busulfan treatment might induce a reduction in percentage of Ph-positive cells in the bone marrow.[32] In vitro studies after intensive chemotherapy demonstrated that Ph-negative hematopoiesis was achieved in some patients and that this was probably due to faster regeneration of normal compared with leukaemic cells.[33]

These findings led to trials to reduce or eliminate the Ph-positive clone by intensive chemotherapy, similar to that used for acute leukaemia. The hope was that the successful treatment of acute leukaemia might translate to CML. Although many patients had more substantial Ph reductions, few became completely Ph-negative. It was, however, again confirmed that, at least early in the course of CML, normal haematopoiesis might still be present in the bone marrow. This knowledge has been of importance for the development of intensive treatment of CML patients, aiming at Ph negativity during IFN-α treatment and mobilizing Ph-negative stem cells for autotransplantation.

The rationale for intensive treatment in general is that minimizing or eliminating the Ph-positive clone and replacing it with normal cells should reduce the rate of secondary genetic changes and thereby postpone blast crisis. Today, intensive therapy consists of high-dose IFN-α and high-dose chemotherapy with or without stem cell support. In this chapter, we shall only discuss the antitumour effect of intensive chemotherapy.

The outcomes of a number of studies of different combinations are shown in Table 10.2.

Table 10.2 Intensive chemotherapy in chronic-phase CML

Drugs[a]	No. of patients	Treatment-related mortality rate (%)	Tumour reduction	Ph response rate[b] (%)	Overall survival	Refs
L-5	37		+	+	?	37,38
ROAP 10	37	3	+	53	?	39
DOAP	32	0	+	60	+(?)	40
ICE	28				?	41
ICE	17		+	80	?	42
mini-ICE	19	0	+	80	?	42
ICE	17 + 6	0	+	60	?	43,44
mini-ICE	10	10	+	80	?	45
DA	107	3	+	>50[c]	?	36
MEA	67	3	+	>50[c]	?	36
Cy	23	0	+	70	?	35
HU[1]	10 + 5 + 14	0	+	+?	?	46–48
HU[2]	18	0	+	70	?	49
I-A[1]	40	5	+	70	?	50
I-A[2]	11	0	+	0	?	51, 52
5 + 2/7 + 3	19	0	+	14	?	45

[a] See Table 10.3.
[b] Partial or complete in bone marrow or peripheral blood.
[c] Patients pretreated with IFN-α to reduce tumour burden.

Table 10.3 Drug combinations used in intensive chemotherapy (see Table 10.2)

L-5	Splenic irradiation, splenectomy, variable doses of Ara-C and thioguanine
ROAP 10	Rubidazone 300 mg/m^2 i.v. day 1 (or daunorubicin 30 mg/m^2/day i.v. days 1–4), Ara-C 80 mg/m^2/day i.v. days 1–10, vincristine 2 mg day 1, and prednisone 100 mg/day p.o. days 1–5
DOAP	Daunorubicin 120 mg/m^2/day i.v. day 1, Ara-C i.v. 80 mg/m^2/day i.v. days 1–10, vincristine 2 mg i.v. day 1, prednisone 100 mg/day p.o. days 1–5
ICE	Ara-C 800 mg/m^2/day i.v. days 1–5, idarubicin 8 mg/m^2/day i.v. days 1–5, etoposide 150 mg/m^2/day i.v. days 1–3
mini-ICE	Ara-C 800 mg/m^2/day i.v. days 1–3, idarubicin 8 mg/m^2/day i.v. days 1–3, etoposide 150 mg/m^2/day i.v. days 1–3
DA	Daunorubicin 50 mg/m^2/day i.v. days 1–3, Ara-C 200 mg/m^2/day i.v. days 1–7
MEA	Mitoxantrone 12 mg/m^2/day i.v. days 1–4, etoposide 100 mg/m^2/day i.v. days 1–4, Ara-C 1 g/m^2 twice daily i.v. days 1–4
Cy	Cyclofosphamide 5 g/m^2 i.v. day 1
Hu^1	Hydroxyurea 3.5 g/m^2/day p.o. days 1–7
Hu^2	Hydroxyurea 2 g/m^2/day p.o. until ANC $\approx 1 \times 10^9$/l
I-A^1	Idarubicin 8, 10, or 20 mg/m^2 i.v. day 1, Ara-C 1 g/m^2/day continuous i.v. infusion days 1–5
I-A^2	Idarubicin 10 mg/m^2/day i.v. days 1–2, Ara-C 100 mg/m^2/day i.v. days 1–5
5 + 2	Idarubicin 12 mg/m^2/day i.v. days 1–2, Ara-C 100 mg/m^2/day by continuous i.v. infusion over 24 h days 1–5
3 + 7	Daunorubicin 50 mg/m^2/day i.v. days 1–3, Ara-C 200 mg/m^2/day by continuous i.v. infusion over 24 h days 1–7

This table only gives rough estimates of the toxicity and the clinical and cytogenetic effects of the different therapy regimens. As well as the choice of drugs, there are many other factors that influence the outcome of treatment. Thus the time from diagnosis to the start of treatment is important. It is easier to achieve major cytogenetic responses in patients diagnosed less than 1 year before treatment compared with those diagnosed later.[34] This is probably due to previous treatment, which could have been toxic to normal stem cells, but it could also be due to tumour cell burden, which increases with time. From studies of IFN-α, we also know that it is easier to achieve Ph negativity in patients with low tumour burden, and there is every reason to believe that the same thing is true for chemotherapy.[35]

Intensive chemotherapy is nowadays usually given to obtain Ph-negative stem cells from blood or from bone marrow, to be used in autologous stem cell transplantation. This is at least the situation for the major parts of the studies reported in Table 10.2, especially in the late 1980s and the 1990s.

It can be seen from Table 10.2 that many different therapies are and have been used, and it seems that – at least when they are really intense – a major Ph response (<35% bone marrow cells Ph-positive) can be observed in up to 80% of chronic-phase CML patients. The duration of Ph negativity in patients who did not go on to autotransplantation was relatively short, usually lasting at most 6–8 months. The toxicity measured as mortality of the regimens seems to be relatively low, most probably because of a positive selection of good-risk patients. Toxicities measured as neutropenia, thrombocytopenia, infections, and bleeding seem to be the same as for the intensive treatment of acute leukaemia. The mortality rate varies between 0% and 10%. In most cases G-CSF was given after the chemotherapy in order to reduce the duration of neutropenia.

The exact Ph effect of treatment with only DA or MEA[36] is not known, since in the studies reported in Table 10.2, the patients were all pretreated with hydroxyurea plus IFN-α for 6 months (DA chemotherapy) or with hydroxyurea plus IFN-α for 6 months and DA (MEA chemotherapy). Each of these regimens, however, resulted in Ph negativity in 30% of the patients. In most of the other studies, the patients had also received different prior regimens, mostly IFN-α, before receiving intensive chemotherapy.

Although it is possible that the intensive treatments may have prolonged survival, only a few comparative studies have been performed to confirm their superiority. One is the study by Kantarjian et al,[40] where 32 patients were given DOAP in three cycles before starting IFN-α treatment. The outcome was compared with that of 62 matched historical controls treated with IFN-α alone. A trend to survival advantage was found in the group receiving chemotherapy ($p = 0.084$) (Figure 10.2). This lack of significance could have been due to too short a follow-up time. In a later report, the same Houston group reports a possible

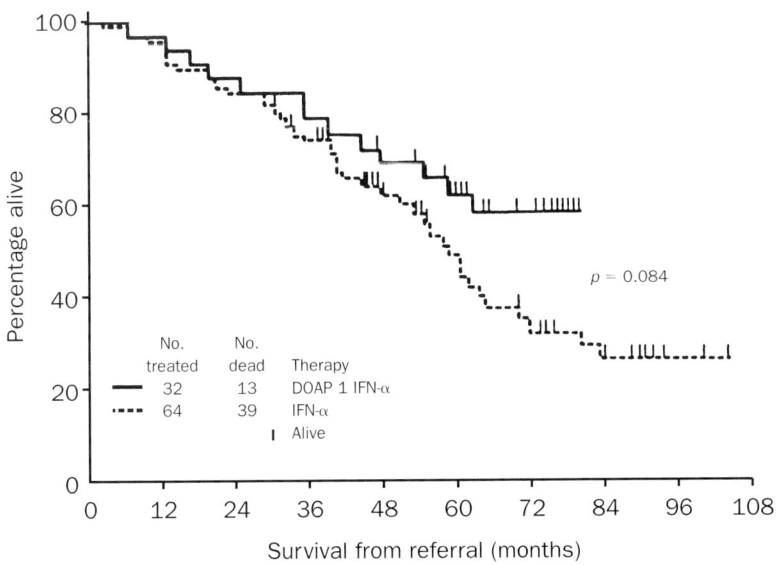

Figure 10.2 Effect of acute-leukaemia-type pretreatment on IFN-α-treated CML patients. Reproduced from reference 40 with permission from *Cancer*.

advantage of adding acute-leukaemia-type chemotherapy to IFN-α treatment.[53]

Another indication of the benefit of very aggressive chemotherapy is with allogeneic bone marrow transplantation (BMT), where many patients seem to be cured. One strong reason for this is certainly the graft-versus-leukaemia (GVL) effect, which is especially pronounced in CML. Gale et al,[54] in a retrospective analysis, reported that 112 patients in relapse after allogeneic BMT had a clear survival advantage compared with a matched historical control group receiving conventional chemotherapy only ($p < 0.0001$). It might therefore be suggested that intensive chemotherapy adds to the GVL effect in allogeneic BMT for CML.

A better way to determine whether the intensive treatment used for transplants cures CML is to analyse results of transplants between genetically identical twins. Here allograft-related immune effects most probably do not operate. The International Bone Marrow Transplant Registry has reported about 60% relapses at 5 years in twin transplant recipients,[55] while in another study,[56] relapses in twins were even less common. These data from twins suggest that about one-third of subjects may be cured by intensive pretransplant chemotherapy and/or radiation. However, since it is unknown whether more relapses would occur were twin grafts T-cell-depleted, we cannot be sure about the effect of chemotherapy. According to Lengfelder and Hehlmann[57], however, non-twin patients undergoing T-cell-depleted transplants have longer survival after relapse compared with controls.

CONCLUSIONS

Chemotherapy alone does not cure CML. The best palliative single-drug chemotherapy at present is hydroxyurea, which, compared with busulfan, prolongs survival by about 1 year. Hydroxyurea is also less toxic than busulfan, and so, for those patients who are not candidates for curative allogeneic stem cell transplantation and who are not suitable for the superior (from a survival point of view) IFN-α treatment, it is the drug of choice.

Many drugs and drug combinations at higher dosages might induce more significant tumour reduction (measured as Ph negativity). This treatment might well prolong survival compared with symptomatic chemotherapy, but at the price of a higher incidence of and more pronounced toxicity.

REFERENCES

1. Minot GR, Buckman TE, Isaacs R, Chronic myelogenous leukemia. Age, incidence, duration and benefit derived from treatment. *JAMA* 1924; **82:** 1489–94.
2. Galton D, Myleran in chronic myeloid leukemia. *Lancet* 1953; **i:** 208–13.
3. Kantarijan HM, Giles FJ, O'Brien SM, Talpaz M, Clinical course and therapy of chronic myelogenous leukemia with interferon-alpha and chemotherapy. *Hematol Oncol Clin North Am* 1998; **12:** 31–80.
4. Hehlmann R, Cytostatic therapy in chronic myelogenous leukemia: review and perspectives. In: *Chronic Myelocytic Leukemia and Interferon* (Huhn D, Hellriegel KP, Niederle N, eds). Berlin: Springer-Verlag, 1988: 102–12.
5. Hehlmann R, Heimpel H, Hasford J et al and the German CML Study Group, Randomized comparison of busulfan and hydroxyurea in chronic myelogenous leukemia (CML). Prolongation of survival by hydroxyurea. *Blood* 1993; **82:** 398–407.
6. Haut A, Abbott WS, Wintrobe MM et al, Busulfan in the treatment of chronic myelocytic leukemia. The effect of long term intermittent therapy. *Blood* 1961; **17:** 1–19.
7. Medical Research Council's Working Party for Therapeutic Trials in Leukaemia, Chronic granulocytic leukaemia: comparison of radiotherapy and busulphan therapy. *BMJ* 1968; **i:** 201–8.
8. Galton DAG, Treatment of the chronic leukaemias. *Br Med Bull* 1959; **15:** 78–85.
9. Vicariot M, Goldman JM, Catovsky D, Galton DAG, Treatment of chronic granulocytic leukaemia with repeated single doses of busulphan. *Eur J Cancer* 1979; **15:** 559–63.
10. Podoll E, Winkler S, Busulfan lung. Report of two cases and review of the literature. *Am J Roentgenol Radium Ther Nucl Med* 1974; **120:** 151–6.

11. Galton DAG, Busulphan (1,4 dimethanesulphonyloxybutane): summary of clinical results. *Ann NY Acad Sci* 1958; **68:** 967–73.
12. Kenis Y, Dustin P, Henry JA, Tagnon HJ, Action du Myleran dans 22 cas de leucémie myeloide chronique. *Rev Fr Etud Clin Biol* 1956; **1:** 435–42.
13. Kyle RA, Schwartz RS, Oliner HL, Dameshek W, A syndrome resembling adrenal cortical insufficiency associated with long term busulfan (Myleran) therapy. *Blood* 1961; **18:** 497–510.
14. Kennedy BJ, Yarbro KW, Metabolic and therapeutic effects of hydroxyurea in chronic myeloid leukemia. *JAMA* 1966; **195:** 1038–43.
15. Daoud MS, Gibson LE, Pittelkow MR, Hydroxyurea dermopathy: a unique lichenoid eruption complicating long-term therapy with hydroxyurea. *J Am Acad Dermatol* 1997; **36**(2 Pt 1): 178–82.
16. Weinlich G, Schuler G, Greil R et al, Leg ulcers associated with long-term hydroxyurea therapy. *J Am Acad Dermatol* 1998; **39**(2 Pt 2): 372–4.
17. Bolin RW, Robinson WA, Sutherland J, Hamman RF, Busulfan versus hydroxyurea in long-term therapy of chronic myelogenous leukemia. *Cancer* 1982; **50:** 1683–6.
18. Chronic Myeloid Leukemia Trialists' Collaborative Group, Hydroxyurea versus busulphan for chronic myeloid leukaemia: an individual patient data meta-analysis of three randomized trials. *Br J Haematol* 2000; **110:** 573–6.
19. Kato N, Kimura K, Yasukawa K, Yoshida K, Hydroxyurea-related leg ulcers in a patient with chronic myelogenous leukemia: a case report and review of the literature. *J Dermatol* 1999; **26:** 56–62.
20. Jackson N, Shukri A, Ali K, Hydroxyurea treatment for chronic myeloid leukaemia during pregnancy. *Br J Haematol* 1993; **85:** 203–4.
21. Cortes JE, Kantarjian H, Chronic leukemias. In: *Cancer Management: A Multidisciplinary Approach*, 2nd edn (Pazdur R, Coia LD, Hoskins WJ et al, eds). Huntington, NY: Publisher Research Management, 1998: 306–15.
22. O'Brien S, Kantarjian H, Keating M et al, Homoharringtonine therapy induces responses in patients with chronic myelogenous leukemia in late chronic phase. *Blood* 1995; **86:** 3322–6.
23. O'Brien S, Kantarjian H, Feldman E, Sequential homoharringtonine and interferon produce high hematologic and cytogenetic response rates in Philadelphia chromosome positive chronic myelogenous leukemia. *Proc Am Soc Clin Oncol* 1995; **14:** 336.
24. Kantarjian H, O'Brien S, Keating M et al, Homoharringtonine (HHT) and low-dose cytosine arabinoside (Ara-C) combination therapy has significant activity in patients (pts) with late phase Philadelphia chromosome (Ph)-positive chronic myelogenous leukemia (CML). *Blood* 1996; **88**(Suppl 1): 578a.
25. Sokal J, Bigner S, Low-dose cytosine arabinoside in early and advanced chronic granulocytic leukemia. *Blood* 1986; **66**(Suppl 1): 233a (Abst 810).
26. Robertson MJ, Tantravahi R, Griffin JD et al, Hematologic remission and cytogenetic improvement after treatment of stable-phase chronic myelogenous leukemia with continuous infusion of low-dose cytarabine. *Am J Hematol* 1993; **43:** 95–102.
27. Aihara M, Sasaki Y, Yoshida Y, Successful therapy of Ph1 positive chronic myelocytic leukemia with oral form of etoposide. *Rinsho Ketsueki* 1990; **10:** 1745–9.
28. Saven A, Piro LD, Lemon RH et al, Complete hematologic remissions in chronic-phase, Philadelphia-chromosome-positive, chronic myelogenous leukemia after 2-chlorodeoxyadenosine. *Cancer* 1994; **12:** 2953–63.
29. Cortes J, Kantarjian H, Talpaz M et al, Treatment of chronic myelogenous leukemia with nucleoside analogs deoxycoformycin and fludarabine. *Leukemia* 1997; **6:** 788–91.
30. Allan NC, Richards SM, Shepherd PC, UK Medical Research Council randomised, multicentre trial of interferon-alpha n1 for chronic myeloid leukaemia: improved survival irrespective of cytogenetic response. *Lancet* 1995; **345:** 1392–7.
31. Goldman JM, Szydlo R, Horowitz MM et al, Choice of pretransplant treatment and timing of transplants for chronic myelogenous leukemia in chronic phase. *Blood* 1993; **82:** 2235–8.
32. Finney R, McDonald GA, Baikie AG et al, Chronic granulocytic leukaemia with Ph1-negative cells in bone marrow and a ten year remission after busulphan hypoplasia. *Br J Haematol* 1972; **23:** 283–8.
33. Goto T, Nishikori M, Arlin Z et al, Growth characteristics of leukemic and normal hematopoietic cells in Ph^1+ chronic myelogenous leukemia and effect of intensive treatment. *Blood* 1982; **59:** 793–808.
34. Carella AM, Frassoni F, ICE, mini-ICE or high-dose hydroxyurea to mobilize Philadelphia (Ph1)-negative PBPC in chronic myelogenous leukaemia. *Br J Haematol* 1996; **95:** 212–16.
35. Hughes TP, Grigg A, Szer J et al, Mobilization of

predominantly Philadelphia chromosome-negative blood progenitors using cyclophosphamide and rHUG-CSF in early chronic-phase chronic myeloid leukaemia: correlation with Sokal prognostic index and haematological control. *Br J Haematol* 1997; **96:** 635–40.
36. Simonsson B, Oberg G, Bjoreman M et al, Intensive chemotherapy of chronic myelogenous leukemia. In preparation.
37. Cunningham I, Gee T, Dowling M et al, Results of treatment of Ph^1+ chronic myelogenous leukemia with an intensive treatment regimen (L-5 protocol). *Blood* 1979; **53:** 375–95.
38. Clarksson B, Chronic myelogenous leukemia: Is aggressive treatment indicated? *J Clin Oncol* 1985; **3:** 135–8.
39. Kantarjian HM, Vellekoop L, McCredie KB et al, Intensive combination chemotherapy (ROAP 10) and splenectomy in the management of chronic myelogenous leukemia. *J Clin Oncol* 1985; **3:** 192–200.
40. Kantarjian HM, Talpaz M, Keating MJ et al, Intensive chemotherapy induction followed by interferon-alpha maintenance in patients with Philadelphia chromosome-positive myelogenous leukemia. *Cancer* 1991; **68:** 1201–7.
41. Carella AM, Podesta M, Frassoni F et al, Collection of 'normal' blood repopulating cells during early hemopoietic recovery after intensive conventional chemotherapy in chronic myelogenous leukemia. *Bone Marrow Transplant* 1993; **12:** 267–71.
42. Carella AM, Lerma E, Celesti L et al, Effective mobilization of Philadelphia-chromosome-negative cells in chronic myelogenous leukaemia patients using a less intensive regimen. *Br J Haematol* 1998; **100:** 445–8.
43. Waller CF, Heinzinger M, Rosenstiel A et al, Mobilization and transplantation of Ph chromosome negative peripheral blood progenitor cells in patients with CML. *Br J Haematol* 1998; **103:** 227–34.
44. Mehta J, Mijovic A, Powles R et al, Myelosuppressive chemotherapy to mobilize normal stem cells in chronic myeloid leukemia. *Bone Marrow Transplant* 1996; **17:** 25–9.
45. Fischer T, Neubauer A, Mohm J et al, Outcome of peripheral blood stem cell mobilization in advanced phases of CML is dependent on the type of chemotherapy applied. *Ann Hematol* 1998; **77:** 21–6.
46. Johnson RJ, Owne RG, Child JA et al, Mobilization of Philadelphia-negative peripheral blood mononuclear cells in chronic myeloid leukaemia using hydroxyurea and G-CSF (filgrastim). *Br J Haematol* 1996; **93:** 863–8.
47. Treleaven J, Powles R, Signhal S et al, High-dose hydroxyurea and G-CSF to collect Philadelphia-negative cells in chronic myeloid leukemia. *Blood* 1995; **86:** 405a (Abst 1608).
48. Kolitz JE, Kempin SJ, Schluger A et al, A phase II pilot trial of high-dose hydroxyurea in chronic myelogenous leukemia. *Semin Oncol* 1992; **19**(3): 27–31.
49. Pratt G, Johnson RJ, Rawstron AC et al, Autologous stem cell transplantation in chronic myeloid leukaemia using Philadelphia chromosome negative blood progenitors mobilised with hydroxyurea and G-CSF. *Bone Marrow Transplant* 1998; **21:** 455–60.
50. Chalmers EA, Franklin IM, Kelsey SM et al, Treatment of chronic myeloid leukaemia in first chronic phase with idarubicin and cytarabine mobilisation of Philadelphia-negative peripheral blood stem cells. *Br J Haematol* 1997; **96:** 627–34.
51. Nielsen H, Nielsen JL, Karle H, Initial cytoreduction by mitoxantrone and cytarabine has no impact on the outcome of interferon-alfa-2b therapy in chronic myelogenous leukemia. *Eur J Haematol* 1992; **49:** 67–70.
52. Fischer T, Neubauer A, Mohm J et al, Chemotherapy-induced mobilization of karyotypically normal PBSC for autografting in CML. *Bone Marrow Transplant* 1998; **21:** 1029–36.
53. Giks FJ, Talpaz H, O'Brien SM et al, Interferon alpha (IFN) and cyclic intensive chemotherapy (CIC) for chronic phase (CP) chronic myelogenous leukemia (CML). *Blood* 1999; **10**(Suppl 1): 274b (Abst 4436).
54. Gale RP, Baccarani M, Horowitz MM, Zhang MJ, Is the course of chronic myelogenous leukemia affected by bone marrow transplantation? An analysis in patients relapsing after bone marrow transplants. *Blood* 1993; **92**(Suppl 1): 167.
55. Gale RP, Goldman JM, Horowitz MM, for the International Bone Marrow Transplant Registry, Identical twin transplants in chronic myelogenous leukemia in chronic phase. *Exp Hematol* 1991; **19:** 573.
56. Fefer A, Cheever MA, Greenberg PD et al, Treatment of chronic granulocytic leukemia with chemoradiotherapy and transplantation of marrow from identical twins. *N Engl J Med* 1982; **306:** 63–8.
57. Lengfelder E, Hehlmann R, Intensive combination chemotherapy in treatment of CML. *Bone Marrow Transplant* 1996; **17**(Suppl 3): 55–7.

11

Interferon-α and Ara-C

Gianantonio Rosti, Elena Trabacchi, Francesca Bonifazi, Antonio de Vivo, Simona Bassi, Sante Tura

CONTENTS • Introduction • Rationale for the use of Ara-C in CML • Observational studies • Randomized controlled trials • Toxicity and compliance • Cytarabine octaphosphate (YNK01)

INTRODUCTION

The superior efficacy of interferon-α (IFN-α) over conventional chemotherapy (hydroxyurea and busulfan) in the treatment of chronic myeloid leukaemia (CML) in first chronic phase has been demonstrated in a number of uncontrolled observational studies[1–8] since the early 1980s and, more importantly, in four randomized controlled trials.[9–12] All of the latter studies indicated significantly longer survival for IFN-α-treated patients compared with control groups. In particular, the 5-year survival rates ranged between 50% and 59% for patients receiving IFN-α, compared with between 29% and 44% for patients assigned to a conventional treatment. As noted by Silver et al,[13] notwithstanding the differences among the designs of randomized controlled trials and imperfections in the way in which they were conducted, there is a bulk of evidence that IFN-α improves survival in CML. The improvement in life expectancy is a median of 20 months. The magnitude of the survival gain is more conspicuous if a cytogenetic response is obtained: on stratifying patients as a function of the IFN-α-related grade of reduction of bone marrow Philadelphia chromosome (Ph)-positive metaphases, the survival gain progressively increases,[9] being maximal for complete responders (100% Ph-negative). The cytogenetic response is considered a surrogate marker of survival.[13] IFN-α is most effective in early chronic-phase patients with low-Sokal-risk disease, without or with minimal pretreatment – but, to a lesser degree, the beneficial effect on outcome is evident for each prognostic category. To confirm more convincingly the beneficial effect of IFN-α over chemotherapy, a meta-analysis[14] pooling the results of the randomized clinical trials definitely showed that the 5-year survival rate of IFN-α-treated patients was 57%, versus 42% for chemotherapy ($p < 0.0001$). These 'IFN-α-based' results constitute the clinical basis and point of comparison for all the new regimens devoted to further improving the survival of CML patients who lack suitable donors or who are ineligible for allogeneic bone marrow transplantation.

The drug most extensively investigated in association with IFN-α is cytosine arabinoside (Ara-C, cytarabine), based on experimental and clinical observations. Recently, an oral formulation of Ara-C (cytarabine octaphosphate, YNK01) has been proposed to improve overall compliance with the drug association.

RATIONALE FOR THE USE OF Ara-C IN CML

Ara-C is an arabinoside nucleoside belonging to the antimetabolite class of antineoplastic drugs.

To exert its activity, the parent drug must be phosphorylated to the active 5′-triphosphate form, deoxy-Ara-CTP, which is incorporated into DNA. The incorporation of deoxy-Ara-CTP into DNA results in defective DNA replication, leading to cell death. The cytotoxic effects of Ara-C are maximized during the S phase of the cell cycle, and therefore its spectrum of activity is restricted to dividing cells. Ara-C is probably the most potent drug in the treatment of acute myeloid leukaemia. The first in vitro experimental observations that lead to the subsequent development of clinical projects on Ara-C or IFN-α plus Ara-C in the treatment of CML were due to Spiro et al[15] and Sokal et al.[16] In particular, Sokal et al studied the effects of 11 antineoplastic drugs on the growth of granulocyte–macrophage colony-forming units (CFU-GM) from normal subjects and Ph-positive CML, attempting to define the concentration of each drug causing growth inhibition over 50% (I_{50}). Colony formation was inhibited regularly by the addition of antileukaemic drugs, but Ara-C showed a preferential, selective inhibition (Figure 11.1). In fact, unlike all the other drugs tested, the median I_{50} values of Ara-C on CML CFU-GM were significantly below the median as compared with 15 experiements on normal CFU-GM. Since the experiments allowed 12 days of exposure to each drug, they did not reflect simply the percentage of S-phase progenitors present in the system but were a real measure of the sensitivity to each drug. In this context, the results for hydroxyurea, another rapidly acting S-phase drug, are particularly significant: with hydroxyurea, the I_{50} values for CML and healthy subjects were roughly the same, in contrast to Ara-C.

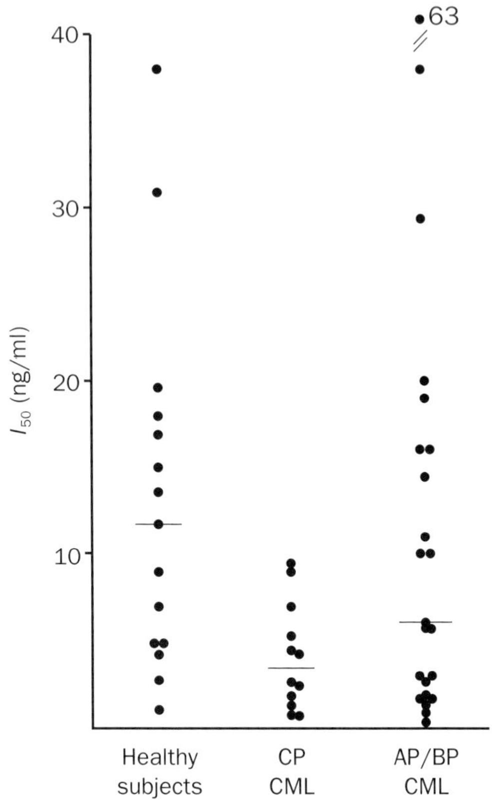

Figure 11.1 I_{50} concentration of Ara-C in studies of 15 normal subjects, 12 patients in the chronic phase of CML (CP CML) and 25 patients with accelerated/blastic disease (AP/BP CML). Horizontal lines represent median values. From Sokal JE, Leong SS, Gomez GA, Preferential inhibition by cytarabine of CFU-GM from patients with chronic granulocytic leukemia. *Cancer* 1987; **59:** 197–202.

Preclinical studies refer mainly to Ara-C alone, and this drug, as demonstrated in the pivotal work of Sokal et al,[16] exerts a preferential effect on Ph-positive progenitors. On the other hand, preclinical data aimed at specifically investigating the activity of Ara-C in association with IFN-α on Ph-positive progenitor cells are very limited: the only record is from Imanishi et al,[17] who showed a possible in vitro synergy between IFN-α and Ara-C on Ph-positive progenitors. A possible explanation of the synergistic effect of IFN-α and Ara-C lies in a putative protective effect of IFN-α on normal CFU-GM. In fact, Richman et al[18] showed in their experimental work that IFN-α may block in G_0/G_1 phase normal progenitors more efficiently than CML ones, with the latter being more subject to the S-phase-linked action of Ara-C.

The first clinical results with Ara-C alone were reported by Sokal et al[19] on a limited number of subjects. They treated 4 patients in late chronic phase with Ara-C, showing that the drug was active in vivo: 2/4 patients achieved a complete haematological response. Robertson et al[20] obtained similar results.

OBSERVATIONAL STUDIES

Pretreated patients and advanced disease

Even more than from laboratory results, the motivation for investigation of IFN-α plus Ara-C in randomized controlled trials has come from observational studies that tested this combination among patients with CML in late chronic phase or even in accelerated phase. The first, large clinical trial was due to the MD Anderson Cancer Center group: Kantarjian et al[21] treated 60 patients with advanced-phase CML: 20 were in accelerated phase (based on cytogenetic clonal evolution in 16 and on other haematological features in the remaining 4), while 40 were in late chronic phase (19 more than three years from diagnosis). A stratification of the patients according to risk of progression at diagnosis was not reported. An unspecified number of patients had been treated with IFN-α with or without other drugs before study entry. The results were compared with a control group of 39 late chronic-phase and 19 accelerated-phase patients treated with IFN-α alone in previous trials at the same institution. The treatment schedule was based on IFN-α (target dose 5 MU/m^2/day) and Ara-C (15 mg/m^2/day for 2 weeks every month until haematological response, then for 1 week every month as maintenance). Haematological response criteria were based on the disappearance of all signs and symptoms of the disease, including palpable splenomegaly, and on the normalization of peripheral blood counts, while a partial response required a decrease by more than 50% of pretreatment levels of white blood cells (WBC) and platelets. The cytogenetic response criteria were based on the rate of reduction of Ph-positive metaphases: complete response 0% Ph-positive, partial response 1–34% Ph-positive, and minor response 35–90% Ph-positive. Late chronic-phase patients had a better complete haematological response rate (22 of 40, i.e. 55%) and a better cytogenetic response rate (2 partial and 4 minor, i.e. 15%) compared with the control group of patients treated with IFN-α alone (same target dose), where the respective figures were 28% and 5% (Table 11.1). The 3-year survival rate was significantly higher in patients treated with IFN-α and Ara-C (75%) compared with historical controls (48%) ($p < 0.01$). The marked asynchronism of the two curves must, however, be considered. Results in accelerated-phase patients were less remarkable: in brief, 10 of 20 (50%) achieved a haematological response and 4 (20%) a cytogenetic response (minimal in 3 and partial in 1). Accelerated-phase patients treated with the study schedule had a trend towards a higher 3-year survival rate compared with historical controls (74% versus 49%; $p = 0.17$); this difference was probably due to the unbalanced presence in the two groups of patients with intrinsically better prognosis, i.e. a diagnosis of accelerated phase based solely on cytogenetic clonal evolution (16 of 20 in the study group and 9 of 19 in the historical control group). Kantarjian et al concluded that these results were encouraging and that the new schedule was worth testing in patients with early, untreated disease.

Early chronic phase

Arthur et al[22] conducted a multicentre open study, collecting 30 patients over 43 months of accrual. They were in early chronic phase (47% low Sokal risk and 53% intermediate or high risk), previously untreated; the schedule adopted was a combination of IFN-α (target dose 9 MU/day) and Ara-C 20 mg/m^2/day for 21 days, every 42 days. The study drugs followed a pretreatment period with hydroxyurea. The response criteria were those adopted by Kantarjian et al.[21] After 12 months, 28 of 30 patients (93%) were in complete haematological response, while 16 (53%) had a partial (7

Table 11.1 Comparison of patient characteristics, treatment response and prognosis in late chronic-phase CML. From Kantarjian HM, Keating J, Elihu H et al, Treatment of advanced stages of Philadelphia chromosome positive chronic myelogenous leukemia with interferon and low-dose cytarabine. *J Clin Oncol* 1992; 10: 772–8.

		Study group (40 patients)		Historical control (39 patients)		
Characteristic	**Category**	**No.**	**%**	**No.**	**%**	***P***
Age (years)	⩾50	18	45	14	36	0.41
Splenomegaly	Palpable	11	27	12	31	0.75
WBC count ($\times 10^3/\mu l$)	⩾50	14	35	11	28	0.52
Platelet count ($\times 10^3/\mu l$)	⩾450	19	47	18	46	0.90
Peripheral blasts (%)	⩾5	3	7	6	15	0.27
Marrow blasts (%)	⩾5	6	15	8	21	0.52
Peripheral basophils (%)	⩾7	5	12	7	18	0.50
Duration of disease from diagnosis (years)	1–3	21	52	24	62	0.42
	>3 years	19	48	15	38	
Response to therapy	CHR[a]	22	55	11	28	0.02
	Ph suppression	6	15	2	5	0.15
3-year survival rate		75%		48%		<0.01

[a] Complete haematological response.

patients) or complete (9 patients) cytogenetic response on at least one occasion. The 53% partial plus complete cytogenetic response rate is an extremely good one, and it would have been very interesting to know the long-term survival figures and risk of progression of this patient population. Unfortunately, the brief median follow-up of 14 months at the time of reporting (extremes 10–53 months) precludes any reasonable conclusions on long-term survival.

The first pilot study of the French CML study group was published in 1989:[23] 24 patients included in this trial received IFN-α (5 MU/m^2/day as target dose) and Ara-C (10–40 mg/day on 10–15 days a month), with 63% of them obtaining a major (>66% Ph-negative) or complete (100% Ph-negative) cytogenetic response; 4/24 were complete responders. Subsequently, the French group will run two large randomized controlled trials. Recently, Kantarjian et al[24] reported the MD Anderson Cancer Center experience with IFN-α (target dose 5 MU/m^2/day) and continuous subcutaneous administration of Ara-C (10 mg/day): 140 patients were entered into the study, 134 of whom were evaluable for response and survival. Their outcomes were compared with two other sequential single-arm studies by the same group with IFN-α and intermittent Ara-C (15 mg/m^2/day for 7 days a month) (46 patients) and IFN-α alone (274 patients).[25] The prognostic score distribution (overall MD Anderson model)[26] did not differ significantly among the three groups, with roughly half in the good-prognosis group and half in intermediate- and poor-risk groups. The study group

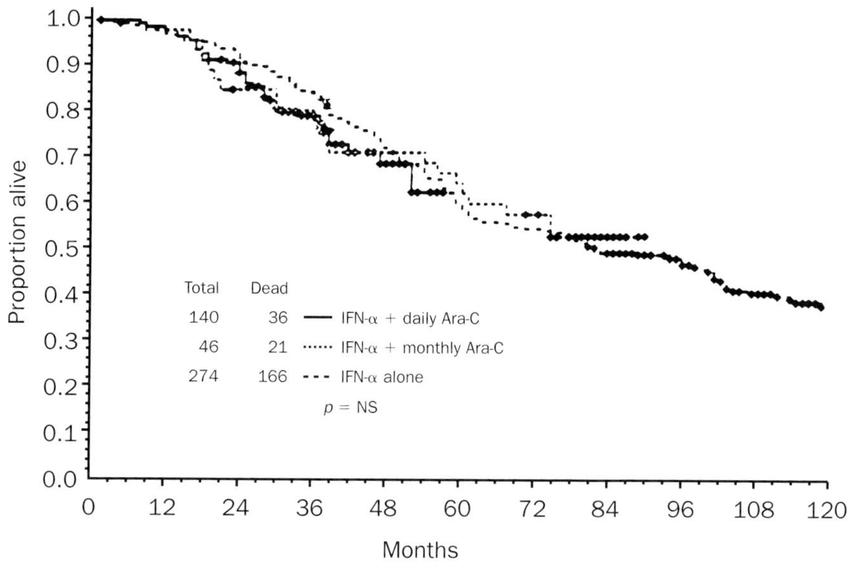

Figure 11.2 Survival with IFN-α plus daily Ara-C, IFN-α plus intermittent Ara-C, and IFN-α alone. From Kantarjian HM, O'Brian S, Smith TL et al, Treatment of Philadelphia chromosome positive early chronic phase chronic myelogenous leukemia with daily doses of interferon and low-dose cytarabine. *J Clin Oncol* 1999; **17:** 284–92.

achieved a higher complete haematological remission rate compared with the others (92% versus 84% versus 80%, respectively; $p = 0.01$) and a significantly higher overall cytogenetic response rate (>10% to 100% Ph negativity): 74% versus 73% versus 50% respectively ($p = 0.003$). However, the proportion of good cytogenetic responders (partial and complete responders of the MD Anderson scoring system) was not significantly different among the three groups (50% versus 38% versus 38%, respectively). As far as survival was concerned, with a median follow-up of 42 months, the estimated 4-year survival rate was 70% and the survival curves were superimposable on those of control groups with IFN-α plus intermittent Ara-C or with IFN-α alone. The survival comparison between different sequential studies gives conflicting results between, on the one hand, a better overall (haematological and cytogenetic) response rate of the study group over controls and, on the other hand, no differences at all in survival expectation (Figure 11.2). The latter observation, as stated by Kantarjian et al, is probably due to a number of known and unperceived differences among sequential non-randomized studies.

The experience of Thaler et al[27] with a multicentre Austrian group is based on 84 patients in early chronic phase receiving induction treatment with hydroxyurea followed (after 3 months) by the study regimen: IFN-α (at a fixed low dose of 3.5 MU/day) and Ara-C 10–20 mg/day. An intrapatient dose modulation was scheduled as a function of poor haematological response. The complete haematological rate was 54%, whereas a minority of patients (25%) were major (66–99% Ph-negative) or complete cytogenetic responders.

Since a systematic developmental plan for Ara-C in CML was not operative, each institution or multicentre network built on clinical trials based on different treatment schedules where Ara-C was given with quite different modalities (Table 11.2). Moreover, some trials scheduled an intrapatient dose escalation or cycle prolongation while others did not, and the schedule was intermittent in some but continuous in others. Other factors that preclude an unbiased comparison among published experiences (at least one suitable to identify a conceivably better schedule) are differences in the accrual of patients, in their risk distribution, in the type and modalities of induction therapy (generally, hydroxyurea-based), and, more importantly, in IFN-α schedule. As far as Ara-C is concerned, the differences among the various studies in terms of Ara-C schedule and the total monthly dose of Ara-C given are noteworthy: the latter value ranges between a minimum of 170 mg (Guilhort et al[28]) to a maximum of 714 mg (Arthur and Ma;[22] see Table 11.2). The results clearly lie in a wide range. For example, Arthur et al[22] had the best cytogenetic response rate (53%). This would conceivably have a positive influence on long-term survival: unfortunately, the very brief observation period (14 months) precludes this fundamental observation. In contrast, Thaler et al[27] had a worse cytogenetic result (25%): their patients received a less intense Ara-C schedule (monthly dose 170 mg) and even less IFN-α (fixed dose 3.5 MU/day). Moreover, a higher proportion of non-low-risk patients was present compared with other studies.

A positive evaluation of the effects of combined treatment on survival is difficult: the studies that reported a survival evaluation have a median observation period ranging between 14 and 42 months that is less than the expected median survival of chronic-phase CML patients treated with an IFN-α-based regimen (reported by Silver et al[13]), which is generally somewhat more than 60 months.

Generally, the clinical results obtained in observational studies have been judged positively by the authors of these studies, and it has been considered worthwhile testing Ara-C in larger randomized controlled trials.

RANDOMIZED CONTROLLED TRIALS

The first randomized controlled trial of the French group (CML 88)[28] was based on a common treatment of 237 chronic-phase CML patients (207 of whom were evaluable) entered into the study: patients were given IFN-α 5 MU/day total dose plus hydroxyurea to haematological response, and, from the third month onwards, responding patients were randomly assigned to maintenance treatment with IFN-α alone at the target dose of 5 MU/m^2 or the same IFN-α schedule plus Ara-C 10 mg/m^2/day for 10 days a month. Briefly, the rate of haematological response (83%) was the same in the two arms; the overall rate of cytogenetic response was the same, although a larger proportion (23%) of patients receiving the combination treatment went on to a complete cytogenetic response, compared with 15% of patients receiving IFN-α alone. This trial showed the feasibility of the combination treatment within a large randomized controlled trial; moreover, the higher proportion of complete cytogenetic responders, even though not statistically significant, prompted further investigation of the therapeutic role of Ara-C at different doses. In fact, based on the results of the CML 88 trial, a second, larger trial was published by the French group in 1997: CML 91. Guilhot et al[29] randomized 721 early chronic-phase patients at diagnosis to receive IFN-α at the target dose 5 MU/m^2/day and Ara-C 40 mg/day 10 days a month (360 patients) or IFN-α alone at the same dose (361 patients). Hence the total dose of Ara-C is more than twice that in CML 88. A second difference from CML 88 is in the total number of days on Ara-C, which could be increased to 15 in the case of poor haematological disease control. Consequently, the total monthly dose of Ara-C in this intermittent schedule varies between 400 and 600 mg. Patients assigned to IFN-α, haematologically refractory after 6 months or still less than 33% Ph-negative after 12 months, could be cross over to receive the combined treatment. Table 11.3 presents the patients' data at diagnosis. Complete haematological responses were achieved by 237 of 360 patients (66%) in the IFN-α plus Ara-C group and 198 of 361 patients (55%) in the IFN-α group. With regard to the major plus complete cytogenetic response rate at 12 months, the superiority of the combined treatment was quite evident: 126 of 311 (41%) evaluable patients receiving IFN-α plus Ara-C achieved this result, compared with 75 of 314 (24%) evaluable patients receiving IFN-α. A detailed analysis of cytogenetic responses is presented in Table 11.4. The differences are in

Table 11.2 IFN-α plus Ara-C in observational and randomized controlled studies

Study	No. of patients	% Sokal low risk	Disease status	IFN-α target dose (MU/day)	Ara-C schedule	Ara-C monthly dose (mg)	CHR (%)	CCR (%)	M+CCR (%)	Median observation period (months)	Estimated survival (months)	Notes
Arthur and Ma[22]	30	47	CP/<12 months from diagnosis	9	20 mg/m^2 for 21 days, every 42 days	~714[a]	93	30	53	14	NR	
Thaler et al[27]	84	39	CP/newly diagnosed	3.5	10–20 mg/m^2/day	170–340	54	18	25	28	65 (at 4 yrs)	
Kantarjian et al[24]	134	53[b]	CP/<12 months from diagnosis	9	10 mg/m^2/day	300	92	31	50	42	70 (at 4 yrs)	Longest observation
Kantarjian et al[25]	46	53	CP	9	15 mg/m^2 for 7 days a month	180	84	20	38	NR	72 (at 4 yrs)	All patients at risk after 72 months
Guilhot et al[28]	103	NR	CP/stable HR after IFN-α + hydroxyurea	9	10 mg/m^2 for 10 days a month	170	NR	23	NR	NR	Median survival 67 months	
Guilhot et al[29]	360	47	Early CP	9	40 mg for 10–15 days a month	400–600	67	15	41	35	87 (at 3 yrs)	
Rosti et al[31]	275	52	Early CP	9	40 mg for 10 days a month	400	87	14	28	24	85 (at 3 yrs)	

Abbreviations: CHR, complete haematological responders; CCR, complete cytogenetic responders; M+CCR, major plus complete cytogenetic responders; CR, chronic phase; NR, not reported; HR, haematological response. The body surface area has been normalized to 1.7 m^2 for all calculations.

[a] 40 mg for 21 days, with 21 days off before the subsequent cycle.

[b] Overall MD Anderson Cancer Center prognostic model.

Table 11.3 Clinical and biological characteristics of the study patients according to treatment assignment. Taken with permission from *The New England Journal of Medicine*, Guilhot F, Guerci A, Fiere D et al, Vol. 337, pp. 223–9, 1997.

Characteristic	**IFN-α + Ara-C (n = 360)**	**IFN-α (n = 361)**
Sex: M/F	195/165	203/158
Age (years):		
Median	50	51
Range	7–71	2–71
Splenomegaly		
No. of patients[a]	164 (46)	188 (52)
Distance below costal margin (cm)[b]	8 ± 6	8±6
WBC count (10^9/l)[b]	120 ± 120.6	131 ± 121.3
Haemoglobin (g/dl)[b]	12.3 ± 1.9	12.1 ± 2.1
Haematocrit (%)[b]	37 ± 6	36 ± 6
Platelet count (10^9/l)[b]	467 ± 336	519 ± 436
Peripheral blood blast cells:		
No. of patients[a]	119 (33)	132 (37)
Percentage of cells[b]	2.25 ± 1.62	2.71 ± 2.42
Sokal risk group: no. of patients:[a]		
Low	168 (47)	144 (40)
Intermediate	142 (39)	151 (42)
High	50 (14)	66 (18)

[a] Percentages in parentheses.
[b] Mean ± SD.

favour of the combined treatment, for both haematological and cytogenetic responses.

With regard to major and complete cytogenetic responses, the results for the IFN-α plus Ara-C arm still remain significantly better after adjusting for Sokal risk distribution: in fact 47% IFN-α plus Ara-C patients were low-risk, as compared with 40% of those receiving IFN-α alone. The superior response rates for the combined treatment lead to a better survival probability: at the time of the first report, with a median observation period of 35 months, the estimated 3-year survival rate was 85.7%, compared with 79.1% (p = 0.02) (Figure 11.4). This difference remained significant, although to an inferior degree (p = 0.03), when patients given allogeneic bone marrow transplantation were censored at the time of transplant. Since the first

Table 11.4 Cytogenetic responses at 12 months according to treatment assignment. Taken with permission from *The New England Journal of Medicine*, Guilhot F, Guerci A, Fiere D et al, Vol. 317, pp. 223–9, 1997. © 1997 Massachusetts Medical Society. All rights reserved.

Response[a]	IFN-α + Ara-C (n = 311)[b]	IFN-α (n = 314)[b]
	No. of patients[c]	
Major:	126 (41)	75 (24)
Complete	46 (15)	28 (9)
Partial	80 (26)	47 (15)
Minor	77 (25)	88 (28)
Treatment failure	53 (17)	78 (25)
Data not available	55 (18)	73 (23)

[a] See text for definitions of response.
[b] Data only for patients with at least 12 months of observation.
[c] Percentages in parentheses.

publication in 1997,[29] the trial has been updated to April 2000: the median observation period of living patients was 61 months and the 5-year survival rate was 71% for IFN-α plus Ara-C (95% confidence intervals (CI) 65 76%) and 59% for IFN-α alone (95% CI 53–64%) (Joseph Tanzer, personal communication).

The crossover scheduled from the IFN-α arm to the IFN-α plus Ara-C arm for patients haematologically refractory at 6 months gave unimpressive results. In fact, only 18 of 118 patients (15%) who crossed over to receive Ara-C achieved a cytogenetic response, which was major in 11 patients and complete in 7. Among the group of patients refractory to IFN-α there are certainly a proportion of 'pure' refractory cases, who are able to tolerate therapeutic doses of IFN-α but are affected by a genuinely unresponsive disease; a second type of unresponsiveness is related more to bad compliance to treatment than to disease resistance. The report of the French study does not present an analytical survey of IFN-α courses and clinical tolerance before crossover; moreover, the 118 hematologically refractory patients are not stratified as a function of risk category. As a consequence, it is not possible to further analyse this group of patients to obtain a better understanding of which variables are related to the failure and success of crossover.

The Italian Cooperative Study Group on CML closed in 1997 a randomized trial based on the same rationale as the French one – the CML 94 protocol: overall, 837 newly diagnosed CML patients were recruited, and 540 eligible patients were randomized 1 : 1 to IFN-α (265 patients, with a target dose of 5 MU/m^2/day) and IFN-α plus Ara-C (275 patients, with a dose of 40 mg/day on 10 days a month). Patients refractory to IFN-α alone could be rescued to response by adding Ara-C at prefixed check points evaluating the degree of haematological

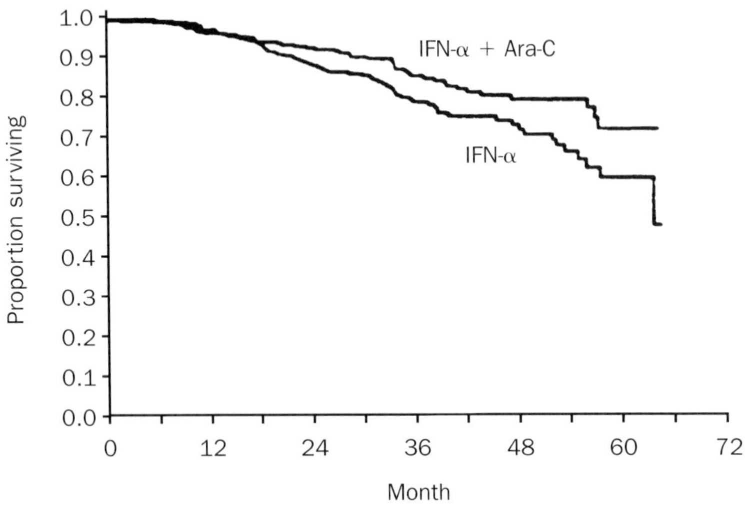

Figure 11.3 Kaplan–Meier estimates of overall survival according to treatment group. $p = 0.02$ for the comparison of the groups by the logrank test. Data are based on an intention-to-treat analysis. Taken with permission from *The New England Journal of Medicine*, Guilhot F, Guerci A, Fiere D et al, Vol. 317, pp. 223–9, 1997.

and cytogenetic response. At 3 years, all responsive patients maintaining at least a minor cytogenetic response (>33% Ph-negative) are newly randomized to the maximum tolerated dose of IFN-α or to low doses (3 MU t.i.w.) in order to evaluate which maintenance IFN-α schedule will be better in the long term. The first interim report[30] showed an early survival advantage for IFN-α plus Ara-C. The study was updated in 1999:[31] with a median observation time of living patients of 25 months, on a strict intention-to-treat basis, a survival advantage for patients receiving the combined treatment was shown (logrank 4.41; $p = 0.03$).

However, the cytogenetic response rate in this study, even though significantly in favour of IFN-α plus Ara-C, shows a less evident difference compared with the results of the French CML 91 study. In fact, the major plus complete cytogenetic response rate, referred to the best result obtained at any time (mainly at 12 months but including later responses too), is 28% (72 of 275 patients) for the IFN-α plus Ara-C arm compared with 19% (50 of 265 patients) for the IFN-α arm. The net difference is then 9%. On the other hand, the major plus complete cytogenetic response rate of the French trial[29] was 41% (126 of 311 patients evaluated) for IFN-α plus Ara-C, compared with 24% (75 of 314 patients evaluated) for IFN-α. The net difference is 17%. This large difference in the cytogenetic response rate in favour of the combined treatment implies a beneficial effect on survival, both with a relatively brief median observation time (35 months in the original paper[29]) and at a longer follow-up (61 months: Joseph Tanzer, personal communication).

In the Italian experience, the difference between the two arms for this surrogate marker of survival is less impressive than in the French CML 91 trial:[29] the previously mentioned positive effect on early survival probability needs to be confirmed in the long term.

After stratification for Sokal risk, the survival

advantage was still present among low-Sokal-risk patients, but not among intermediate- or high-risk ones.

TOXICITY AND COMPLIANCE

The positive effects on general outcome of the IFN-α plus Ara-C combination should be weighted against the number and degree of additional adverse effects of the two agents compared with compliance with the gold standard treatment, IFN-α alone, at comparable doses.

None of the published studies was specifically designed to answer the quality-of-life issue – either for IFN-α plus Ara-C or in a comparative way between the two schedules.

When one considers the published results of the observational studies it is clear that it is difficult to draw definite conclusions about the toxicity and acceptability of IFN-α plus Ara-C combinations, owing to the differences among the various schedules (see Table 11.2) and the absence of direct comparisons with previous experiences with IFN-α alone. Moreover, it is often difficult to determine which drug is responsible for a specific adverse event. For example, both IFN-α and Ara-C contribute to mucositis, and there is also an additive effect of the two agents together. The same is probably true for chronic side-effects such as fatigue, depression, weight loss, and liver toxicity, as well as for dose-limiting haematological changes. A few side-effects are clearly related to just one of the drugs (for example, bone and muscle pains and autoimmune phenomena are linked to IFN-α). However, some useful observations can be made – at least with regard to the most frequent side-effects. Kantarjian et al,[24] for example, found in their experience with daily Ara-C (10 mg/day), that fatigue and neurotoxicity were the most significant side-effects, the former being more likely attributable to both drugs and the latter to IFN-α. Overall, fatigue was reported in 44% of cases (although only 11% of these were WHO grade 3–4), whereas neurological changes occurred in 25%. Mucositis was not specifically reported: diarrhoea was noted in 7% of cases, oral ulcers in 4%, and nausea and vomiting in 5%.

On the other hand, Arthur and Ma,[22] with a different Ara-C schedule (20 mg/m^2/day for 21 days every 42 days), had a higher incidence of mucositis (53% of cases), diarrhoea (20%), and nausea and vomiting (56% and 23% respectively). Stratification according to WHO grading was not reported. The French CML 91 trial[29] showed that Ara-C as single agent was responsible for significant side-effects in 85 patients. Nausea, vomiting, diarrhoea, and mucositis were those more frequently reported.

In summary, Ara-C causes a significant amount of additive side-effects; the target organ is, not unexpectedly, the gastrointestinal tract. It is not possible to state to what degree Ara-C worsens treatment compliance compared with IFN-α alone, and consequently how much the quality of life is affected.

CYTARABINE OCTAPHOSPHATE (YNK01)

Cytarabine octaphosphate (YNK01) is an active precursor of Ara-C that is administered orally and after absorption is metabolized in the liver into active Ara-C. In phase I repeated-dose studies over 5 consecutive days (100–900 mg/day) the dose-limiting toxicity was thrombocytopenia and the maximum tolerated dose was 700–900 mg/day. The half-life of YNK01 is 21 hours, and the plasma levels in steady state are comparable with those achieved following continuous perfusion of Ara-C at low doses (20 mg/m^2). The oral administration of YNK01 should improve the compliance of CML patients with prolonged treatment with a drug that otherwise would have to be administered parenterally and on a daily basis only. YNK01 has been tested in phase I and II trials in acute myeloblastic leukaemia, myelodysplastic syndromes, and non-Hodgkin's lymphomas with different schedules: the main reported side-effects were gastrointestinal, including nausea and diarrhoea, particularly with daily dosage of 600 mg or more.

The French study group enrolled 98 patients with previously untreated or minimally pretreated PH-positive CML in a study of IFN-α and YNK01.[32] The median age was 54 years (range 18–74 years); 46% of cases were low-Sokal-risk, 35% were intermediate-risk, and 19% were high-risk. IFN-α was given at a dose of 3 MU/m^2/day in the first week and 5 MU/m^2/day thereafter. YNK01 was given at a dose of 600 mg/day from day 1 to day 14 of each month. A complete haematological response was obtained in 64% of cases after 3 months and in 72% of cases after 6 months. A cytogenetic response (major plus complete, ⩾65% Ph-negative) was achieved in 16 cases (21% of evaluable and 16% of enrolled cases) between the 6th and 12th months. A minimal plus minor cytogenetic response (5–65% Ph-negative) was obtained in 34 cases (44% of evaluable and 35% of enrolled cases). In summary, the overall cytogenetic response (based on intention-to-treat) was 40 of 98 (41%). The mean administered dose of IFN-α was 3.8 MU/m^2/day. The mean dose of YNK01 decreased from 600 to 350 mg/day. Of 98 patients, 18 abandoned the treatment protocol for an allogeneic bone marrow transplant. Of the remaining 80 cases, 32 went off-treatment for side-effects and another 6 for other reasons. One fatal adverse event (a case of sudden death) was registered. Grade 1 WHO toxicity was observed in 70 of 98 cases (71%). Grade 2 or 3 toxicity was observed in 17 of 98 cases (17%). The toxic or side-effects were the following: fatigue with a performance score of 70–80% in 67% of cases, a 'flu-like' syndrome in 63% of cases, minor neurological symptoms in 24% of cases, minor psychiatric troubles (mainly depression) in 21% of cases, skin changes or reaction in 35% of cases, with alopecia in 9%, cardiac troubles (arrhythmia) in 3% of cases, gastrointestinal symptoms in 81% of cases, with nausea and vomiting in 52%, diarrhoea in 51%, and a significant (⩾10%) weight loss in 36% of cases. Since in this study IFN-α and YNK01 were administered simultaneously, it was difficult to attribute the toxic or side-effects to either drug with certainty, but the chairman of the study (F Guilhot, personal communication) reports that all the investigators agree that weight loss and gastrointestinal side-effects were mainly secondary to YNK01 and were the main cause of treatment discontinuation.

The Italian Cooperative Study Group on CML has undertaken a study identical to the French one. This study is identified as protocol CML 97/IFN/LDAC ORAL. As in the French study, treatment was IFN-α 5 MU/m^2/day and YNK01 600 mg/day from day 1 to day 14 of every month, and the treatment duration was 12 months. In this study, 86 new cases of Ph-positive CML, median age 51 years, range 20–74 years, were enrolled over a 12-month period (1998). The case distribution by risk was 40% low, 43% intermediate, and 16% high. To date, all 86 patients have been followed for at least 6 months, while information on the whole treatment period (12 months) is still limited to 57 of these cases. The complete haematological response rate at 6 months is 50% (95% CI 40–60%) based on intention-to-treat (43 of 86) and 75% (95% CI 63–85%) based on cases evaluable for the response (43 of 57). The cytogenetic response rate (minor plus major plus complete, >33% Ph-negative) at 12 months is 31%. The mean daily dose of YNK01 decreased from 567 mg (month 1) to 315 mg (month 6). The gastrointestinal toxicity, which was attributed mainly to YNK01 as in the French study, during the first 3 months ranged from 49% for nausea and vomiting to 29% for diarrhoea, with a significant (>10%) weight loss in 34% of cases. Nausea, vomiting, and diarrhoea were grade >2 in all but seven cases. If these data are compared with the last interim analysis of the protocol CML 94 (the IFN-α plus Ara-C arm),[30] the cytogenetic and haematological response rates of this study are in the same range, while gastrointestinal toxicity is at least twice as high.

Both studies suggested that YNK01 can substitute for low-dose subcutaneous Ara-C, but revealed that a dose of YNK01 of 600 mg/day is poorly tolerated, mainly owing to gastrointestinal toxicity, so that the performance status of the patients is significantly affected and up to 30% of patients do not comply with treatment and abandon it. The main conclusion of these studies is that the combination of IFN-α and YNK01 should be exploited further, testing different YNK01 doses and schedules.

REFERENCES

1. Talpaz M, McCredie KB, Mavlight GM et al, Leukocyte interferon-induced myeloid cytoreduction in chronic myelogenous leukemia. *Blood* 1983; **62:** 689–97.
2. Silver RT, Benn P, Verma RS et al, Recombinant gamma-interferon has activity in chronic myeloid leukemia. *Am J Clin Oncol* 1990; **13:** 49–56.
3. Talpaz M, Kantarjian HM, McCredie KB et al, Hematologic remission and cytogenetic improvement induced by recombinant human interferon alpha in chronic myelogenous leukemia. *N Engl J Med* 1986; **314:** 1065–73.
4. Talpaz M, Kantarjian HM, McCredie KB et al, Clinical investigation of human alpha interferon in chronic myelogenous leukemia. *Blood* 1987; **69:** 1280–5.
5. Ozer H, George SL, Schiffer CA et al, Prolonged subcutaneous administration of recombinant alpha2b interferon in patients with previously untreated Philadelphia chromosome-positive chronic-phase chronic myelogenous leukemia: effect on remission duration and survival. Cancer and Leukemia Group B Study 8583. *Blood* 1993; **82:** 2975–82.
6. Fernandez-Ranada J, Lavilla E, Odriozola J et al, Interferon alpha 2a in the treatment of chronic myelogenous leukemia in chronic phase: results of the Spanish Group. *Leuk Lymphoma* 1993; **11:** 175–84.
7. Alimena G, Morra E, Lazzarino M et al, Interferon alpha-2b as therapy for Ph-positive chronic myelogenous leukemia: a study of 82 patients with intermittent or daily administration. *Blood* 1988; **72:** 642–9.
8. Manstruct M, Mahon FX, Faberes C et al, Response to recombinant interferon alpha in patients with chronic myelogenous leukemia in a single center: results and analysis of predictive factors. *Leukemia* 1995; **9:** 1997–2004.
9. Italian Cooperative Study Group on Chronic Myeloid Leukemia, Interferon alpha-2a as compared with conventional chemotherapy for the treatment of chronic myeloid leukemia. *N Engl J Med* 1994; **330:** 820–6.
10. Allan NC, Richards SM, Sheperd PCA et al, United Kingdom Medical Research Council randomised multicentre trial of interferon-alfa for chronic myeloid leukemia: improved survival irrespective of cytogenetic response. *Lancet* 1995; **345:** 1392–9.
11. Hehlmann R, Heimpel H, Hasford et al, The German CML Study Group. Randomized comparison of interferon-alpha with busulfan and hydroxyurea in chronic myelogenous leukemia. *Blood* 1994; **84:** 4064–71.
12. Ohnishi BK, Ohno R, Tomonaga M et al, A randomized trial comparing interferon alpha with busulphan for newly diagnosed chronic myelogenous leukemia. *Blood* 1995; **86:** 906–13.
13. Silver RT, Woolf ST, Helmann R et al, An evidence-based analysis of the effect of busulphan, hydroxyurea, interferon and allogeneic bone marrow transplantation in treating the chronic phase of chronic myeloid leukemia: developed for the American Society of Hematology. *Blood* 1999; **94:** 1517–36.
14. Chronic Myeloid Leukemia Trialist' Collaborative Group. Interferon alfa versus chemotherapy for chronic myeloid leukemia: a meta-analysis of seven randomized trials. *J Natl Cancer Inst* 1997; **89:** 1616–20.
15. Spiro TE, Mattelaer MA, Efira A et al, Sensitivity of myeloid progenitor cells in healthy subjects and patients with chronic myeloid leukemia to chemotherapeutic agents. *J Natl Cancer Inst* 1981; **66:** 1053–9.
16. Sokal JE, Leong SS, Gomez GA, Preferential inhibition by cytarabine of CFU-GM from patients with chronic granulocytic leukemia. *Cancer* 1987; **59:** 197–202.
17. Imanishi J, Tanaka A, Kuramoto A et al, Experimental research into clinical applications of interferons. *Gan To Kagaku Ryoho* 1984; **11:** 53–9.
18. Richman CM, Slapak CA, Toh B, Interferon protects normal human granulocyte/macrophage colony-forming cells from Ara-C cytotoxicity. *J Biol Response Mod.* 1990; **9:** 570–5.
19. Sokal J, Beininger SH, Low-dose cytosine arabinoside by subcutaneous infusion in early and advanced chronic granulocytic leukemia. *Blood* 1986; **68:** 233a.

20. Robertson MJ, Tantravahi R, Gitman JD et al, Hematologic remission and cytogenetic improvement in treatment of stable-phase chronic myelogenous leukemia with continuous infusion of low-dose cytarabine. *Am J Hematol* 1993; **43:** 95–102.
21. Kantarjian HM, Keating J, Elihu H et al, Treatment of advanced stages of Philadelphia chromosome positive chronic myelogenous leukemia with interferon and low-dose cytarabine. *J Clin Oncol* 1992; **10:** 772–8.
22. Arthur CK, Ma DDF, Combined interferon alfa-2a and cytosine arabinoside as first-line treatment for chronic myeloid leukemia. *Acta Hematol* 1993; **89**(Suppl 1): 15–21.
23. Guilhot F, Dreyfus B, Desmarest MC et al, Combined therapy with interferon and chemotherapy in chronic myelogenous leukemia. *Nouv Rev Fr Hematol* 1989; **31:** 171–3.
24. Kantarjian HM, O'Brien S, Smith TL et al, Treatment of Philadelphia chromosome positive early chronic phase chronic myelogenous leukemia with daily doses of interferon and low-dose cytarabine. *J Clin Oncol* 1999; **17:** 284–92.
25. Kantarjian HM, O'Brien S, Smith TL et al, Prolonged survival in chronic myelogenous leukemia following cytogenetic response to alpha interferon therapy. *Ann Intern Med* 1995; **122:** 254–61.
26. Kantarjian HM, Keating MJ, Smith TL et al, Proposal for a simple synthesis prognostic staging system in chronic myelogenous leukemia. *Am J Med* 1990; **88:** 1–8.
27. Thaler J, Hilbe W, Apfelbeck U et al, Interferon-alpha-2c and LD Ara-C for the treatment of patients with CML: results of the Austrian multicenter phase II study. *Leuk Res* 1997; **21:** 75–80.
28. Guilhot F, Guerci A, Fiere D et al, The treatment of chronic myelogenous leukemia by interferon and cytosine-arabinoside: rational and design of the French Trials. *Bone Marrow Transplant* 1995; **17**(Suppl 3): 29–31.
29. Guilhot F, Chastang C, Michallet M et al, Interferon alfa-2b combined with cytarabine versus interferon alone in chronic myelogenous leukemia. *N Engl J Med* 1997; **337:** 223–9.
30. Tura S, Cytarabine increases karyotypic response in alpha-IFN treated chronic myeloid leukemia patients: results of a national prospective randomized trial. *Blood* 1998; **92**(Suppl 1): Abst 1299.
31. Rosti G, Bonifazi F, De Vivo A et al, Cytarabine increases karyotypic response and survival in alpha-interferon in treated chronic myelogenous leukemia patients: results of a national prospective randomized trial of the Italian Cooperative Study Group on CML. *Blood* 1999; **94**(Suppl 1): Abst 2669.
32. Guilhot F, Harousseau JL, Fiere D et al, Phase I/II trial of Ara-C prodrug YNK01 in chronic myelogenous leukemia patients: hematologic and cytogenetic responses. *Proc Am Soc Clin Oncol* 1996; **15:** Abst 149.

12

Prognostic factors

Joerg Hasford, Markus Pfirrmann, Rüdiger Hehlmann, Patricia CA Shepherd, François Guilhot, François X Mahon, Josef Thaler, Juan L Steegmann, Hanneke C Kluin-Nelemans, Andries Louwagie, Kazunori Ohnishi, Otto Kloke

CONTENTS • Introduction • Methodology • Prognostic scores in CML • The CML Collaborative Prognostic Factors Project and the New CML score • Conclusions and outlook

> 'It appears to me a most excellent thing for the physician to cultivate prognosis ... by seeing and announcing beforehand those who will live and those who will die, he will thus escape censure.'
>
> Hippocrates, *Aphorisms* II.19

INTRODUCTION

Prognostic factors are continuous or discrete variables helping to assess a certain development in advance. They are measured at baseline, i.e. prior to initiation of treatment, or at specified time points during or after treatment, and allow a reliable discrimination in the course of disease and in treatment outcomes. Well-known examples are the relationship between age and sex and expected lifetime. Usually, more than one variable with discriminating power can be identified, and thus prognostic models or scores combining the relevant variables, mostly by an accumulated function, are constructed.

Prognostic models suit a variety of important tasks in modern medicine.

The prediction of the course of disease for individual patients and patient groups
Many patients would like to know what to expect. Health and life insurers need such data, too.

The development and administration of prognosis-adjusted treatments
As most treatments are accompanied by dose-dependent adverse drug reactions, each patient should ideally receive only as much treatment as necessary to successfully fight his or her disease. For such an individualized treatment, the prognosis of a patient has to be known, and appropriate prognosis-adjusted treatment regimens have to be tested for efficacy and safety.

An improved understanding of aetiology and the natural history of disease
Although a given prognostic factor does not necessarily play a *causal* role, prognostic models may help to elucidate aetiology or explain the natural history of disease, for example the presence or absence of the Philadelphia chromosome in chronic myeloid leukaemia (CML) patients.

The assessment of the quality of health care
Outcome quality is usually evaluated by comparing outcomes either among hospitals, physi-

cians, regions, and health care systems or in relation to a standard. Reliable data on outcome quality of a particular health care provider can only be achieved if an adjustment with regard to the prognostic profile of the patients was considered. Otherwise, hospitals that mainly take care of seriously sick patients and thus generate correspondingly rather poor outcomes may falsely be alleged to provide poor quality.

The promotion of an economical use of resources

Many – sometimes expensive – treatments work only in a subgroup of patients. Especially in the area of secondary preventive treatments, the number needed to treat to avoid an event such as myocardial infarction or stroke may be as high as several hundred patients. Valid knowledge about prognosis will help to determine those patients who will most likely benefit from a particular treatment, thus allowing a saving of unnecessary treatment costs. In CML, there is evidence that for high-risk patients, interferon-α (IFN-α) has no additive therapeutic value when compared with hydroxyurea. Hence, one may save the more expensive IFN-α without doing harm to the patient.

The improvement of trial design and analysis

Prognostic models will allow stratified allocation to randomized trials so that prognosis-adjusted treatments can be properly evaluated. In addition, validated prognostic models may serve the adjustment of statistical tests in case of heterogeneities between treatment groups and a more precise estimation of the size of treatment effect.

The possibility of a sound comparative interpretation of the results of clinical trials and studies

As the differences in effect size are quite often bigger between different prognostic groups than between different treatments, for proper interpretation of the results of various trials it is absolutely essential to know the prognostic profile of the patients. This is even more important for uncontrolled therapeutic studies, which are still common in the USA.[1–3]

There is no doubt that prognostic models are used for extremely important tasks and highly sensible decisions which may adversely impact upon patients' lives if based on flawed models, and thus the greatest care has to be taken in constructing and validating prognostic models. Although the basic methodology for the analysis and validation of prognostic models is available, the procedures are not yet widely known and in real life often not easily well performed. That is one reason for the estimate by Wyatt and Altman in 1995 that only a few of the hundreds of prognostic models published every year are routinely used to inform difficult clinical decisions.[4] Therefore we first want to discuss the basic requirements and statistical techniques that allow for valid and clinically credible and useful prognostic models. To support a better understanding, we shall outline some procedures of the CML Prognostic Factors Project (CPFP),[5] whose updated results will be presented in the last part of this chapter.

METHODOLOGY

As for all good quality research, it is highly advisable to write a detailed research plan. In general, the typical structure and contents of a clinical trial protocol as formulated in the Appendix of the EU-GCP[6] give some guidance if interpreted appropriately in the context of prognostic factor analysis.

To start with, the inception cohort of patients has to be defined in detail. All clinically relevant variables should be included, and patient data should be provided with exact and widely accepted definitions of these variables.[4]

Rationale and objectives of the study

The relevant literature should be summarized, and the conclusions should lead to the explicitly stated objectives of the study:

> The current prognostic scores for CML (in 1994) allow to differentiate fairly well the prognosis of

chemotherapy patients, but not of patients treated with IFN. This is particularly unsatisfactory as IFN therapy seems to work in a (yet unknown) subgroup of patients very well. Thus, it is still impossible to select the best therapy for a particular patient.

It is our aim to establish a large data bank of patients with CML treated in prospective studies according to a uniform protocol in Europe, North America, and Japan. The major objectives of the subsequent statistical analyses are:

- the extraction and validation of prognostic factors of CML patients treated with IFN alone or in combination with chemotherapy;
- the validation of published prognostic scores;
- the evaluation of haematological and cytogenetic response as time-dependent prognostic factors.

Selection of studies and patients

Inclusion and exclusion criteria for patients and/or studies are needed to assess the focus and generalizability of the subsequent analyses and results. Patients treated within prospective studies should be aimed for. Great care has to be taken to specify the disease and the permitted treatment regimens, and sufficient time should have passed for observation and follow-up to observe the outcomes of interest. Thus the relevant section of our research plan stated:[5]

> The patients have to fulfil the following criteria:
>
> Well confirmed diagnosis of Ph-positive or bcr/abl-positive CML; no treatment prior to study treatment unless well documented and for less than 6 months after diagnosis; treatment according to a uniform protocol in a prospective study; therapy with interferon, either alone or in combination with chemotherapy; date of diagnosis known; initiation of treatment between 01/01/1980 and 31/12/1994.

The inception cohort of patients has thus been defined in detail, and all clinically relevant patient data with exact and widely accepted definitions of the variables should be considered.

Definition of outcome variables

As in clinical trials, outcome variables have to be specified in detail together with the methods of their measurement. Within the CPFP, we applied the following definition of survival time:[5]

> Survival will be calculated as time from start of therapy to death, irrespective of the cause of death as it might be difficult in such a multinational project to have a uniform assessment of causes of death. Patients having received bone marrow transplantation in first chronic phase will be censored at the time of bone marrow transplantation (bmt).

Great care has to be taken that patients are censored only when there is no hint that the reason for censoring bears any relationship to the outcome variable under investigation. Otherwise, the analyses may be flawed. In the CPFP, only patients who received bone marrow transplantation (BMT) in first chronic phase were censored, since a BMT in second chronic phase, accelerated phase, or blastic phase resembles a salvage treatment.

Whereas the definition of survival time usually does not present major problems, softer outcome variables such as accelerated phase or haematological or cytogenetic remission may do so. Although no standard definitions are available, one is well advised to sensibly choose among those that have already been published. Regarding haematological remission, for instance, we applied the definition given by Talpaz et al[7] For cytogenetic remission, it is recommended that one specifies a minimum number of analysed metaphases (20 in our project), since it makes a relevant difference in validity whether a complete remission has been diagnosed by investigation of 40 metaphases or of only 5.

Selection of learning and validation samples

As a rather often neglected matter of fact, prognostic models cannot be constructed and validated using the same data set. Most commonly, there will be no a priori hypothesis referring to a specific prognostic model; thus the extraction of a prognostic model has to be regarded as a hypothesis-generating exploratory statistical procedure whose results have to be validated, i.e. confirmed, before the prognostic model can claim credibility and validity. There are a number of different approaches that safeguard increasing degrees of validity.[8]

Resubstitution

By the method of resubstitution, the prognostic model developed within the inception cohort is applied to the baseline characteristics of each patient to obtain his or her predicted or theoretical survival time. Provided that factors with prognostic value exist and that both the factors and the model were properly selected, this method of testing performance is biased in favour of good prediction because the model is developed within and applied to the same data.[8] Resubstitution checks the internal validity of the analysis only.

Half-sample replication

Here one draws a random sample of half of the total sample size, constructs a prognostic model in the first sample, and resubstitutes it in the second sample, and vice versa. Applying a model to a different data set enhances its credibility in comparison with resubstitution, but it has to be kept in mind that both samples contain patient data collected under the same protocol, i.e. the two samples are not really independent. The jack-knife technique can be considered as an extension of the method of half-sample replication, with subsets based on excluding one patient instead of half the patients.

Cross-sample validation

By the method of cross-sample validation, the prognostic model is developed employing data of patients from one study or a group of studies, and then the discriminating power of this model is tested in patients of a truly independent study or group of studies. This type of confirmatory testing of a prognostic model provides the most substantive evidence of its validity. The real-life problem usually is that patient data from truly independent studies are not available. This problem can be overcome by collaborative projects with many study groups working together, such as in the CPFP.

The methods used for validation should be stated in the research plan. To increase the power of detecting the prognostic value of a variable and to reliably estimate model parameters, the learning sample is usually kept larger than the validation sample by a factor of 2 or 3 : 1.

The CPFP group decided that for the extraction and validation of the prognostic model, studies with all their patients were either randomly drawn for the learning sample, which finally consisted of approximately 75% of all patients, or for the validation sample, with about 25% of all patients.

Quality control

As in clinical trials, great care has to be taken that the data are complete, accurate, and unbiased. Various checks for logical sequence, causes of data outliers, and unexplained values with categorical variables should be pursued. Calendar dates have to be examined for their natural order and completeness, and the contents of directly dependent items and the reasons for missing values closely scrutinized. All quality control procedures have to be terminated prior to the statistical analyses. Only after the file-closing procedure may prognostic modelling begin.

Statistical analyses

The statistical analyses and the construction of a prognostic model do not strictly follow a 'cookbook recipe' as is available for the classical intent-to-treat analysis of a phase III clinical trial, but require close cooperation between biostatisticians and clinicians, a methodologically guided guess (experience), understanding of the disease, lots of tolerance towards frustration, and some luck. Thus, one should not expect such a highly detailed analysis plan as is common for clinical trials.

The first step is the selection of those variables that are to be included in the multiple model (Figure 12.1). There are two approaches: a purely statistical one and the one based on previous publications and medical reasoning. Mostly, both approaches are combined. The statistical approach tests descriptively whether there is an association between a particular baseline variable and the outcome variable. Regarding survival time, continuous baseline variables such as age or white blood cell count are analysed using the Cox model; categorical data are analysed using the logrank test. Continuous data can be categorized, either by a biometric procedure (e.g. the median split) or by medical reasoning. The variables found to be statistically significant in univariate analyses will be included in the multiple analyses. The same applies to variables that are considered to be relevant from a medical point of view or have already been published as being of prognostic value. It is common to select for multiple analyses all variables that show a statistically significant association with the outcome variable at a significance level of $2\alpha = 0.1$ to avoid too early a removal of a possibly prognostic factor.

Of course, there may be multicolinearities between some variables. Criteria for the selec-

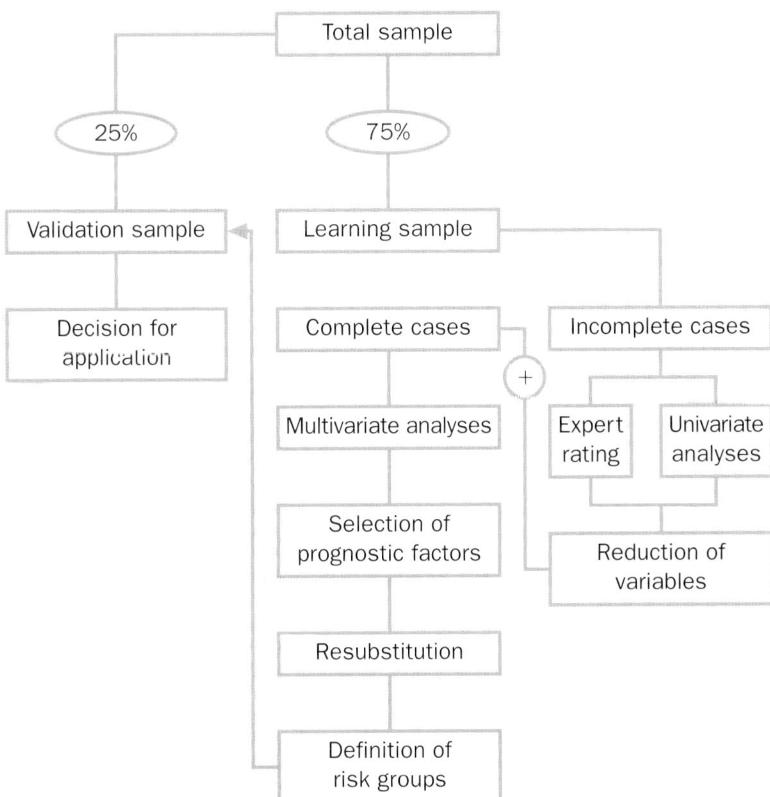

Figure 12.1 Scheme for extracting and validating the New CML score.

tion of those to be included in the final model are easiness to measure, reliability and validity of measurement, biological plausibility, and completeness. The selection of the multiple model depends on the kind of outcome variable. For survival time or other time-to-event variables, such as duration of chronic phase or time to cytogenetic response, the Cox model is usually applied. For qualitative outcome variables such as haematological response within the first 9 months or cytogenetic response within the first 21 months, a stepwise logistic regression model has to be fitted. Selection procedures for the best final model are given for instance by Collett[9] and Hosmer and Lemeshow[10] respectively.

The value of the resulting prognostic model will be calculated for each patient. The distribution of prognostic score values can then be divided into distinct risk groups using the minimal *p*-value approach.[11] This approach helps to find the cutpoints of the prognostic score values, which statistically separate the outcome variable best. In a resubstitution analysis, the *internal* validity of the model is checked. Only if the result is satisfying, for example if the survival curves are statistically significantly as well as clinically relevantly different, will the model be applied to the validation sample.

The Cox model has the advantage that it is a widely accepted method: plenty of experiences, publications, and software packages are available. It is semiparametric in the sense that it allows us to estimate the effect of each factor on the outcome variable.

Classification and regression tree (CART) method

A more recent approach in the analysis of prognostic factors is the classification and regression tree (CART) method.[12] CART is a non-parametric tool to investigate correlations between variables and to identify subgroups of patients, which, with regard to the outcome variable, are internally as homogeneous and externally as different as possible.

At each step, the baseline variables are checked for the cut-off point (split) that maximally discriminates the outcome variable. The selection of this 'best' split is based on a goodness-of-split test statistic. This will be a chi-squared test in the case of categorical outcome variables and a logrank test for survival data. A terminal node is reached when no further split is significant or the number of events at this node is less than a predefined minimum. The terminal nodes of the tree indicate the prognostic subgroups that could be ranked by prognostic profile. In a resubstitution analysis, survival probabilities for the patients will be calculated and survival curves plotted according to terminal subgroups.

As a non-parametric method, a tree-structured classification technique can deal with all kinds of variables and distributions. With the first split at the root node, CART identifies a most influential main factor; all other nodes reveal conditional interactions. Variables with a skewed distribution or only a few different realizations have, however, little chance to be selected at lower steps. The final prognostic groups are straightforward to interpret, in particular for non-statisticians.

CART and Cox may be considered as complementary techniques. It makes sense first to use CART to identify relevant interactions and then to test interactions in a Cox model.

Time-dependent prognostic factors

The most interesting time-dependent prognostic factors such as haematological and cytogenetic response or tumour remission appear only after treatment has been initiated. Time-dependent prognostic factors (TDPFs) perform two relevant tasks:

1. They provide additional clinically useful information, and may improve the precision of prognosis; for example, the prognosis of a low-risk CML patient varies considerably depending whether or not he or she achieves cytogenetic response.
2. As medical treatment becomes more effective – for example, the median survival time

for CML patients treated with IFN-α is now about six years – it takes more and more time to assess the value of new treatment options with clinical endpoint trials. However, CML patients do not have so much time. Thus, there is an urgent search for valid surrogate measures allowing a much faster assessment of treatment success. Such surrogate measures are quite often nothing other than TDPFs. However, a critical point here is that surrogate measures such as cytogenetic remission might be valid for CML patients with low risk but not for those with high risk, i.e. their validity may be risk-group or treatment-dependent too.

From a statistical point of view, TDPFs require more sophisticated techniques, since they have to cope with the so-called 'time-till-response bias',[13] i.e. a patient has to survive for at least some time to have a chance of haematological or cytogenetic response at all. In this case, a naive evaluation of Kaplan–Meier curves is not suitable. Appropriate methods are Simon–Makuch curves of graphical representation and the Mantel–Byar test for confirmatory analysis. In some situations, the application of landmark analysis and a logrank test at the chosen landmark is justifiable.[14]

PROGNOSTIC SCORES IN CML

Owing to the evident relevance of knowing prognostic factors, several CML study groups have already worked in this area. Tura et al[15] were surely among the first to publish prognostic factors in CML, later followed by Cervantes et al,[16] Sokal et al,[17] Kantarjian et al,[18,19] Thiele et al,[20] and Hehlmann et al.[21,22] In recent years, the need for valid prognostic factors became more urgent with the introduction of IFN-α into treatment regimens for CML. The Sokal score achieved widespread use, and works well as a prognostic discriminator for survival in patients treated with chemotherapy (e.g. busulfan or hydroxyurea). Ohnishi et al,[23] Hasford et al,[24] and Ozer et al[2] reported, however, that the Sokal score does not work well with patients treated with IFN-α. Administered either alone or combined with hydroxyurea or Ara-C, IFN-α became accepted as the best available conservative treatment for patients with chronic-phase CML. Allogeneic bone marrow transplantation is still regarded as the only curative therapy, but carries a considerable risk of early death and chronic graft-versus-host disease (GVHD). Hence, there is a need to find out which treatment might be more appropriate for a particular patient. In addition, since most CML studies in the USA have no control group, one needs a valid prognostic model to be able to properly interpret their results.

Cross-sample validation of CML prognostic models

As we did not want to develop a new prognostic model while already-published ones were still performing well, we first of all examined various prognostic models within our CPFP data set of chronic-phase CML patients treated with IFN-α. Details of data collection, quality control, and baseline characteristics have been published elsewhere.[5]

To the best of our knowledge, Tura et al[15] were the first to publish a prognostic model, as early as 1981. Six variables had a statistically significant impact: splenomegaly, hepatomegaly, blast cells, leukocytosis, thrombocytopenia (respectively thrombocytosis), and a rise in granulated precursor cells. According to the number of risk factors present, Tura et al suggested three prognostic groups:

- low-risk group: up to one risk factor present;
- intermediate-risk group: two or three risk factors;
- high-risk group: more than three risk factors.

Of 1400 IFN-α-treated CML patients in our data bank, 834 provided all data required by this model. The median survival times were 77, 65, and 55 months, and the survival curves of the

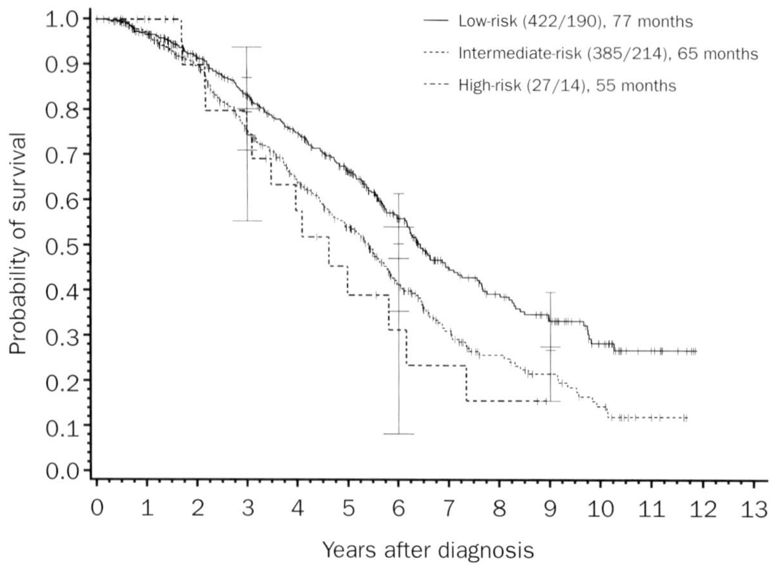

Figure 12.2 Cross-sample validation: the Tura score applied to 834 patients with early-stage CML treated with IFN-α. The notation '(422/190), 77 months' indicates that of 422 patients, 190 died, and that the median survival time was 77 months (similarly for the intermediate-risk and high-risk groups). Confidence intervals for probability of survival are given at 3, 6, and 9 years for each risk group.

intermediate-risk and high-risk groups did not separate well (Figure 12.2).

Cervantes and Rozman[16] found splenomegaly, hepatomegaly, erythroid precursors in blood, and over 5% marrow myeloblasts to be statistically significant in a multiple Cox model. Again, three prognostic groups were identified:

- low-risk group: up to one factor present;
- intermediate-risk group: two factors;
- high-risk group: three or four factors.

Only 449 patients of our sample provided complete information with regard to the score's variables. The median survival times were 78, 65, and 50 months (Figure 12.3). As with the Tura score, the intermediate-risk and high-risk groups did not separate well – findings that were also reported by Kantarjian et al.[19] In their publication, Kantarjian et al introduced the so-called simple Synthesis Prognostic Staging System. Its performance was evaluated prior to the development of the New CML score. Neither the simple Synthesis Prognostic Staging System nor the established Sokal score[17] could provide a satisfying differentiation of survival curves.[5] Even though we varied the two cut-points of the Sokal score, the separation of intermediate-risk and high-risk patients did not improve.

All these prognostic models were developed with CML patients treated with various chemotherapy regimens, frequently including splenectomy and occasionally even radiation. Interestingly, most scoring systems exhibited serious problems in separating intermediate-risk and high-risk patients. Thiele's prognostic models[20] include variables that are not routinely collected: data on pseudo-Gaucher cells, a prognostic factor of his Model I, were available for only two patients of our international data set, and, mainly because of megakaryocytes and fibrosis in bone marrow, just 14 patients had complete data with regard to Model II.

Thus, there was no doubt about the necessity to develop a new prognostic model for CML patients treated with an IFN-α-based therapy, since, in comparison with chemotherapy, IFN-α seems to influence the natural course of the disease in a substantially different way.

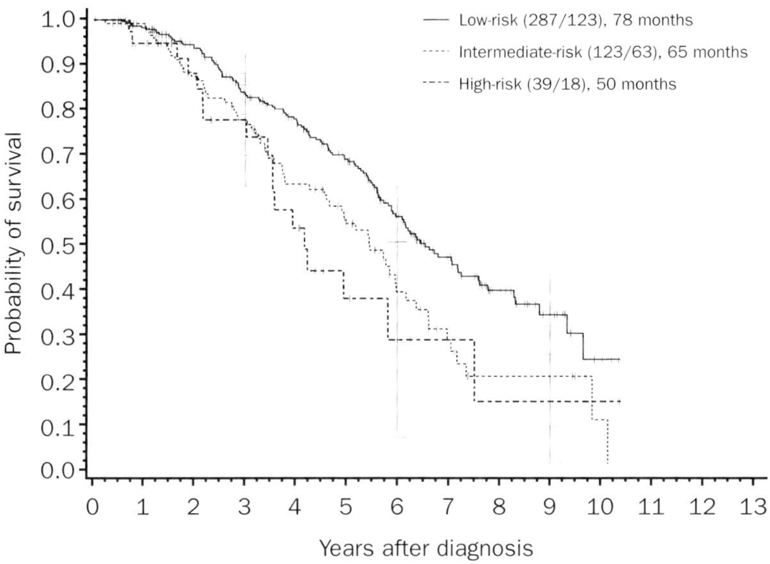

Figure 12.3 Cross-sample validation: the Cervantes score applied to 449 patients with early-stage CML treated with IFN-α. The notation '(287/123), 78 months' indicates that of 287 patients, 123 died, and that the median survival time was 78 months (similarly for the intermediate-risk and high-risk groups). Confidence intervals for probability of survival are given at 3, 6, and 9 years for each risk group.

THE CML COLLABORATIVE PROGNOSTIC FACTORS PROJECT AND THE NEW CML SCORE

The CPFP received data from 14 studies involving 12 centres from Austria, Belgium, The Netherlands, Luxembourg, France, Germany, the UK, Italy, Japan, Spain and the USA. Details of the research plan have been mentioned above and published elsewhere.[5] Six prognostic variables were identified by multiple Cox regression. From their prognostic score, three statistically significantly distinct prognostic groups could be extracted by application of the minimal *p*-value approach. All analyses were restricted to a learning sample consisting of 981 patients from 11 studies. The newly suggested risk groups were then examined in the validation sample consisting of 322 patients from three studies that were completely independent of score development.

The New CML score is calculated as follows:

New CML score = (0.6666 × age [0 when age <50 years; 1, otherwise] + 0.0420 × spleen size [cm below costal margin] + 0.0584 × blasts [%] + 0.0413 × eosinophils [%] + 0.2039 × basophils [0 when basophils <3%; 1, otherwise + 1.0956 × platelet count [0 when platelets $<1500 \times 10^9$/l; 1 otherwise]) × 1000

The score showed almost identical characteristics in both learning and validation samples. After the most recent update in 1999, the logrank test resulted in a p-value < 0.0001 for both samples. Combining the two samples in one, the median survival times in the three prognostic groups, currently 1400 patients altogether, were 100, 69, and 45 months (Figure 12.4). The 95% confidence intervals do not overlap, at 3, 6, or 9 years after start of treatment. The 10-year survival rates are 42%, 18%, and 5% respectively. Of the patients, 42% belong to the low-risk group, 45% to the intermediate-risk group, and 13% to the high-risk group. A program for the calculation of the score is accessible by Internet (www.pharmacoepi.de). It is possible to download the program on a PC.

Comparison between the Sokal score and the New CML

Although the Sokal score could not clearly distinguish between survival curves for the intermediate-risk and high-risk groups in the large sample of the CPFP group,[5] there seems to be some concern about the application of the New CML score, since the percentage of patients supposed to be at high risk is considerably

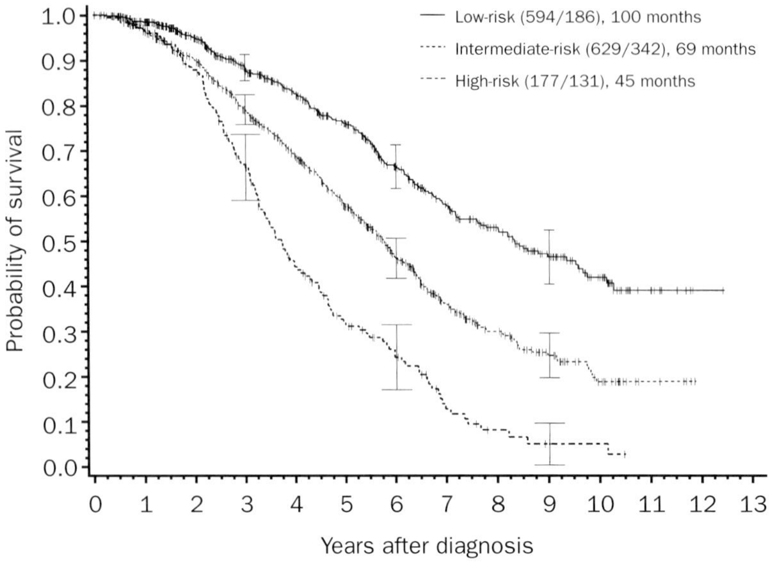

Figure 12.4 The New CML score applied to 1400 patients with early-stage CML treated with IFN-α. The notation '(594/186), 100 months' indicates that of 594 patients, 186 died, and that the median survival time was 100 months (similarly for intermediate-risk and high-risk groups). Confidence intervals for probability of survival are given at 3, 6, and 9 years for each risk group.

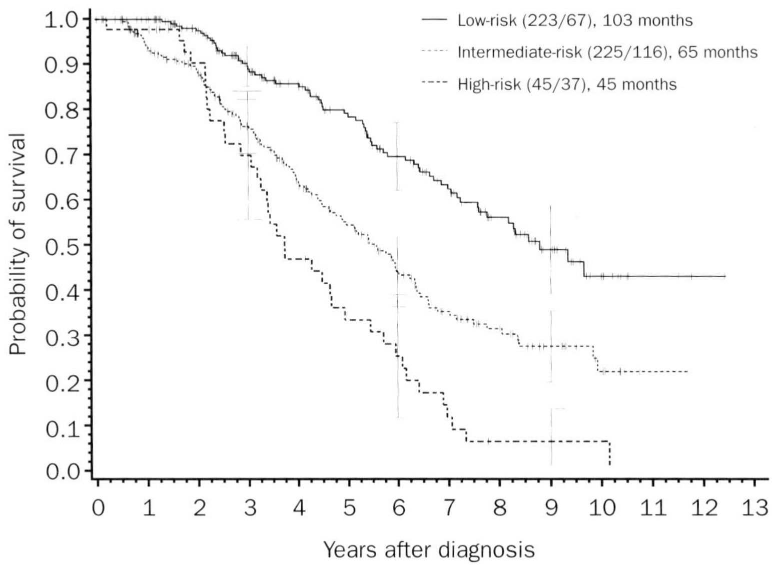

Figure 12.5 Cross-sample validation: the New CML score applied to 493 patients with early-stage CML treated with IFN-α. The notation '(223/67), 103 months' indicates that of 223 patients, 67 died, and that the median survival time was 103 months (similarly for the intermediate-risk and high-risk groups). Confidence intervals for probability of survival are given at 3, 6, and 9 years for each risk group. Logrank test: $p < 0.0001$.

lower with the New CML score than with the Sokal score. Hence, the question was raised whether all these patients with a Sokal score of 'high risk' really are at high risk.

To tackle this question, we compared the Sokal score[17] and the New CML score by cross-sample validation with an investigated sample of 493 patients who were not included in the learning sample when extracting the multiple Cox model for the New CML score, i.e. all were independent of the score's development.

Owing to the greater number of patients and the longer follow-up, the identification of three risk groups with statistically significantly different survival ($p < 0.0001$) was even more obvious than in the original validation sample[5] (Figure 12.5). In contrast, the Sokal score was not able to differentiate between intermediate-

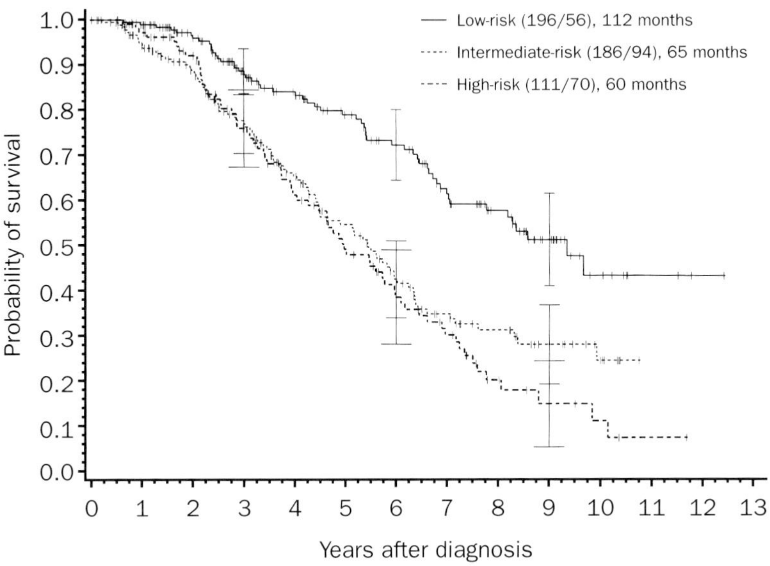

Figure 12.6 Cross-sample validation: the Sokal score applied to 493 patients with early-stage CML treated with IFN-α. The notation '(196/56), 112 months' indicates that of 196 patients, 56 died, and that the median survival time was 112 months (similarly for the intermediate-risk and high-risk groups). Confidence intervals for probability of survival are given at 3, 6, and 9 years for each risk group.

risk and high-risk patients at all (Figure 12.6). To investigate these findings in more detail, we looked especially at those patients whom the two scores put into different risk groups.

Comparison of high-risk groups

Whereas 111 of 493 patients (23%) were allocated to the high-risk group by the Sokal score, only 45 patients (9%) were high-risk according to the New CML score (Table 12.1). Of the 111 patients at high risk according to the Sokal score, only 38 patients (34%) were given the same prognosis with the New CML score – most (63, i.e. 57%) were rather classified as intermediate-risk and 10 (9%) even as low-risk. Because of the small sample size of the latter group, we focused on the comparison between the intermediate-risk and high-risk groups. Although only 101 patients were in either group, survival curves for intermediate risk and high risk according to the New CML score were statistically significantly different ($p = 0.0105$) (Figure 12.7). The 63 patients at intermediate risk according to the New CML score but high risk according to the Sokal score had a median survival of 67 months, which is 24 months more than the patients allocated to the high-risk group by both scores (median survival 43 months) and about the same median survival (65 months) as the intermediate-risk group of the learning sample on which the New CML score was developed.[5] This means that of the patients placed in the high-risk group according to the Sokal score, two-thirds obviously should not be there. Only 7 patients were classified as intermediate-risk by the Sokal score and as high-risk by the New CML score (Figure 12.8). As these were only 16% of all high-risk patients according to the New CML score, large numbers would be needed to investigate whether differences to the group at high risk according to both scores could be identified; however, there was no indication for this.

Comparison of intermediate-risk groups

Of the 186 patients at intermediate risk according to the Sokal score, at least 51 (27%) seemed to have a more favourable risk (Figure 12.9). There might also be a trend recognizable for the aforementioned 7 patients at high risk according to the New CML score to actually be high-risk patients, but again numbers were too low for any firm conclusions to be drawn. The 51 patients at low risk according to the New CML

Table 12.1 Risk group distribution of the Sokal score in comparison with the New CML score when applied to 493 patients of the CPFP data base – all patients independent of any score development

	Sokal score				
New CML score	**<0.8 (low-risk)**	**0.8–1.2 (intermediate-risk)**	**>1.2 (high-risk)**	**Total of cell percents (row): distribution of New CML score**	
≤780 (low-risk)					
n	162	51	10	*n* (row)	223
Cell percent	33	10	2	percent (row)	45
Row percent	73	23	4		
Column percent	83	27	9		
>780–1480 (intermediate-risk)					
n	34	128	63	*n* (row)	225
Cell percent	7	26	13	percent (row)	46
Row percent	15	57	28		
Column percent	17	69	57		
>1480 (high-risk)					
n	0	7	38	*n* (row)	45
Cell percent	0	1	8	percent (row)	9
Row percent	0	16	84		
Column percent	0	4	34		
Total of cell percents (column): distribution of Sokal score				Total number of investigated patients:	
n (column)	196	186	111	*n* = 493	
Percent (column)[a]	40	38	23		

[a] These percentages sum to 101% owing to rounding error.

score had a significantly better survival ($p = 0.0128$) than the 128 patients at intermediate risk according to both scores. As for its high-risk group, the Sokal score showed a statistically significant failure in the allocation of patients into a risk group that was homogeneous with regard to survival. The above 128 patients were only 57% of the 225 patients with intermediate risk also according to the New CML score (Figure 12.10). The previously described 63 patients at high risk according to the Sokal score (28% of 225) had a better survival (median survival 67 months versus 59 months) than the patients at intermediate risk according to both scores; i.e. the actual order of the two risk groups was reversed – an alarmingly poor result for the 'prognostic system' Sokal score. The 34 patients at low risk according to the Sokal score had no statistically signifi-

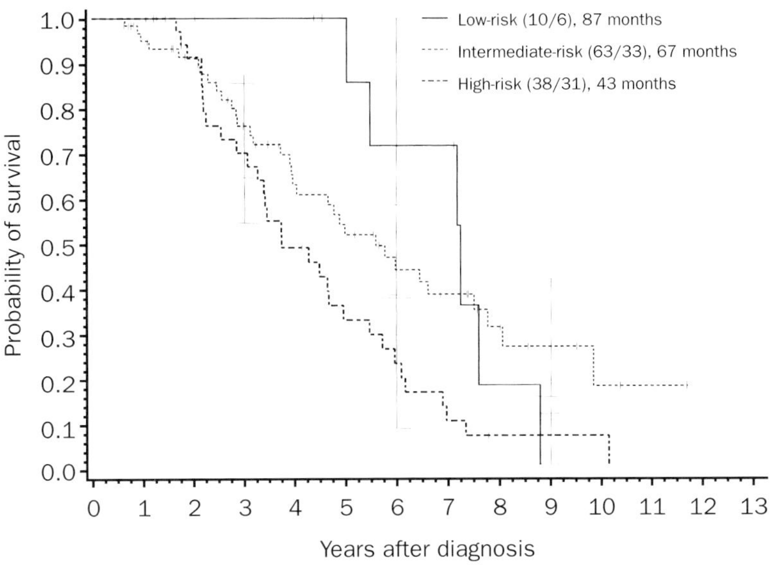

Figure 12.7 The New CML score applied to 111 patients with early-stage CML treated with IFN-α. All patients were classified as high-risk patients by the Sokal score. The notation '(10/6), 87 months' indicates that of 10 patients, 6 died, and that the median survival time was 87 months (similarly for the intermediate-risk and high-risk groups). If applicable, confidence intervals for probability of survival are given at 3, 6, and 9 years for each risk group. Logrank test between intermediate-risk and high-risk patients according to the New CML score: $p = 0.0105$.

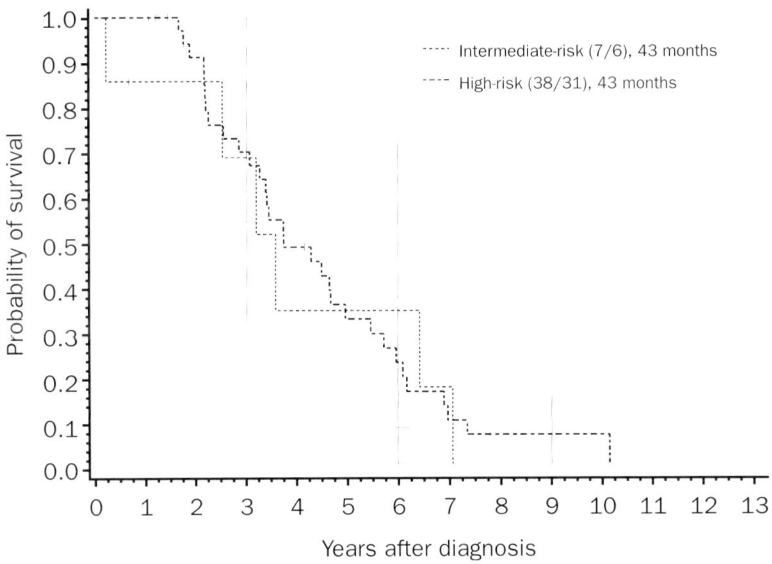

Figure 12.8 The Sokal score applied to 45 patients with early-stage CML treated with IFN-α. All patients were classified as high-risk patients by the New CML score. The notation '(7/6), 43 months' indicates that of 7 patients, 6 died, and that the median survival time was 43 months (similarly for the high-risk group). If applicable, confidence intervals for probability of survival are given at 3, 6, and 9 years for each risk group.

cantly better survival than either of the other two Sokal risk groups.

Comparison of low-risk groups

With regard to low-risk patients, the differences between the two scores were less prominent (Figures 12.11 and 12.12). The combination of low risk according to both scores identified a patient group with a particularly good prognosis. However, omitting from consideration the small group of 10 patients at high risk according to the Sokal score, neither the 51 patients at low risk according to the New CML score and intermediate risk according to the Sokal score nor the 34 where it was the other way round had a statistically significantly different

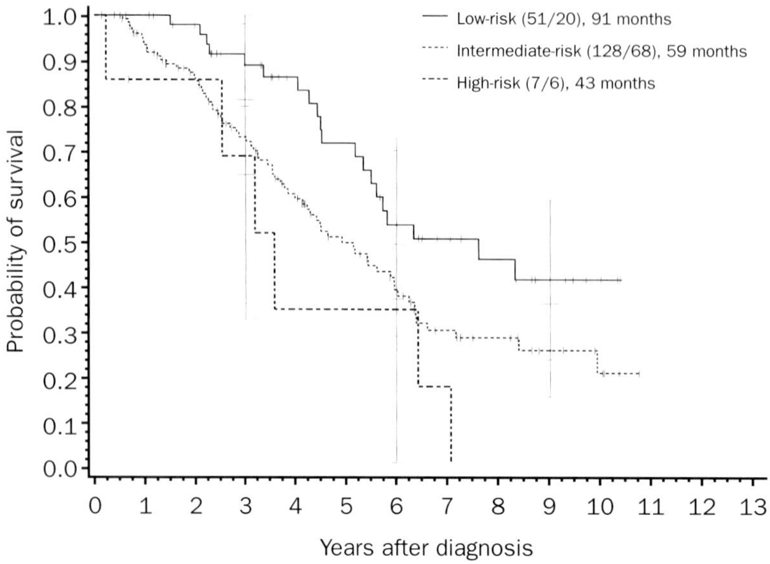

Figure 12.9 The New CML score applied to 186 patients with early-stage CML treated with IFN-α. All patients were classified as intermediate-risk patients by the Sokal score. The notation '(51/20), 91 months' indicates that of 51 patients, 20 died, and that the median survival time was 91 months (similarly for the intermediate-risk and high-risk groups). If applicable, confidence intervals for probability of survival are given at 3, 6, and 9 years for each risk group. Logrank test between low-risk and intermediate-risk patients according to New CML score: $p = 0.0128$.

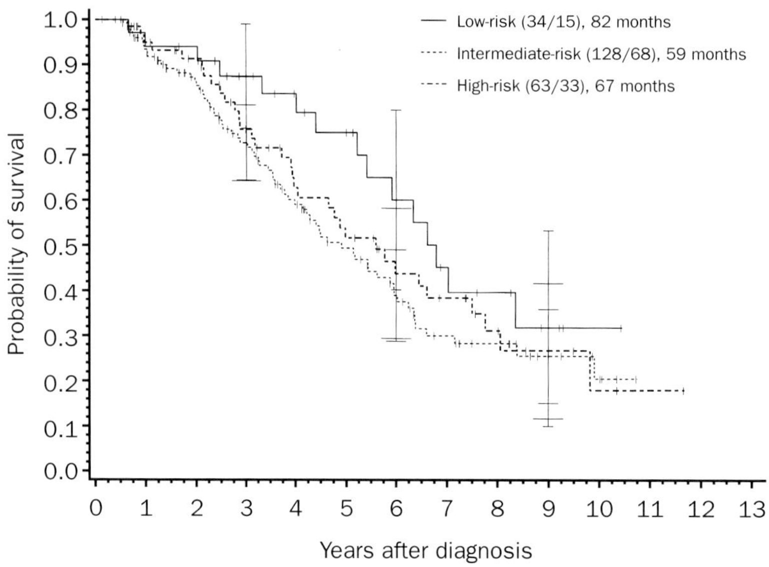

Figure 12.10 The Sokal score applied to 225 patients with early-stage CML treated with IFN-α. All patients were classified as intermediate-risk patients by the New CML score. The notation '(34/15), 82 months' indicates that of 34 patients, 15 died, and that the median survival time was 82 months (similarly for the intermediate-risk and high-risk groups). If applicable, confidence intervals for probability of survival are given at 3, 6, and 9 years for each risk group. Logrank test between low-risk and intermediate-risk patients according to the Sokal score as well as logrank test between low-risk and high-risk patients according to the Sokal score were not significant.

survival from the group at low risk according to both scores.

Conclusions from the comparison of the Sokal score and the New CML score

With the New CML score, patients are no longer as evenly distributed over risk groups as clinicians might like, but it seems that the New CML score simply depicts reality: there *actually do seem to be only about 9–15% patients who are at high risk when undergoing IFN-α-based therapy.* We have statistically significant evidence that

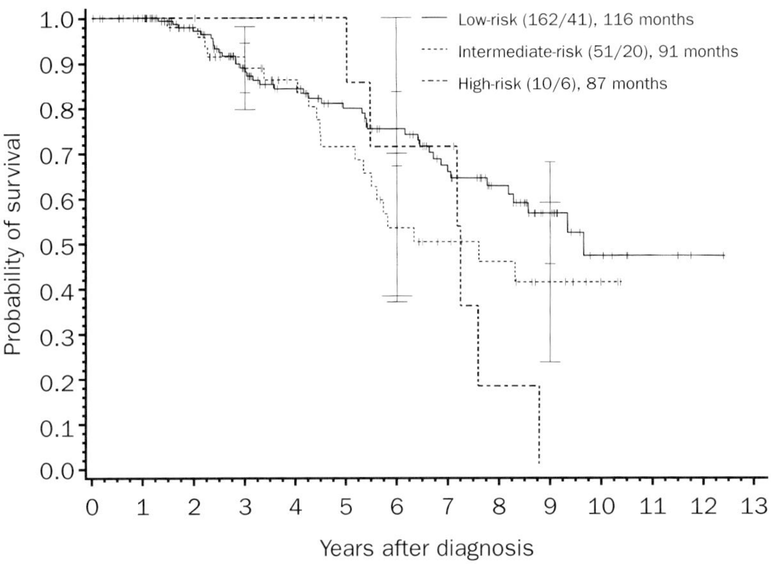

Figure 12.11 The Sokal score applied to 223 patients with early-stage CML treated with IFN-α. All patients were classified as low-risk patients by the New CML score. The notation '(162/41), 116 months' indicates that of 162 patients, 41 died, and that the median survival time was 116 months (similarly for the intermediate-risk and high-risk groups). If applicable, confidence intervals for probability of survival are given at 3, 6, and 9 years for each risk group. Logrank test between low-risk and intermediate-risk patients according to the Sokal score was not significant.

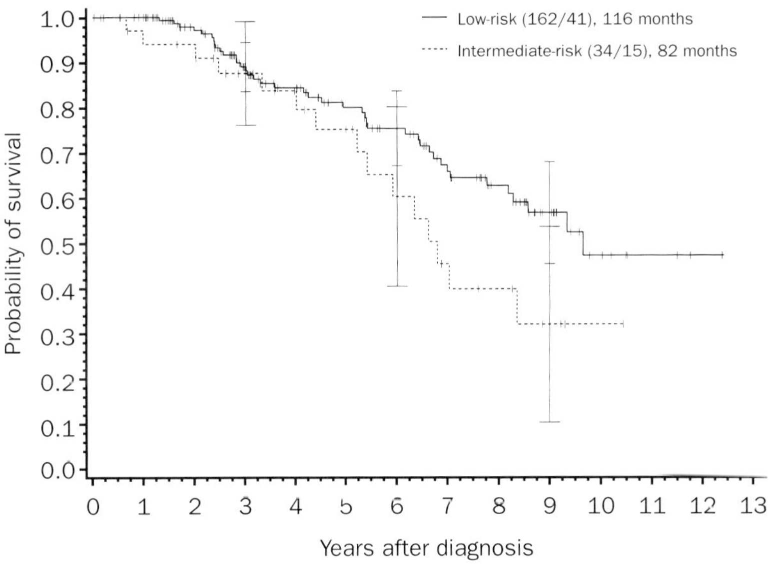

Figure 12.12 The New CML score applied to 196 patients with early-stage CML treated with IFN-α. All patients were classified as low-risk patients by the Sokal score. The notation '(162/41), 116 months' indicates that of 162 patients, 41 died, and that the median survival time was 116 months (similarly for the intermediate-risk group). If applicable, confidence intervals for probability of survival are given at 3, 6, and 9 years for each risk group. Logrank test between low-risk and intermediate-risk patients according to the New CML score was not significant.

haematological and cytogenetic responders in the low-risk and the intermediate-risk groups according to the New CML score have a better survival than non-responders with respect to either criterion (results not yet published). According to our data, haematological responders within 9 months of IFN-α therapy had a median survival of 76 months, median survival for cytogenetic responders has not yet been reached, and the 5-year survival rate is 79%. Looking in particular at patients who are intermediate-risk and high-risk according to the New CML score, not only do the prognostic factors at baseline distinguish two groups with statistically significantly different survivals but also time-dependent response criteria appear to have a different influence. Therefore, for patients treated with IFN-α, it is not appropriate to

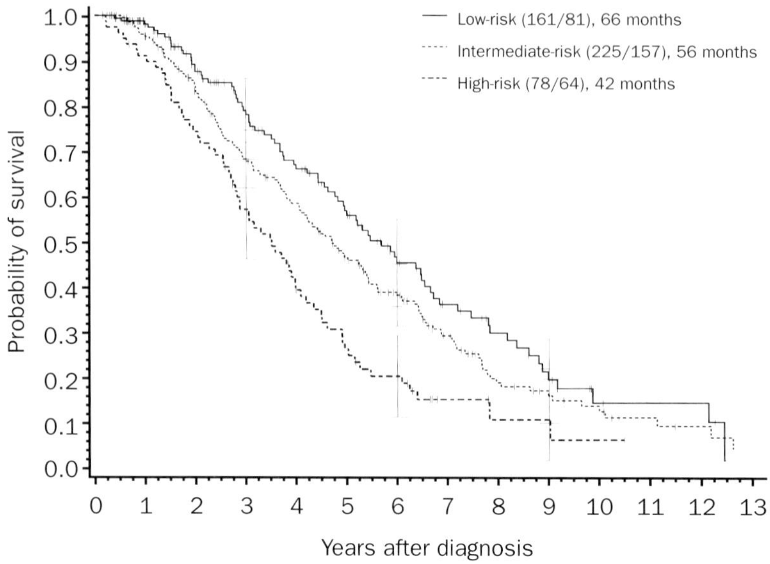

Figure 12.13 Cross-sample validation: the New CML score applied to 464 patients with early-stage CML treated with hydroxyurea only. The notation '(161/81), 66 months' indicates that of 161 patients, 81 died, and that the median survival time was 66 months (similarly for the intermediate-risk and high-risk groups). If applicable, confidence intervals for probability of survival are given at 3, 6, and 9 years for each risk group. Logrank test: $p < 0.0001$.

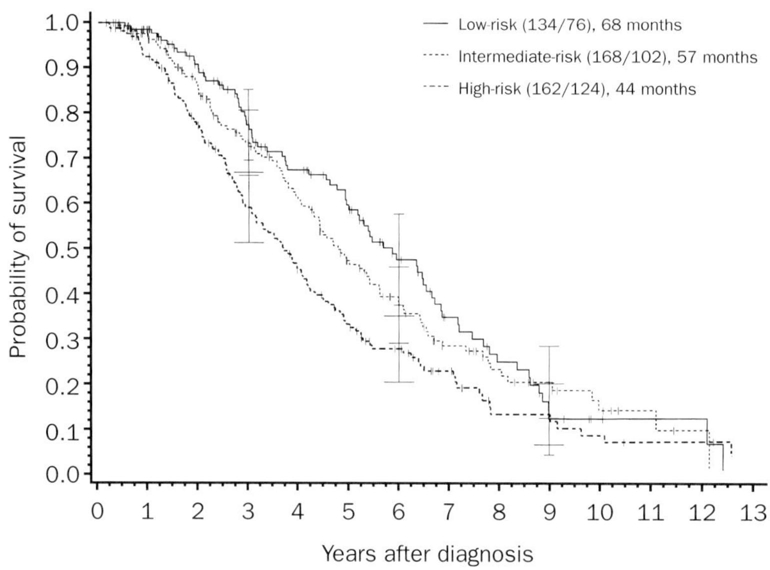

Figure 12.14 Cross-sample validation: the Sokal score applied to 464 patients with early-stage CML treated with hydroxyurea only. The notation '(134/76), 68 months' indicates that of 134 patients, 76 died, and that the median survival time was 68 months (similarly for the intermediate-risk and high-risk groups). If applicable, confidence intervals for probability of survival are given at 3, 6, and 9 years for each risk group. Logrank test: $p = 0.0025$.

combine intermediate-risk and high-risk patients in a so-called 'non-low'-risk group.

In summary, if a clinician considers the application of evidence-based treatment selection, he or she omit to administer a therapy including IFN-α to an intermediate-risk group patient with the potential to become a haematological or cytogenetic responder just because he or she has mistakenly relied on the wrong high-risk group classification of the Sokal score. This may be harmful to the patient. Further use of the Sokal score for patients mainly (to be) treated with IFN-α carries the risk of wrong risk-group stratification, and thus increases the

Table 12.2 Median survival time and 5-year survival rate stratified for therapy and risk group according to New CML score

Therapy and risk group	Median survival time (months)	5-year survival rate (±2 SD)
IFN-α (+chemotherapy) New CML score: ≤780 ⇒ low risk	100	0.76 (±0.04)
Hydroxyurea New CML score: ≤780 ⇒ low risk	66	0.55 (±0.10)
IFN-α (+chemotherapy) New CML score: >780–1480 ⇒ intermediate risk	69	0.57 (±0.04)
Hydroxyurea New CML score: >780–1480 ⇒ intermediate risk	56	0.46 (±0.07)
IFN-α (+chemotherapy) New CML score: >1480 ⇒ high risk	45	0.31 (±0.07)
Hydroxyurea New CML score: >1480 ⇒ high risk	42	0.25 (±0.10)

probability of non-optimal treatment selection for individual patients.

Further features of the New CML score

The New CML score also discriminates between survivals for patients treated with hydroxyurea or IFN-α plus Ara-C. Hence, for conventional therapies, there is no longer any need to use another prognostic model for patients with CML. Looking in particular at the 464 patients in our data base who were only treated with hydroxyurea, survival curves had a similar appearance whether patients were stratified according to the New CML score (Figure 12.13) or the Sokal score (Figure 12.14). Again, the validity of the typically large high-risk group featured by the Sokal score might be at question.

With its application also to patients treated with chemotherapy, the New CML score gives support when deciding on prognosis-adjusted treatment (Table 12.2). On comparing IFN-based treatments with hydroxyurea and stratifying for prognostic groups, it is evident that patients in the low-risk group benefit most from treatment with IFN-α. The median survival time is 100 months with IFN-α, compared with 66 months with hydroxyurea, and the 5-year survival rates are 76% and 55% respectively. In the high-risk group, however, survival curves are almost identical, with median survival times of 45 and 42 months. Thus, physicians might consider applying new experimental approaches to high-risk patients with CML or, alternatively, carrying on treating high-risk patients with hydroxyurea, which causes fewer adverse reactions, is more convenient to handle, and is considerably less expensive than IFN-α.

CONCLUSIONS AND OUTLOOK

Without valid prognostic models, modern medicine cannot perform as well as required. Validation of a model on independent samples is an absolute necessity, and close collaboration between major research groups is needed. The CML Collaborative Prognostic Factors Project has achieved this.

The New CML score, generating three distinct prognostic groups, has been validated in independent studies and works well for patients treated with IFN-α, IFN-α plus hydroxyurea, IFN-α plus Ara-C, or hydroxyurea alone. As new treatments (e.g. STI571) may have different modes of action, validation remains a constant obligation. The New CML score already allows decisions to be made about prognosis-adjusted treatments, and will hopefully be accepted as a starting point for providing the possibility for every CML patient to receive individually optimized treatment. The next challenge is to develop a rational strategy for deciding who should opt for BMT or for conventional treatment as first-line treatment.

ACKNOWLEDGEMENT

We would like to thank the following investigators who also contributed data to the CPFP data base: The Italian Cooperative Study Group on CML (represented by Prof Dr S Tura, Bologna, and Prof Dr M Baccarani, Udine), Prof Dr G Alimena (Rome), Dr MJ Moro (Castilla-León), and Prof Dr L Dabich (Ann Arbor).

REFERENCES

1. Talpaz M, Kantarjian H, Kurzrock R et al, Interferon-alpha produces sustained cytogenetic responses in chronic myelogenous leukemia Philadelphia chromosome-positive patients. *Ann Intern Med* 1991; **114:** 532–8.
2. Ozer H, George SL, Schiffer CA et al, Prolonged subcutaneous administration of recombinant α2b interferon in patients with previously untreated Philadelphia chromosome-positive chronic-phase chronic myelogenous leukemia: effect on remission duration and survival: Cancer and Leukemia Group B Study 8583. *Blood* 1993; **82:** 2975–84.
3. Schofield JR, Robinson WA, Murphy JR et al, Low doses of interferon-α are as effective as higher doses in inducing remissions and prolonging survival in chronic myeloid leukemia. *Ann Intern Med* 1994; **121:** 736–44.
4. Wyatt JC, Altman DG, Commentary: Prognostic models: clinically useful or quickly forgotten? *BMJ* 1995; **311:** 1539–41.
5. Hasford J, Pfirrmann M, Hehlmann R et al, A new prognostic score for survival of patients with chronic myeloid leukemia treated with interferon alfa. *J Natl Cancer Inst* 1998; **90:** 850–8.
6. EC-CPMP Working Party on Efficacy of Medicinal Products. *Note for Guidance: Good Clinical Practice for Trials on Medicinal Products in the European Community*. Brussels, 1990.
7. Talpaz M, Kantarjian HM, McCredie KB et al, Clinical investigation of human alpha interferon in chronic myelogenous leukemia. *Blood* 1987; **69:** 1280–8.
8. Peduzzi PN, Detre KM, Chan YK et al, Validation of a risk function to predict mortality in a VA population with coronary artery disease. *Controlled Clin Trials* 1982; **3:** 47–60.
9. Collett D, *Modelling Survival Data in Medical Research*. London: Chapman & Hall, 1994.
10. Hosmer DW, Lemeshow S, *Applied Logistic Regression*. New York: Wiley, 1989.
11. Altman DG, Lausen B, Sauerbrei W et al, Dangers of using 'optimal' cutpoints in the evaluation of prognostic factors. *J Natl Cancer Inst* 1994; **86:** 829–35.
12. Breiman L, Friedman JH, Olshen RA et al, *Classification and Regression Trees (CART)*. Belmont, CA: Wadsworth, 1984.
13. Simon R, Makuch RW, A non-parametric graphical representation of the relationship between

survival and the occurrence of an event: application to responder versus non-responder bias. *Stat Med* 1984; **3:** 35–44.

14. Anderson JR, Cain KC, Gelber RD, Analysis of survival by tumor response. *J Clin Oncol* 1983; **1:** 710–19.
15. Tura S, Baccarani M, Corbelli G and The Italian Cooperative Study Group on Chronic Myeloid Leukaemia, Staging of chronic myeloid leukaemia. *Br J Haematol* 1981; **47:** 105–19.
16. Cervantes F, Rozman C, A multivariate analysis of prognostic factors in chronic myeloid leukemia. *Blood* 1982; **60:** 1298–304.
17. Sokal JE, Cox EB, Baccarani M et al, Prognostic discrimination in 'good-risk' chronic granulocytic leukemia. *Blood* 1984; **63:** 789–99.
18. Kantarjian HM, Smith TL, McCredie KB et al, Chronic myelogenous leukemia: a multivariate analysis of the associations of patient characteristics and therapy with survival. *Blood* 1985; **66:** 1326–35.
19. Kantarjian HM, Keating MJ, Smith TL et al, Proposal for a simple synthesis prognostic staging system in chronic myelogenous leukemia. *Am J Med* 1990; **88:** 1–8.
20. Thiele J, Kvasnicka HM, Zankovich R et al, Parameters of predictive value in chronic myeloid leukemia – the prognostic impact of histopathological variables in a multivariate regression analysis. *Leuk Lymphoma* 1991; **4:** 63–74.
21. Hehlmann R, Heimpel H, Kolb HJ et al, The German CML-Study, comparison of busulfan vs. hydroxyurea vs. interferon alpha and establishment of prognostic score 1. *Leuk Lymphoma* 1993; **11**(Suppl 1): 159–68.
22. Hehlmann R, Ansari H, Hasford J et al, Comparative analysis of the impact of risk profile and of drug therapy on survival in CML using Sokal's index and a new score. *Br J Haematol* 1997; **97:** 76–85.
23. Ohnishi K, Ohno R, Tomonaga M et al, A randomized trial comparing interferon-α with busulfan for newly diagnosed chronic myelogenous leukemia in chronic phase. *Blood* 1995; **86:** 906–16.
24. Hasford J, Ansari H, Pfirrmann M et al, Analysis and validation of prognostic factors for CML. *Bone Marrow Transplant* 1996; **17**(Suppl 3): S49–54.

13

Evidence-based guidelines for the treatment of chronic-phase chronic myeloid leukemia

Richard T Silver

CONTENTS • Introduction • What are evidence-based clinical practice guidelines? • Why the CML guidelines were established by the American Society of Hematology • Chemotherapy with busulfan and hydroxyurea • Interferon • Allogeneic bone marrow transplantation • Patient preferences • Recommendations • Conclusions • Epilogue • Disclaimer

INTRODUCTION

In this chapter, I shall review evidence-based clinical practice guidelines (EB-CPGs) in general, discuss how they apply to chronic myeloid leukemia (CML) in particular, and emphasize the importance of shared decision-making. In closing, I shall discuss the effect of the new signal transduction inhibitor STI571 on the process to date.

WHAT ARE EVIDENCE-BASED CLINICAL PRACTICE GUIDELINES?

EB-CPGs provide physicians who have neither the time, nor the expertise, nor the interest to evaluate a vast quantity of evidence bearing on the data affecting major medical decisions. They afford a convenient and rational path to consistency in clinical decision making, hopefully improving outcomes and reducing inappropriate care.[1–5] Evidence-based guidelines should be sharply differentiated from guidelines and recommendations originating from managed care organizations, pharmaceutical companies, and other organizations that have a financial stake in decisions made by physicians. EB-CPGs not only provide clinical recommendations but also make explicit the methods and value judgments applied in evaluating the evidence.[6] In addition, they explain where evidence has not fully resolved clinical questions, and include explanations and caveats to help clinicians adapt recommendations unique to their patients.[2,6,7] This concern for methodology is important to those who use the guidelines, as their value is directly related to how well they were assembled.[1,7–11]

Evidence-based guidelines are usually produced by a panel of experts who have different points of view and areas of expertise but, rather than relying upon their own biases, evaluate evidence using strict, previously established rules. Thus, EB-CPGs should also be distinguished from guidelines, consensus statements, and other reviews that are founded upon *expert opinion* rather than a systematic review of evidence.[6]

Evaluating the medical literature may be associated with many methodologic difficulties. For example, several clinical trials may purport to examine a single procedure, even though different experimental techniques were used by the researchers. For another example, trials may apply different criteria to the exclusion of patients because of age, comorbidity, and coincidental drugs administered. Although case studies may provide information important for the guideline panel, the weight given to such information must be specified.[1,7] Because the evidence upon which they are based often does not eliminate all uncertainty, EB-CPGs should differentiate between recommendations made with great confidence and those carrying less weight. The quality of evidence supporting each recommendation should be stated.[9–13]

Some have unfairly stated that the use of EB-CPGs is 'cookbook medicine.' However, only the clinician is capable of assessing how evidence-derived recommendations can benefit the individual patient. Only the clinician can guarantee that recommendations made in guidelines on the basis of evidence current at the time of publication are modified because of the latest research. And only the clinician can use the information contained in the evidence-based guideline to educate patients and elicit patient preferences. Applied flexibly and with care, guidelines are tools to strengthen the physician's hand in formulating recommendations and educating patients and their families.[5]

WHY THE CML GUIDELINES WERE ESTABLISHED BY THE AMERICAN SOCIETY OF HEMATOLOGY

Experts differ on the best treatment for patients in the chronic phase of CML. Options include busulfan, hydroxyurea, or interferon-based regimens, or bone marrow transplantation (BMT). Until a few years ago, allogeneic BMT was the treatment of choice for all eligible patients, since it was the only treatment that appeared to change the natural course of the disease. Therefore, randomized studies comparing transplantation with chemotherapy (hydroxyurea or busulfan) were not feasible, and follow-up reports of observational studies were not deemed necessary. The situation changed when interferon-based regimens were shown to influence the natural course of CML by also prolonging survival.

In order to place these two radically different treatment regimens in perspective, an Expert Panel on Chronic Myeloid Leukemia was convened by the American Society of Hematology. The panel published its findings in September 1999.[14]

The panel members included hematologists and oncologists from the USA, UK, France, Germany, and Italy, a practice guidelines methodologist, and a biostatician. Because of the importance of the subject, one panelist was a designated representative of the American Society of Clinical Oncology.[14]

Only the presence of the Philadelphia (Ph) chromosome and/or chimeric *BCR/ABL* gene was considered adequate for the diagnosis of CML. The efficacy and tolerability of several distinct approaches to the treatment of patients in the chronic phase of chronic myeloid (myelogenous, myelocytic, granulocytic) leukemia were studied. The scope of this chapter is similar to that of the earlier publication. The reader is referred to that document for a more complete statement of methods.[14]

These guidelines summarize benefits and adverse effects associated with long-term treatment with busulfan, hydroxyurea, and interferon-based regimens, as well as those associated with allogeneic BMT, and comment upon new data employing the tyrosine kinase inhibitor STI571. Their purview excludes consideration of other chemotherapeutic agents, busulfan compared with any therapy other than hydroxyurea, high-dose combination chemotherapy, BMT other than that involving allogeneic transplants using matched sibling and unrelated donors, radiation, splenectomy, experimental therapies, and regimens and protocols for preventing graft-versus-host disease (GVHD).[14]

Treatment efficacy was evaluated primarily by means of life expectancy (survival rate). Although intermediate outcomes including evidence of hematologic or cytogenetic remission were taken into consideration, these were considered to be less persuasive than survival. Potential adverse effects of treatment were considered to be of considerable interest. Because there were inadequate data on treatment costs, this factor did not figure in the guidelines. Randomized controlled trials were generally held to provide a stronger class of evidence than observational studies. The literature search was documented, and criteria established for evaluating the quality of evidence were cited.[14]

In brief, a total of 2423 studies on 'chronic myelogenous leukemia' were retrieved in 1996 using a computerized literature search of the Medline database; 960 of these addressed treatments of interest, while 207 met criteria for further evaluation. Relevant articles, including those on chronic myeloid, myelogenous, myelocytic, and granulocytic leukemia, were added in the years 1997 and 1998,[14] and additionally in 1999 and 2000.

Both the internal and external validity of studies were judged using explicit criteria. At the conclusion of the evaluation process, the designs, results, and limitations of studies were assembled systematically in five evidence tables which included studies of recombinant interferon alfa (rIFN-α) only, observational studies of rIFN-α combined with other drugs, randomized trials comparing rIFN-α with chemotherapy, incidence of IFN-induced acute, subacute, or chronic clinical toxicity, and studies of survival in chronic-phase CML patients undergoing allogeneic BMT with matched related donors. Recommendations made in the guidelines were formulated in accordance with explicit predetermined and stated criteria (Table 13.1). The panel generally avoided making recommendations where there were no data that met these criteria[14] – a concept continued in this chapter.

CHEMOTHERAPY WITH BUSULFAN AND HYDROXYUREA

A major randomized controlled trial has demonstrated the superiority of hydroxyurea over busulfan, with median survivals of 58 and 45 months, respectively, and 5-year survival rates of 44% and 32%, respectively.[15] A meta-analysis of five other trials also supported a survival advantage for hydroxyurea over busulfan. Furthermore, although hydroxyurea is associated with adverse effects, busulfan causes more frequent and serious complications of irreversible cytopenia and pulmonary, hepatic, and cardiac fibrosis than hydroxyurea.[16]

INTERFERON

The following comments relate only to rIFN-α 2a, 2b, and 2c, not to human leukocyte interferon or to rIFN-β. rIFN-γ is relatively ineffective in CML,[17] and is not reviewed here.

The preponderance of the evidence for the effectiveness of rIFN-α as therapy for chronic-phase CML derives from approximately 30 uncontrolled observational studies.[18] Although important, these studies provide inadequate proof of the advantages of rIFN-α over chemotherapy, since there are serious methodologic problems involving varying definitions of hematologic and cytogenetic remission, differences in patient case mix, and inadequate description of patient characteristics. Furthermore, such observational studies may include a disproportionately large number of patients predisposed to experience particularly favorable or unfavorable outcomes. Other methodologic problems with these studies include inadequate length of follow-up and the existence of inconsistent data in reports of a single cohort. Most of the studies did not use survival rate as the primary outcome measure. This is a serious problem, since such intermediate outcomes as hematologic or varying degrees of cytogenetic remission do not always translate into increased survival. Life expectancy, disease-specific mortality, and quality of life – the outcomes that matter most to patients – are the best measures of therapeutic success (or failure), although many observational studies have not measured them.

Table 13.1 Decision rules for issuing recommendations for the CML analysis[1]

1. Recommendations can be made only if there is direct scientific evidence of improved health outcomes, not because a panel member believes there is benefit or because it is accepted practice in CML. When such evidence is lacking, the results of the analysis should state that there is insufficient evidence to make a recommendation.

2. The analysis will not result in recommendation for one intervention over another unless there is evidence from a controlled study (internal controls) or from dramatic findings in an uncontrolled study that patients treated with that intervention experience better outcomes (e.g. higher survival) than those treated by the alternative. The outcomes that matter most are those that patients experience (e.g. lengthened survival) – not intermediate outcomes for which the linkage to health outcomes is less certain (e.g. cytogenetic remission).

3. When extrapolations of evidence are made from one patient population to another to infer effectiveness, the analysis should make this explicit and discuss the implications.

4. Claims of *proof* should be accompanied by full disclosure of the limitations of the evidence.

5. Claims about *benefit* should clarify the magnitude of benefit, preferably in absolute terms rather than as relative benefit. These claims should be accompanied by a description of potential adverse effects, preferably by estimating the probability of these adverse effects. Confidence intervals should be used to clarify the range of uncertainty about the estimates.

6. When there are complex tradeoffs between benefits and adverse effects such that patients might have different views about the best choice depending on personal preferences, the analysis should not make categorical recommendations but should instead advise shared decision-making based on the values patients assign to potential outcomes.

[1]From Table 1 in Silver RT, Woolf SH, Hehlmann R et al, An evidence-based analysis of the effect of busulfan, hydroxyurea, interferon, and allogeneic bone marrow transplantation in treating the chronic phase of chronic myeloid leukemia; developed for the American Society of Hematology. *Blood* 1999; **94:** 1517–36.

Randomized controlled trials of rIFN-α

Four prospective randomized controlled trials, with a total of more than 1400 patients, provide the most compelling evidence that rIFN-α is more efficacious than chemotherapy.[19–22] In these trials, 5-year survival rates for rIFN-α were 50–59% versus 29–44% for busulfan and hydroxyurea, respectively. It should be noted that, because these were prospective trials, selection bias was reduced, that each included a comparison group, and that each measured survival rate as an outcome. Nevertheless, imperfections in design and conduct included:

- selective exclusion of patients from treatment post randomization;

- less than perfect adherence to a standardized protocol;
- different inclusion criteria and differences in treatment intensity among trials;
- variability in treatment regimens;
- changes in treatment assignments that make it difficult to formulate explicit inferences about the magnitude of benefit attributable to specific treatments;
- problems related to crossover from rIFN-α to chemotherapy.

In addition, survival estimates may have been imprecise.

The value of combining rIFN-α with cytarabine (cytosine arabinoside, Ara-C) was first suggested by observational studies,[23–28] and has received support from a recent French multicenter randomized controlled trial involving more than 700 patients.[29] Comparing regimens of rIFN-α and hydroxyurea (as part of induction) combined with cytarabine (20 mg/m^2/day × 10 days) versus rIFN-α and hydroxyurea alone, researchers reported 3-year survival rates of 85% versus 79%, respectively; and complete hematologic and cytogenetic remissions of 66% versus 55% and 15% versus 9%, respectively. However, a recent Italian randomized controlled trial comparing rIFN-α and cytarabine versus rIFN-α alone did not confirm additional benefit (G Rosti and S Tura, personal communication). Such differences may be related to dose intensity and duration of cytarabine.

Summary of benefits with rIFN-α

It is clear that the evidence from clinical trials of the efficacy of therapy with rIFN-α for patients with chronic-phase CML is not without distinct limitations. Nevertheless, randomized controlled trials comparing rIFN-α with busulfan or hydroxyurea demonstrate, on balance, that rIFN-α therapy extends life expectancy in patients with favorable features: no or minimal prior treatment, relatively normal hemoglobin levels and platelet counts, less than 10% blasts in the blood, and treatment commencing early (particularly within 6 months of diagnosis). Effects may be enhanced when rIFN-α is coupled with hydroxyurea or cytarabine. The issue with cytarabine has not been completely resolved.

Regardless of the risk category of the patient (low, intermediate, or high) rIFN-α confers greater benefit than chemotherapy during early chronic-phase disease, although the magnitude of the benefit varies. Continuing rIFN-α therapy through the chronic phase leads to better outcomes than discontinuing the therapy.[16] The survival advantages associated with rIFN-α therapy achieve statistical significance, insofar as this can be ascertained. The pooled 5-year survival rates as seen in a meta-analysis are 57% for rIFN-α and 42% for chemotherapy ($p < 0.0001$).[16] Thus, rIFN-α increases life expectancy by a median of approximately 20 months, according to controlled trials involving busulfan or hydroxyurea. The overall probability that patients will live at least 5 years following treatment is 50–59% – an improvement over the 29–44% seen with chemotherapy. Of importance, the evidence of survival benefit from rIFN-α derives only from trials in which it was combined with other drugs, especially hydroxyurea.[14]

Significantly, although the aforementioned conclusions reflect pooled data, prolonged survival is likely for patients achieving major cytogenetic response, as landmark analysis has shown. (In a landmark analysis, a fixed time is selected after the initiation of therapy as a landmark for conducting the analysis. Patients still on study at the landmark time are separated into two response categories according to whether they have responded before that time, while patients removed from protocol before the time of landmark evaluation are excluded from the analysis. Patients are then followed forward in time to ascertain whether survival from the landmark depends on the patient's response status at the landmark, regardless of any subsequent shifts in response status. Thus, probability estimates and statistical tests are conditional on the response status of patients at the landmark time.)

Adding cytarabine to rIFN-α *may* confer added benefit, but unquestionably increases toxicity, and the differences between the French and Italian data are not yet resolved. For patients in the later stages of chronic phase, or more than 1 year from diagnosis, or with more than 10–30% blasts in peripheral blood, there is no adequate evidence from randomized controlled trials that indicates survival advantages of rIFN-α compared with hydroxyurea.

Summary of adverse effects with rIFN-α

Retrospective observational studies and reports from general clinical experience are the source of evidence regarding the adverse effects of rIFN-α therapy. Such issues as differences in patient selection and definition of complications (e.g. acute, subacute, or chronic) lead to wide variations in reported complication rates.

Therapy with rIFN-α leads to constitutional side-effects in virtually all patients. The frequency of toxicity with rIFN-α is greater than with busulfan or hydroxyurea. Between 4% and 18% of patients discontinue treatment because of toxicity, compared with 1% for hydroxyurea.[14] In one observational study, side-effects were such that patients received only 60% of the target dose.[30] Acute symptoms are mild to moderate in most patients, although a wide constellation of other more severe acute reactions and chronic complications have been documented.[14] The incidence of adverse effects is usually dose- and duration-dependent.

ALLOGENEIC BONE MARROW TRANSPLANTATION

The projected actuarial 3-year to 5-year survival rates for patients receiving allogeneic BMT range from 38% to 80%. These data come from uncontrolled observational and retrospective studies; survival is probably better at more experienced centers. Most studies report 50–60% 3-year to 5-year survival rates, and slightly lower rates for disease-free survival.[14] Relapse rates within 3–5 years are less than 20% in most studies. That allogeneic BMT may offer eligible patients (especially young adults with a genetically HLA-identical sibling donor) a prospect for cure is indicated by the projected survival curve after 3–7 years.

Concerns regarding interpretation of BMT trials

Most studies are retrospective, most provide few details on methods of patient selection, and many apply varying definitions of relapse. Furthermore, since study designs are heterogenous, it is unclear to which specific intervention(s) the reported outcome can be attributed. The statistical problems include the mean duration of follow-up, which may be undocumented, and the relatively small samples of patients employed in the calculations, for example those who have lived more than 7 years. Another problem is that many patients enter transplant studies after having tried and failed treatment with rIFN-α.

Concerns regarding the comparison of BMT with rIFN-α therapy

Considering all patients as a group, there is currently no unequivocal evidence that BMT is necessarily more effective than rIFN-α-derived regimens as first-line treatment for *all* patients with CML. In general, there *is* a continuous relapse rate over time for rIFN-α-treated patients, with the curves of rIFN-α and BMT crossing at about 7–8 years, yielding a survival advantage for BMT. This pattern is frequently cited as evidence that BMT 'cures' CML. The implied superiority of BMT just cited, given the data on which the curves are based, is derived from patients with differing clinical presentations, lengths of follow-up, and analytic methods. These differences have been discussed in detail elsewhere.[14] Attempts to control for these differences were made by comparing patients from the International Bone

Marrow Transplant Registry (IBMTR) with a German randomized trial of patients who received either rIFN-α or hydroxyurea. Although the data presented supported the view that BMT produces better long-term outcomes, many concerns have been raised regarding the definitive evidence.[14] The primary data suffer from fundamental design problems, including selection biases, the reliance on observational data supplied by BMT registries, and the small numbers and uncertain censorship criteria affecting survival estimates at the trial end of the curves. In this regard, the probability estimates of the critical 8-year endpoint of the analysis were based on only 15 patients! When the data were stratified by Sokal score, the differences in survival rate between transplant patients and the patients with the lowest risk score who received rIFN-α did not achieve statistical significance. This observation is important, since recent analysis at 10 years of the Italian Cooperative Group CML Study indicates that the low-risk group of patients treated with rIFN-α survived as well as did patients who had received BMT. The recently inaugurated study of the German Chronic Myeloid Leukemia Study Group attempting to randomize patients in a prospective fashion between rIFN-α-based therapy and BMT[31] will be most important in resolving these issues.

Potential adverse effects of BMT

If in fact BMT is proven to increase the overall chances of long-term survival in comparison to rIFN-α, the magnitude of the increase in benefits must be compared with the potential for serious harm (e.g. GVHD) and death that may accompany the procedure, especially in the short term.

Death rate

Transplant-related mortality is 20–40%, although this statistic hides a wide range of values: significantly higher when mismatched or unrelated donors are involved, and considerably lower when matched siblings and modern regimens for the prevention of opportunistic infections and GVHD are used. The *preparatory regimen* produces toxic effects in virtually all patients. BMT is often accompanied by GVHD, opportunistic infections, and other complications, including interstitial pneumonitis, veno-occlusive disease, and secondary malignancies. Each of these complications presents serious problems with BMT. For example, interstitial pneumonitis is the cause of death for between 4% and 32% of patients receiving BMT.

Variables likely to improve BMT outcomes

Factors associated with improved BMT outcomes and a more advantageous tradeoff between benefits and adverse effects have been identified. Patients between 20 and 30 years of age have higher overall and disease-free survival and lower transplant-related mortality than older patients, although modern methods of GVHD prophylaxis may reduce this relative benefit. Outcomes also improve when BMT is performed within 1–2 years of diagnosis and when the marrow transplant comes from an HLA-matched sibling or other relative, although newer technology such as DNA rather than serologic typing is improving outcomes for matched unrelated donors. Unfortunately, the more precise the genomic typing of class 1 HLA alleles, the lower the number of acceptable unrelated donors.

Conditioning and pretransplant regimens

The optimal conditioning regimens and protocols reducing the risk of GVHD have produced conflicting results. Patients who received busulfan before BMT tend to have lower survival than those who received hydroxyurea.[32,33] T-cell depletion reduces the risk of GVHD, but increases the risk of relapse and lowers survival.[34–37] Studies are currently underway to attempt to select the T cells that reduce GVHD but help prevent relapse (J Ritz, personal communication). It is clear that prior treatment with rIFN-α does not appear to affect matched *related* transplants[38,39] if the interferon is stopped approximately 90 days prior to the transplant.[40] Results from one center suggest that for patients treated with matched *unrelated* donors and with rIFN-α administered for more than 6 months pre-transplant have an increased risk of acute GVHD and mortality.[41]

PATIENT PREFERENCES

In the treatment of CML with either rIFN-α or BMT, *objective* clinical variables (e.g. patient age and comorbid conditions) help to some extent to determine which decisions should be made, and yet much depends upon *subjective* views expressed by patients. For one patient, improved survival at any cost may be paramount. For another patient, avoiding potentially severe side-effects and complications, balancing short-term risks and long-term benefits, and relying exclusively on evidence from controlled studies may be important. Recent research on the physician–patient relationship has confirmed the intuitive observation that the clinical encounter itself can be therapeutic. Important components of the physician–patient interview include empathetic listening, negotiating priorities and expectations, providing explanations, presenting information, and offering hope.[42–45]

In all cases, the physician should educate the patient regarding the benefits and harms associated with each treatment option and the quality of the evidence that supports each option. Detailed information about the place of shared decision-making in complex clinical interactions appears elsewhere.[44,45]

RECOMMENDATIONS

rIFN-α

Items 1–10 apply only to patients in the early stage of chronic-phase CML.

1. Evidence provided by randomized controlled trials indicates that patients with good prognostic factors are the ones who have the highest probability of survival if given rIFN-α. It is still unclear the degree to which added chemotherapy (e.g. hydroxyurea or cytarabine) provides additional benefit. This recommendation may not apply to patients who suffer from major comorbidity or from conditions that contraindicate the use of rIFN-α.
2. Patients should understand that the previous treatment recommendation adds a median of about 20 months on average to life expectancy for rIFN-α compared with chemotherapy alone. A careful and complete explanation of the most serious potential adverse effects of rIFN-α, their frequency, and their effect on quality of life should be presented. Achieving a major cytogenic response, however, may lead to more prolonged survival, and should be clearly presented. Such education permits patients to assess for themselves whether the benefit they may receive outweighs the increased risk of adverse effects.
3. Monotherapy with rIFN-α, as shown by one observational trial, provides no survival benefit over hydroxyurea. The clinical trials in which rIFN-α has been shown to be more effective than chemotherapy combined it with other agents such as hydroxyurea, busulfan or cytarabine, and included fewer patients with advanced disease.
4. The starting dose for rIFN-α in trials in which improved survival was achieved was 3–5 MU/m^2/day. After 2–3 weeks, doses were gradually increased to a dose of 9–12 MU/day (or the maximally tolerated dose) to achieve a satisfactory hematologic response (i.e. a white blood cell count of 2000–4000/μl and a platelet count of approximately 50 000/μl) or until signs of toxicity necessitated dose reduction.
5. The optimal duration of rIFN-α therapy has not been determined. All studies continued rIFN-α until disease progression or toxicity was observed, and in most trials the time

from initiation of rIFN-α therapy to complete cytogenetic remissions ranged from 6 to 60 months.

6. Adding cytarabine (20 mg/m^2/day × 10 days monthly) to rIFN-α increased the probability of survival, but also increased the risk of toxicity, according to the findings of a French controlled trial. A recent Italian trial employing rIFN-α in a slightly different fashion did not confirm the therapeutic results.
7. A major or complete cytogenetic response increases the likelihood of prolonged survival. Conflicting evidence prevents a decision of how long to continue rIFN-α treatment either in patients who have achieved a complete response or, alternatively, in patients whose hematologic or cytogenetic responses are unsatisfactory. If observational studies can be relied upon, then complete cytogenetic remissions require approximately 6 months to 4 years of therapy.
8. Evidence from controlled trials is inadequate to provide an upper age limit to rIFN-α therapy. In clinical trials, using an age cut-off, patients were excluded if they were older than 70–75 years.
9. Evidence supports therapy with hydroxyurea for patients who realize that this course of action may result in reduced survival benefits in comparison with rIFN-α therapy, although toxicity is reduced. Hydroxyurea is more likely than busulfan to improve survival, and less likely to produce serious toxicity, based upon evidence from one randomized controlled trial and several observational studies.
10. Based on controlled trials, survival data do not permit a recommendation of rIFN-α over chemotherapy for patients in advanced chronic-phase CML, including those with symptomatic disease or abnormal physical and laboratory findings (e.g. unexplained fatigue, weight loss, fever, progressive organomegaly, treatment-resistant leukocytosis, thrombocytosis, over 10% blasts and promyelocytes in the differential count, and/or extramedullary manifestations of blast phase disease).

Allogeneic BMT

1. Since prospective randomized controlled trials with internal controls have not been performed, it is not possible to state with assurance whether BMT either as first-line treatment or after initial treatment with chemotherapy or rIFN-α is superior to non-transplant therapy for *all* patients. Uncontrolled observational studies suggest survival advantages for BMT following chemotherapy compared with non-transplant approaches, and BMT appears to increase the likelihood of long-term remission, although selection bias and methodologic factors may account for these conclusions. Nor is it certain that the benefits of BMT will be as great in normal practice conditions as they are in studies reported in the literature.
2. There is a high risk of immediate complications and transplant-related mortality associated with BMT. Thus, any actual benefit to BMT treatment over the long term may be offset by short-term morbidity and mortality.

The following recommendations should be entertained only by physicians and patients willing to consider transplantation despite the inadequacy of available evidence from randomized controlled trials.

3. Allogeneic BMT is a reasonable option if there is a suitable HLA-matched sibling or other relative and if the patient's health status will permit her or him to tolerate the procedure. BMT performed with marrow from 'matched' unrelated donors tends to be inferior, although outcomes vary, depending on patient selection, transplant methods, typing techniques, the expertise of participating centers, and the definition of accelerated- and blast phase disease.
4. Patients with high Sokal or Hasford scores should be warned that they have a reduced

chance of success with rIFN-α and that early BMT might be a preferable option.

5. The patient should understand the relative risks and benefits of BMT, and should grasp the concept of a tradeoff between potential long-term benefits and increased immediate risks, perhaps involving both complications and mortality. It should be clear to the patient that the outcome estimates presented may not fully take account of age, the duration of illness, whether or not there is an HLA-matched donor, and the experience of the transplant center. The patient should also realize that to delay the procedure or to use a matched unrelated donor might adversely affect the potential outcomes. All risks should be evaluated in terms of the patient's own priorities and life plans.
6. Uncontrolled observational studies suggest that BMT outcomes are better if the procedure is performed within 1–2 years of diagnosis. Delay of more than 1 year following diagnosis might encourage a reevaluation of the relative risks and benefits of transplant.
7. Allogeneic BMT provides greater benefit to younger patients. However, there is insufficient evidence to suggest an exact upper age limit beyond which the procedure should not be offered, although most centers certainly favor transplantation for younger patients.
8. Administration of busulfan chemotherapy prior to transplantation may decrease the likelihood of benefit from the procedure, according to evidence from uncontrolled observational studies. Little evidence reflects upon the possible benefit of prior cytoreduction with hydroxyurea or rIFN-α before early transplantation. Observational evidence suggests that with matched-related donors, prior treatment with rIFN-α does not compromise results, although there are deleterious effects with matched unrelated donors. Whether the patient's hematologic or cytogenic response to rIFN-α reliably predicts the success of allogeneic BMT remains uncertain.

CONCLUSIONS

An orderly approach to treatment decisions for patients with chronic-phase CML is recommended, although proposing an algorithm to represent a pathway of choices is inappropriate given the limitations of current evidence and the degree of physician skill and art required to adapt available evidence to patient variability. The logical sequence of decisions for physician and patient are as follows:

1. It must first be decided whether BMT is a viable option. This entails an orderly assessment of the patient's age and health status and of the availability of a marrow donor, either matched-related or unrelated.
2. For the patient whose treatment will not include BMT, a decision must be made as to the best options for drug therapy. For example, will rIFN-α be administered and, if so, at what dose and duration and in combination with which other agents?
3. A systematic plan should be prepared for the evaluation of degree and duration of cytogenetic and molecular response.
4. The options and tradeoffs favored by the physician should be presented to the patient. The physician should do so understanding that it is appropriate for a clinical negotiation to take place and that 'control-sharing' may be a useful negotiating strategy, even if the patient can control nothing more than, for example, whether or not the physician will make a telephone call to explain the options to the patient's spouse or child or, for another, the scheduling of treatment sessions.[45]

EPILOGUE

The development of a potent signal transduction inhibitor, STI571 (Glivec; Gleevec), now undergoing clinical trials throughout the world, is discussed in detail in Chapters 33 and 34. Currently, studies are underway comparing rIFN-α with STI571 in newly diagnosed patients with CML, and investigating the use of STI571 in those who are intolerant or who have not responded to rIFN-α.[46–48] The effect of transplantation on the response to subsequent STI571 is also being evaluated. In the coming years, information will be available regarding the effect of STI571 on survival, the development of toxicity, and long-term toxicity. Hopefully, the guideline process elaborated in this chapter will provide the principles and framework for the evaluation of this exciting drug, and others surely to follow, for treating CML. In this fashion, the mistakes we have made in designing studies and interpreting their results will not be continually repeated in the future.

DISCLAIMER

The recommendations given in this chapter represent a range of approaches to the management of CML by this author. They are not intended to serve either as inflexible rules or as the unequivocal truth. Others may clearly disagree with the advice offered. Adhering to the recommendations will not automatically assume a successful outcome, nor will not following the guidelines necessarily end in a poor result. The final decision regarding the treatment of CML for the individual patient must be made by that individual together with the participating physician.

REFERENCES

1. Brook RH, Using scientific information to improve quality of health care. *Ann NY Acad Sci* 1993; **703:** 74–84.
2. Mosteller F, Some evaluation needs. *Ann NY Acad Sci* 1993; **703:** 12–17.
3. Hayward RSA, Wilson MC, Tunis SR et al, Users' guides to the medical literature: VIII. How to use clinical practice guidelines: are the recommendations valid? *JAMA* 1995; **274:** 570–4.
4. Woolf SH, Practice guidelines, a new reality in medicine: II. Methods of developing guidelines. *Arch Intern Med* 1992; **152:** 946–52.
5. Sackett DL, Rosenberg WM, Gray JAM et al, Evidence based medicine: what it is and what it isn't. *BMJ* 1996; **312:** 71–2.
6. Antman EM, Lau J, Kupelnick B et al, A comparison of results of meta-analyses of randomized control trials and recommendations of clinical experts: treatments for myocardial infarction. *JAMA* 1992; **268:** 240–8.
7. Haynes RB, Some problems in applying evidence in clinical practice. *Ann NY Acad Sci* 1993; **703:** 210–24.
8. Chalmers I, The Cochrane Collaboration: preparing, maintaining, and disseminating systematic reviews of the effects of health care. *Ann NY Acad Sci* 1993; **703:** 156–62.
9. Friedland DJ, *Evidence-Based Medicine: A Framework for Clinical Practice.* Stamford, CT: Appleton & Lange, 1998: 1–8.
10. Sackett DL, Richardson WS, Rosenberg W, Haynes RB, *Evidence-based Medicine: How to Practice and Teach EBM.* New York: Churchill Livingstone, 1997.
11. Chalmers I, Dickersin K, Chalmers T, Getting to grips with Archie Cochrane's agenda. *BMJ* 1992; **305:** 786–7.
12. Wilson MC, Hayward RSA, Tunis SR et al, Users' guides to the medical literature: VII. How to use clinical practice guidelines: B. What are the recommendations and will they help you in caring for your patients? *JAMA* 1995; **274:** 1630–2.
13. Haynes A, Feder G, Guidance on guidelines: writing them is easier than making them work. *BMJ* 1992; **305:** 785–6.
14. Silver RT, Woolf SH, Hehlmann R et al, An evidence-based analysis of the effect of busulfan, hydroxyurea, interferon, and allogeneic bone marrow transplantation in treating chronic phase of chronic myeloid leukemia: developed for the American Society of Hematology. *Blood* 1999; **94**(Suppl 1): 1517–36.
15. Hehlmann R, Heimpel H, Hasford J et al, Randomized comparison of busulfan and hydroxyurea in chronic myelogenous leukemia: prolongation of survival by hydroxyurea. *Blood* 1993; **82:** 398–407.
16. Chronic Myeloid Leukemia Trialists' Collaborative Group, Interferon alfa versus chemotherapy for chronic myeloid leukemia: a meta-analysis of seven randomized trials. *J Natl Cancer Inst* 1997; **89:** 1616–20.
17. Silver RT, Benn P, Verna RS et al, Recombinant gamma-interferon has activity in chronic

myeloid leukemia. *Am J Clin Oncol* 1990; **12:** 49–54.
18. Alimena G, Morra E, Lazzarino M et al, Interferon alpha-2b as therapy for Ph′-positive chronic myelogenous leukemia: a study of 82 patients treated with intermittent or daily administration. *Blood* 1988; **72:** 642–7.
19. Hehlmann R, Heimpel H, Hasford J et al, The German CML Study Group. Randomized comparison of 1 interferon-alpha with busulfan and hydroxyurea in chronic myelogenous leukemia. *Blood* 1994; **84:** 4064–77.
20. Italian Cooperative Group on Chronic Myeloid Leukemia, Interferon alfa-2a as compared with conventional chemotherapy for the treatment of chronic myeloid leukemia. *N Engl J Med* 1994; **330:** 820–5.
21. Allan NC, Richards SM, Shepherd PCA et al, UK Medical Research Council randomized, multicentre trial of interferon-alpha for chronic myeloid leukemia: improved survival irrespective of cytogenetic response. *Lancet* 1995; **345:** 1392–7.
22. Ohnishi BK, Ohno R, Tomonaga M et al, A randomized trial comparing interferon-alpha with busulfan for newly diagnosed chronic myelogenous leukemia in chronic phase. *Blood* 1995; **86:** 906–16.
23. Henic H, Preudhomme C, Noel M et al, Frequency of molecular elimination of Ph1 clone in chronic myelogenous leukemia (CML) with interferon alpha. *Leukemia* 1996; **10:** 185.
24. Silver RT, Benn P, Szatrowski TP et al, Infusional cytosine arabinoside (Ara-c) and recombinant interferon alpha (r-IFN-alpha) for the treatment of chronic myeloid leukemia. *Proc Am Soc Clin Oncol* 1990; **9:** 209.
25. Guihot F, Dreyfus B, Brizard A et al, Cytogenetic remission in chronic myelogenous leukemia using interferon alpha-2a and hydroxyurea with or without low-dose cytosine arabinoside. *Leuk Lymphoma* 1991; **4:** 49.
26. Kantarjian HM, Keating MJ, Estey EH et al, Treatment of advanced stages of Philadelphia chromosome-positive chronic myelogenous leukemia with interferon-alpha and low-dose cytarabine. *J Clin Oncol* 1992; **10:** 772–8.
27. Freund M, Hild F, Grote-Metke A et al, Combination of chemotherapy and interferon alpha-2b in the treatment of chronic myelogenous leukemia. *Semin Hematol* 1993; **30**(Suppl 3): 11–13.
28. Silver RT, Szatrowski TP, Peterson B et al, Combined α-interferon (rIFNα-2b) and low dose cytosine arabinoside for Ph(+) chronic phase chronic myeloid leukemia. *Blood* 1996; **88**(Suppl 1): 638a.
29. Guilhot F, Chastang C, Michallet M et al, Interferon alfa-2b combined with cytarabine versus interferon alone in chronic myelogenous leukemia. French Chronic Myeloid Leukemia Study Group. *N Engl J Med* 1997; **337:** 223–9.
30. Ozer H, George SL, Schiffer CA et al, Prolonged subcutaneous administration of recombinant alpha2b interferon in patients with previously untreated Philadelphia chromosome-positive chronic-phase chronic myelogenous leukemia: effect on remission duration and survival. Cancer and Leukemia Group B Study 8583. *Blood* 1993; **82:** 2975–84.
31. Hehlmann R, Berger U, Hochhaus A et al, Randomized comparison of allogeneic bone marrow transplantation and IFN based drug treatment in CML: early results. *Proc Am Soc Clin Oncol* 2000; **19:** 5a (Abst 10).
32. Brodsky I, Biggs JC, Szer J et al, Treatment of chronic myelogenous leukemia with allogeneic bone marrow transplantation after preparation with busulfan and cyclophosphamide (BuCy2): an update. *Semin Oncol* 1993; **20**(Suppl 4): 27–31.
33. Goldman JM, Szydio R, Horowitz MM et al, Choice of pretransplant treatment and timing of transplants for chronic myelogenous leukemia in chronic phase. *Blood* 1993; **82:** 2235–8.
34. Goldman JM, Gale RP, Horowitz MM et al, Bone marrow transplantation for chronic myelogenous leukemia in chronic phase: increased risk for relapse associated with T-cell depletion. *Ann Intern Med* 1988; **108:** 806–14.
35. Wagner JE, Zahurak M, Piantadosi S et al, Bone marrow transplantation of chronic myelogenous leukemia in chronic phase: evaluation of risks and benefits. *J Clin Oncol* 1992; **10:** 779–89.
36. Devergie A, Reiffers J, Vernant JP et al, Long-term follow-up after bone marrow transplantation for chronic myelogenous leukemia: factors associated with relapse. *Bone Marrow Transplant* 1990; **5:** 379–86.
37. Aschan J, Ringden O, Sundberg B et al, Increased risk of relapse in patients with chronic myelogenous leukemia given T-cell depleted marrow compared to methotrexate combined with cyclosporine or monotherapy for the prevention of graft-versus-host disease. *Eur J Haematol* 1993; **50:** 269–74.

38. Zuffa E, Bandini G, Bonini A et al, Prior treatment with alpha-interferon does not adversely affect the outcome of allogeneic BMT in chronic phase chronic myeloid leukemia. *Haematologica* 1998; **83:** 231–6.
39. Tomas JF, Lopez-Lorenzo JL, Requena MJ et al, Absence of influence of prior treatment with interferon on the outcome of allogeneic bone marrow transplantation for chronic myeloid leukemia. *Bone Marrow Transplant* 1998; **22:** 47–51.
40. Hehlmann R, Hochhaus A, Kolb H et al, Interferon alpha before allogeneic bone marrow transplantation in chronic myelogenous leukemia does not affect outcome adversely as long as it is discontinued at least 90 days before the procedure. *Blood* 1999; **94:** 3668–77.
41. Morton AJ, Gooley T, Hansen JA et al, Association between pretransplant interferon-alpha and outcome after unrelated donor marrow transplantation for chronic myelogenous leukemia in chronic phase. *Blood* 1998; **92:** 394–401.
42. Lazare A, Putnam SM, Lipkin M Jr, Three functions of the medical interview. In: *The Medical Interview: Clinical Care, Education, and Research* (eds Mack Lipkin Jr., Samuel M Putnam, Aaron Lazare). New York: Springer-Verlag, 1995: 3–19.
43. Lazare A, The interview as a clinical negotiation. In: *The Medical Interview: Clinical Care, Education, and Research.* New York: Springer-Verlag, 1995: 50–63.
44. Novack DH, Therapeutic aspects of the clinical encounter. In: *The Medical Interview: Clinical Care, Education, and Research.* New York: Springer-Verlag, 1995: 32–49.
45. Woolf SH, Shared decision-making: the case for letting patients decide which choice is best. *J Fam Pract* 1997; **45:** 205.
46. Talpaz M, Silver RT, Druker B et al, A phase II study of STI-571 in adult patients with Philadelphia chromosome positive chronic myeloid leukemia in accelerated phase. *Blood* 2000; **96:** 469a (Abst 2021).
47. Kantarjian H, Sawyers C, Hochhaus A et al, Phase II study of STI-571, a tyrosine kinase inhibitor, in patients (pts) with resistant or refractory Philadelphia chromosome-positive chronic myeloid leukemia (Ph + CML). *Blood* 2000; **96:** 470a (Abst 2022).
48. Shah NP, Snyder DS, Nicoll JM et al, PCR-negative molecular remissions in chronic-, accelerated-, and blast crisis-phase CML patients treated with STI-571, an ABL-specific kinase inhibitor. *Blood* 2000; **96:** 471a (Abst 2026).

Part 3

Allogeneic haematopoietic stem cell transplantation for chronic myeloid leukaemia

14

Donor selection in allogeneic bone marrow transplantation

Andrea L Pay, Ann-Margaret Little, J Alejandro Madrigal

CONTENTS • HLA diversity and matching in BMT • Source of HLA-matched donors • Non-HLA factors in donor selection • Summary

HLA DIVERSITY AND MATCHING IN BMT

Bone marrow transplantation (BMT) between individuals is now a routine treatment for a variety of haematological diseases, including chronic myeloid leukaemia (CML). The main drawback of this therapeutic procedure, however, is rejection of either the host tissue by the graft, or of graft tissue by the host.[1] The ensuing allogeneic response is stimulated by both major and minor genetic differences between the donor and the recipient, and is mediated by the human leukocyte antigens (HLA) encoded by the major histocompatibility complex (MHC). HLA molecules can be divided into two groups – class I and II – based on their expression and function. The primary function of HLA class I molecules is to present peptides generated from proteins produced within the cell to cytotoxic T cells that express the CD8 co-receptor. These peptides are predominantly either of self origin and will initiate no immune response, since T cells will be tolerant to them, or of viral origin and their presentation will initiate a T-cell response in order to eliminate the virus-infected cell. HLA class II molecules present peptides from exogenously produced proteins, which have been internalized and broken down within the cell. These class II molecules interact with helper T cells expressing the CD4 co-receptor.

The outstanding feature of HLA molecules is their extensive polymorphism. Currently, over 1100 alleles that encode HLA molecules have been defined[2] (see Table 14.1). Polymorphism within HLA molecules has been shown to locate to the functional sites of the molecules such that different HLA molecules bind and present different sets of peptides to the immune system.[3] Thus, HLA polymorphism within the human population is considered an advantage for the species, since variety in the ability to generate immune responses between different individuals should ensure the capacity of the species to survive exposure to different pathogens. However, it is this polymorphism that is a major barrier to successful allogeneic transplantation of both solid organs and stem cells. HLA disparity between donor and patient can result in the mismatched HLA molecules forming targets for alloreactive T-cell responses in graft rejection and graft-versus-host disease (GVHD). In simple terms, if there is a mismatch between the HLA molecules of the patient and donor, donor-derived T cells can recognize the mismatched patient antigen-presenting HLA molecules as being non-self. This interaction can lead to T-cell-mediated attack on the recipient's tissue, causing a graft-versus-host response, leading to tissue destruction in areas such as the skin and gut.[4] Such a response is referred to as direct antigen recognition. Indirect antigen recognition may also occur in an HLA-matched scenario, whereby donor-derived T cells may recognize patient-derived peptides presented by the patient's identical HLA molecules as foreign, and this can again lead to immune response against the patient's tissue. Peptides that initiate such a response are called minor histocompatibility antigens (mHA).[5] Indirect antigen presentation can also occur through the HLA molecules of the donor by presentation of peptides broken down from mismatched antigens of the patient to the donor's own T cells. Graft rejection may also be mediated by the reverse response of GVHD, where the patient's T cells react against the transplanted donor bone marrow cells; however, since most patients are treated with a combination of immunosuppressive irradiation and chemotherapy pre-transplant, the risk of graft rejection is minimal.

Thus the optimum choice of donor for allogeneic bone marrow transplantation depends on the degree of HLA identity between potential donor and recipient, with HLA-identical sibling donors being preferred, since they are more likely to share genetic polymorphisms additional to HLA. As mentioned previously, over 1100 alleles that encode HLA molecules have been defined. This diversity is divided between several genetic loci.[6] There are three classical HLA class I loci: HLA-A, -B, and -C, whose protein products all function in antigen presentation to T cells. Additionally, HLA class I molecules function in determining immune responses by natural killer (NK) cells. There are also three different types of antigen-presenting class II molecules: HLA-DR, -DQ, and -DP.

As the possible different combinations of alleles that could be present on a haplotype exceeds the total number of living human beings, and as each individual possesses two haplotypes, the number of different HLA types in existence is potentially enormous. This means that it would be very difficult to identify a potential donor outside the patient's immediate family. However, in reality, not all of

Table 14.1 Number of HLA serological specificities and DNA-defined HLA alleles: numbers of HLA alleles officially assigned by the WHO Nomenclature Committee for Factors of the HLA System given for each locus on 6 December 1999[2]

	Serological specificities	Alleles
HLA class I		
A	24	168
B	49	332
C	9	90
HLA class II		
DRB1/3/4/5/6/7	20	298
DQB1	7	44
DPB1	6	88

these possible combinations exist, owing to linkage disequilibrium within the MHC, which results in certain HLA alleles from different loci being found on the same haplotype at higher frequency than expected from random association. A common haplotype in the Caucasoid population is HLA-A*0101 (allele frequency 15%), −B*0801 (allele frequency 13.7%), and – DRB1*0301 (allele frequency 12.4%), with the expected haplotype frequency being 0.25%.[7] However, the actual frequency of this haplotype in the Caucasoid population is 6.4%, owing to the lack of recombination between these loci. Due to the genetic proximity of HLA-B and -C alleles on chromosome 6, there tends to be tighter association between HLA-B and -C types.[8] Thus, for many individuals who share identical HLA-B type, it is likely that they share HLA-C type. However, the application of high-resolution DNA-based typing methods for HLA typing has demonstrated that the association between HLA-B and -C is not necessarily as strong as previously thought, with many HLA-B-matched donors and patients being mismatched for HLA-C, and therefore potential donors and patients should be typed for HLA-C as well as HLA-B.[9,10] The association between HLA-DR loci and HLA-DQ loci is also strong, with many HLA-DR and -DQ alleles being in linkage disequilibrium. However, this association does not extend to the HLA-DP loci, since the presence of a recombinatorial hotspot between HLA-DP and -DQ has resulted in very little linkage disequilibrium.[11,12] This means that it is more difficult to find an HLA-DP-matched donor when searching outside a patient's immediate family. The presence of linkage disequilibrium within the MHC means that patients possessing common haplotypes are more likely to find an HLA-matched donor, whereas patients possessing rare haplotypes are less likely to.

Traditionally, HLA polymorphism was detected using allo-antibodies, usually obtained from multiparous women, where the pattern of reactivity between antibodies and polymorphic epitopes on the HLA molecules defines the HLA type. Using this methodology, a number of different HLA specificities can be defined (see Table 14.1). However, the application of DNA-based methodologies, specifically polymerase chain reaction (PCR)-based methods, has allowed the identification of many more specificities (see Table 14.2), and as a result allows higher-resolution matching between donors and patients.[13] Despite the increased resolution that can be achieved using DNA-based methods, such methods are not always applied in matching donors and patients, and several studies have highlighted the loss of apparent HLA identity that can be detected if high-resolution methodologies are used.[14,15]

Diversity also exists at the population level. The frequency and number of alleles expressed varies between human populations from different geographical locations, and it is believed that this is the result of local pathogen-driven selection at HLA loci. Some populations, North European Caucasoids for example, show greater diversity while others, such as specific Amerindian populations, have a relatively limited number of different alleles.[16] This is probably a reflection of a greater degree of admixing within the Caucasoid population than that which has occurred in the more isolated Amerindian populations. Alternatively, a recent genetic bottleneck within the Amerindian populations may be responsible for the reduced number of alleles, with only those 'advantageous' alleles being present in the present-day population. Thus variation in the HLA types of individuals from different populations can pose a problem when looking for an unrelated donor, particularly for patients with mixed-ethnicity parentage.

As many of the HLA alleles that have been defined only differ by a single amino acid residue in the encoded HLA molecule, this then raises the question of how well matched a patient and donor have to be for a successful transplant outcome. Unfortunately, there is no clear-cut answer to this question. We know that the outcome for HLA-identical sibling transplants is overall better than for HLA-identical unrelated donor transplants, and this may be due to the additional non-HLA differences that exist between unrelated donors and patients.

Table 14.2 Techniques currently utilized for HLA typing

Technique	Features	Resolution
Serology	Defines protein epitopes	Low to medium
Sequence-specific oligonucleotide probing (SSOP)	One PCR reaction, but the use of multiple probes makes the assay tedious; heterozygous ambiguities are a problem that requires further resolution	Low to high
Sequence-specific primers (SSP)	Multiple PCR reactions with different primer pairs are required – not good for high throughput	Low to high
Sequence-based typing	Heterozygous ambiguities need further resolution	High
Reference-strand conformation analysis (RSCA)	RSCA determines HLA type based on differences in the conformation of DNA molecules that have different sequences – no heterozygous ambiguities, since alleles are determined individually	High

However, another possibility is that supposed HLA-identical unrelated donor and patient pairs may really be mismatched, and that it is this unrecognized mismatch that leads to a poorer outcome for the unrelated transplants. We and others have demonstrated that many HLA mismatches can be identified if high-resolution HLA typing is performed on patient and donor pairs.[9,14,15] The next question is to find out if particular mismatches are more detrimental than others, and this can only be done by performing high-resolution typing for multiple HLA loci and correlating the results with transplant outcome. Several recent studies have highlighted the role of accurate HLA matching in achieving improved transplant outcome. A retrospective high-resolution HLA typing analysis of 440 donor and patient pairs (39% CML) transplanted in Japan demonstrated that incompatibility for HLA-A and HLA-C was associated with increased risk of GVHD (grades III–IV).[17] Mismatching for HLA-A was also associated with an increased risk of death. Interestingly, HLA-C matching was associated with an increased risk of relapse of leukaemia. This finding suggests a role for HLA-C mismatching in averting relapse through a graft-versus-leukaemia (GVL) pathway that would coincide with the increase in GVHD. In contrast to the HLA class I data, mismatching for HLA class II loci was not identified as a significant risk factor for either acute GVHD or death.

In a separate HLA typing study performed on 300 CML patient–donor pairs, an association between HLA class I mismatching and graft failure was found, whereas HLA class II mismatching was associated with GVHD (grades III–IV).[18]

Although the overall results of these two most recent studies differ, they share the finding that better matching is associated with better outcome. The differences in terms of the role of individual loci may be attributed to other differences in the patient populations and in pre- and post-transplant regimes, and to variation in the HLA polymorphism found in the two populations studied.

We are currently undertaking a multicentre study at the Anthony Nolan Research Institute, where we are retrospectively HLA typing all donor and patient pairs, where the donor has been provided by the Anthony Nolan Bone Marrow Trust Register and the patient is transplanted within the UK. To date, 138 transplant pairs have been analysed for HLA-A, -B, -C, -DRB1, -DQB1, and -DPB1 compatibility using a high-resolution HLA typing method: reference strand conformation analysis (RSCA). All pairs were originally typed by serology for HLA-A and -B (some were also typed by DNA methods), and by molecular techniques for HLA-DRB1 and -DQB1. Although the numbers studied fully are relatively small and only univariate analysis has been performed, our data support the previous findings that HLA class I mismatching is as detrimental as HLA class II mismatching (Figure 14.1).

Thus, to answer the question as to which HLA mismatches are most detrimental, and which are acceptable requires the continued analysis of transplanted pairs to build up a database of known HLA-mismatched transplanted pairs that can eventually be analysed with respect to mismatching of individual loci. A large cohort of patients and donors is required in

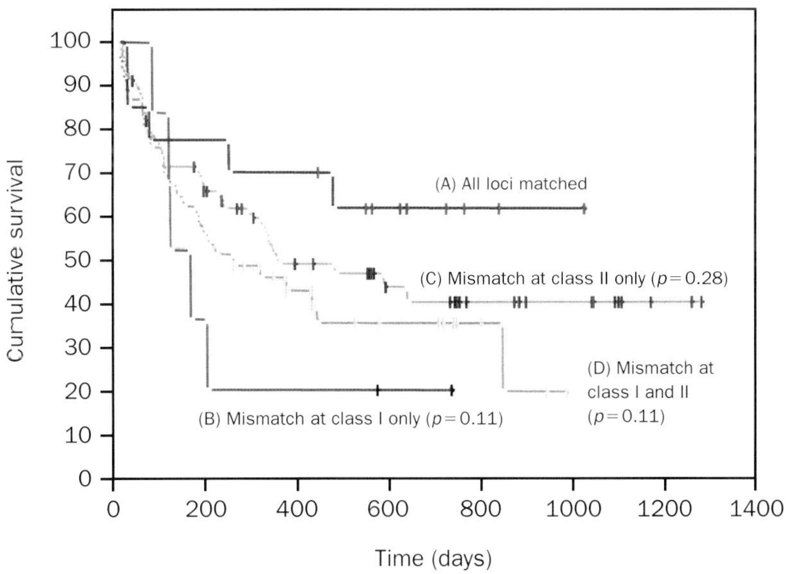

Figure 14.1 The effect of HLA matching on overall survival post unrelated bone marrow transplant. A Kaplan–Meier survival plot showing cumulative survival against time in days post transplant. The survival of individuals who were completely matched with their donors (A) was compared with those who had mismatches at class I only (B), class II only (C) and class I with class II (D). Significance was calculated using the Log Rank Statistic in a pair-wise comparison with sex matched transplants (A). Tick marks represent individuals who were alive at the time of final analysis.

order to carry out studies where pairs are matched for all non-genetic factors that can independently affect the outcome of BMT.

SOURCE OF HLA-MATCHED DONORS

As mentioned previously, the optimum allogeneic bone marrow donor for a patient is an HLA-matched sibling, and therefore the first step in identifying a donor involves the HLA typing (usually for HLA-A, -B, and -DR) of the patient's immediate family, including parents, to identify haplotypes. The chance of two siblings sharing HLA identity is 25% (when the parents have no common haplotypes), and typical figures quoted for patients are 20–30% success rates of finding an HLA-matched sibling donor. If a sibling is found to be HLA-identical, the transplant can be performed if the sibling donor fulfils other medical requirements (and is willing!). If the sibling donor is a monozygotic twin, this is a syngeneic transplant, since the sibling is not only HLA-matched, but also matched for virtually all other genetic loci. If a related donor with only one HLA difference is identified, the transplant may be performed with this donor, despite the risk of GVHD.

For those patients who do not have an HLA-identical sibling, there are other options. The establishment of HLA-typed volunteer unrelated donor registries has allowed transplantation of bone marrow between unrelated individuals. The first volunteer unrelated donor registry was established in the UK in 1974 by Mrs Shirley Nolan, the mother of Anthony, who suffered from Wiskott–Aldrich syndrome. There were no sibling donors for Anthony, and although the field of unrelated BMT was in its infancy, this did not prevent Mrs Nolan from establishing the Anthony Nolan Bone Marrow Trust Register. Unfortunately, Anthony died before a donor was found, but the efforts to recruit volunteer donors continued, and currently over 300 000 volunteer HLA-typed individuals are registered with the Anthony Nolan Bone Marrow Trust. The pioneering work of Mrs Nolan inspired the establishment of other volunteer bone marrow donor registries throughout the world, and currently there are 44 registers listed with Bone Marrow Donors Worldwide (BMDW),[19] with more than 6 million potential donors registered.

Initially, an unrelated bone marrow donor search is performed within the patient's home country. If a donor is not found, an international donor search is then performed via the Bone Marrow Donors Worldwide (BMDW) database, which allows the transplant centre to evaluate the probability of finding a donor, and determine which registries in the world have suitable HLA-matched donors. The donor selection procedure is detailed in Figure 14.2.

Despite there being over 6 million potential volunteer bone marrow donors, not all donor searches are successful, and for many patients an appropriate donor may still never be identified. However, new registries emerging from countries within Asia and Latin America will increase the availability of donors with different HLA types for patients all over the world.

Although bone marrow donation is a common practice now for the provision of stem cells to leukaemia (and other) patients, stem cells can also be provided from other sources, one of which is human umbilical cord blood. Cord blood transplantation (CBT) has become increasingly useful as a substitute for, or in addition to, BMT. Cord blood is an ideal source of stem cells, since it contains many more naive progenitor cells, giving less chance of a graft-versus-host response. The cord blood is also more readily available, and does not require the donor to undergo surgery with a general anaesthetic. However, there are several controversial issues surrounding the use of CBT.[20] Originally, the placenta and umbilical cord were thought of as 'discarded tissues', and the consent of the mother was not required for them to be used for research or clinical purposes; however, this view has now changed, and it is a legal requirement to obtain maternal informed consent acting on behalf of the child.[21] Problems also lie with ownership of the cord blood, which may be stored for many years. What happens if the cord blood donor himself later in life develops a

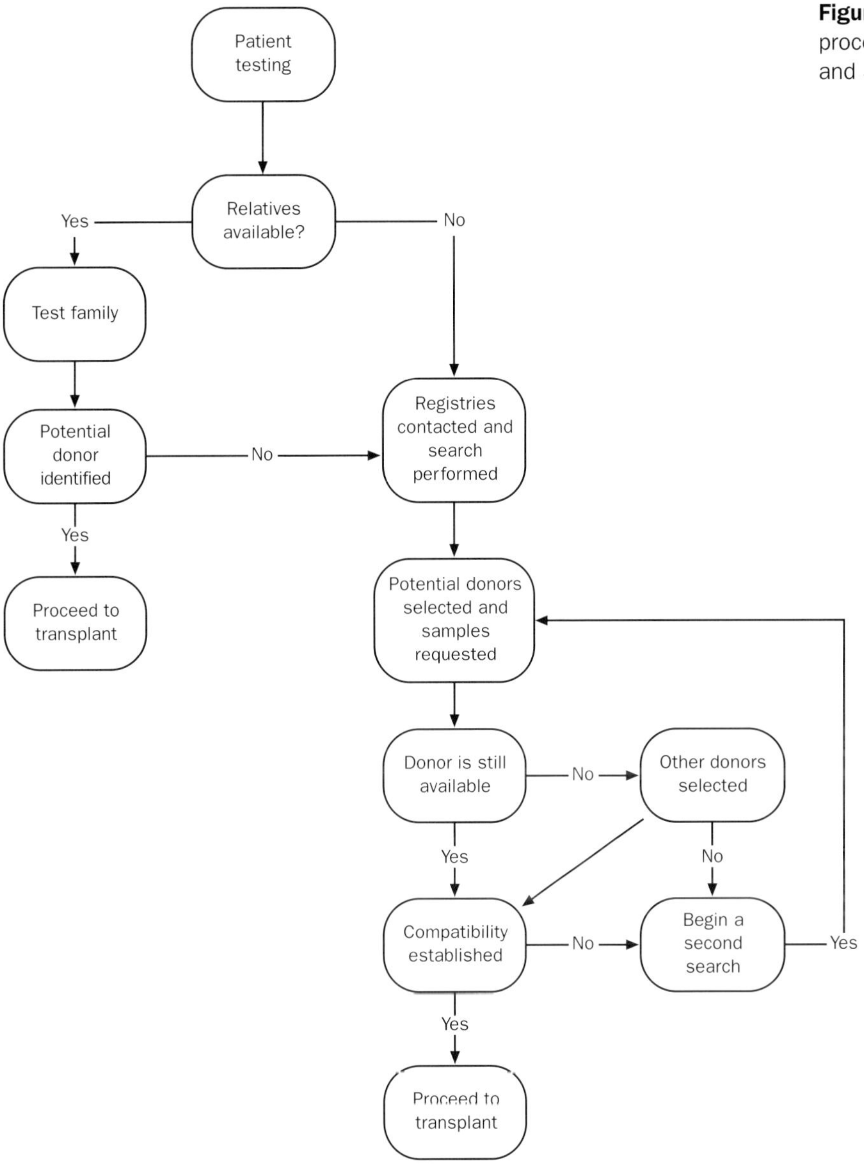

Figure 14.2 Donor selection procedure. (Adapted from Little and Sinnott.[39])

haematological disease curable by CBT? Consent clauses now require mutual anonymity of donor and recipient and non-commitment to autotransplantation.[22] Also, because of the low numbers of cells available from the cord blood graft (the number of cells obtained varies for different cords), this option may only be available to recipients with a body weight less than 40 kg (since the number of nucleated cells needs to be greater than 3×10^7/kg for successful engraftment).[23] Cord blood banks have been established, although funding is a problem since it costs between $1000 and $2000 to test, collect, and freeze a sample, even without the cost of storing it for many years.[20] Despite all these controversies, CBT is still a viable option, and has proved to be successful.[24,25]

Stem cells may also be provided through

peripheral blood stem cell transplantation (PBSCT) from an HLA-matched donor. In order to boost the number of stem cells ($CD34^+$) in circulation, the donor is treated with granulocyte colony-stimulating factor (G-CSF). The advantages of PBSCT are that the donor does not need to undergo surgery or a hospital stay or take prolonged leave from work. Although this approach has been used for related donors, it is not yet widely used in unrelated donations since the long-term effects of G-CSF mobilization are still to be addressed.[26]

Other types of transplant available to a patient who has had an unsuccessful search for an HLA-matched donor are autologous transplantation with the patient's own stem cells taken in remission. The patient's cells are stored and reinfused into the patient after high-dose chemotherapy.[27] The problem with this procedure is that the cells may still be leukaemic and lead to disease relapse.

Haploidentical related bone marrow and cord blood transplants have been carried out for chronic leukaemia patients, although the successful outcome of the transplant depends upon the degree of HLA identity between the individuals.[28] Because of this problem, a haploidentical sibling transplant with more than two HLA antigen mismatches will usually only be carried out as a last resort.[29]

NON-HLA FACTORS IN DONOR SELECTION

HLA identity is not the only factor to consider when selecting a bone marrow donor. The sex of the donor may also influence graft outcome, with male donors being preferred, since studies show that male patients who receive marrow from female donors have a higher incidence of GVHD than when male donors are used.[30] One possible explanation for this is the generation of minor histocompatibility peptides from proteins encoded by the Y chromosome. Thus T cells from a female donor, which will not have encountered Y-specific peptides (as presented by HLA molecules), may react against the male tissue to give a graft-versus-host response. One such Y-specific antigenic peptide has been defined (H-Y), and H-Y-specific cytotoxic T lymphocytes have been found in male patients with GVHD post BMT from a female donor.[31]

Patient and donor age can also influence transplant outcome, with younger donors and patients having a more successful transplant.[32] This may partly be due to younger, stronger individuals being able to cope with the transplantation process better than an older person. However, the ageing process of the immune system may also have a significant impact. In mouse studies, the use of younger marrow donors has also been shown to give a better transplant outcome; this could be due to the better immunological function of the graft compared with that of older donors.[33,34] As will be discussed in Chapter 16, the timing of the transplant is also important with respect to the stage of disease and the interval from diagnosis to transplant. It has been shown that survival post allogeneic transplant is greater when patients with CML are transplanted in chronic phase, with the transplant occurring within one year of diagnosis.[35] Manipulation of the graft can also lead to improved outcome, although there are conflicting views on the subject. When a donor has a known mismatch with the recipient and GVHD is likely to occur, the graft can be T-cell-depleted in order to try and remove the T cells that would mediate the response. Although T-cell depletion of the graft is associated with decreased GVHD, it is also associated with decreased engraftment and increased disease relapse. Different protocols are now aiming towards less complete depletion, with specific depletion of the alloreactive cell populations that mediate the GVHD effect.[36] Additional donor- and patient-related factors that influence outcome include viral infections pre and post transplantation. The most common viral problem post BMT comes from cytomegalovirus (CMV).[37] This can be due to CMV reactivation of a seropositive patient through immunosuppression, or by infection from a seropositive donor. Some centres will always choose a seronegative donor if possible, or match patient and donor for CMV status.[38]

SUMMARY

Haematopoietic stem cell transplantation has had a significant impact on the treatment of patients with leukaemia and other haematological disorders, and for many patients a stem cell transplant is the only chance of survival. The formation of HLA-typed volunteer unrelated bone marrow donor registry and more recently cord blood registries has greatly aided those patients who do not have a suitable related donor. Advances in the technology used to define the HLA types of both donors and patients have significantly improved the degree of matching that can be performed, and it is clear that better matching is associated with improved transplant outcome. However, not every patient in need of a stem cell transplant will be able to find a perfect match, and not all mismatched transplants are unsuccessful. Therefore future improvements in the use of allogeneic stem cell transplants will be achieved as more data are analysed to determine which mismatches are acceptable versus those that are not acceptable.

REFERENCES

1. Szydlo R, Goldman JM, Klein JP et al, Results of allogeneic bone marrow transplants for leukemia using donors other than HLA-identical siblings. *J Clin Oncol* 1997; **15:** 1767–77.
2. Marsh SGE, *The IMGT/HLA Database* – http://www.ebi.ac.uk/imgt/hla/.
3. Falk K, Rotzschke O, Stevanovic S et al, Allele-specific motifs revealed by sequencing of self-peptides eluted from MHC molecules. *Nature* 1991; **351:** 290–6.
4. Hings I, Severson R, Filipovich AH et al, Treatment of moderate and severe acute GVHD after allogeneic bone marrow transplantation. *Transplantation* 1994; **58:** 437–42.
5. Martin PJ, Increased disparity for minor histocompatibility antigens as a potential cause of increased GVHD risk in marrow transplantation from unrelated donors compared with related donors. *Bone Marrow Transplant* 1991; **8:** 217–23.
6. Little A-M, Parham P, Polymorphism and evolution of HLA molecules. *Rev Immunogenet* 1999; **1:** 105–23.
7. Imanishi T, Akaza T, Kimura A et al, Allele and haplotype frequencies for HLA and complement loci in various ethnic groups. In: *HLA 1991 – Proceedings of the Eleventh International Histocompatibility Workshop and Conference* (Tsuji K, Aizawa M, Sasazuki TJ, eds). Oxford: Oxford University Press, 1992: 1065–220.
8. Bunce M, Barnardo MCNM, Proctor J et al, High resolution HLA-C typing by PCR-SSP: identification of allelic frequencies and linkage disequilibria in 604 unrelated random UK Caucasoids and a comparison with serology. *Tissue Antigens* 1996; **48:** 680–91.
9. Petersdorf EW, Stanley JF, Martin PJ, Hansen A, Molecular diversity of the HLA-C locus in unrelated marrow transplantation. *Tissue Antigens* 1994; **44:** 93–9.
10. Prasad V, Heller G, Kernan N et al, The probability of HLA-C matching between patient and unrelated donor at the molecular level: estimations based on the linkage disequilibrium between DNA typed HLA-B and HLA-C alleles. *Transplantation* 1999; **68:** 1044–50.
11. Baisch JM, Capra JD, Linkage disequilibrium within the HLA complex does not extend into HLA-DP. *Scand J Immunol* 1993; **37:** 499–503.
12. Howell WM, Evans PR, Devereux SA et al, Absence of strong HLA-DR/DQ-DP linkage disequilibrium in the British and French Canadian Caucasoid populations. *Eur J Immunogenet* 1993; **20:** 363–71.
13. Little A-M, Marsh SGE, Madrigal JA, HLA typing: current methodologies utilised for bone marrow donor selection. *Curr Opin Hematol* 1998; **5:** 419-28.
14. Scott I, O'Shea J, Bunce M et al, Molecular typing shows a high level of HLA class I incompatibility in serologically well matched donor/patient pairs: implications for unrelated bone marrow donor selection. *Blood* 1998; **92:** 4864–71.
15. Arguello JR, Little AM, Bohan E et al, A high resolution HLA class I and class II matching method for bone marrow donor selection. *Bone Marrow Transplant* 1998; **22:** 527–34.
16. Belich MP, Madrigal JA, Hildebrand WH et al, Unusual HLA-B alleles in two tribes of Brazilian Indians. *Nature* 1992; **357:** 326–9.
17. Sasazuki T, Juji T, Morishima Y et al, Effect of matching of class I HLA alleles on clinical outcome after transplantation of hematopoietic stem cells from an unrelated donor. Japan Marrow Donor Program. *N Engl J Med* 1998; **339:** 1177–85.
18. Petersdorf EW, Gooley TA, Anasetti C et al,

Optimizing outcome after unrelated marrow transplantation by comprehensive matching of HLA class I and II alleles in the donor and recipient. *Blood* 1998; **92:** 3515–20.

19. BMDW, www.BMDW.ORG (1999).
20. Burgio GR, Locatelli F, Transplant of bone marrow and cord blood hematopoietic stem cells in pediatric practice, revisited according to the fundamental principles of bioethics. *Bone Marrow Transplant* 1997; **19:** 1163–8.
21. Sazama K, Cord blood stem cells belong to the infant, not to the mother. *Transfusion* 1995; **35:** 967–8.
22. Gluckman E, Wagner J, Hows J et al, Cord blood banking for hematopoietic stem cell transplantation: an international cord blood transplant registry. *Bone Marrow Transplant* 1993; **11:** 199–200.
23. Spencer A, Szydlo RM, Brookes PA et al, Bone marrow transplantation for chronic myeloid leukemia with volunteer unrelated donors using ex vivo or in vivo T-cell depletion: major prognostic impact of HLA class I identity between donor and recipient. *Blood* 1995; **86:** 3590–7.
24. Gluckman E, Rocha V, Boyer-Chammard A et al, Outcome of cord-blood transplantation from related and unrelated donors. Eurocord Transplant Group and the European Blood and Marrow Transplantation Group. *N Engl J Med* 1997; **337:** 373–81.
25. Kline RM, Bertolone SJ, Umbilical cord blood transplantation: providing a donor for everyone needing a bone marrow transplant? *South Med J* 1998; **91:** 821–8.
26. Dini G, Arcese W, Barbanti M et al, Peripheral blood stem cell collection from G-CSF-stimulated unrelated donors for second transplant. *Bone Marrow Transplant* 1998; **22:** S41–5.
27. McGlave P, Unrelated donor and autologous marrow transplant therapy of chronic myelogenous leukemia (CML). *Leukemia* 1993; **7:** 1082–3.
28. Speiser DE, Hermans J, van Biezen A et al, Haploidentical family member transplants for patients with chronic myeloid leukaemia: a report of the Chronic Leukaemia Working. *Bone Marrow Transplant* 1997; **19:** 1197–203.
29. Bishop MR, Henslee-Downey PJ, Anderson JR et al, Long-term survival in advanced chronic myelogenous leukemia following bone marrow transplantation from haploidentical related donors. *Bone Marrow Transplant* 1996; **18:** 747–53.
30. Gratwohl A, Hermans J, Apperley J et al, Acute graft-versus-host disease: grade and outcome in patients with chronic myelogenous leukemia. Working Party Chronic Leukemia of the European Group for Blood and Marrow Transplantation. *Blood* 1995; **86:** 813–18.
31. Rufer N, Wolpert E, Helg C et al, HA-1 and the SMCY-derived peptide FIDSYICQV (H-Y) are immunodominant minor histocompatibility antigens after bone marrow transplantation. *Transplantation* 1998; **66:** 910–16.
32. Gluckman E, Barrett AJ, Arcese W et al, Bone marrow transplantation in severe aplastic anaemia: a survey of the European Group for Bone Marrow Transplantation (E.G.B.M.T.). *Br J Haematol* 1981; **49:** 165–73.
33. Jacobsen N, Badsberg JH, Lonnqvist B et al, Graft-versus leukaemia activity associated with CMV-seropositive donor, post-transplant CMV infection, young donor age and chronic graft-versus-host disease in bone marrow allograft recipients. The Nordic Bone Marrow Transplantation Group. *Bone Marrow Transplant* 1990; **5:** 413–18.
34. Gorczynski RM, Chang MP, Peripheral (somatic) expansion of the murine cytotoxic T lymphocyte repertoire. II. Comparison of diversity in recognition repertoire of alloreactive T cells in spleen and thymus of young or aged DBA/2J mice transplanted with bone marrow cells from young or aged donors. *J Immunol* 1984; **133:** 2381–9.
35. Goldman JM, Szydlo R, Horowitz MM et al, Choice of pretransplant treatment and timing of transplants for chronic myelogenous leukemia in chronic phase. *Blood* 1993; **82:** 2235–8.
36. Koh MB, Prentice HG, Lowdell MW, Selective removal of alloreactive cells from haematopoietic stem cell grafts: graft engineering for GVHD prophylaxis. *Bone Marrow Transplant* 1999; **23:** 1071–9.
37. Meyers JD, Flournoy N, Thomas D, Risk factors for cytomegalovirus infection after human marrow transplantation. *J Infect Dis* 1986; **153:** 478–88.
38. Webster A, Blizzard B, Pillay CD et al, Value of routine surveillance cultures for detection of CMV pneumonitis following bone marrow transplantation. *Bone Marrow Transplant* 1993; **12:** 477–81.
39. Little A-M, Sinnott P, HLA typing for bone marrow transplantation. *CPD Bulletin for Immunology and Allergy* 1999, **1:** 47–50.

15

Risk assessment for allogeneic transplantation

Alois Gratwohl

CONTENTS • Introduction • General principles • Factors influencing outcome • Conclusions

INTRODUCTION

This chapter addresses the problem of risk assessment prior to allogeneic haematopoietic stem cell transplantation (HSCT) for patients with chronic myeloid leukaemia (CML). It lists the many points to be considered in a careful risk analysis, summarizes the similarities with HSCT for other indications as well as the special situation in CML, and should serve as a basis for patient counselling on an individualized level. At a time of general availability of 'all information' for any patient, nothing can replace a personalized assessment between the patient, his or her partner, and the responsible physician. This is particularly true for CML, where an allogeneic HSCT is always associated with initial risk of increased mortality but with hope for improved survival in the long run (Figure 15.1). Depending on the different prognostic factors, the risk of early death as a result of HSCT is higher or lower. The content of this chapter should serve as a starting platform for decision-making.

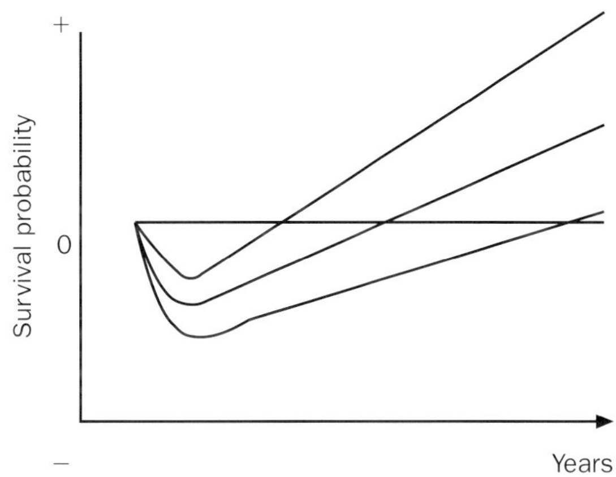

Figure 15.1 Survival curves for patients with CML treated with HSCT or conventional therapy show different patterns and intersect at a given time point. This is associated initially with excess mortality (left part) and a survival advantage thereafter (right part of figure) for HSCT patients. The magnitude of initial risk is lowest in patients with poor-risk disease factors and low risks for transplant-related mortality (upper curve); it is highest for patients with low-risk disease factors but high risks for transplant-related mortality (lower curve). Adapted from Gale et al.[50]

GENERAL PRINCIPLES

The result of the first successful allogeneic HLA-identical sibling transplant was published more than 30 years ago, and an estimated number of over 200 000 autologous and allogeneic HSCT have since been performed worldwide.[1,2] A few general principles can be established based on these figures. The outcome of any HSCT depends on *fixed* factors given at the time of transplant, related to disease, patient, and transplant (donor), as well as on *variable* factors, which can be influenced by the transplant team, such as conditioning, prevention of graft-versus-host disease (GVHD), and treatment or supportive care. The latter aspects are discussed in detail in other chapters; this chapter concentrates on the former. Knowledge of both is essential in order to tailor the approach on an individualized patient basis.

Outcome following HSCT is assessed by four main endpoints: survival, leukaemia-free survival (LFS), relapse incidence (RI), and transplant-related mortality (TRM).[3] This simple approach designed very early in the history of HSCT was sufficient until recently. Relapse of the disease after HSCT was uniformly associated with progressive disease and severe TRM with lethal outcome. This is no longer the case today. Patients with relapse have a possibility of ongoing long-term survival. Similarly, single organ failure as a long-term consequence of conditioning (e.g. sterility or growth retardation) can be compatible with survival, but may influence treatment choice. Both elements need to be considered. Still, the four endpoints adequately describe the main influence of prognostic factors.

The discussion is further complicated by two elements, namely the need for a prolonged follow-up for true assessment of novel approaches and the reciprocal effects of many interventions on outcome measures. Although 30 years have elapsed since the first HSCT for CML patients,[4] few have such a long follow-up. Large numbers of transplants have been performed only during the last decade. New interventions, such as low-intensity conditioning approaches, were introduced only a few years ago and have no follow-up at all. Most of the therapeutic interventions in the context of HSCT have opposite impacts on TRM and RI. For example, increasing the intensity of the conditioning regimen reduces RI but increases the risk of TRM, and vice versa; increase in GVHD prevention or treatment reduces TRM but increases RI, and vice versa. Hence we still lack several elements for optimal decision analysis. Still, correct assessment of individualized risk means today that different approaches should be selected for a patient with a high risk for TRM but a low risk for relapse, compared with a patient with a low risk for TRM but a high risk for relapse.

FACTORS INFLUENCING OUTCOME

The major factors influencing outcome are listed in Table 15.1. They relate to disease, patient and transplant. They are discussed here for patients with CML, but are valid independently of the type of HSCT and the disease for which it is performed.

Disease-specific factors

The strongest predictor for outcome is the stage of disease at the time of transplant.[1,5–11] This was recognized early in the history of HSCT, and holds true for all disease indications. It even led to the speculation at one time that different forms of leukaemia represent different facets of the same disease.[12] Clearly, patients with advanced CML (accelerated phase or blast crisis) have a worse outcome than patients transplanted in first chronic phase (Table 15.2). More than 50% of all patients transplanted in first chronic phase can be expected to be alive at more than 10 years post HSCT. This figure decreases to about 25% for patients transplanted in accelerated phase and to about 15% for those transplanted in blast crisis. The same differences between these stages have been observed in single-centre series, and national and international registries. Similarly, the influence of stage holds for all donor types and stem cell sources. This decrease in survival for advanced disease is related to higher risk of both RI and TRM. The latter is still poorly understood. It remains a matter of speculation whether prior therapy or the disease sensitizes to more toxicity and complications or whether intrinsic cellular changes trigger the cytokine cascade.

Table 15.1 Factors influencing the outcome of HSCT

	RI	TRM	LFS	Survival
Disease-specific factors[a]				
Stage: AP/BC vs CP	↑	↑	↓	↓
Chronic-phase patients only				
Basophil count (>3%)	↑		↓	↓
Sokal score (higher)	(↑)	↑	↓	↓
Leukocyte count (higher)	↑		↓	↓
Time interval (>12 mths)		↑	↓	↓
Pretreatment busulfan		↑	↓	↓
Pretreatment interferon-α		↑	↓	
Patient-specific factors				
Age (higher)	?	↑	↓	↓
Sex (male)		↑	↓	↓
Race	?	?	?	?
Viral status (CMV positivity)		↑	↓	↓
Donor/transplant-specific factors				
Histocompatibility:				
Identical twin	↑	↓	↓	↑
Unrelated	↓	↑	?	?
Mismatched	↓	↑	↓	↓
Sex				
Female donor for male recipient	↓	↑	↓	↓
Viral status				
CMV positivity	?	↑	↓	↓
Cell content (higher CFU-GM)	?	↓	↑	↑

[a]AP, accelerated phase; BC, blast crisis; CP, chronic phase.

Within the subgroup of patients with chronic phase, the same factors are important as in conventional treatment and summarized in the Sokal score (age, spleen size, platelet count, and percentage of blasts)[13,14] or the Hasford score (age, spleen size, platelet count, blast count, and eosinophil and basophil count).[15] This statement is based on indirect evidence – no conclusive study has been done to date, and some have had conflicting results. This is related to the fact that larger registries have no information on the Sokal index at the time of diagnosis; in contrast, comprehensive study groups, which collect all disease-specific information at diagnosis, do not have enough transplant patients for appropriate analysis. Retrospective analyses of the registries have shown that high leukocyte count or high basophil count (>3%) at

Table 15.2 Outcome of transplants depending on risk factors (EBMT analysis 1999)[a]

	No. of patients		Probabilities at 10 years[b] (%)			
Category	**Initial**	**At 10 years**	**Survival**	**LFS**	**TRM**	**RI**
All	6628	263	33	35	44	38
By stage:[c]						
1st CP	4634	215	52	41	39	33
AP	954	30	25	21	57	52
BC	288	4	15	10	70	67
By histocompatibility:						
HLA-identical sibling	3489	197	54	42	37	34
Non-identical family member	295	3	43	42	48	19
Twin	37	5	85	41	3	57
Unrelated	804	10	38	38	50	24
By time interval:						
1st CP[c]; HLA-identical only	2987		59	45	35	31
<12 months	1779		63	48	31	31
>12 months	1208		53	41	42	30
By age:						
<20 years	202		70	55	22	30
20–40 years	1704		63	48	32	29
>40 years	1081		50	38	44	32

[a] Based on a preliminary, unpublished analysis by the European Group for Blood and Marrow Transplantation (EBMT) Chronic Leukemia Working Party.
[b] According to Kaplan–Meier.
[c] CP, chronic phase; AP, accelerated phase; BC, blast crisis.

the time of diagnosis predict a higher risk of relapse. The issue is complicated by the additional impact of the time interval from diagnosis to transplant. The Seattle group were the first to show that patients transplanted early in their disease had a better survival.[16] Initially, these data were disputed.[17] This was due in part to the inverse correlation between signs of prognosis and the time from diagnosis to transplant. Patients with poor-risk features at the time of diagnosis as reflected by their high leukocyte counts were referred to transplantation earlier than patients with initially low leukocyte counts, as illustrated in Figure 15.2.[9] This trend was reversed in the most recent years, and recent analyses from the European Group for Blood and Marrow Transplantation (EBMT) have repeatedly confirmed the

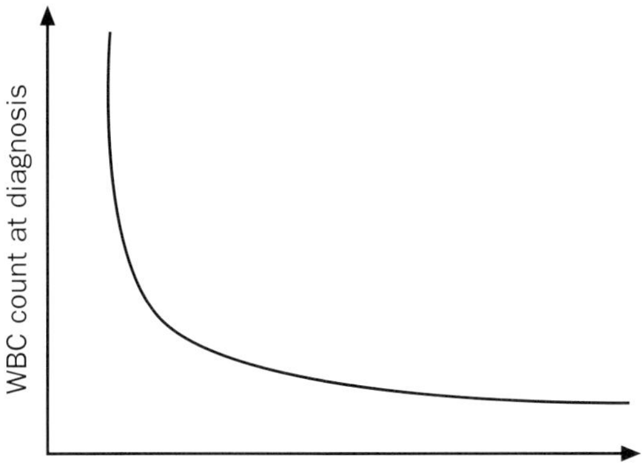

Figure 15.2 Inverse correlation between white blood cell (WBC) count at diagnosis and the interval from diagnosis to transplant in a cohort of patients reported to the EBMT in the 1980s. Adapted from Gratwohl et al.[9]

increased risk of TRM when the transplant is performed more than one year after diagnosis (Table 15.2).[10,18]

Pretreatment plays an essential role, and must be taken into consideration, since all patients with CML have some form of treatment prior to transplant. Initially, debulking of the disease in the form of splenectomy or splenic irradiation was considered essential for eradication of the disease.[5] Retrospective studies failed to show an advantage of either form of pretreatment with regard to survival, TRM, or RI.[19] In a prospective randomized controlled study the EBMT confirmed the lack of benefit of additional splenic irradiation of 10 Gy to the spleen immediately prior to transplant. Both groups of 114 and 113 patients were stratified for risk factors, and showed survival rates at 6 years of 62% and 57% respectively ($p = 0.70$).[20,21] However, the debate still continues as to whether additional spleen treatment remains of value for a selected subgroup of patients.[22] It is clearly of no benefit for patients at high risk for relapse (e.g. T-cell-depleted transplants), and nor is it possible to show an advantage for patients with very low risk for relapse. In a subgroup of intermediate-risk patients (patients with chronic phase, receiving non-T-cell-depleted HSCT but with a basophil count of over 3% at diagnosis), a statistically significant higher RI was observed in patients without prior spleen treatment (15% at 6 years versus 32%; $p = 0.05$). The debate goes on as to whether splenic irradiation should be reconsidered for selected patients.[23] It can certainly help patients with poor engraftment after HSCT.[24]

Busulfan and hydroxyurea were the treatments of choice for patients with CML in the early 1980s.[25] An International Bone Marrow Transplant Registry (IBMTR) analysis clearly showed a disadvantage for patients pretreated with busulfan. These patients ($n = 158$) had a LFS rate at 3 years of 45%, compared with 61% for those pretreated with hydroxyurea ($n = 292$) ($p < 0.001$). They suffered from a higher incidence of transplant-related complications, in particular interstitial pneumonitis.[26] Busulfan should not be given to any patient who is a potential candidate for an allogeneic HSCT. The introduction of interferon-α (IFN-α) has changed the situation. Theoretical considerations suggest a negative impact. IFN-α can trigger the cytokine cascade, and this should increase TRM. The Essen group first examined a group of 133 consecutive patients, and showed a higher increase of graft failure in unrelated or mismatched transplants (7/17 versus 0/13) pretreated with IFN-α, and more fatal complications in patients with donors other than HLA-identical siblings and IFN-α treatment for more than one year. This was mainly attributable to a 3.1-fold higher relative risk of fatal infections in IFN-α-pretreated patients.[27] A similar higher TRM rate was reported by the Seattle group for a group of 184 unrelated transplants. Pretransplant IFN-α for more than 6 months was associated with an increased risk of severe acute GVHD (relative risk 3.0) and increased mortality (relative risk 2.1). Increased GVHD mortality occurred between 100 and 365 days post transplant.[28] A clue came from Holler et al,[29] who observed a higher TRM mainly in patients treated with IFN-α within the 3 months prior to HSCT. Although five groups failed to confirm an impact of IFN-α pretreatment, their results can now be explained: they had incomplete information on the history of IFN-α treatment. A recent analysis by the German CML Study Group has clarified the situation. Based on the randomized CML studies I and II, which compared IFN-α with chemotherapy and included 197 transplant patients, IFN-α pretreatment had a negative impact.[30] This was restricted to patients who had received IFN-α in the last three months preceding transplant. The 5-year survival rate was 46% for the 50 patients who received IFN-α within the last 90 days before HSCT and 71% for the 36 patients who did not ($p < 0.001$). The difference in survival was due to a higher TRM within the first 100 days in the group given IFN-α up to HSCT. When IFN-α was stopped 90 days prior to HSCT, results no longer differed between patients with or without IFN-α in their pretransplant history. These data support the current concept that patients with a donor and a clear indication for an allogeneic transplant should be transplanted without delay and without pretreatment with IFN-α.[25] In contrast, patients on IFN-α who become candidates for HSCT treatment should be taken off IFN-α 3 months prior to the planned HSCT whenever possible.

Patient factors

Besides stage of disease, *age* was recognized early on as a very important factor for outcome.[5–9] Children at comparative stages of the disease always had better outcomes than adult patients. Many teams had age limits based on personal experience. Over the last decade, age limits have disappeared and have been replaced by more individualized assessment. Although some studies have challenged the concept of age as a factor increasing TRM, registry analyses looking at large numbers of patients show an almost-linear increase of TRM with increasing age, when other factors are adjusted in multivariate analyses. As illustrated in Table 15.2, TRM increases by about 5% with each decade. There is no cutoff when age is no longer important, and nor is there an age above which transplants can no longer be performed. Older patients with few other risk factors can undergo transplantation with reasonable success.

The influence of *sex* on outcome per se is controversial. It plays a significant role when minor histocompatibility antigens are considered in the setting of a female donor for a male recipient. It remains a question of debate for the individual patient. In the EBMT long-term analysis, female patients had better outcome due to lower TRM, independent of other risk factors.[10] The reasons are unknown, and need to be defined. It is interesting to note in this context that women also have a lower TRM in multiple myeloma.[31]

Few other patient factors have been analysed carefully enough in CML patients. General well-being, assessed by Karnofsky score, WHO score, ECOG score, etc., is probably of importance. Poor general health signals a higher risk for TRM in general in HSCT studies.[1] It has not been addressed in CML series.

Similarly, viral status of the patient is significant. Several studies have shown that patients with cytomegalovirus (CMV) positivity are at high risk for CMV reactivation and transplant-related complications.[32–34] This has been clearly shown for patients with CML undergoing unrelated HSCT. This may hold true for the viral status and viral load in general. In a study of 379 leukaemia patients, seropositivity for more than three herpesviruses of the recipient or donor was correlated with more acute GVHD of grade II or higher and with greater TRM.[35]

Donor–transplant factors

Several donor factors have prognostic relevance; they are related to histocompatibility, age, sex, ABO blood group, viral status, and stem cell source.

Histocompatibility between donor and recipient is the second most important factor besides stage.[1] This is best illustrated by the difference in outcome when identical-twin results are compared with mismatched transplants (Table 15.2). Absence of histoincompatibility, as in identical-twin transplants, abrogates the risks of rejection and GVHD, and hence reduces TRM. In contrast, absence of histoincompatibility also reduces the graft-versus-leukaemia effect and increases RI. Survival is always influenced by the net sum. Since options for retreatment remain open for patients with identical-twin transplants and relapse, survival but not LFS is best in recipients of such transplants (Table 15.2).[36,37]

The role of major and minor histocompatibility antigens in related or unrelated HSCT for CML is discussed in other chapters of the book. As a general principle and guide in the decision analyses,[1,33] it can be assumed that any mismatch increases the likelihood of TRM and decreases the risk of RI.[1,33,34,38–40] So far, in most instances, the increase in TRM has not been balanced by a gain in RI. It remains unanswered whether 'perfectly matched' unrelated transplants will decrease RI without increased TRM, and whether one day we will be able to determine 'permissible' mismatches in the unrelated setting and to identify selection criteria for mismatching prior to transplant.

The question of the role of ABO in compatibility between donor and recipient is unresolved. So far, no large series has received careful analysis. There are preliminary indications that a minor ABO barrier may increase the risk of TRM. This could be an additional factor when a selection is to be made between several, otherwise identical, unrelated donors. Similarly, there are suggestions that older donors, independent of recipient age, increase the risk of TRM.[33]

The viral status of the donor is as relevant as that of the patient. CMV-positive donors represent a risk for CML-negative recipients.[32] Similarly, the total number of herpesviruses for which there is positivity correlates with an increased risk for TRM (see above).[35]

Two main stem cell sources are available today: bone marrow (BM) and peripheral blood (PB).[2] Cord blood is still at an experimental stage, since the majority of patients with CML are adults. Preliminary data show that PB provides a higher number of $CD34^+$ cells and granulocyte–macrophage colony-forming units (CFU-GM), but also a higher number of T cells.[41] Theoretically, there is a risk of a higher incidence of GVHD, but also a better antileukaemic efficacy. So far, data from retrospective analyses and preliminary data from prospective randomized trials show that the incidence and severity of acute GVHD are similar with the two sources.[41–43] There is a trend towards more chronic GVHD with PB.[44] In one retrospective series, there was a trend towards reduced risk of relapse with PB. In this retrospective analysis, the Essen group described an incidence of molecular relapse of CML of 44% at 4 years in 62 BM recipients, compared with 7% in 29 PB transplant recipients.[45] Whether this holds true in larger series remains to be seen in the next few years.

Risk score analysis

Based on the selection of risk factors from previous studies, the EBMT Chronic Leukemia Working Party has developed a simple standardized risk score for patients with CML.[18] The selection is restricted to the five main pretransplant risk factors: donor type, stage of disease at time of transplant, recipient age, donor–recipient sex combination, and interval from diagnosis to transplant. Each risk factor contributes 0 to 2 points to the final risk score (Table 15.3). As the risk score for an individual patient, the sum of the risk points is chosen (Table 15.3). The lowest possible score on this scale is 0, which applies to a patient who receives a graft from an HLA-identical sibling donor within 12 months of diagnosis, in first chronic phase, below the age of 20 years, and who is not male with a female donor. The highest possible score on the scale is 7, which applies to a male patient over the age of 40 years who receives a graft in blast crisis from an unrelated female donor beyond 12 months from diagnosis. On the basis of 3142 patients transplanted for CML between 1989 and 1999, the

Table 15.3 EBMT risk score

Donor type	
HLA-identical sibling	0
Unrelated/non-identical	1
Stage of disease	
Chronic phase	0
Accelerated phase	1
Blast crisis	2
Age	
<20 years	0
20–40 years	1
>40 years	2
Donor–recipient sex combination	
Other	0
Female donor for male recipient	1
Time interval between diagnosis and transplantation	
<12 months	0
>12 months	1

Each of the five risk factors contributes 0, 1, or 2 points. The sum indicates the individual risk score (see Gratwohl et al[18]).

final scoring system was highly predictive for LFS and TRM. This is illustrated in Figure 15.3 and Table 15.4.

This study clearly shows that the identified risk factors are cumulative. It gives an estimate of the price paid in increased TRM if the transplant is delayed beyond 12 months from diagnosis, or if the disease progresses. This analysis provides a rational basis for counselling, and suggests that risk-adapted treatment for patients with CML should be possible.

Prognostic factors at relapse

Patients with CML who relapse after first allogeneic HSCT still have a chance for long-term survival.[46] There are four treatment options: donor lymphocyte infusion (DLI), retransplant, treatment with IFN-α, or intensive chemotherapy. Each of these approaches has its specific advantages and disadvantages. Currently, DLI is the treatment option of choice for patients with early disease.[47] Results at later stages are less convincing. In order to assess the value of the individual therapeutic options, the EBMT was interested to learn about the inherent factors predicting outcome.[48] Five hundred patients who relapsed between 1980 and 1996 were updated in 1999 with a minimum follow-up of 3 years. These data clearly show that survival after relapse is significantly related to four factors: disease phase at time of first transplant, disease stage at time of relapse, time from transplant to relapse, and donor type. Patients transplanted initially in first chronic phase have better outcome than others, patients with cytogenetic relapse or relapse in chronic phase have a better chance than those with advanced-phase relapse, patients with a time interval of more than one year between first transplant and relapse have better survival, and patients transplanted from an HLA-identical sibling do better. Again, these risk factors are cumulative. The probability of survival at 10 years post relapse is optimal and above 40% for 140 patients with no factors, 28% for 140 patients with one factor, 10% for 94 patients with two factors, and zero for 70 patients with three and four factors. These elements should be taken into account when the results of salvage therapies are compared and treatment options are being discussed.

Currently, the EBMT Chronic Leukemia Working Party is evaluating in a prospective comparative setting the values of DLI, and IFN-α therapy for low-risk relapse patients, as well as highly aggressive approaches, including double-transplant approaches for patients with advanced relapse of disease.[49]

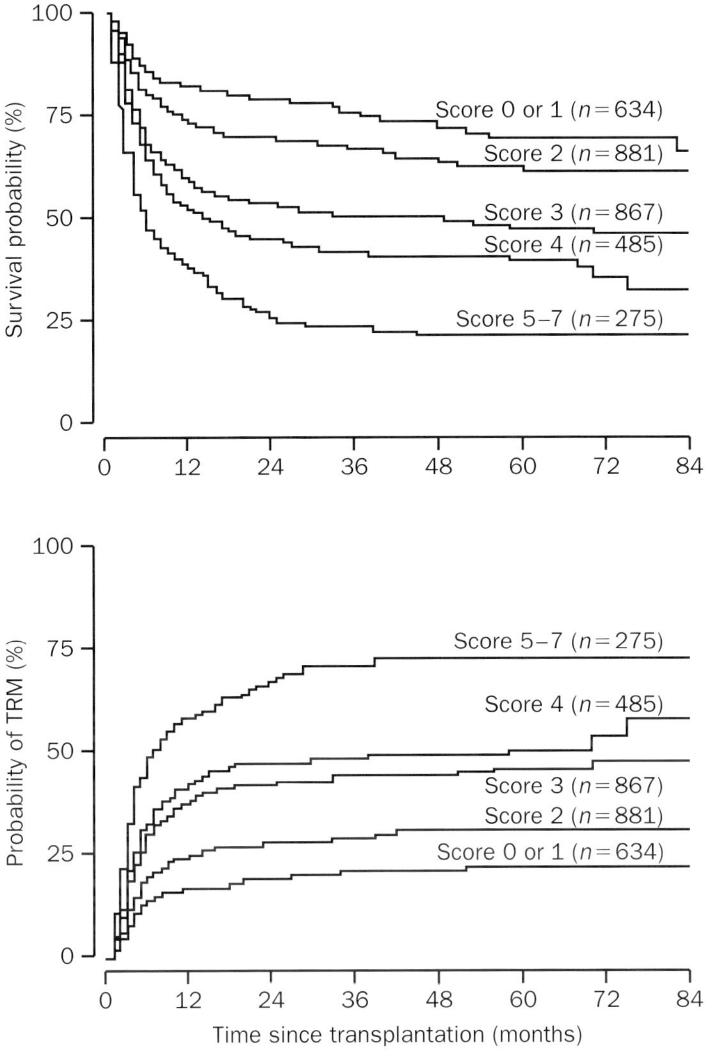

Figure 15.3 Survival and TRM of CML patients transplanted in Europe and reported to the EBMT according to their risk score (see text).[18] Reproduced with permission from Ref. 18.

CONCLUSIONS

At the present time, HSCT remains associated with an intrinsic risk of failure due to relapse after disease or transplant-related complications. For the individual patient, it may seem erratic and rather a lottery. This is not the case, and the situation can be assessed. The risk associated with HSCT is a continuum, and ranges from about 10% TRM to close to 80%. The main risk factors associated with it are known, highly predictive, and cumulative. Today, we can discuss the personal risk profile with a patient and evaluate the chances as well as risk of failure of HSCT compared with alternative therapeutic approaches. Depending on the personal situation, immediate transplant or deferment for a predetermined time will be appropriate. Adaptation of the techniques on an individualized level should ultimately improve the outcome of the whole cohort. The very near future will show whether these expectations will be met.

Table 15.4 Influence of risk score on outcome

	Patients		Probabilities at 10 years[a] (%)			
Risk score	No.	%	Survival	LFS	TRM	RI
0	65	2	72	60	20	26
1	569	18	70	60	23	23
2	881	28	62	43	31	32
3	867	28	48	37	46	31
4	485	15	40	35	51	28
5	214	7	18	15	71	41
6	57	2	22	16	73	32
7	4	0.1	—	—	—	—

[a] According to Kaplan–Meier.

REFERENCES

1. Thomas ED, Blume KG, Forman SJ (eds), *Hematopoietic Stem Cell Transplantation*, 2nd edn. Oxford: Blackwell Science, 1999.
2. Gratwohl A, Passweg J, Baldomero H, Hermans J, Special report: Blood and marrow transplantation activity in Europe 1997. *Bone Marrow Transplant* 1999; **24:** 231–5.
3. Clift R, Goldman J, Gratwohl A, Horowitz M, Proposals for standardized reporting of results of bone marrow transplantation for leukaemia. *Bone Marrow Transplant* 1989; **4:** 445–8.
4. Fefer A, Cheever MA, Thomas ED et al, Disappearance of Ph-1 positive cells in four patients with chronic myeloid leukemia after chemotherapy, irradiation and marrow transplantation from an identical twin. *N Engl J Med* 1979; **300:** 353–7.
5. Speck B, Bortin MM, Champlin R et al, Allogeneic bone marrow transplantation for chronic myelogenous leukaemia. *Lancet* 1984; **i:** 665–8.
6. Goldman JM, Apperley J, Jones L et al, Bone marrow transplantation for patients with chronic myeloid leukemia. *N Engl J Med* 1986; **314:** 202–7.
7. Clift RA, Appelbaum FR, Thomas ED, Treatment of chronic myeloid leukemia by marrow transplantation. *Blood* 1993; **82:** 1954–6.
8. Armitage JO, Bone marrow transplantation. *N Engl J Med* 1994; **330:** 827–38.
9. Gratwohl A, Hermans J, Niederwieser D et al, for the Chronic Leukemia Working Party of the European Group for Bone Marrow Transplantation, Bone marrow transplantation for chronic myeloid leukemia: long-term results. *Bone Marrow Transplant* 1993; **12:** 509–16.
10. van Rhee F, Szydlo RM, Hermans J et al, Long-term results after allogeneic bone marrow transplantation for chronic myelogenous leukemia in chronic phase: a report from the Chronic Leukemia Working Party of the European Group for Blood and Marrow Transplantation. *Bone Marrow Transplant* 1997; **20:** 553–60.
11. Savage DG, Szydlo RM, Chase A et al, Bone marrow transplantation for chronic myeloid leukaemia: the effects of different criteria for defining chronic phase on probabilities of survival and relapse. *Br J Haematol* 1997; **99:** 30–5.
12. Gratwohl A, Hermans J, Barrett AJ et al, Report from the Working Party on Leukaemia, European Group for Bone Marrow Transplantation: Allogeneic bone marrow transplantation for leukaemia in Europe. *Lancet* 1998; **352:** 1379–82.
13. The Italian Cooperative Study Group on Chronic Myeloid Leukemia, Prognostic factors in chronic

myeloid leukemia. Relationship with interferon and bone marrow transplantation. *Leuk Lymphoma* 1993; **11**(Suppl 1): 67–71.
14. Sokal JE, Cox EB, Baccarani M et al, Prognostic dissemination in 'good risk' chronic granulocytic leukemia. *Blood* 1984; **63:** 789–99.
15. Hasford J, Pfirrmann M, Hehlmann R et al, A new prognostic score for survival of patients with chronic myeloid leukemia treated with interferon alfa. Writing Committee for the Collaborative CML Prognostic Factors Project Group. *J Natl Cancer Inst* 1998; **90:** 850–8.
16. Thomas ED, Clift RN, Fefer A et al, Marrow transplantation for the treatment of chronic myelogenous leukemia. *Ann Intern Med* 1986; **104:** 155–61.
17. Goldman JM, Gale RP, Horowitz MM et al, Bone marrow transplantation for chronic myeloid leukemia in chronic phase. Increased risk of relapse associated with T-cell depletion. *Ann Intern Med* 1988; **108:** 806–14.
18. Gratwohl A, Hermans J, Goldman JM et al, for the Chronic Leukemia Working Party of the European Group for Blood and Marrow Transplantation (EBMT), Risk assessment for patients with chronic myeloid leukaemia before allogeneic blood or marrow transplantation. *Lancet* 1998; **352:** 1087–92.
19. Gratwohl A, Gluckman E, Goldman J, Zwaan F, Effect of splenectomy before bone-marrow transplantation on survival in chronic granulocytic leukemia. *Lancet* 1985; **ii:** 1290–1.
20. Gratwohl A, Hermans J, v Biezen A et al, for the Chronic Leukaemia Working Party of the European Group for Bone Marrow Transplantation, No advantage for patients who receive splenic irradiation before bone marrow transplantation for chronic myeloid leukaemia: results of a prospective randomized study. *Bone Marrow Transplant* 1992; **10:** 147–52.
21. Gratwohl A, Hermans J, v Biezen A et al, Splenic irradiation before bone marrow transplantation for chronic myeloid leukemia. *Br J Haematol* 1996; **95:** 494–500.
22. Jabro G, Koc Y, Boyle T et al, Role of splenic irradiation in patients with chronic myeloid leukemia undergoing allogeneic bone marrow transplantation. *Biol Blood Marrow Transplant* 1999; **5:** 173–5.
23. Gratwohl A, van Biezen A, Hermans J et al, Role of splenic irradiation in patients with chronic myeloid leukemia undergoing allogeneic bone marrow transplantation. *Biol Blood Marrow Transplant* 2000; **6:** 211–13.
24. von Bueltzingsloewen A, Bordigoni P, Dorvaux Y et al, Splenectomy may reverse pancytopenia occurring after allogeneic bone marrow transplantation. *Bone Marrow Transplant* 1994; **14:** 339–40.
25. Silver RT, Woolf SH, Hehlmann R et al, An evidence-based analysis of the effect of busulfan, hydroxyurea, interferon, and allogeneic bone marrow transplantation in treating the chronic phase of chronic myeloid leukemia: developed for the American Society of Hematology. *Blood* 1999; **94:** 1517–36.
26. Goldman JM, Szydlo R, Horowitz MM et al, Choice of pretransplant treatment and timing of transplants for chronic myelogenous leukemia in chronic phase. *Blood* 1993; **82:** 2235–8.
27. Beelen DW, Graeven U, Elmaagacli AH et al, Prolonged administration of interferon alpha in patients with chronic phase Philadelphia positive chronic myelogenous leukemia before allogeneic bone marrow transplantation may adversely affect transplant outcome. *Blood* 1995; **85:** 2981–90.
28. Morton AJ, Gooley T, Hansen JA et al, Association between pretransplant interferon and outcome after unrelated donor marrow transplants for chronic myeloid leukemia in chronic phase. *Blood* 1998; **92:** 394–8.
29. Holler E, Schleuning M, Ledderose G et al, Interferon alpha prior to allogeneic BMT in patients with chronic myeloid leukemia. *Ann Haematol* 1996; **73:** A96.
30. Hehlmann R, Hochhaus A, Kolb HJ et al, Interferon-alpha before allogeneic bone marrow transplantation in chronic myelogenous leukemia does not affect outcome adversely, provided it is discontinued at least 90 days before the procedure. *Blood* 1999; **94:** 3668–77.
31. Gahrton G, Svensson H, Björkstrand B et al, Syngeneic transplantation in multiple myeloma – a case-matched comparison with autologous and allogeneic transplantation. *Bone Marrow Transplant* 1999; **24:** 741–5.
32. Spencer A, Szydlo RM, Brookes PA et al, Bone marrow transplantation for chronic myeloid leukemia with volunteer unrelated donors using ex vivo or in vivo T-cell depletion: major prognostic impact of HLA class I identity between donor and recipient. *Blood* 1995; **86:** 3590–7.
33. Hansen JA, Gooley TA, Martin PJ et al, Bone

marrow transplants from unrelated donors for patients with chronic myeloid leukemia. *N Engl J Med* 1998; **338:** 962–8.
34. Sierra J, Storer B, Hansen JA et al, Transplantation of marrow cells from unrelated donors for treatment of high risk acute leukemia: the effect of leukemia cell burden, HLA-matching and marrow cell dose. *Blood* 1997; **89:** 4226–35.
35. Bostrom L, Ringden O, Gratama JW et al, A role of herpes virus serology for the development of acute GvHD. *Bone Marrow Transplant* 1990; **5:** 321–6.
36. Frassoni F, van Biezen A, Beelen D et al, Long-term disease free survival after identical twin transplant in chronic myeloid leukemia: graft-versus-tumor or reduction of leukemic burden? Submitted.
37. Barrett AJ, Ringdén O, Zhang M-J et al, Effect of nucleated cell dose on relapse and survival in identical twin transplants for leukemia. *Blood* 2000; **95:** 3323–7.
38. Devergie A, Apperley JF, Labopin M et al, for the Chronic Leukemia Working Party of the European Group for Blood and Marrow Transplantation, European results of matched unrelated donor bone marrow transplantation for chronic myeloid leukemia. Impact of HLA class II matching. *Bone Marrow Transplant* 1997; **20:** 11–19.
39. Szydlo R, Goldman JM, Klein JP et al, Results of allogeneic bone marrow transplants for leukemia using donors other than HLA-identical siblings. *J Clin Oncol* 1997; **15:** 1767–77.
40. Przepiorka D, Khouri I, Thall P et al, Thiotepa, busulfan and cyclophosphamide as a preparative regimen for allogeneic transplantation for advanced chronic myelogenous leukemia. *Bone Marrow Transplant* 1999; **23:** 977–81.
41. Russell N, Gratwohl A, Schmitz N, Annotation: The place of blood stem cells in allogeneic transplantation. *Br J Haematol* 1996; **93:** 747–53.
42. Schmitz N, Bacigalupo A, Labopin M et al, Transplantation of peripheral blood progenitor cells from HLA-sibling donors. European Group for Blood and Marrow Transplantation (EBMT). *Br J Haematol* 1996; **95:** 715–23.
43. Champlin RE, Schmitz N, Horowitz MM et al, Blood stem cells versus bone marrow as a source of hematopoietic cells for allogeneic transplantation. *Blood* 2000; **95:** 3702–9.
44. Ustun C, Arslan O, Beksac M et al, A retrospective comparison of allogeneic peripheral blood stem cell and bone marrow transplantation results from a single center: a focus on the incidence of graft-vs.-host disease and relapse. *Biol Blood Marrow Transplant* 1999; **5:** 28–35.
45. Elmaagacli AH, Beelen DW, Opalka B et al, The risk of residual molecular and cytogenetic disease in patients with Philadelphia-chromosome positive first chronic phase chronic myelogenous leukemia is reduced after transplantation of allogeneic peripheral blood stem cells compared with bone marrow. *Blood* 1999; **94:** 384–9.
46. Arcese W, Goldman JM, D'Arcangelo E et al, Outcome for patients who relapse after allogeneic bone marrow transplantation for chronic myeloid leukemia. Chronic Leukemia Working Party. European Bone Marrow Transplantation Group. *Blood* 1993; **82:** 3211–19.
47. Kolb HJ, Donor leukocyte transfusions for treatment of leukemic relapse after bone marrow transplantation. EBMT Immunology and Chronic Leukemia Working Parties. *Vox Sang* 1998; **74**(Suppl 2): 321–9.
48. Guglielmi C, Arcese W, Hermans J et al, Risk assessment in patients with Ph+ CML at first relapse after allogeneic BMT. An EBMT retrospective analysis. *Blood* 2000; **95:** 3328–34.
49. Passweg JR, Hoffmann T, Tichelli A et al, Double allogeneic peripheral stem cell transplants for patients at high risk of relapse. *Bone Marrow Transplant* 1998; **22:** 321–4.
50. Gale RP, Hehlmann R, Zhang MJ et al, Survival with bone marrow transplantation versus hydroxyurea or interferon for chronic myelogenous leukemia. The German CML Study Group. *Blood* 1998; **91:** 1810–19.

16

The decision whether to allograft a patient with CML

John M Goldman

CONTENTS • **Introduction** • **Prediction of survival with conventional therapy** • **Definitions of cure** • **Prognostic factors for survival after transplantation** • **Therapeutic strategy for the newly diagnosed patient** • **Allografting for a patient in the advanced phase of CML** • **Conclusions**

INTRODUCTION

The decision whether to proceed to an allogeneic stem cell transplant (SCT) for a given patient with CML and the timing of the transplant have become very much more complex since allogeneic SCT was introduced into clinical practice in the early 1980s. This complexity reflects the fact that whereas survival without SCT has improved to a certain degree in the last 20 years, the results of SCT have also improved during this time. Moreover the development of the new tyrosine kinase inhibitor STI571 (Glivec) offers the prospect of further still unquantifiable improvement in non-transplant therapy. Thus it is difficult to provide for a new patient with CML an accurate estimate of the probability of survival with or without a transplant. To this uncertainty must be added the fact that some patients have strong views as to whether they do or do not wish to submit themselves to a transplant procedure regardless of the recommendation they may receive from their haematologist. In this chapter, I briefly review the factors influencing the probability of survival with conventional therapy or after allogeneic SCT, and discuss the possible policies that the clinician may adopt in advising an individual patient with newly diagnosed CML. I also discuss the place of allogeneic SCT for a patient with advanced-phase CML.

Prediction of survival with conventional therapy

It was known during most of the 20th century that the duration of survival from diagnosis varied very considerably for individual patients with CML, but the basis for this heterogeneity was and still remains largely unexplained. In 1984, Sokal and colleagues[1] developed a prognostic index based on age, spleen size, percentage of blasts in the blood, and platelet count at diagnosis. They divided patients into three broad categories with relatively good, intermediate, and relatively poor survival respectively, but the 'Sokal index' is a relatively crude method of predicting survival for individual patients and there are many examples of patients who have survived for much longer or shorter periods than their Sokal index would have suggested. A number of other attempts have been made to predict survival at the time of diagnosis, but none has entirely superseded the Sokal method (see Chapter 12).

Useful information may be obtained in certain circumstances if the clinician can observe a patient's response to treatment. Galton[2] observed in the 1950s that the leukocyte doubling time differed in different patients and that those with slower disease could be treated with lower doses of busulfan. Moreover, the amount of busulfan administered to individual patients in the first year after diagnosis was inversely related to the duration of survival.[3] More recently, it has become apparent that a patient's response to treatment with interferon-α (IFN-α) correlates relatively well with the duration of survival. Thus patients who obtain a durable haematological response to IFN-α tend to survive longer than those who do not, and those who achieve major or complete cytogenetic remissions with IFN-α treatment clearly survive longer than cytogenetic non-responders.[4,5] It is particularly interesting to note that a small minority of patients who achieve a complete cytogenetic response and who then stop taking IFN-α can remain in cytogenetic remission for a number of years.

Though there is little doubt that IFN-α can prolong survival for a given cohort of patients in comparison with the hypothetical survival for the same patients if they had been treated with a conventional cytotoxic drug[6] such as hydroxyurea – a speculation that is almost impossible to prove or refute in individual cases – the highly variable response to IFN-α must to some degree reflect the intrinsic heterogeneity of the disease in different patients, and can thus be regarded as an 'operational' prognostic index. In other words, one might postulate that the patient who responds rapidly to IFN-α has a better overall prognosis with IFN-α treatment (or with other non-transplant therapy) than the patient who responds less well (and vice versa), and one could use this knowledge to recommend proceeding to or deferring a transplant procedure. If this general principle were accepted, it may transpire that response to STI571 is an even better discriminant for a cohort of CML patients than response to IFN-α.

Since the Sokal index was based predominantly on studies of patients treated with busulfan, the question arises whether an analogous study of patients treated with IFN-α would yield comparable results. Hasford and colleagues[7] analysed data on 1303 patients treated with IFN-α in 14 separate studies, and devised a new scoring system based on patient age, spleen size, blast cell count, platelet count, eosinophil count, and basophil count. It is possible that the combined use of the Hasford scoring system together with an initial trial of IFN-α for a finite period could identify a cohort of patients predicted to have a survival better than average if treated with IFN-α. This issue is discussed in more detail below.

Definitions of cure

The primary objective of treatment for all types of haematological malignancy must be to cure the disease, and many patients are rightly dissatisfied with any treatment that does not offer the prospect of cure. However, in CML, as in other types of malignancy where relapse may occur after prolonged periods of 'remission', the precise definition of cure is not entirely straightforward. Thus one may propose somewhat simplistically that cure is achieved when all CML cells have been eradicated from a patient's body. This definition leads immediately to obvious problems – how could one possibly study a patient's whole body during life? Further, if occasional leukaemia cells persisted in a patient's body but lacked pluripotentiality and were thus incapable of regenerating the disease or if occasional 'pluripotential' leukaemia cells persisted in a patient's body but were fully restrained by a graft-versus-leukaemia (GVL) effect, would this not be tantamount to cure?

The introduction of highly sensitive reverse-transcriptase polymerase chain reaction (RT-PCR) techniques to identify and quantitate small numbers of leukaemia-specific transcripts in the blood or marrow of patients in complete cytogenetic remission after treatment with IFN-α or allogeneic SCT has been very informative.[8] Thus the great majority of the patients who achieve complete cytogenetic remission during treatment with IFN-α continue to have *BCR/ABL* transcripts detectable in their peripheral blood, albeit at much lower concentration than those who do not achieve cytogenetic remission.[9] Occasional IFN-α-treated patients are negative by PCR studies, but this negativity is not usually maintained. These observations contrast with results of RT-PCR studies after allogeneic SCT. The majority of patients who survive an allograft performed in chronic phase are continuously negative when studied by RT-PCR, and some such patients have now survived more than 20 years since SCT. It is reasonable to regard such patients as genuinely 'cured', although occasional patients show evidence of *BCR/ABL* transcripts in their blood 5–10 years after SCT,[10] and one patient in our experience relapsed 14 years after allografting.[11]

Thus, for the present, one may conclude that allogeneic SCT is the only therapeutic approach that offers a real possibility of 'cure'. Patients for whom a 'cure' is the only objective may be prepared to consider undergoing an allogeneic SCT even when the probability of transplant-related mortality seems high. Conversely, others may consider that the risk of mortality within the first year of SCT is unacceptable, however low it appears to be, and will thus prefer a more conventional approach to treatment. This topic is further complicated by the possibility that STI571, either alone or in combination with other agents, may increase the chance of 'cure' or at least of long-term freedom from clinical evidence of leukaemia.[12,13]

Prognostic factors for survival after transplantation

The factors that influence the probability of survival after allogeneic SCT for CML are now reasonably well characterized, and are well reflected in the study reported from the European Group for Blood and Marrow Transplantation in 1998.[14] These workers studied a cohort of 2275 patients transplanted in all phases of CML with matched sibling or phenotypically HLA-'matched' alternative donors, and identified five major factors that appeared to impact on the probability of survival during the ensuing 6 years. These were patient age, disease phase, degree of histocompatibility between donor and recipient, duration of chronic phase, and gender match of patient and donor. They ascribed to each transplant a score of 0 if the prognostic factor was thought to indicate a favourable outcome and a score of 1 or 2 if the particular factor was unfavourable. On this basis they could show that patients with five favourable factors had a probability of survival at 5 years post SCT of 70–80%, whereas for patients with many poor prognostic factors the comparable figure was 15–20%. Clearly this approach to assessing the probability of success for a given transplant can greatly assist the haematologist in advising a particular patient. The study is described in greater detail in Chapter 15.

The notion that patients transplanted in advanced phases of CML (accelerated phase or blastic transformation) have a higher transplant-related mortality (TRM) and also a higher risk of relapse than those transplanted in chronic phase is well documented in studies reported from the Seattle group[15] and retrospective analyses reported by the International Bone Marrow Transplant Registry (IBMTR).[16] It is therefore reasonable to assume that for a patient with a suitably matched sibling or alternative donor, the transplant should be performed while the patient is still in the chronic phase of his or her disease. The chance that a patient's chronic-phase disease will progress to a more advanced phase is difficult to calculate accurately, but may be 10–15% in the first year after diagnosis and higher in subsequent years.[17] This by itself would be an argument for performing the transplant soon after diagnosis. There is also evidence that the TRM for both matched sibling transplants[18] and transplants using matched unrelated donors[19] is higher in patients transplanted more than one year from diagnosis than in patients transplanted within one year. The reason for this adverse effect of delayed transplant is not clear, but it may be related to the cumulative harmful effects of treatment with busulfan or IFN-α. Whether the use of STI571 for more than one year will have a similar adverse effect on TRM remains to be seen.

There are other factors that must be taken into account when attempting to predict the probability of survival for a given patient contemplating treatment by SCT: CMV serostatus, prior IFN-α treatment, stem cell source, T-cell depletion, and intensity of conditioning.

CMV serostatus

Patients who have never been exposed to infection with cytomegalovirus (CMV) and who received a SCT from a CMV-negative donor have a negligible probably of developing CML infection, whereas CMV-seropositive patients not infrequently reactivate CMV, which may cause clinically significant infection. This can usually be treated successfully in the context of an HLA-sibling transplant, but CMV-seropositive patients allografted with T-cell-depleted donor stem cells may have an increased risk of mortality from viral infections generally,[20] and this may apply especially to CMV-seropositive patients receiving stem cells from matched unrelated donors.[21,22]

Prior treatment with IFN-α

It has been suggested in recent years that the administration of IFN-α before allogeneic SCT may adversely impact on the probability of survival. The Essen group reported that TRM was higher in patients who had received IFN-α for one year or more before allografting than in those not treated with IFN-α.[23] Similar conclusions were reached in a study reported from Seattle.[24] Conversely, no adverse effect of prior IFN-α treatment could be detected in a large series of patients analysed by the IBMTR. A study from the German CML Multi-Centre Study Group concluded that administration of IFN-α within 90 days preceding the allograft did significantly increase the TRM; however, if patients treated with IFN-α had their IFN-α discontinued more than 90 days before the allograft, no such adverse effect could be identified.[25] For the present, it seems reasonable to conclude that the possible deleterious effect of prior IFN-α is small or negligible if the drug is stopped three or more months before the patient proceeds to allografting. This conclusion is relevant to the suggestion that some patients should receive a 'trial' of IFN-α before the decision whether or not to proceed to an allograft is made (see below).

Blood or marrow as source of stem cells?

It is now clear that leukaemia patients allografted with HLA-identical blood-derived stem cells engraft more rapidly than those who received comparable transplants with marrow-derived stem cells. Conversely, chronic graft-versus-host disease (GVHD) seems to be increased in recipients of blood-derived stem cells. It is not currently clear whether the use of blood-derived stem cells for allografting patients with CML in chronic phase offers any long-term advantage over the use of marrow-derived stem cells.[26] In CML, the putative increased risk of GVHD might be offset by T-cell depletion. This topic is discussed in greater detail in Chapter 18.

T-cell depletion of donor mononuclear cells

Though the majority of centres where transplants are performed for patients with CML in chronic phase take no steps to deplete donor marrow or blood cells of T cells as prophylaxis for GVHD, this approach is used in some centres.[27] There is no doubt that T-cell depletion greatly increases the risk of relapse, but this of course can be treated with a high degree of success with subsequent transfusion of donor T cells. In some cases, the use of T-cell depletion of donor marrow has resulted in a reduction in TRM.

Reduced-intensity-conditioning allogeneic stem cell transplants

There has been great interest in the last few years in the possibility that allogeneic SCT performed with low-dose chemotherapy and/or low-dose chemoradiotherapy as conditioning, in conjunction with relatively high numbers of $CD34^+$ and together with donor-derived T cells, may establish full donor chimerism with eradication of leukaemia while reducing the TRM associated with a conventional transplant. This approach, also referred to as non-myeloablative SCT, has been used in a small number of patients with CML in chronic phase, some of whom have achieved complete donor chimerism and eradication of cytogenetic and molecular evidence of leukaemia.[28–31] It is too early to say whether this approach offers distinct advantages over a conventional transplant in terms of reduced TRM and comparable disease eradication.

THERAPEUTIC STRATEGY FOR THE NEWLY DIAGNOSED PATIENT

There are at least two possible approaches to deciding whether and when to recommend an allogeneic SCT to a patient with newly diagnosed CML in chronic phase.

(1) Early decision in favour of or against allografting (Figure 16.1)

One approach is to try to decide within 4–8 weeks of diagnosis whether or not a given patient is a candidate for allografting. This decision should take into account on the one hand the best estimate of the patient's expected survival with non-transplant therapy and on the other the probability of survival (and of relapse) after allogeneic transplantation. If one assumes the patient is newly diagnosed and in chronic phase, two at least of the prognostic factors considered by Gratwohl et al[14] will be 'favourable'. It remains then to identify the best available donor, who ideally would be an HLA-identical sibling, and to set an upper age limit for transplantation. For sibling transplants, this is variously set at 50, 55, or 60 years in different transplant units; for alternative donor transplants the upper age limits are often somewhat lower. If then the estimated TRM is below an arbitrary level, which may be set as high as 30%, the clinician may recommend that the patient undergoes the transplant procedure. Patients with a higher projected TRM would be offered treatment by other methods. Clearly the final decision of whether or not to proceed to transplant must be made by the patient in collaboration with appropriate family members.

(2) Trial of therapy before allografting (Figure 16.2)

The alternative approach is try to place the newly diagnosed patient into one of three categories: (a) a candidate for early allografting; (b) not a candidate for transplant; (c) an intermediate group where the advisability of allografting is unclear. These categories will again be defined on the basis of criteria specified in (1) above, but patient age and the degree of histocompatibility between patient and donor will be of paramount importance. For example, a 25-year-old man with an HLA-identical brother would be offered an early allograft in most specialist centres, whereas a 55-year-old man for whom the best available donor was a volunteer mismatched for one DRB1 allele would in most centres not be considered for transplant. But what of the 55-year-old man with an HLA-identical sibling or the 35-year-old woman with a molecularly 10-antigen-matched unrelated donor? Or the patient with a suitable donor who is reluctant to consider a transplant soon after diagnosis? The patients may fit into the intermediate group, for whom it may be reasonable to initiate a trial of non-transplant therapy with the intention of categorizing the patient as 'good risk' or 'poor risk' (with conventional therapy) on the basis of response to therapy in the short term.

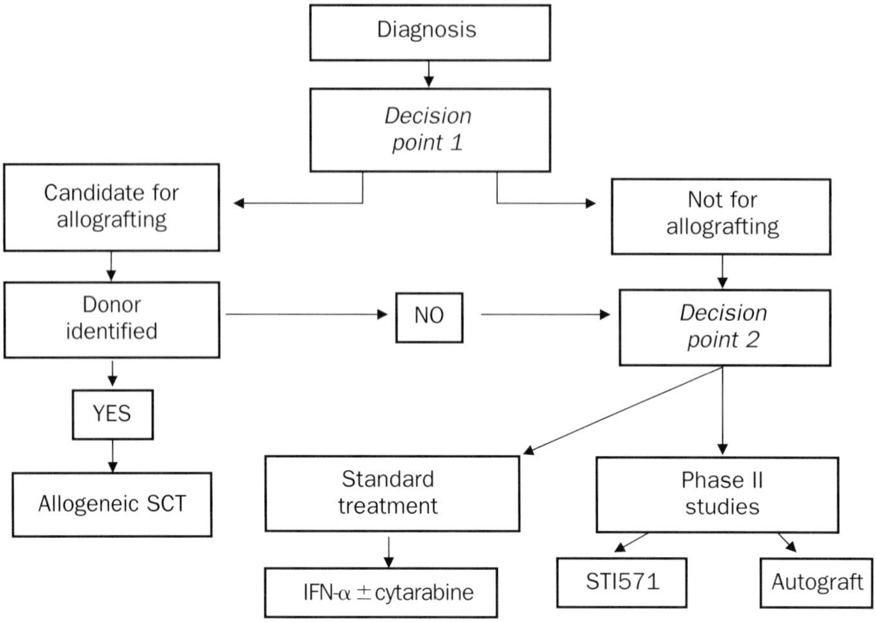

Figure 16.1
Algorithm based on the assumption that a transplant for a patient in chronic phase should ideally be performed within 6 months of diagnosis or not at all. Thus the option for a trial of treatment with IFN-α or STI571 in the 'intermediate group' has been omitted from this scheme.

The best approach for a trial of non-transplant therapy is not entirely clear. Until recently, it would have been reasonable to offer the patient a trial period of treatment with IFN-α. The problem would have been to set firm criteria by which to judge the success or failure of the trial. One might, for example, start a patient on treatment with 5 MU/m^2 of IFN-α and decide that any patient who failed to achieve a haematological response within 3 months or any patient who failed to achieve a degree of cytogenetic response within 6 months should be judged to have failed the trial. By implication, any patient who did not fail the trial would continue treatment with IFN-α. In practice, this approach does have a number of disadvantages, such as the continued risk of disease transformation during the trial period, the arbitrary nature of the definitions of success or failure, and the uncertainty as to how long the IFN-α should be continued in a patient who appears at first to respond cytogenetically and then loses his or her response.

However, the suggestion that the combination of IFN-α plus cytarabine (cytosine arabinoside, Ara-C) may prolong life in comparison with IFN-α alone strengthens the argument in favour of the 'trial of therapy before allografting' approach.[32] Moreover, the early results with the use of STI571,[12,13] and the possibility that STI571 in conjunction with other agents may be better than STI alone, strongly support the notion that for patients who are not obvious candidates for early allografting (category (a) above), some trial of non-transplant therapy should be considered. The precise details of this trial will not be easy to specify.

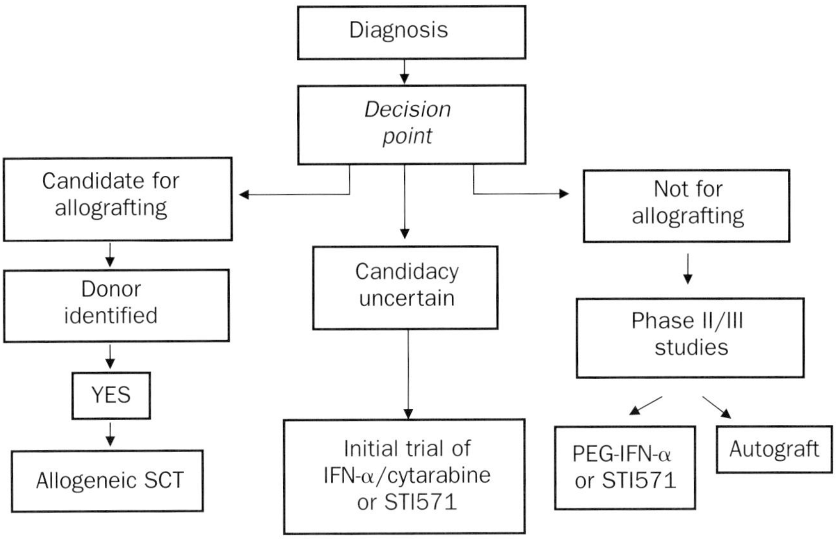

Figure 16.2
Algorithm showing a possible programme for treating a newly diagnosed patient with CML in chronic phase, assuming that one can define one category of patients for whom early transplant is advisable and another category for whom transplant cannot be advised. The intermediate group for whom the advisability of early transplant is uncertain can then be offered a trial of treatment with IFN-α (with or without cytarabine) or, in the future, with STI571 alone or in combination with other agents. For patients not deemed eligible for allografting, an autograft or the use of pegylated IFN-α (PEG-IFN-α) or STI571 can be considered as primary treatment.

ALLOGRAFTING FOR A PATIENT IN THE ADVANCED PHASE OF CML

The precise role of allogeneic SCT in the management of patients with CML in advanced phase is still unresolved. One obvious problem is the definition of advanced-phase disease. When the results of allografting for patients with CML in chronic phase defined by the current Hammersmith criteria were revisited using stricter criteria proposed by the IBMTR, notably by excluding from acceptance as chronic-phase patients those with platelet counts in excess of $1000 \times 10^9/l$, the actuarial curve for survival was substantially 'improved'.[33] This said, the definition of blastic transformation is reasonably well agreed,[34] and it is certain that the results of allografting for patients in blastic transformation are substantially inferior to the results of allografting in chronic phase. Results of allografting for patients in the so-called accelerated phase are in general intermediate between the results of allografting in chronic phase and the results achieved in transformation.[15,16]

In summary, one may speculate that the allograft should ideally be performed while a patient is still in the chronic phase of his or her disease. If this is not possible – either because the patient is reluctant to consider an allograft while the prospect of survival for a few years without transplant seems reasonable or because the risk of transplant-related mortality in chronic phase seems to be unduly high – then it is reasonable to consider a transplant once the patient has entered the accelerated phase. For patients in frank blastic transformation, one could consider an allograft as primary treatment, but it seems generally preferable to treat such patients first with chemotherapy appropriate to lymphoid or myeloid blastic transformation and to assess the response thereafter. Patients in whom the blast cell population cannot be suppressed with aggressive chemotherapy are extremely unlikely to fare well after allografting. Conversely, patients who can be restored to 'second chronic phase' may have a reasonably good chance of surviving the transplant, and some will be proved eventually to have been cured by the procedure.[35]

CONCLUSIONS

It is today more important than ever before that the clinician confronted with a new patient with CML recommends a treatment programme that attempts to balance the patient's likely survival with conventional cytotoxic drugs against the probability of cure after allogeneic SCT. This already complex picture has recently become even more complicated by the advent of STI571, which may prove to prolong survival in comparison with IFN-α or IFN-α plus cytarabine. Moreover, the identification of putative targets for an allogeneic GVL effect could lay the foundations for immunotherapy in the autologous setting. One might then speculate that the best treatment for CML patients might be a combination of STI571 with other drugs, followed by immunotherapy to eradicate residual disease. The next few years are likely to see further fundamental changes in our approach to the management of this fascinating disease.

REFERENCES

1. Sokal JE, Cox EB, Baccarani M et al, Prognostic discrimination in 'good risk' chronic granulocytic leukemia. *Blood* 1984; **63:** 789–99.
2. Galton DAG, Treatment of the chronic leukaemias. *Br Med Bull* 1959; **15:** 79–86.
3. Wareham NJ, Johnson SA, Goldman JM, Relationship of the duration of the chronic phase in chronic granulocytic leukaemia to the need for treatment during the first year after diagnosis. *Cancer Chemother Pharmacol* 1982; **8:** 205–10.
4. Talpaz M, Kantarjian HM, McCredie KB et al, Hematologic remission and cytogenetic improvement induced by recombinant human interferon alpha A in chronic myelogenous leukemia. *N Engl J Med* 1986; **314:** 1065–9.
5. Kantarjian HM, Smith TL, O'Brien S et al, Prolonged survival in chronic myelogenous leukemia after cytogenetic response to interferon-α therapy. *Ann Intern Med* 1995; **122:** 254–61.
6. CML Trialists Collaborative Group, Interferon alfa versus chemotherapy for chronic myeloid leukemia: a meta-analysis of seven randomized trials. *J Natl Cancer Inst* 1997; **89:** 1616–20.
7. Hasford J, Pfirrmann J, Hehlmann R et al, A new prognostic score for survival of patients with chronic myeloid leukemia treated with interferon alfa. *J Natl Cancer Inst* 1998; **90:** 850–8.
8. Cross NCP, Lin F, Chase A et al, Competitive PCR to estimate the number of BCR–ABL transcripts in chronic myeloid leukemia patients after bone marrow transplantation. *Blood* 1993; **82:** 1929–36.
9. Hochhaus A, Reiter A, Sausele S et al, Molecular heterogeneity in compete cytogenetic responders after interferon-α therapy for chronic myelogenous leukaemia: low levels of minimal residual disease are associated with continuing remission. *Blood* 2000; **85:** 62–6.
10. Olavarria E, Kanfer E, Szydlo R et al, Early detection of BCR/ABL transcripts by quantitative RT-PCR predicts outcome after allogeneic stem cell transplantation for chronic myeloid leukaemia. *Blood* 2001; **97:** 1560–5.
11. Yong A, Goldman JM, Relapse of chronic myeloid leukaemia 14 years after allogeneic bone marrow transplantation. *Bone Marrow Transplant* 1999; **23:** 827–8.
12. Druker BJ, Talpaz M, Resta DJ et al, Efficacy and safety of a specific inhibitor of the BCR-ABL tyrosine kinase in chronic myeloid leukemia. *N Engl J Med* 2001; **344:** 1031–7.
13. Goldman JM, Melo JV, Targeting the BCR-ABL tyrosine kinase in chronic myeloid leukemia. *N Engl J Med* 2001; **344:** 1084–6.
14. Gratwohl A, Hermans J, Goldman JM et al, Risk assessment for patients with chronic myeloid leukaemia before allogeneic blood or marrow transplantation. *Lancet* 1998; **352:** 1087–92.
15. Thomas ED, Clift RA, Fefer A et al, Marrow transplantation for the treatment of chronic

myelogenous leukemia. *Ann Intern Med* 1986; **104:** 155–63.
16. Speck B, Bortin MM, Champlin R et al, Allogeneic bone marrow transplantation for chronic myeloid leukaemia. *Lancet* 1984; **i:** 665–8.
17. Sokal JE, Prognosis in chronic myeloid leukemia: biology of the disease vs. treatment. *Baillière's Clin Haematol* 1987; **1:** 907–29.
18. Goldman JM, Szydlo R, Horowitz MM et al, Choice of pretransplant treatment and timing of transplants for chronic myelogenous leukemia in chronic phase. *Blood* 1993; **82:** 2235–8.
19. Hansen JA, Gooley TA, Martin PJ et al, Bone marrow transplantation from unrelated donors for patients with chronic myeloid leukemia. *N Engl J Med* 1998; **338:** 962–8.
20. Broers AEC, van der Holt R, van Esser JWJ et al, Increased transplant related morbidity and mortality in CMV-seropositive patients despite highly effective prevention of CMV disease after allogeneic T-cell depleted stem cell transplantation. *Blood* 2000; **95:** 2240–5.
21. McGlave PB, Shu XO, Wen W et al, Unrelated donor marrow transplantation for chronic myelogenous leukemia: 9 years' experience of the National Marrow Donor Program. *Blood* 2000; **95:** 2219–25.
22. Craddock C, Szydlo RM, Dazzi F et al, Cytomegalovirus seropositivity adversely influences outcome after T-depleted unrelated donor transplant in patients with chronic myeloid leukemia: the case for tailored GVHD prophylaxis. *Br J Haematol* 2001; **112:** 228–36.
23. Beelen DW, Graeven U, Elmaagacli AH et al, Prolonged administration of interferon-α in patients with chronic-phase Philadelphia chromosome-positive chronic myelogenous leukemia before allogeneic bone marrow transplantation may adversely affect transplant outcome. *Blood* 1995; **85:** 2981–90.
24. Morton AJ, Gooley T, Hansen JA et al, Association between pretransplant interferon-α and outcome after unrelated donor marrow transplantation for chronic myelogenous leukemia in chronic phase. *Blood* 1998; **92:** 394–401.
25. Hehlmann R, Hochhaus A, Kolb H-J et al, Interferon-α before allogeneic bone marrow transplantation in chronic myelogenous leukemia does not affect outcome adversely, provided it is discontinued at least 90 days before the procedure. *Blood* 1999; **94:** 3668–77.
26. Elmaagacli AH, Beelen DW, Opalka B et al, The risk of residual molecular and cytogenetic disease in patients with Philadelphia chromosome positive chronic phase myelogenous leukemia is reduced after transplantation of allogeneic peripheral blood stem cells. *Blood* 1999; **94:** 384–9.
27. Drobyski WR, Hessner MJ, Klein JP et al, T-cell depletion plus salvage immunotherapy with donor leukocyte infusions as a strategy to treat chronic phase chronic myelogenous leukemia patients undergoing HLA-identical sibling marrow transplantation. *Blood* 1999; **94:** 434–41.
28. Slavin S, Nagler A, Naparstek E et al, Nonmyeloablative stem cell transplantation with cell therapy as an alternative to conventional bone marrow transplantation with lethal cytoreduction for the treatment of malignant and nonmalignant hematologic diseases. *Blood* 1998; **91:** 756–63.
29. Giralt S, Estey E, Albitar M et al, Engraftment of allogeneic hematopoietic progenitor cells with purine analog-containing chemotherapy: harnessing graft-versus-leukemia without myeloablative therapy. *Blood* 1997; **89:** 4531–6.
30. Childs R, Epperson D, Bahceci E et al, Molecular remission of chronic myeloid leukaemia following a non-myeloablative allogeneic peripheral blood stem cell transplant: in vivo and in vitro evidence for a graft versus leukaemia effect. *Br J Haematol* 1999; **107:** 396–400.
31. Raiola AM, van Lint MT, Lamparelli T et al, Reduced intensity thiotepa–cyclophosphamide conditioning for allogeneic haemopoietic stem cell transplants (HSCT) in patients up to 60 years of age. *Br J Haematol* 2000; **109:** 716–21.
32. Guilhot F, Chastang C, Michallet M et al, Interferon alpha 2b combined with cytarabine versus interferon alone in chronic myelogenous leukemia. *N Engl J Med* 1997; **337:** 223–9.
33. Savage DG, Szydlo RM, Chase A et al, Bone marrow transplantation for chronic myeloid leukaemia: the effects of differing criteria for defining chronic phase on probabilities of survival and relapse. *Br J Haematol* 1997; **99:** 30–5.
34. Karanas A, Silver RT, Characteristics of the terminal phase of chronic granulocytic leukemia. *Blood* 1968; **32:** 445–9.
35. Visani G, Rosti G, Bandini G et al, Second chronic phase before transplantation is crucial for improving survival of blastic phase chronic myeloid leukaemia. *Br J Haematol* 2000; **109:** 722–8.

17

Conditioning regimens and T-cell depletion

Charles Craddock

CONTENTS • Introduction • Biology of stem cell engraftment and its relevance to the design of conditioning regimens • Myeloablative conditioning regimens in allogeneic transplantation • Clinical development of myeloablative conditioning regimens • Prospects for the development of reduced-intensity conditioning regimens • T-cell depletion and CD34 selection

INTRODUCTION

Allogeneic stem cell transplantation (SCT) remains the only curative therapeutic option in patients with CML. Using myeloablative conditioning regimens, long-term disease-free survival rates of up to 70% can be achieved in young patients who are fortunate enough to have an HLA-identical sibling donor. Until recently, it was believed that a myeloablative conditioning regimen played a critical role in the success of allografting – first by securing stem cell engraftment and secondly by eradicating malignant host haematopoiesis. However, such regimens are associated with substantial immediate and long-term toxicity, which, in addition to prejudicing transplant outcome in 'good-risk' patients, precludes their extension to older patients or those with significant co-morbidities. The increased realization of the importance of a graft-versus-leukaemia (GVL) effect in CML has led to the proposal that it may be possible to improve the outcome of allografting by reducing the intensity of the conditioning regimen with the aim of harnessing a GVL effect as the main antileukaemic strategy. Preliminary results using such non-myeloablative clinical protocols confirm that sustained engraftment of allogeneic stem cells can be achieved with a marked reduction in the immediate toxicity of transplantation. The extent to which this radically different transplant strategy allows the delivery of a sustained antileukaemic effect is unclear at present, but it is likely that this approach will make an important contribution to allogeneic SCT in the future.

BIOLOGY OF STEM CELL ENGRAFTMENT AND ITS RELEVANCE TO THE DESIGN OF CONDITIONING REGIMENS

Molecular basis of stem cell engraftment

The establishment of donor haematopoiesis after SCT is dependent upon two critical steps: the initial homing or lodgement of transplanted haematopoietic progenitors (HP) and their subsequent proliferation within the bone marrow microenvironment. The molecular pathways mediating the migration of HP from the peripheral blood to the bone marrow microenvironment are not fully understood. Although a number of cytoadhesion molecules, including the integrin VLA-4, CD44, and members of the selectin family, mediate the adhesion of HP to cultured bone marrow stroma, their contribution to progenitor trafficking in vivo was unclear until the recent development of a model of HP homing. Using this model, in which the effect of blocking antibodies on the distribution of HP shortly after transplantation is examined, it has been shown that VLA-4, through an interaction with its cognate ligand, VCAM-1, plays a central role in the homing of transplanted HP in vivo.[1] Data from other studies have provided evidence that CD44 and P- and E-selectin also contribute to stem cell lodgement.[2,3] In addition to classical cytoadhesion molecules, there is evidence that the chemokine SDF-1 mediates a component of stem cell homing, since antibodies both to SDF-1 and to its receptor CXCR4 block the homing of transplanted human progenitors in a NOD/SCID mouse model.[4] It is therefore likely that homing is a combinatorial process mediated through a number of different cytoadhesion pathways. Intriguingly, stem cell factor (SCF) and interleukin-6 (IL-6) upregulate the expression of SDF on bone marrow stroma and augment stem cell homing, raising the possibility that it may be possible to manipulate the early stages of stem cell engraftment in a clinical setting. The proliferation of HP once they have homed can be influenced by the administration of cytokines such as granulocyte colony-stimulating factor (G-CSF) and thrombopoietin, which can be employed to hasten neutrophil or platelet engraftment.

Determinants of allogeneic stem cell engraftment

It has previously been assumed that the durable engraftment of allogeneic stem cells is dependent upon two properties of a myeloablative conditioning regimen: the creation of 'space' within the bone marrow cavity and the prevention of rejection of transplanted allogeneic stem cells. The importance of creating 'niches' for incoming stem cells has been challenged by Storb's demonstration, in a dog model, that durable stem cell engraftment can be achieved using a non-myeloablative dose (200 cGy) of total-body irradiation (TBI), provided that post-transplant immunosuppression is delivered.[5] The observation that non-myeloablative doses of TBI facilitate engraftment despite marrow shielding confirms the importance of immunosuppression as opposed to any effect of low-dose radiation on the bone marrow microenvironment. An independent predictor of stem cell engraftment relates to the total number of stem cells transplanted. In murine models, major barriers to engraftment, such as MHC disparity and T-cell depletion (TCD), can be overcome by increasing the stem cell dose alone.[6] These observations have had a major impact on the development of clinical protocols for three reasons. First, they argue against myeloablation being a primary requirement of a conditioning regimen. Secondly, they emphasize the importance of host immunosuppression. Finally, they stress the benefit of optimizing the size of the stem cell inoculum, particularly if the intensity of the conditioning regimen is reduced (Table 17.1). In experimental models, a number of reduced-intensity regimens have been developed that aim to deliver sufficient immunosuppression to ensure engraftment. These include the use of low-dose TBI coupled with post-transplant immunosuppression and the use of thymic irradiation in combination with anti-T-cell antibodies. Recent advances in our understanding of the mechanism of T-cell activation have suggested that more-specific strategies may be developed to manipulate host-versus-graft (HVG) reactions in future, such as blockade of T-cell activation through disruption of the second signal mediated by the CD28/B7 pathway or CD40 ligand.[7]

Mechanism of graft failure in recipients of T-cell-depleted allografts

Depletion of donor T cells from the stem cell inoculum is associated with an increased risk of graft failure. Although the defect in stem cell engraftment associated with TCD can be compensated for by increasing the intensity of conditioning therapy, graft failure remains a significant complication of TCD, particularly after unrelated-donor transplantation. The cellular mechanisms mediating primary graft

Table 17.1 Future strategies for optimizing allogeneic stem cell engraftment

Approach	Method
1. Increased stem cell dose	Novel mobilizing agents: • Flt3 ligand • anti-VLA-4
2. Augmented stem cell homing	Upregulation of cytoadhesion molecules on: • haematopoietic progenitors, e.g. SDF-1 • Microenvironment, e.g. VCAM-1
3. Induction of tolerance	• CD28/B7 blockade • CD40-ligand modulation

rejection have not been fully delineated, but it is clear that alloreactive host $CD4^+$ and $CD8^+$ T cells as well as natural killer (NK) cells play an important role.[8] In murine models, using doubly mutant perforin-deficient or Fas-ligand-defective mice, the generation of alloreactive cytotoxic $CD8^+$ T cells capable of graft rejection can be shown to be mediated through both perforin- and Fas-ligand-dependent pathways.[9] The increased risk of graft failure in TCD allografts has been ascribed to the absence of alloreactive donor T cells that inhibit an HVG reaction. However, the demonstration that non-alloreactive donor T cells can facilitate engraftment provides evidence that T cells may act through alternative pathways such as cytokine release or the modulation of cytoadhesion molecule expression on HP.[10] A population of $CD8^+$ donor T cells that are αβ-receptor-negative and that facilitate engraftment of allogeneic and xenogeneic cells has recently been characterized.[11] Further characterization of the mechanism by which T cells facilitate engraftment may be of value in the design of low-intensity conditioning regimens that incorporate TCD.

MYELOABLATIVE CONDITIONING REGIMENS IN ALLOGENEIC TRANSPLANTATION

The pioneering work that demonstrated that allogeneic transplantation using HLA-identical sibling donors was capable of producing long-term disease-free survival in patients with CML employed a conditioning regimen consisting of a combination of cyclophosphamide and TBI.[12,13] It was subsequently shown that busulfan could be substituted for TBI with broadly similar results.[14] These two regimens have remained the most frequently used in patients undergoing allografting using both sibling donors and volunteer unrelated donors (VUDs), and remain the 'gold standard' by which novel reduced-intensity regimens must be judged. The impetus behind the recent development of non-myeloablative conditioning regimens reflects, to a large extent, the toxicity of current conditioning regimens. The steady improvement in outcome after allogeneic transplantation has led to an increased realization of the incidence and severity of late conditioning-related toxicities in patients in whom long-term disease-free survival can now be confidently predicted. The long-term complications of the currently used regimens reflect, to a large extent, the individual toxicities of the individual components of each conditioning regimen as discussed below.

Total-body irradiation

TBI exerts an important immunosuppressive and antileukaemic effect when administered in myeloablative doses. The degree of immunosuppression achieved is related to the TBI dose,[15] and increasing the dose of radiation overcomes the increased incidence of graft failure associated with TCD or the use of an unrelated donor.[16] TBI also plays an important role in determining the outcome of an allograft through its antileukaemic effect. Leukaemic cells from the malignant clone in CML are highly radiosensitive, and increased doses of TBI are associated with increased rates of leukaemic cell killing, although the clinical benefits of an increased TBI dose must always be balanced against the concomitant increase in regimen-related toxicity.

Administration of TBI in a myeloablative dose is associated with significant toxicity, which contributes to both immediate and delayed transplant-related mortality (TRM). The complications associated with a TBI-containing conditioning regimen manifest themselves as immediate, intermediate, or late toxicities. The immediate side-effects of nausea, vomiting, diarrhoea, and parotitis can usually be managed adequately with symptomatic therapy. The most significant intermediate-term complications are pneumonitis and veno-occlusive disease (VOD) of the liver. Radiobiological principles predict that the pulmonary toxicity of TBI can be reduced by either decreasing the overall dose of radiation administered or reducing the dose rate.[17] The possibility of reducing the incidence of interstitial pneumonitis (IP) by delivering TBI in a fractionated form is supported by a number of retrospective studies, although interpretation of these data is complicated by differences in the definition of IP and possible biases in treatment delivery. Although the benefit of fractionated TBI in terms of reducing IP has not been confirmed by a prospective randomized study, its use was associated with improved overall survival, and it is now the policy of most units to employ this form of delivery.[18,19] The magnitude of the TBI dose has also been implicated in the pathogenesis of VOD after allogeneic transplantation. Major long-term complications of TBI include cataract formation, endocrine disturbance, and infertility. The incidence of cataract formation after TBI has been substantially reduced from approximately 80% to 20–30% since the introduction of fractionated TBI, but it should be remembered that there is also a risk of cataract formation using non-TBI-containing regimens, which may reflect other factors associated with allogeneic transplantation, such as steroid exposure.[20] In children, the major endocrine toxicity, in addition to overt or compensated hypothyroidism, is growth failure, associated with decreased growth hormone production, although there is evidence that this effect may be abrogated by the use of fractionated TBI.[21] Infertility is highly likely after the use of a TBI-containing regimen, although the possibility of ovarian and testicular recovery exists.

The challenge of how to increase the antileukaemic effect of TBI while decreasing the associated organ toxicity is being addressed using radiolabelled immunoconjugates, which allow radiation to be targetted to the marrow using antibodies with a specificity for haematopoietic tissue. A number of antibodies are currently being investigated, including anti-CD20 and anti-CD45. Recent data from the Seattle group, using antibody to CD45 conjugated with ^{131}I, suggest that such an approach is feasible and allows a three- to fourfold increase in the dose of radiation delivered to haematopoietic tissue compared with organs such as liver and kidney.[22] Provisional data using this approach to intensify the conventional busulfan/cyclophosphamide conditioning regimen in patients with acute myeloid leukaemia in second complete remission are encouraging both in terms of limiting toxicity and decreasing relapse.[23]

Cyclophosphamide

High-dose cyclophosphamide is a component of both commonly used myeloablative conditioning regimens in CML. In common with TBI, it possesses both immunosuppressive and antileukaemic properties. Cyclophosphamide is a prodrug that must be metabolized by the P450 system in the liver to produce its metabolically active derivatives, including phosporamide mustard, which exert their antimetabolite activity through the production of interstrand and intrastrand DNA links. Pharmacological studies suggest that there may be a number of previously unrecognized interactions between cyclophosphamide and other components of conditioning regimens, such as busulfan, that increase cyclophosphamide clearance.[24] The two major complications of cyclophosphamide at the doses employed in allogeneic transplantation (120–200 mg/kg) are haemorrhagic cystitis and cardiac toxicity. The former can be substantially reduced by the use of the thiol sodium 2-mercaptoethanesulfonate (mesna), while the latter is very rare at doses of cyclophosphamide below 150 mg/kg.

Busulfan

The combination of busulfan and cyclophosphamide was originally chosen in order to design a conditioning regimen that did not require irradiation facilities. Busulfan was at the time widely used as an oral alkylating drug in the management of chronic-phase CML, but its potent in vivo activity against normal and malignant haematopoietic stem cells led to its adoption in both allogeneic and autologous transplantation. The major complications of busulfan therapy are VOD of the liver, pulmonary and CNS toxicity, and infertility. Busulfan is highly lipophilic, with very little protein binding, and is eliminated principally by the liver. The pharmacokinetics of busulfan have come under scrutiny in the last decade, and it is now recognized that there is considerable interpatient variability, which appears to contribute significantly to its toxicity.[25] In patients receiving busulfan-containing regimens, multivariate analysis shows that the busulfan area under the curve (AUC) is a predictor of the risk of developing severe VOD and survival.[26,27] In addition, it has been shown that a low busulfan AUC is associated with an increased risk of relapse in adults allografted for CML.[28] By using pharmacokinetic data obtained during the first day of busulfan administration, it is possible to adjust subsequent dosages with the aim of reducing the risk of VOD and improving the drug's therapeutic index. A recently developed intravenous formulation of busulfan is associated with less interpatient variation in the AUC and more predictable drug levels.[29] The other major side-effects of busulfan are seizures (which can be effectively prevented using prophylactic phenytoin or diazepam), pulmonary fibrosis, and infertility. Busulfan is associated with gonadal failure in both sexes, and recovery of normal function is rare, particularly in women.

CLINICAL DEVELOPMENT OF MYELOABLATIVE CONDITIONING REGIMENS

A number of randomized studies have addressed the question of whether there is an optimal conditioning regimen in patients undergoing transplantation from an HLA-identical sibling. Two of the studies were restricted to patients with CML in first chronic phase, and both demonstrated equivalence of the regimens in terms of overall survival (OS) and leukaemia-free survival (LFS)[30,31] (Figure 17.1). Two other studies compared outcome in patients with acute leukaemia or CML using either busulfan/cyclophosphamide or a TBI-based regimen (cyclophosphamide/TBI or etoposide/TBI).[32,33] Both studies demonstrated equivalence of outcome in patients with CML, although the Nordic study found improved survival in patients with advanced leukaemia using a TBI-based regimen. The other issue affecting the choice of myeloablative conditioning regimen is whether there is any clinical benefit to be gained from intensifying the conditioning regimen. The only prospective study to have addressed this issue comes from Seattle, where the effect of increasing the TBI dose to 15.75 Gy (compared with 12 Gy) was examined in patients undergoing a cyclophosphamide/TBI-conditioned sibling allograft for CML in first chronic phase.[34] Although the use of the higher TBI dose was associated with a reduced relapse rate, there was no improvement in overall survival, because of a concomitant increase in non-relapse mortality (Figure 17.2). No subsequent studies have been able to demonstrate that the decreased risk of leukaemic relapse associated with intensification of the conditioning regimen translates into improved overall survival, although encouraging single-centre data have been reported with the combination of etoposide and a cyclophosphamide/TBI regimen. This is also true in patients with accelerated-phase disease or blast crisis, where the increased risk of disease relapse has led to a search for more aggressive conditioning regimens. The most promising development in these patients is the development of radiolabelled immunotherapy, which offers the possibility of dose intensification without increased toxicity.[35]

The optimal conditioning regimen in patients undergoing SCT from a VUD is unresolved. The increased degree of HLA disparity attendant upon the use of such a donor is associated with an increased risk of graft failure compared with results obtained using a sibling donor.[36] The risk of primary graft failure is higher in patients with CML than in those with acute leukaemia, perhaps because of the absence of an immunosuppressive effect of prior intensive chemotherapy. The largest single-centre experience of VUD allografting in CML, from the Seattle group, using a cyclophosphamide/TBI regimen and no TCD, reports a 6% incidence of primary graft failure compared with the incidence of less than 1% in patients undergoing transplantation from an HLA-identical sibling.[37] In order to facilitate engraftment, most groups elect to use a cyclophosphamide/TBI regimen, although it has not been formally established whether a TBI-based regimen is necessary. Indeed, a number of investigators have reported similar rates of engraftment of T-cell-replete marrow using a busulfan/cyclophosphamide regimen.[38,39] No formal comparison of the two regimens has been reported in this setting. Future strategies to improve engraftment after VUD transplanta-

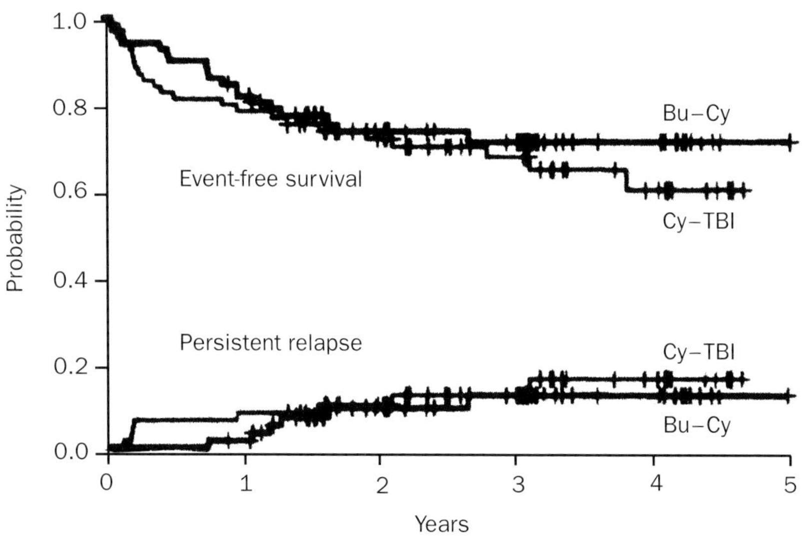

Figure 17.1 The probabilities of event-free survival and of developing persistent cytogenetic relapse for patients transplanted after the cyclophosphamide/TBI (Cy–TBI) or busulfan/cyclophosphamide (Bu–Cy) regimens are shown. Reproduced, with permission, from Clift et al (1994).[30]

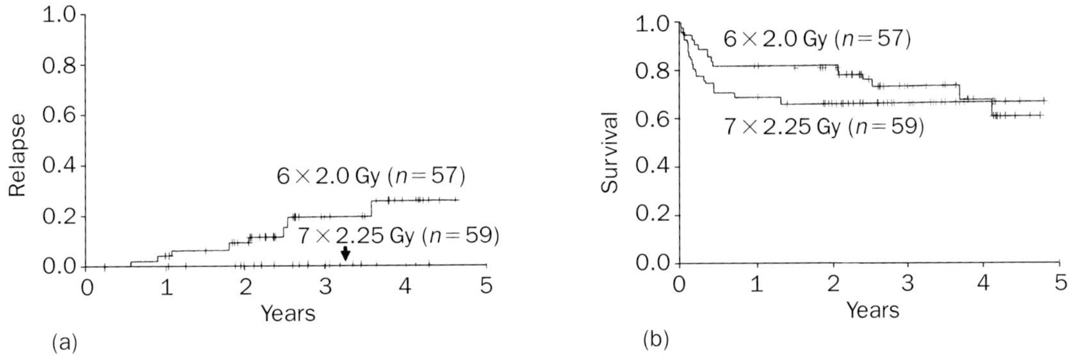

Figure 17.2 Probability of relapse (a) and survival (b) undergoing allogeneic transplantation from HLA-identical siblings using two irradiation regimens (12 Gy versus 15.75 Gy). Reproduced with permission, from Clift et al (1991).[34]

tion, particularly in the setting of TCD, are likely either to incorporate the use of a more intensely immunosuppressive conditioning regimen, with drugs such as fludarabine, or to increase the stem cell dose through the use of G-CSF-mobilized peripheral blood stem cells (PBSC).[40]

CLINICAL DEVELOPMENT OF NON-MYELOABLATIVE CONDITIONING REGIMENS

The growing realization of the importance of a GVL effect, coupled with the demonstration that a myeloablative conditioning regimen is not required to achieve durable stem cell engraftment, has led to the suggestion that the toxicity of allografting might be reduced by decreasing the intensity of the conditioning regimen. This approach, which dispenses with intensive chemoradiotherapy and utilizes the GVL effect of an allograft as the primary antileukaemic strategy, is of particular interest in diseases such as CML, where there is a well-documented GVL effect. The current approaches to the development of reduced-intensity conditioning regimens can be considered by classifying them according to the conditioning regimen employed.

Fludarabine-based regimens

Fludarabine, a highly immunosuppressive purine analogue, has been used by a number of centres in conjunction with non-myeloablative doses of alkylating drugs such as busulfan, melphalan, or cyclophosphamide to achieve engraftment of allogeneic stem cells. Giralt and Slavin and co-workers were the first to report durable engraftment of allogeneic peripheral blood stem cells using a fludarabine-based conditioning regimen.[41,42] Both studies were distinguished by the low TRM in patients with advanced malignancies who had been deemed unsuitable for a myeloablative conditioning regimen. The transplant procedure was well tolerated, with minimal mucositis, and engraftment was reported in all patients. The major complication was severe (grade 3–4) acute GVHD, which occurred in more than 20% of patients. Similar excellent rates of donor engraftment coupled with reduced toxicity have been reported using a preparative regimen combining cyclophosphamide with fludarabine by groups in Bethesda and Genoa.[43,44]

Low-dose TBI-based regimens

An alternative approach to delivering a non-myeloablative but highly immunosuppressive conditioning regimen has been developed by Storb's group based on data obtained in a canine model. In these studies, it has been shown that a non-myeloablative dose of TBI (200 cGy), in combination with post-transplant cyclosporin and mycophenolate mofetil, allows the generation of stable mixed chimeras with minimal toxicity.[5] This approach has been successfully translated into a clinical protocol. Forty-four patients with haematological malignancies, conditioned with 200 cGy TBI, cyclosporin and mycophenolate mofetil, have undergone transplantation using PBSC harvested from HLA-identical siblings.[45] The transplant procedure was well tolerated and in some cases performed on an outpatient basis. Non-fatal graft rejection was observed in approximately 20% of patients, particularly those with CML who had not received prior intensive chemotherapy. Clinically significant GVHD (grade 2–4) developed in 39% of patients. A major disease response was observed in 70% of patients. Of 8 patients with CML, 4 achieved a cytogenetic response and 3 a molecular response.

Regimens based on thymic irradiation and T-cell-depleting antibodies

Sykes and colleagues[46] have demonstrated, in a murine model, that the combination of thymic irradiation and in vivo TCD allows the engraftment of MHC-mismatched bone marrow cells and the acquisition of donor-specific tolerance. In an extension of this work, the Boston group has developed a protocol in which patients are conditioned using cyclophosphamide, antithymocyte globulin (ATG), and thymic irradiation.[47] This conditioning regimen permits the establishment of durable multilineage mixed chimerism after bone marrow transplantation from HLA-identical siblings or HLA-mismatched family members. GVHD has been observed, but is reported to be controllable with conventional therapy. In preliminary studies in 5 patients with refractory non-Hodgkin's lymphoma undergoing bone marrow transplantation, 3 showed evidence of response to therapy and 1 patient entered complete remission.

PROSPECTS FOR THE DEVELOPMENT OF REDUCED-INTENSITY CONDITIONING REGIMENS

Preliminary experience with reduced-intensity conditioning regimens confirms their ability to secure the engraftment of allogeneic stem cells, while significantly reducing regimen-related toxicity. This achievement has given rise to the hope that it may be possible to substantially improve the safety and tolerability of allografting in standard-risk patients, in addition to allowing its extension to patients in whom it is currently contraindicated. A number of unresolved questions remain to be answered before the use of reduced-intensity conditioning regimens can be viewed as standard therapy in CML. First, the ability of such regimens to deliver a sustained antileukaemic effect remains unclear. Although proof of principle has been demonstrated in a small number of patients with CML who achieved a molecular remission using such a regimen,[45,48] it remains unclear whether such an effect is durable and how often it is achievable. Secondly, it appears that these protocols are still associated with a significant risk of acute and chronic GVHD, limiting their application and effectiveness, particularly in elderly patients. In addition, the presence of active GVHD prevents the timely application of donor lymphocyte infusion (DLI). It will therefore be of importance to define whether strategies such as TCD or prolonging the duration of cyclosporin administration can reduce the risk of GVHD without compromising engraftment or GVL.[49] This will be of particular importance in the design of non-myeloablative protocols in which VUDs will be used as the source of stem cells, where preliminary data suggest that there is a high risk of severe GVHD. Thirdly, although there is an association between the acquisition of full donor lymphoid chimerism and the delivery of a sustained GVL effect in patients with CML when using a myeloablative conditioning regimen,[50] it has not been established whether this remains true when using a reduced-intensity regimen. Careful studies correlating chimerism status with disease response will therefore be critical in designing DLI schedules.[51] Similarly, although escalating schedules allowing the administration of DLI with minimal toxicity after myeloablative conditioning have been established,[52,53] the toxicity and consequent feasibility of lymphocyte infusion early after transplantation remain to be determined. Thus research into approaches that maximize the effective dose of lymphocytes administered while minimizing the risk of GVHD are central to the success of these programmes. Lastly, few data are available concerning the medium- and long-term toxicity of these protocols. Data concerning the nature of immune reconstitution will be important in view of the intensely immunosuppressive nature of some of the conditioning therapies. Despite these caveats, preliminary experience with these protocols gives grounds for hope that our increased understanding of the biology of stem cell engraftment and the mechanism of the GVL effect will in the future be translated into the development of increasingly effective and safe protocols for allogeneic transplantation.

T-CELL DEPLETION AND CD34 SELECTION

GVHD remains the most important preventable cause of morbidity and mortality after allogeneic SCT. However, although depletion of T cells from the donor stem cell inoculum has the capacity to reduce both the incidence and severity of acute and chronic GVHD, enthusiasm for this approach has been tempered by the increased risk of leukaemic relapse and graft failure associated with this approach. However, the demonstration by Kolb and colleagues that DLI is effective in restoring remission in patients who relapse after allogeneic SCT for CML has led to a revival of interest in TCD in CML.[54]

Methods of T-cell depletion

On average, a bone marrow harvest contains approximately 10^9 T cells, resulting in an infused T-cell dose in the region of $(1–2) \times 10^7$ T cells/kg. The corresponding figures in patients undergoing transplantation using a PBSC harvest are approximately 1 log higher. A number of investigators have attempted to define the number of infused T cells below which the likelihood of developing significant acute GVHD is unlikely. Although such studies need to be interpreted with caution given the impact of other factors such as donor and patient age, degree of HLA disparity, and intensity of the conditioning therapy, there appears to be a very low risk of severe acute GVHD when the T-cell dose is less than 1×10^5 T cells/kg.[55,56]

A number of strategies have been designed to reduce the number of T cells in the donor stem cell inoculum.[57] Broadly speaking, these can be divided into ex vivo methods in which the stem cell product is manipulated prior to infusion or in vivo TCD where antibodies that bind to infused T cells are administered to the patient prior to transplantation of an unmanipulated product. Initial approaches to ex vivo TCD employed antibodies with specificity against T-cell epitopes, which, when incubated with donor marrow in the presence of complement, resulted in a 2–3 log reduction in T-cell number. Later studies used antibodies with a broader specificity, such as Campath antibodies, which recognize the CD52 antigen on T and B lymphocytes and monocytes. Both approaches are successful in reducing the incidence of both acute and chronic GVHD. The increasing use of mobilized PBSC in allogeneic SCT, coupled with the development of efficient $CD34^+$ cell selection systems, has allowed the development of passive methods of TCD. Such an approach allows consistent engraftment of donor stem cells with minimal acute GVHD using both myeloablative and non-myeloablative conditioning regimens, and permits easy manipulation of the T-cell dose administered.[58] Campath antibodies have also been used successfully in the setting of in vivo

TCD, and reduce the incidence and severity of acute and chronic GVHD.[59] However, while such an approach eliminates the need to manipulate the stem cell graft and is simple to perform, it is difficult to quantitate or control the numbers of T cells infused using this approach.

Results with TCD

Early studies of TCD, using ex vivo treatment of marrow with Campath-1M, in patients undergoing allogeneic SCT for CML demonstrated that, although effective in reducing the incidence of GVHD, it was associated with a marked increase in the risk of leukaemic relapse compared with a group of historical controls.[60] This was confirmed by an International Bone Marrow Transplant Registry (IBMTR) survey demonstrating a 5.4 relative risk for relapse in patients with CML who had undergone TCD compared with T-cell-replete controls.[61] In VUD transplants, the increased HLA disparity has been reported to compensate for the reduced GVL effect produced by TCD, although this does not appear to be the case in patients receiving in vivo TCD.[59,62] The disparity is likely to reflect the differing degrees of TCD achieved. The increased risk of relapse associated with TCD can be compensated for by intensifying the conditioning regimen by adding cytosine arabinoside or thiotepa to the conventional cyclophosphamide/TBI conditioning regimen. Although this has been reported to decrease the risk of relapse in some series, it appears to come at the expense of increased regimen-related toxicity.

In common with the experience gained in other diseases, the use of TCD in patients allografted for CML has been associated with an increased risk of primary graft failure and delayed immune reconstitution. A number of reports have demonstrated a correlation between TBI dose and engraftment, and increasing the intensity of the conditioning regimen has been shown to improve engraftment in the setting of TCD.[63] An alternative approach is to increase the number of haematopoietic progenitors transplanted by using peripheral blood rather than bone marrow as the stem cell source.[58] Impaired immune reconstitution remains a major complication of TCD. This appears to be a particular problem in cytomegalovirus (CMV)-positive patients, where, in addition to an increased risk of CMV reaction, there is also an independent increase in TRM.[64]

Future approaches to TCD in conditioning regimens

The demonstration that DLI can salvage the majority of patients who relapse after allogeneic SCT for CML, coupled with the development of safer DLI regimens, has led to a revival of interest in the role of TCD in CML. A retrospective analysis from two transplant groups in Boston confirmed the ability of TCD to decrease the incidence of GVHD while demonstrating that the increased risk of relapse (62% versus 24%) could be mitigated by the prompt administration of donor lymphocytes.[65] Selective depletion of $CD6^+$ and $CD8^+$ T-cell subsets has been explored as an approach that allows retention of a GVL effect while achieving a reduction in the risk of GVHD.[66,67] In addition, the ability to achieve efficient transduction of lymphocytes with transgenes such as the herpes simplex virus thymidine kinase (HSV-Tk) gene raises the possibility of exploiting a GVL effect while retaining the ability to control clinically significant GVHD. Alternative approaches include the selective depletion of alloreactive T cells by incubation of the stem cell inoculum ex vivo.[68] The rational development of such strategies is, however, dependent on further understanding of the cellular basis of the GVL effect. It is to be hoped that progress in this area, coupled with a clearer understanding of the contribution of infused T cells to both stem cell engraftment and post-transplant immune reconstitution, will allow the rational development of cellular therapies for the treatment of CML.

REFERENCES

1. Papayannopoulou T, Craddock C, Nakamoto B et al, The VLA4/VCAM-1 adhesion pathway defines contrasting mechanisms of lodgement of transplanted murine hemopoietic progenitors between bone marrow and spleen. *Proc Natl Acad Sci USA* 1995; **92:** 9647–51.
2. Frenette J, Subbarao S, Mazo I et al, Endothelial selectins and vascular cell adhesion molecule-1 promote hematopoietic progenitor homing to bone marrow. *Proc Natl Acad Sci USA* 1998; **95:** 14423–8.
3. Vermeulen V, Le Pesteur F, Gagenerault M et al, Role of adhesion molecules in the homing and mobilization of murine hematopoietic stem and progenitor cells. *Blood* 1998; **92:** 894–900.
4. Peled A, Petit I, Kollet O et al, Dependence of human stem cell engraftment and repopulation of NOD/SCID mice on CXCR4. *Science* 1999; **283:** 845–8.
5. Yu C, Storb R, Mathey B et al, DLA-identical bone marrow grafts after low-dose total body irradiation: effects of high dose corticosteroids and cyclosporine on engraftment. *Blood* 1995; **86:** 4376–81.
6. Bacher-Lustig E, Rachamim N, Li H et al, Megadose of T cell-depleted bone marrow overcomes MHC barriers in sublethally irradiated mice. *Nature Med* 1995; **1:** 1268–73.
7. Guinan E, Boussiotis V, Neuberg D et al, Transplantation of anergic histoincompatible bone marrow grafts. *N Engl J Med* 1999; **340:** 1701 14.
8. Martin P, Akatsuka Y, Hahne M, Sale G, Involvement of donor T-cell cytotoxic effector mechanisms in preventing allogeneic marrow graft rejection. *Blood* 1998; **92:** 2177–81.
9. Baker M, Riley R, Podack E et al, Graft-versus-host-disease-associated lymphoid hypoplasia and B cell dysfunction is dependent upon donor T cell-mediated Fas-ligand function, but not perforin function. *Proc Natl Acad Sci USA* 1997; **94:** 1366–70.
10. Fowler D, Whitfield B, Livingston M et al, Non-host reactive donor CD8+ T cells of Tc2 phenotype potently inhibit marrow graft rejection. *Blood* 1998; **91:** 4045–50.
11. Kaufman C, Colson Y, Wren SM et al, Phenotypic characterisation of a novel bone marrow derived cell that facilitates engraftment of allogeneic stem cells. *Blood* 1994; **84:** 2436–46.
12. Goldman J, Apperley J, Jones L et al, Bone marrow transplantation for patients with chronic myeloid leukaemia. *N Engl J Med* 1986; **314:** 202–7.
13. Thomas E, Clift R, Fefer A et al, Marrow transplantation for the treatment of chronic myelogenous leukemia. *Ann Intern Med* 1986; **105:** 155–63.
14. Tutschka P, Copelan E, Klein J et al, Bone marrow transplantation for leukemia following a new busulfan and cyclophosphamide regimen. *Blood* 1987; **70:** 1382–8.
15. Down J, Tarbell N, Thames H et al, Syngeneic and allogeneic bone marrow engraftment after total body irradiation: dependence on dose, dose rate and fractionation. *Blood* 1991; **71:** 661–9.
16. Champlin R, Ho W, Mitsuyasu R et al, Graft failure and leukemic relapse following T-lymphocyte depleted bone marrow transplantation: effect of intensification of immunosuppressive conditioning. *Transplant Proc* 1987; **19:** 2616–19.
17. Peters L, Withers H, Cundiff J et al, Radiobiological considerations in the use of total-body irradiation for bone-marrow transplantation. *Radiology* 1979; **131:** 243–7.
18. Thomas E, Clift R, Hersman J et al, Marrow transplantation for acute nonlymphocytic leukemia in first remission using fractionated or single dose irradiation. *Int J Radiat Oncol Biol Phys* 1982; **8:** 817–21.
19. Deeg H, Sullivan K, Buckner C et al, Marrow transplantation for acute non lymphoblastic leukemia in first remission: toxicity and long term follow up of patients conditioned with single dose or fractionated total body irradiation. *Bone Marrow Transplant* 1986; **1:** 151–7.
20. Deeg H, Flournoy N, Sullivan K, Cataracts after total body irradiation and marrow transplantation: a sparing effect of dose fractionation. *Int J Radiat Oncol Biol Phys* 1984; **10:** 957–64.
21. Sanders J, Late effects in children receiving total body irradiation for bone marrow transplantation. *Radiother Oncol* 1990; **18**(Suppl 1): 82–7.
22. Appelbaum FR, Is there a better way to deliver total body irradiation? *Bone Marrow Transplant* 1992; **10**(Suppl 10)**:** 77–81.
23. Matthews DC, Appelbaum FR, Eary JF et al, Development of a marrow transplant regimen for acute leukaemia using targeted hematopoietic irradiation delivered by ^{131}I-labeled anti-CD45 antibody, combined with cyclophosphamide and total body irradiation. *Blood* 1995; **85:** 1122–31.

24. Slattery J Kalhorn T, McDonald J et al, Conditioning regimen-dependent disposition of cyclophosphamide and hydroxycyclophosphamide in human marrow transplantation patients. *J Clin Oncol* 1996; **14:** 1484–94.
25. Hassan M, Ljungman P, Bolme P et al, Busulfan bioavailability. *Blood* 1994; **84:** 2144–50.
26. Grochow L, Jones R, Brundrett R et al, Pharmacokinetics of busulfan: correlation with veno-occlusive disease in patients undergoing bone marrow transplantation. *Cancer Chemother Pharmacol* 1989; **25:** 55–61.
27. Dix S, Wingard J, Mullins R et al, Association of busulfan area under the curve with veno-occlusive disease following BMT. *Bone Marrow Transplant* 1996; **17:** 225–30.
28. Slattery J, Clift R, Buckner C et al, Marrow transplantation for chronic myeloid leukemia: the influence of plasma busulfan levels on the outcome of transplantation. *Blood* 1997; **89:** 3055–60.
29. Andersson B, McWilliams K, Tran H et al, IV busulfan, cyclophosphamide and allogeneic hemopoietic stem cells for chronic myeloid leukemia. *Blood* 1999; **92:** 285a.
30. Clift R, Buckner C, Thomas E et al, Marrow transplantation for chronic myeloid leukaemia: a randomized study comparing cyclophosphamide and total body irradiation with busulfan and cyclophosphamide. *Blood* 1994; **84:** 2036–43.
31. Devergie A, Blaise D, Attal M et al, Allogeneic bone marrow transplantation for chronic myeloid leukaemia in first chronic phase: a randomised trial of busulfan–Cytoxan versus Cytoxan–total body irradiation as preparative regimen: a report from the French Society of Bone Marrow Graft (SFGM). *Blood* 1995; **85:** 2263–8.
32. Ringden O, Ruutu T, Remberger M et al, A randomised trial comparing busulfan with total body irradiation as conditioning in allogeneic bone marrow transplant recipients with leukemia: a report from the Nordic Bone Marrow Transplant Group. *Blood* 1994; **83:** 2723–30.
33. Blume K, Kopecky K, Henslee-Downey J et al, A prospective randomised comparison of total body irradiation–etoposide versus busulfan–cyclophosphamide as preparatory regimens for bone marrow transplantation in patients with leukemia who were not in first remission. *Blood* 1993; **81:** 2187–93.
34. Clift R, Buckner CD, Appelbaum FR et al, Allogeneic marrow transplantation in patients with chronic myeloid leukemia in the chronic phase: a randomised trial of two irradiation regimens. *Blood* 1991; **77:** 1660–5.
35. Appelbaum FR, Radioimmunotherapy and hematopoietic cell transplantation. In: *Hematopoietic Cell Transplantation* (Thomas ED, Blume KG, Forman SJ, eds). Cambridge, MA: Blackwell Scientific, 1999: 168–74.
36. McGlave PB, Shu XO, Wen W et al, Unrelated donor marrow transplantation for chronic myelogenous leukemia: 9 years experience of the National Marrow Donor Program. *Blood* 2000; **95:** 2219–25.
37. Hansen J, Gooley T, Martin P et al, Bone marrow transplants from unrelated donors for patients with chronic myeloid leukemia. *N Engl J Med* 1998; **338:** 962–8.
38. Topolsky D, Crilley P, Styler M et al, Unrelated donor bone marrow transplantation without T cell depletion using a chemotherapy only conditioning regimen: low incidence of failed engraftment and severe acute GVHD. *Bone Marrow Transplant* 1995; **15:** 361–5.
39. Bertz H, Potthoff K, Mertesmann R, Finke J, Busulfan/cyclophosphamide in volunteer unrelated donor (VUD) BMT: excellent feasibility and low incidence of treatment-related toxicity. *Bone Marrow Transplant* 1997; **19:** 1169–73.
40. Ringden O, Remberger M, Runde V et al, Peripheral blood stem cell transplantation from unrelated donors: a comparison with marrow transplantation. *Blood* 1999; **94:** 455–64.
41. Giralt S, Estey E, Albitar M et al, Engraftment of allogeneic hematopoietic progenitor cells with purine analog-containing chemotherapy: harnessing graft-versus-leukemia without myeloablative therapy. *Blood* 1997; **89:** 4531–6.
42. Slavin S, Nagser A, Naparstet E et al, Nonmyeloablative stem cell transplantation and cell therapy as an alternative to conventional bone marrow transplantation with lethal cytoreduction for the treatment of malignant and nonmalignant hematologic diseases. *Blood* 1998; **91:** 756–63.
43. Carella A, Lerma E, Dejana A et al, Engraftment of HLA-matched sibling hematopoietic stem cells after immunosuppressive conditioning regimen in patients with hematologic neoplasias. *Haematologica* 1998; **83:** 904–9.
44. Childs R, Clave E, Bahceci E et al, Non-

myeloablative allogeneic peripheral blood stem cell transplants (PBSCT) for malignant diseases reduces transplant-related mortality. *Blood* 1998; **92:** 552a.

45. McSweeney P, Shizuru J, Bensinger W et al, Outpatient PBSC allografts using immunosuppression with low dose TBI before and cyclosporine and mycophenolate mofetil after transplant. *Blood* 1998; **92:** 519a.
46. Sykes M, Szot G, Swenson K et al, Induction of high levels of allogeneic hematopoietic reconstitution and donor-specific tolerance without myelosuppressive conditioning. *Nature Med* 1997; **3:** 783–7.
47. Sykes M, Preffer F, McCaffey S et al, Mixed lymphohaemopoietic chimerism and graft-versus-lymphoma effects after non-myeloablative chemotherapy and HLA-mismatched bone marrow transplantation. *Lancet* 1999; **353:** 1755–9.
48. Childs T, Epperson D, Bahceci E et al, Molecular remission of chronic myeloid leukaemia following a non-myeloablative allogeneic peripheral blood stem cell transplant: in vivo and in vitro evidence for a graft-versus-leukaemia effect. *Br J Haematol* 1999; **107:** 396–400.
49. Craddock C, Bardy P, Kreiter S et al, Engraftment of T-cell-depleted allogeneic haematopoietic stem cell using a reduced intensity conditioning regimen. *Br J Haematol* 2000; **111:** 797–800.
50. Mackinnon S, Barnett L, Heller G et al, Minimal residual disease is more common in patients who have mixed T-cell chimerism after bone marrow transplantation for chronic myelogenous leukemia. *Blood* 1994; **83:** 3409–16.
51. Childs R, Clave E, Bahceci E et al, Kinetics of engraftment in non-myeloablative allogeneic peripheral blood transplantation: an analysis of hematopoietic-lineage chimerism. *Blood* 1998; **92:** 520a.
52. Mackinnon S, Papadopoulos E, Carabasi M et al, Adoptive immunotherapy evaluating escalating doses of donor leucocytes for relapse of chronic myeloid leukemia after bone marrow transplantation: separation of graft-versus-leukemia effect from graft-versus-host disease. *Blood* 1995; **86:** 1261–8.
53. Dazzi F, Szydlo R, Craddock C et al, Comparison of single-dose and escalating-dose regimens of donor lymphocyte infusions for relapse after allografting for chronic myeloid leukemia. *Blood* 2000; **95:** 67–71.
54. Kolb H, Schattenberg A, Goldman J et al, Graft-versus-leukemia effect of donor lymphocyte transfusions in marrow grafted patients. *Blood* 1995; **86:** 2041–50.
55. Kernan N, Collins N, Juliano L et al, Clonable lymphocytes in T-cell depleted bone marrow transplants correlate with the development of graft versus host disease. *Blood* 1986; **68:** 770–3.
56. Verdonck L, de Gast G, van Heugten H et al, A fixed low number of T cells in HLA-identical allogeneic bone marrow transplantation. *Blood* 1990; **75:** 776–80.
57. Martin P, Kernan N, T cell depletion for the prevention of graft-versus-host disease. In: *Graft versus Host Disease: Research and Clinical Management*. 1996: 615–37.
58. Urbano-Ispizua A, Rozman C, Martinez C et al, Rapid engraftment without significant graft-versus-host-disease after allogeneic transplantation of CD34[+] selected cells from peripheral blood. *Blood* 1997; **89:** 3967–73.
59. Spencer A, Szydlo R, Brookes P et al, Bone marrow transplantation for chronic myeloid leukemia with volunteer unrelated donors using ex vivo or in vivo T-cell depletion: major prognostic impact of HLA class I identity between donor and recipient. *Blood* 1995; **86:** 3590–7.
60. Goldman J, Gale R, Horowitz M, Bone marrow transplantation for chronic myelogenous leukemia in chronic phase. Increased risk of relapse associated with T cell depletion. *Ann Intern Med* 1988; **108:** 806–14.
61. Horowitz M, Rowlings P, Passweg J et al, Allogeneic bone marrow transplantation for CML: a report from the International Bone Marrow Transplant Registry. *Bone Marrow Transplant* 1996; **17** (Suppl 3)**:** S5–6.
62. Enright H, Davies S, De Fon T et al, Relapse after non T cell depleted allogeneic bone marrow transplantation for chronic myelogenous leukemia: early transplantation, use of an unrelated donor and chronic graft versus host disease are protective. *Blood* 1996; **88:** 714–20.
63. Martin P, Hansen J, Torok-Storb B et al, Graft failure in patients receiving T cell depleted HLA-identical allogeneic marrow transplants. *Bone Marrow Transplant* 1988; **3:** 445–56.
64. Broers A, van der Holt R, van Esser J, Increased transplant-related morbidity and mortality in CMV-seropositive patients despite highly effective prevention of CMV disease after allogeneic T-cell-depleted stem cell transplantation. *Blood* 2000; **95:** 2240–5.

65. Sehn L, Alyea E, Weller E et al, Comparative outcomes of T-cell-depleted and non-T-cell depleted allogeneic bone marrow transplantation for chronic myelogenous leukemia: impact of donor lymphocyte infusion. *J Clin Oncol* 1999; **17:** 561–70.
66. Champlin R, Ho W, Gajewski J et al, Selective depletion of CD8+ T lymphocytes for prevention of graft-versus-host disease after allogeneic bone marrow transplantation. *Blood* 1990; **76:** 418–23.
67. Soiffer R, Fairclough D, Robertson M et al, CD60 depleted allogeneic bone marrow transplantation for acute leukaemia in first complete remission. *Blood* 1997; **89:** 3039–47.
68. Koh M, Prentice H, Lowdell M et al, Selective removal of alloreactive cells from haematopoietic stem cell grafts: graft engineering for GVHD prophylaxis. *Bone Marrow Transplant* 1999; **23:** 1071–9.

18

Blood versus marrow stem cells

Peter Dreger, Norbert Schmitz

CONTENTS • Introduction • PBSC harvesting and donor-related considerations • Reconstitution of haematopoiesis • Reconstitution of the immune system • Acute GVHD • Chronic GVHD • Alternative donors and GVHD • GVL effects • Reduced-intensity conditioning • Graft engineering and cell component therapy • Conclusions

INTRODUCTION

At present, allogeneic stem cell transplantation (SCT) is the only curative treatment for chronic myeloid leukaemia (CML), and CML is one of the most important indications for allogeneic SCT. Whereas bone marrow (BM) was the only source of allogeneic stem cells for over two decades, peripheral blood stem cells (PBSC) mobilized by growth factors have increasingly been used for allogeneic transplantation during recent years. After the first series of patients successfully allografted with granulocyte colony-stimulating factor (G-CSF)-mobilized PBSC were reported in the early 1990s,[1–3] allogeneic PBSC transplantation (PBSCT) instead of allogeneic bone marrow transplantation (BMT) rapidly gained worldwide acceptance; in Europe already by 1998, PBSCT accounted for 36% of all allogeneic stem cell transplants performed (compared with less than 1% in 1993).[4]

The purpose of this chapter is to give a concise and clinically oriented overview of current results and perspectives for allogeneic PBSCT in general, with particular focus on reconstitution of haematopoiesis and the immune system, acute and chronic graft-versus-host-disease (GVHD), graft-versus-leukaemia (GVL) effects, and approaches to manipulate the functional components of PBSC grafts ex vivo ('graft engineering'). Owing to the crucial role of immune-mediated mechanisms in the therapeutic effects of allogeneic SCT in CML, the latter two issues are of particular importance in the context of allogeneic SCT for the treatment of this disease.

PBSC HARVESTING AND DONOR-RELATED CONSIDERATIONS

Although basically PBSC grafts can be obtained without mobilization (i.e. during 'steady-state' haematopoiesis), the circulating stem cell pool should be expanded by exogeneous stimulation prior to stem cell harvesting to ensure reasonable collection efforts and adequate graft quality. Agents used for PBSC mobilization are:

- haematopoietic growth factors,
- cytotoxic chemotherapy, or
- a combination of both.

For obvious reasons, PBSC mobilization employing chemotherapy is not suitable for healthy donors. Thus, mobilization regimens employed for allogeneic stem cell donation are restricted to cytokines alone. To date, G-CSF and granulocyte–macrophage colony-stimulating factor (GM-CSF) are the only growth factors that have been used for the priming of healthy individuals for harvesting of mobilized PBSC.

Both cytokines can be used for expansion of the peripheral blood progenitor cell pool in patients with cancer as well as in healthy donors.[5–11] G-CSF is routinely used for this purpose because of its superior mobilization efficacy,[7,8] and, more importantly, because it is the safest among the agents available for PBSC priming. The use of G-CSF for PBSC mobilization in healthy donors is usually associated with mild to moderate bone pain. More severe adverse events have been observed very rarely;[12] however, individual cases of life-threatening complications have been reported, mainly involving thromboembolic incidents, including myocardial infarction,[13] cerebrovascular disorders,[11] splenic rupture,[14] and anaphylactoid reactions.[15]

In contrast, GM-CSF has a higher risk of inducing systemic adverse effects. Another disadvantage of GM-CSF is that it must be administered for a longer period of time until the PBSC peak is reached.[16]

Additional growth factors, including interleukin-3 (IL-3), IL-8, thrombopoietin, and Flt3 ligand (FL), may have some stem cell-mobilizing capacity when administered alone.[17–21] Because there is as yet no evidence that any of these agents is superior to G-CSF in terms of efficacy and safety, and because the use of all of these cytokines for mobilization is still experimental, they may not be utilized outside clinical trials.

Based on the data currently available, mobilization should be performed with G-CSF 10–16 μg/kg divided into two aliquots.[22] Leukapheresis should start on day 4 or 5 of G-CSF administration, and should not be continued after day 7 of G-CSF administration. Although long-term adverse effects cannot be definitely ruled out at this point of time, G-CSF has been administered safely to large cohorts of patients and healthy donors for the treatment of neutropenia or for PBSC mobilization. The available data do not suggest that the incidence of malignancy might be increased in individuals exposed to G-CSF. Altogether, the risks of G-CSF priming and leukapheresis in healthy donors appear to be acceptable if compared with those of BM collection.

In conclusion, PBSC harvesting from healthy donors is not a trivial procedure without any risk, but appropriate selection of donors should allow one to avoid serious complications. The joint 'ad hoc' Workshop of the International Bone Marrow Transplant Registry (IBMTR), the European Group for Blood and Marrow Transplantation (EBMT) and the National Marrow Donor Program (NMDP) has identified a number of conditions that do not appear to be perfectly compatible with PBSC donation. These include cardiovascular risk factors, a history of thromboembolic events, inflammatory or autoimmune disorders, a history of malignancy, and poor peripheral veins.[11] Furthermore, all efforts should be undertaken to ensure long-term monitoring of healthy donors of both PBSC and BM via national and international transplant registries.

RECONSTITUTION OF HAEMATOPOIESIS

Numerous studies have demonstrated that all subsets of progenitor cells or stem cell equivalents that can be assayed in vitro or in vivo are present in G-CSF-mobilized PBSC products, and there is no evidence that components essential for engraftment are lacking or critically reduced in PBSC grafts obtained from healthy donors.[23–26] In particular, the numbers of cells expressing the CD34 antigen have been found (similar to observations in the autologous setting[27]) to be more than twofold higher in peripheral blood allografts than in marrow grafts.[6,28–30] As a consequence of this, and bearing in mind the striking advantages of autologous PBSC over marrow grafts in terms of speed of engraftment, one of the main expectations that prompted investigators to pursue allogeneic PBSCT was the possibility of accelerating haematopoietic recovery with mobilized blood grafts.

The initial experience with identical twins

did indeed confirm that primary transplantation of G-CSF-primed PBSC consistently resulted in rapid and sustained restoration of haematopoiesis, which was considerably faster compared with the engraftment of historical controls from the same centre receiving syngeneic BM.[31,32] The speed of haematopoietic recovery after allogeneic PBSCT, however, turned out to be much more variable than what is seen after syngeneic or autologous transplantation. The main reason for this seems to be the genetic difference between graft and recipient, which may delay engraftment per se, may cause complications such as GVHD or viral infections, and may necessitate the use of cytotoxic drugs such as methotrexate. Nevertheless, the reconstitution of haematopoiesis after allogeneic PBSCT tended to be more rapid than in historical BM controls.[1–3] These first data were confirmed by randomized trials and matched-pair analyses reported very recently. Table 18.1 lists the results of the eight prospective randomized studies published to date,[33–40] demonstrating that PBSCT results in acceleration of neutrophil recovery by 2–6 days and platelet recovery by 5–8 days. The IBMTR and the EBMT compared the engraftment data of 288 patients with leukaemia who were allografted with PBSC from an HLA-identical sibling donor with the results of 536 matched recipients of BM. Similar to the randomized trials, a highly significant difference in favour of the PBSC group was found with regard to neutrophil and platelet engraftment ($p < 0.001$ for both).[41]

An important factor adversely affecting engraftment is the use of methotrexate post transplant,[42] while a striking correlation between the speed of engraftment and the number of $CD34^+$ cells infused could not be shown. Although unaffected engraftment was seen with $CD34^+$ cell numbers less than 2×10^6/kg, a dose of more than $(4–5) \times 10^6$/kg is currently regarded as the minimum target to ensure engraftment.[43,44]

The engraftment of allogeneic PBSC is durable, as shown by molecular analysis of chimerism and blood group typing.[1,2,45] The strong haematopoietic capacity of G-CSF-mobilized PBSC is also underlined by successful PBSC rescue of patients with non-engraftment after BMT.[46–49]

RECONSTITUTION OF THE IMMUNE SYSTEM

Compared with values observed in allogeneic marrow grafts, PBSC harvests contain about one log more T cells.[6,30,50] Not only is this important with regard to potential GVH and GVL activities of the graft, but it also has implications for the reconstitution of the immune system post transplant. Recent studies suggest that early T-cell regeneration in adult recipients after myeloablative treatment is mainly determined by the amount of mature T cells contained in the graft.[51–54] Thus, allogeneic PBSCT may be associated with acceleration of both haematopoietic and immune engraftment. Two consecutive studies from a single centre indicated that the recovery of T-cell numbers and function after allogeneic PBSCT is indeed faster than after BMT, resulting in a normalization of the CD4 : CD8 ratio as early as 6 months after transplant.[45,55] Accelerated lymphocyte recovery after PBSCT in comparison to BMT was also seen by the majority of other investigators dealing with this issue; however, immunoglobulin recovery does not appear to be faster in recipients of PBSC.[36,56–58] Although a lower rate of fatal infections after PBSCT was observed in one large randomized study,[35] and was also suggested by the IBMTR matched-pair analysis (at least in subgroups of patients),[41] it is not clear at present if the enhanced immune reconstitution may translate into a reduction of infectious complications post transplant.

Similar to the situation after BMT, the natural killer (NK)-cell compartment is the first lymphocyte subset recovering to normal levels after PBSC graft infusion. In spite of this, NK-cell function may be impaired for prolonged periods of time post transplant. Whether this has to do with the reduced functional capacity of the NK cells present in mobilized PBSC collection products that has been found by different investigators remains to be determined.[57,59]

Table 18.1 Haematopoietic recovery after stem cell transfusion: results of randomized studies with HLA-identical siblings

Investigators	No. of patients evaluable	Day ANC $>0.5 \times 10^9$/l		Day platelets $>20 \times 10^9$/l	
		PBSC	BM	PBSC	BM
Vigorito et al (1998)[33,a]	37	+16	+18	+12	+17[e]
Mahmoud et al (1999)[34,a]	30	+8	+16[e]	+11[f]	+18[e]
Bensinger et al (2001)[35,b]	172	+16	+21[e]	+13	+19[e]
Powles et al (2000)[36,c]	39	+18	+23[e]	+11	+18[e]
Blaise et al (2000)[37,b]	111	+15	+21[e]	+13[f]	+21[e,f]
Heldal et al (2000)[38,d]	61	+17	+23[e]	+13	+21[e]
Simpson et al (2000)[39,b]	228	+18	+22[e]	+16	+22[e]
Schmitz et al (2000)[40,b]	350	+12	+15[e]	+15	+20[e]

[a]Single-centre, open-label randomized study.
[b]Multicentre, open-label randomized study.
[c]Single-centre, double-blind randomized study.
[d]Single-centre, open-label randomized study with 5 one-antigen-mismatched family donors in the PBSC group versus 1 in the BM group.
[e]$p < 0.05$.
[f]Recovery to 25×10^9/l.

ACUTE GVHD

Since T cells are the effector cells of both acute and chronic GVH reactions, it was a major concern that the large numbers of T cells contained in PBSC grafts might give rise to an increased incidence or severity of GVHD. However, the initial impression was that the incidence of acute GVHD was lower rather than higher compared with allogeneic BMT.[1–3] With higher patient numbers, it became evident that with standard immunosuppression, there is no striking difference between PBSCT and BMT in terms of acute GVHD. However, in seven of the eight randomized studies summarized in Table 18.2, acute GVHD tended to be more frequent in recipients of PBSC, although this difference was statistically significant only in the largest trial the (EBMT study[40]). Grade II–IV disease was observed in 21–52% of PBSC recipients, compared with 10–39% of BM recipients.[33–39] The IBMTR/EBMT matched-pair analysis also demonstrated a trend for a greater incidence of acute grade II–IV GVHD after allogeneic PBSCT (40% versus 35%; p not significant).[41] Altogether, it seems that PBSCT results in an increased incidence of acute GVHD, although the difference from BMT is not very striking.

It is not understood why the large amounts of T cells infused with the PBSC grafts are not associated with a tremendous enhancement of acute GVH reactions. However, it has been shown that the absolute number of T cells in an allogeneic graft may not be the crucial factor determining the severity of GVHD.[50,60] Thus, provided that a critical number of T cells is present in the graft, the quality (i.e. specificity) rather than the quantity of donor T cells seems to be the more important determinant influencing GVHD frequency and severity.

Another explanation may be that the T cells contained in PBSC products are not only quantitatively but also qualitatively different from T cells contained in BM grafts: murine studies have demonstrated that the T cells in G-CSF-mobilized PBSC grafts express predominantly a Th2 cytokine pattern (IL-4 production), whereas the majority of peripheral blood T cells of mice not exposed to G-CSF show a Th1 pattern (IL-2/interferon-γ (IFN-γ) production).[61] Interestingly, Th2 cells can attenuate acute GVH reactions after allogeneic BMT.[62] Reduced Th1 function and predominance of L-selectin expression patterns associated with decreased alloreactivity were also observed in G-CSF-mobilized blood from humans.[63–65] Moreover, the development of GVH reactions may be modulated by regulatory T-cell subsets or other bystander cells predominating in G-CSF-mobilized PBSC grafts, such as type 2 dendritic cells.[65–67]

CHRONIC GVHD

There is increasing evidence that chronic GVHD occurs in a significantly higher proportion of recipients of unmanipulated PBSC compared with marrow recipients.[68] Vigorito et al[33] reported that 71% of patients allografted with PBSC developed extensive chronic GVH reactions, which was significantly more than the 27% incidence in the marrow recipients. This observation was confirmed in the much larger EBMT trial,[40] as well as in the French study,[37] and is supported by a trend for a greater incidence of chronic GVHD in all the other randomized studies listed in Table 18.2. Similarly, the relative risk of developing chronic GVHD was significantly increased after PBSCT also in the IBMTR/EBMT registry series (cumulative probability 66% at 12 months post transplant).[41] Additional randomized studies are necessary to understand the cause and extent of excess chronic GVHD occurring after allogeneic PBSCT.

ALTERNATIVE DONORS AND GVHD

Experience with transplantation of unmanipulated allogeneic PBSC from donors other than HLA-identical siblings is still limited. The Essen group reported 24 PBSC recipients allografted from zero- to two-antigen-mismatched related donors. As expected, the cumulative probability of grade II–IV acute GVHD was significantly higher in the 19 patients receiving mismatched grafts than in 41 control recipients of HLA-matched PBSC (86% versus 25%; $p < 0.003$). Similar differences were observed in terms of chronic GVHD, although exact figures for this were not reported. There was no influence of donor match, however, on treatment-related mortality, event-free survival, or overall survival.[45]

Owing to the complex ethical and regulatory implications, G-CSF-mobilized PBSC have been used less frequently in the setting of stem cell transplantation from unrelated donors. In 1997, 12% of all unrelated volunteer donor transplants

Table 18.2 Acute and chronic GVHD: results of randomized studies with HLA-identical siblings

Investigators	No. of patients evaluable	Grade II–IV/III–IV acute GVHD (%)		Overall/extensive chronic GVHD (%)	
		PBSC	BM	PBSC	BM
Vigorito et al (1998)[33,a]	37	27/13	19/13	71/71[e]	53/27
Mahmoud et al (1999)[34,a]	30	7[f]	45	NA	NA
Bensinger et al (2001)[35,b]	172	64/15	57/12	NA/46	NA/35
Powles et al (2000)[36,c]	39	68[f]	58	44/NA	40/NA
Blaise et al (2000)[37,b]	111	45/17	42/23	55/34[e]	30/8
Heldal et al (2000)[38,d]	61	21/NA	10/NA	56/15	27/7
Simpson et al (2000)[39,b]	228	NA	NA	NA/45	NA/35
Schmitz et al (2000)[40,b]	350	52/28[e]	39/16	74/NA[e]	53/NA

[a]Single-centre, open-label randomized study.
[b]Multicentre, open-label randomized study.
[c]Single-centre, double-blind randomized study.
[d]Single-centre, open-label randomized study with 5 one antigen-mismatched family donors in the PBSC group versus one in the BM group.
[e]$p < 0.05$.
[f]Acute GVHD of any grade.
NA, not available

were performed with mobilized blood. The first larger series of unrelated PBSC transplants was described by Ringden and co-workers.[30] Acute and chronic GVHD, treatment-related mortality, and overall survival were not significantly different between 45 recipients of unmanipulated PBSC and a matched cohort of patients grafted with marrow. Although acute and chronic GVHD were virtually eliminated, relapse incidence and overall survival did not differ in 18 additional patients receiving T-cell-depleted PBSC from unrelated donors.

GVL EFFECTS

Since the antileukaemic activities of allogeneic stem cell grafts are mediated predominantly by T cells and NK cells,[69,70] the infusion of the large lymphocyte numbers conferred with PBSC allografts may result in increased GVL effects after primary PBSCT. Although it is far too early for definite conclusions to be drawn, recent data observed in patients with CML suggest that complete disease eradication as revealed by *BCR/ABL* polymerase chain reaction (PCR) may indeed occur more often after PBSCT than after BMT.[71] In this series by Elmaagacli and co-workers, the 29 patients with PBSCT also had a superior outcome in terms of freedom from cytogenetic or clinical relapse. This is in accordance with our own experience obtained in a mouse model comparing the GVL activity of PBSC and BM allografts respectively: in an MHC-matched setting, transplantation of unmanipulated PBSC into lethally irradiated recipients who had been injected with cells from the B-lymphoblastic leukaemia A20 resulted in a reduction of the relapse rate to 29%, which was significantly better than the leukemia incidence observed after identical numbers of unmanipulated marrow cells (60%; $p < 0.05$).[25]

Clinical data on the relapse incidence are available for five of the eight randomized studies mentioned. Whereas no difference between BMT and PBSCT becomes evident from the EBMT and French trials, which were both restricted to standard-risk leukaemia, including chronic-phase CML, three studies with broader inclusion criteria found more relapses in BM recipients. This difference reached statistical significance in two of these trials (Table 18.3), and was associated with a benefit in terms of overall survival in the Seattle study, which was, however, exclusively due to the much better outcome of PBSC recipients in the subgroup of patients with advanced disease (Table 18.4). Moreover, preliminary analysis disclosed a better leukaemia-free survival for PBSC recipients in certain unfavourable subgroups of the IBMTR/EBMT registry series, although no decreased incidence of relapse after PBSCT was seen.[41] On the other hand, the Essen group found a signifcantly lower relapse rate after PBSCT compared with BMT for standard-risk but not for poor-risk disease in a recent analysis of 485 non-randomized patients.[72]

The US National Institutes of Health (NIH) group found a strong correlation between the number of $CD34^+$ cells infused and relapse incidence in 31 patients with chronic-phase or accelerated-phase CML: whereas 48% of the patients receiving less than 3×10^6 $CD34^+$ cells/kg relapsed, the probability of disease recurrence in recipients of more than 3×10^6 $CD34^+$ cells/kg was only 14% ($p = 0.05$). Interestingly, the group receiving more than 3×10^6 $CD34^+$ cells/kg consisted almost exclusively of PBSC recipients (PBSC 90%/BM 10%), while the majority of patients in the group receiving fewer $CD34^+$ cells were BM recipients (PBSC 16%/BM 84%).[73] Taken together, the information available to date suggests that unmanipulated PBSC under certain conditions might have advantages over BM in terms of GVL activity in particular in CML, but much more work has to be done before clear-cut conclusions can be drawn on this issue.

Another line of evidence for stronger antitumour activities of PBSC allografts comes from studies aiming at treatment of leukaemia relapse after BMT using allogeneic PBSC boosts. In comparison with the infusion of unmobilized donor leukocytes (DLI), the potential advantages of PBSC are (1) rapid recovery of donor haematopoiesis without prolonged cytopenias; (2) the possibility of reducing patient's tumour cell load by myelosuppressive chemotherapy prior to PBSC infusion; (3) a possible competition of donor-derived progenitor cells with the malignant clone;[74] (4) a reduction in DLI-associated GVH reactions as a result of immune-modulating effects of G-CSF during mobilization.[61] Preliminary data obtained by us and others indicate that durable remissions can indeed be achieved after transfusion of donor-derived mobilized PBSC in patients relapsing with CML or acute myeloid leukaemia (AML) after allogeneic BMT. Even in patients who received additional chemotherapy, extensive cytopenias as observed after conventional DLI could be largely avoided, whereas devastating GVH reactions did not occur.[36,75] The GVL activity of mobilized peripheral blood may be further increased by activation of effector cells with appropriate cytokines.[76]

Table 18.3 Relapse incidence and disease-free survival: results of randomized studies with HLA-identical siblings

	Relapse incidence		Disease-free survival rate	
Investigators	**PBSC**	**BM**	**PBSC**	**BM**
Bensinger et al (2001)[35,a]	14%	25%[d]	65%	45%
Powles et al (2000)[36b]	0%	37%[d]	NA	NA
Blaise et al (2000)[37,a]	6%	11%	67%	66%
Heldal et al (2000)[38,c]	1/28	9/30	82%	66%
Simpson et al (2000)[39,a]	No difference		NA	NA
Schmitz et al (2000)[40,a]	No difference		No difference	

[a]Multicentre, open-label randomized study.
[b]Single-centre, double-blind randomized study.
[c]Single-centre, open-label randomized study with 5 one-antigen-mismatched family donors in the PBSC group versus 1 in the BM group.
[d]$p<0.05$.
NA, not available.

Altogether, these observations suggest that mobilized allogeneic PBSC products are a promising tool for immunotherapy approaches in patients with diseases sensitive to GVL effects, such as CML.

REDUCED-INTENSITY CONDITIONING

A straightforward approach taking advantage of this concept is attempting immune-mediated elimination of residual neoplastic cells by transfusing mobilized PBSC products after conditioning that is not myeloablative per se ('minitransplants'). During the past three years, various strategies to reduce the preparative regimen's toxicity while preserving its immunosuppressive effect have been developed. Investigators at the Fred Hutchinson Cancer Research Center (Seattle) and at the University of Leipzig used low-dose total-body irradiation (TBI) (4 Gy) as preparative regimen and mycophenolate mofetil/cyclosporine as GVHD prophylaxis.[77] Others have focused on regimens containing fludarabine in combination with an alkylating agent. Preliminary data suggest that complete lymphohaematopoietic chimerism and durable remissions can be achieved by these strategies in a considerable proportion of patients even after failure of autografting, implying that GVL activity is responsible for the antitumour effects observed.[77–80] It is not surprising that this approach seems to work best in indolent lymphohaematopoietic neoplasias with known sensitivity to GVL effects, such as low-grade lymphoma and CML, while resistant and rapidly growing tumours are less good candidates for reduced-dose conditioning.[81–83]

Table 18.4 Overall survival: results of randomized studies with HLA-identical siblings

	Overall survival rate (%)	
Investigators	**PBSC**	**BM**
Bensinger et al (2001):[35,a]		
Early-stage patients (92)	75	72
Advanced-stage patients (80)	57	33[d]
Powles et al (2000)[36,b]	70	63
Blaise et al (2000)[37,a]	67	65
Heldal et al (2000)[38,c]	82	74
Simpson et al (2000)[39,a]	70	56[d]
Schmitz et al (2000)[40,a]	No difference	

[a]Multicentre, open-label randomized study.
[b]Single-centre, double-blind randomized study.
[c]Single-centre, open-label randomized study with 5 one-antigen-mismatched family donors in the PBSC group versus 1 in the BM group.
[d]$p < 0.05$.

However, low-intensity regimens can be associated with relevant complications, and should not be administered uncritically. In particular, acute and chronic GVHD continue to be a problem. Ex vivo or in vivo T-cell depletion might be a solution to this, but may be associated with detrimental effects on engraftment, immune reconstitution, and GVL activity.[84,85] Thus, controlled prospective trials are warranted to assess whether allogeneic SCT with reduced-dose conditioning can indeed improve the outcome for patients.

GRAFT ENGINEERING AND CELL COMPONENT THERAPY

Successful attempts to manipulate allogeneic stem cell grafts for eliminating GVH-reactive cells were undertaken in the 1970s.[86] In the clinical situation, however, T-cell depletion (TCD) of marrow grafts has been hampered by two major drawbacks, which are responsible for its overall disappointing results: the reduction of mortality due to GVHD was offset by (1) a dramatic rise in the incidence of engraftment failure and (2) a strongly increased relapse rate,[87] due respectively to non-specific stem cell loss and elimination of GVL activity from the graft.

The use of PBSC can be expected to avoid these problems because of the 'unlimited' numbers of stem cells and GVH/GVL effector cells that can be harvested from mobilized blood as opposed to BM. This hypothesis was confirmed by a recent retrospective study that compared haematopoietic recovery after TCD PBSCT and BMT respectively, showing that TCD PBSC engrafted significantly faster and more completely than TCD marrow.[88] Thus, in conjunction with the recent progress in cell separation technology, PBSC appear to be the perfect source for ex vivo graft engineering.

Soon after we had reported for the first time that 3–4 log of T cells can be depleted from PBSC grafts by $CD34^+$ selection,[89] a number of investigators reported clinical results on HLA-identical recipients of PBSC products that were T-cell-depleted by $CD34^+$ selection using either the Ceprate immunadsorption system (Cellpro, Bothell, WA) or the immunomagnetic Isolex system (Nexell Therapeutics, Irvine, CA). Although immunoselection reduced the median T-cell content of the grafts by 2.5–4 log to $1 \times 10^5 - 1 \times 10^6$/kg, the incidence of grade II–IV acute GVHD was surprisingly high if GVHD prophylaxis consisted of TCD only (with or without cyclosporine).[90–92] With the addition of methotrexate or steroids, however, elimination of both acute and chronic GVHD could be largely achieved in the HLA-identical but not in the mismatched setting if TCD was accomplished with the early Ceprate or Isolex systems[90,93–95]

It was concluded from these results that in the mismatched situation, more vigorous TCD might be neccessary for effective GVHD prevention: the Perugia group employed a double TCD combining E-rosetting with Ceprate $CD34^+$ selection, and achieved a TCD efficacy of more than 4 log. Fifty-three haploidentical patients were reinfused with extensively TCD PBSC containing a mean of only 3.5×10^4 $CD3^+$ T cells/kg in addition to TCD marrow. With the only additional GVHD prophylaxis consisting of pretransplant antithymocyte globulin (ATG), both acute and chronic GVHD were virtually completely eliminated.[96] Although the incidence of primary graft failure was low in this preliminary trial (5%), the overall outcome was affected by frequent life-threatening opportunistic infections, suggesting that immune recovery is critically impaired after heavily TCD SCT in adults, where T-cell regeneration after BMT is largely dependent on the number of mature T cells present in the graft.[51,52]

Another approach to 'Mega' TCD relies on the use of more effective $CD34^+$ selection devices, such as the Clinimacs system (Miltenyi Biotech, Bergisch Gladbach, Germany) or newer versions of the Isolex300i system (Nexell), which both allow highly efficient purification of progenitor cell preparations with fewer than 1×10^5 residual $CD3^+$ T cells/kg.[97] Taken together, modern cell separation systems allow the preparation of PBSC grafts devoid of GVHD effector cells, which can be successfully used for allografting of three-loci-mismatched recipients, but the problem of insufficient restoration of the immune system remains to be settled.

Another unsolved issue regarding TCD allografts is the increased incidence of leukaemia relapse, which will obviously not be overcome with the use of $CD34^+$-selected PBSC alone, although recent reports postulate an inverse correlation between the $CD34^+$ cell dose of allografts and the risk of relapse.[98] However, the large quantities of lymphocytes that can be segregated from PBSC grafts might be used for adding GVL activity to the haematopoietic potential conferred with the isolated $CD34^+$ cells. Along this line, Beelen and co-workers[99] allografted 10 chronic-phase CML patients with Clinimacs-purified PBSC after myeloablative conditioning without standard post-transplant immunosuppression. All patients achieved molecular remission. With a median follow-up of 16 months, four patients have experienced molecular relapse but responded to DLI. Severe acute GVHD did not occur. These preliminary data suggest that this kind of 'pre-emptive' immunotherapy might work in CML by controlling the neoplastic clone without critical risk of GVHD. Similar to GVL activity, specific immunity against critical infectious agents may be restored by addition of appropriate T-cell clones.[100,101]

CONCLUSIONS

Transplantation of allogeneic PBSC has become an attractive alternative to allogeneic BMT. Controlled trials suggest that engraftment is faster than after allogeneic BMT. There is mounting evidence that chronic and – in constrast to the initial impression – also acute GVH reactions are increased after unmanipulated PBSCT, but this may translate into enhanced GVL activity and (so far) appears to have a beneficial rather than detrimental effect on survival, in particular in diseases with high sensitivity to GVL, such as CML. However, the presently available results of the large randomized studies are not sufficient to allow definite conclusions to be drawn on this issue. Regardless of the features of unmanipulated PBSC in comparison with marrow grafts, a major advantage of allogeneic PBSC over BM is their excellent suitability for graft engineering, such as T-cell depletion with consecutive generation of GVL effector cells. With regard to CML, leukaemia-specific target structures for effector T cells have been identified and might be used for CML-specific immunotherapy in the context of allogeneic PBSCT in the near future.[102,103]

REFERENCES

1. Schmitz N, Dreger P, Suttorp M et al, Primary transplantation of allogeneic peripheral blood progenitor cells mobilized by filgrastim (G-CSF). *Blood* 1995; **85:** 1666–72.
2. Körbling M, Przepiorka D, Engel H et al, Allogeneic blood stem cell transplantation for refractory leukemia and lymphoma: potential advantage of blood over marrow allografts. *Blood* 1995; **85:** 1659–65.
3. Bensinger WI, Weaver CH, Appelbaum FR, Buckner CD, Transplantation of allogeneic peripheral blood stem cells mobilized by recombinant human granulocyte colony-stimulating factor (rh G-CSF). *Blood* 1995; **85:** 1655–8.
4. Gratwohl A, Passweg J, Baldomero H et al, Hemopoietic stem cell transplantation in Europe 1998. *Hematol J* 2000; **1:** 333–50.
5. Sheridan WP, Begley CG, Juttner CA et al, Effect of peripheral-blood progenitor cells mobilized by filgrastim (G-CSF) on platelet recovery after high-dose chemotherapy. *Lancet* 1992; **339:** 640–4.
6. Dreger P, Haferlach T, Eckstein V et al, G-CSF-mobilized peripheral blood progenitor cells for allogeneic transplantation: safety, kinetics of mobilization, and composition of the graft. *Br J Haematol* 1994; **87:** 609–13.
7. Fritsch G, Fischmeister G, Haas OA et al, Peripheral blood hematopoietic progenitor cells of cytokine-stimulated healthy donors as an alternative for allogeneic transplantation. *Blood* 1994; **83:** 3420–21.
8. Lane TA, Law P, Maruyama M et al, Harvesting and enrichment of hematopoietic progenitor cells mobilized into the peripheral blood of normal donors by granulocyte–macrophage colony-stimulating factor (GM-CSF) or G-CSF: Potential role in allogeneic marrow transplantation. *Blood* 1995; **85:** 275–82.
9. Dreger P, Schmitz N, Stem cell mobilization in healthy donors: current status. *Infusionsther Transfusionsmed* 1999; **26:** 92–5.
10. Hohaus S, Voso MT, Haas R, The role of cytokines in the mobilization of blood stem cells. In: *Blood Stem Cell Transplantation* (Reiffers J, Goldman J, Armitage JO, eds). London: Martin Dunitz, 1998: 37–54.
11. Anderlini P, Korbling M, Dale D et al, Allogeneic blood stem cell transplantation: considerations for donors. *Blood* 1997; **90:** 903–8.
12. Murata M, Harada M, Kato S et al, Peripheral blood stem cell mobilization and apheresis: analysis of adverse events in 94 normal donors. *Bone Marrow Transplant* 1999; **24:** 1065–71.
13. Bensinger WI, Buckner CD, Rowley S et al, Treatment of normal donors with recombinant growth factors for transplantation of allogeneic blood stem cells. *Bone Marrow Transplant* 1996; **17**(Suppl 2): S19–21.
14. Becker PS, Wagle M, Matous S et al, Spontaneous splenic rupture following administration of granulocyte colony-stimulating factor (G-CSF): occurrence in an allogeneic donor of peripheral blood stem cells. *Biol Blood Marrow Transplant* 1997; **3:** 45–9.
15. Adkins DR, Anaphylactoid reaction in a normal donor given granulocyte colony-stimulating factor. *J Clin Oncol* 1998; **16:** 812–13.
16. Haas R, Ho AD, Bredthauer U et al, Successful

autologous transplantation of blood stem cells mobilized with recombinant human granulocyte–macrophage colony-stimulating factor. *Exp Hematol* 1990; **18:** 94–8.
17. Rosenfeld CS, Bolwell B, LeFever A et al, Comparison of four cytokine regimens for mobilization of peripheral blood stem cells: IL-3 alone and combined with GM-CSF or G-CSF. *Bone Marrow Transplant* 1996; **17:** 179–83.
18. Laterveer L, Lindley IJD, Heemskerk DPM et al, Rapid mobilization of hematopoietic progenitor cells in rhesus monkeys by a single intravenous injection of interleukin-8. *Blood* 1996; **87:** 781–8.
19. Rasko JE, Basser RL, Boyd J et al, Multilineage mobilization of peripheral blood progenitor cells in humans following administration of PEG-rHuMGDF. *Br J Haematol* 1997; **97:** 871–80.
20. Sudo Y, Shimazaki C, Ashihara E et al, Synergistic effect of FLT-3 ligand on the granulocyte colony-stimulating factor-induced mobilisation of hematopoietic stem cells and progenitor cells into blood in mice. *Blood* 1999; **89:** 3186–91.
21. To LB, Haylock DN, Simmons PJ, Juttner CA, The biology and clinical uses of blood stem cells. *Blood* 1997; **89:** 2233–58.
22. Kröger N, Renges H, Krüger W et al, A randomized comparison of once versus twice daily RHG-CSF for stem cell mobilisation in healthy donors for allogeneic transplantation. *Onkologie* 2000; **23**(Suppl 7): 38 (abst).
23. Harada M, Nagafuji K, Fujisaki T et al, G-CSF-Induced mobilization of peripheral blood stem cells from healthy adults for allogeneic transplantation. *J Hematother* 1996; **5:** 63–71.
24. Varas F, Bernard A, Bueren JA, Granulocyte colony-stimulating factor mobilizes into peripheral blood the complete clonal repertoire of hematopoietic precursors residing in the bone marrow of mice. *Blood* 1996; **88:** 2495–501.
25. Glass B, Uharek L, Zeis M et al, Allogeneic peripheral blood progenitor cell transplantation in a murine model: evidence for an improved graft-versus-leukemia effect. *Blood* 1997; **90:** 1694–700.
26. Theilgaard-Mönch K, Raaschou-Jensen K, Andersen H et al, Single leukapheresis products collected from healthy donors after the administration of granulocyte colony-stimulating factor contain tenfold higher numbers of long-term reconstitutung hematopoietic progenitor cells than conventional bone marrow allografts. *Bone Marrow Transplant* 1999; **23:** 243–49.
27. Dreger P, Klöss M, Petersen B et al, Autologous progenitor cell transplantation: prior exposure to stem cell-toxic drugs determines yield and engraftment of peripheral blood progenitor cell but not of bone marrow grafts. *Blood* 1995; **86:** 3970–8.
28. Schmitz N, Bacigalupo A, Hasenclever D et al, Allogeneic bone marrow transplantation vs filgrastim-mobilised peripheral blood progenitor cell transplantation in patients with early leukaemia: first results of a randomised multicentre trial of the European Group for Blood and Marrow Transplantation. *Bone Marrow Transplant* 1998; **21:** 995–1003.
29. Ringden O, Hagglund H, Runde V et al, Faster engraftment of peripheral blood progenitor cells compared to bone marrow from unrelated donors. *Bone Marrow Transplant* 1998; **21**(Suppl 3): S81–4
30. Ringden O, Remberger M, Runde V et al, Peripheral blood stem cell transplantation from unrelated donors: a comparison with marrow transplantation. *Blood* 1999; **94:** 455–64.
31. Weaver CH, Bensinger W, Longin K et al, Syngeneic transplantation with peripheral blood mononuclear cells collected after the administration of recombinant human granulocyte colony-stimulating factor. *Blood* 1993; **82:** 1981–4.
32. Fefer A, Cheever MA, Thomas ED, Bone marrow transplantation for refractory acute leukemia in 34 patients with identical twins. *Blood* 1981; **57:** 421–30.
33. Vigorito AC, Azevedo WM, Marques JFC et al, A randomized, prospective comparison of allogeneic bone marrow and peripheral blood progenitor cell transplantation in the treatment of haematological malignancies. *Bone Marrow Transplant* 1998; **22:** 1145–51.
34. Mahmoud H, Fahmy OA, Kamel A et al, Peripheral blood vs bone marrow as a source for allogeneic hematopoietic stem cell transplantation. *Bone Marrow Transplant* 1999; **24:** 355–8.
35. Bensinger WI, Martin P, Clift RA et al, A prospective, randomised trial of peripheral blood stem cells (PBSC) or marrow for patients undergoing allogeneic transplantation for hematologic malignancies. *N Engl J Med* 2001; **344:** 175–81.
36. Powles R, Mehta J, Kulkarni S et al, Allogeneic

blood and bone-marrow stem cell transplantation in haematological diseases: a randomized trial. *Lancet* 2000; **355:** 1231–7.
37. Blaise D, Kuentz M, Fortanier C et al, Randomized trial of bone marrow versus lenograstim-primed blood cell allogeneic transplantation in patients with early-stage leukemia: a report from the Societe Francaise de Greffe de Moelle. *J Clin Oncol* 2001; **18:** 537–46.
38. Heldal D, Tjonnfjord G, Brinch L et al, A randomised study of allogeneic transplantation with stem cells from blood or bone marrow. *Bone Marrow Transplant* 2000; **25:** 1129–36.
39. Simpson DR, Couban S, Bredeson C et al, A randomized study comparing peripheral blood and bone marrow in patients undergoing matched sibling transplants for myeloid malignancies. *Int J Hematol* 2000; **72**(Suppl 1): 52 (abst).
40. Schmitz N, Beksac M, Hasenclever D et al, A randomized study from the European Group for Blood and Marrow Transplantation comparing allogeneic transplantation of filgrastim-mobilised peripheral blood progenitor cells with bone marrow transplantation in 350 patients with leukemia. *Blood* 2000; **96**(Suppl 1): (abst).
41. Schmitz N, Klein JP, Gratwohl A et al, Prognostic factors for survival after allogeneic peripheral blood progenitor cell transplantation. *Blood* 1998; **92:** (abst).
42. Bensinger WI, Buckner CD, Storb R et al, Transplantation of allogeneic peripheral blood stem cells. *Bone Marrow Transplant* 1996; **17**(Suppl 2): S56–7.
43. Bensinger WI, Appelbaum FR, Demirer T et al, Transplantation of allogeneic peripheral blood stem cells. *Stem Cells* 1995; **13**(Suppl 3): 63–70.
44. Russell NH, Gratwohl A, Schmitz N, The place of blood stem cells in allogeneic transplantation. *Br J Haematol* 1996; **93:** 747–53.
45. Beelen DW, Ottinger HD, Elmaagacli A et al, Transplantation of filgrastim-mobilized peripheral blood stem cells from HLA-identical sibling or alternative family donors in patients with hematologic malignancies: a prospective comparison on clinical outcome, immune reconstitution, and hematopoietic chimerism. *Blood* 1997; **90:** 4725–35.
46. Dreger P, Suttorp M, Haferlach T et al, Allogeneic G-CSF-mobilised peripheral blood progenitor cells for treatment of engraftment failure after bone marrow transplantation. *Blood* 1993; **81:** 1404–7.
47. Arseniev L, Tischler H-J, Battmer K et al, Treatment of poor marrow graft function with allogeneic CD34+ cells immunoselected from G-CSF-mobilized peripheral blood progenitor cells of the marrow donor. *Bone Marrow Transplant* 1994; **14:** 791–7.
48. Molina L, Chabannon C, Viret F et al, Granulocyte colony-stimulating factor-mobilized allogeneic peripheral blood stem cells for rescue of graft failure after allogeneic bone marrow transplantation in two patients with acute myeloblastic leukemia in first complete remission. *Blood* 1995; **85:** 1678–9.
49. Redei I, Waller EK, Holland HK et al, Successful engraftment after primary graft failure in aplastic anemia using G-CSF mobilized peripheral stem cell transfusions. *Bone Marrow Transplant* 1997; **19:** 175–7.
50. Körbling M, Huh YO, Durett A et al, Allogeneic blood stem cell transplantation: Peripheralization and yield of donor-derived primitive hematopoietic progenitor cells (CD34+ Thy-1) and lymphoid subsets, and possible predictors of engraftment and graft-versus-host disease. *Blood* 1995; **86:** 2842–8.
51. Mackall CL, Granger L, Sheard MA et al, T-cell regeneration after bone marrow transplantation: differential CD45 isoform expression on thymic-derived versus thymic-independent progeny. *Blood* 1993; **82:** 2585–94.
52. Roux E, Helg C, Dumont GF et al, Analysis of T-cell repopulation after allogeneic bone marrow transplantation: significant differences between recipients of T-cell depleted and unmanipulated grafts. *Blood* 1996; **87:** 3984–92.
53. Bomberger C, Singh-Jairam M, Rodey G et al, Lymphoid reconstitution after autologous PBSC transplantation with FACS-sorted CD34+ hematopoietic progenitors. *Blood* 1998; **91:** 2588–600.
54. Dreger P, Viehmann K, von Neuhoff N et al, Autografting of highly purified peripheral blood progenitor cells following myeloablative therapy in patients with lymphoma: a prospective study of the long-term effects on tumor eradication, reconstitution of hematopoiesis and immune recovery. *Bone Marrow Transplant* 1999; **24:** 153–61.
55. Ottinger HD, Beelen DW, Scheulen B et al, Improved immune reconstitution after allo-

transplantation of peripheral blood stem cells instead of bone marrow. *Blood* 1996; **88:** 2775–9.

56. Storek J, Witherspoon RP, Maloney DG et al, Improved reconstitution of CD4 T cells and B cells but worsened reconstitution of serum IgG levels after allogeneic transplantation of blood stem cells instead of marrow. *Blood* 1997; **89:** 3891–3.
57. Pavletic ZS, Joshi SS, Pirruccello SJ et al, Lymphocyte reconstitution after allogeneic blood stem cell transplantation for hematologic malignancies. *Bone Marrow Transplant* 1998; **21:** 33–41.
58. Behringer D, Bertz H, Schmoor C et al, Quantitative lymphocyte subset reconstitution after allogeneic hematopoietic transplantation from matched related donors with CD34+ selected PBPC grafts, unselected PBPC grafts or BM grafts. *Bone Marrow Transplant* 1999; **24:** 295–302.
59. Miller JS, Prosper F, McCullar V, Natural killer (NK) cells are functionally abnormal and NK cell progenitors are diminished in granulocyte colony-stimulating factor-mobilized peripheral blood progenitor cell collections. *Blood* 1997; **90:** 3098–105.
60. Jansen J, Goselink HM, Veenhof WFJ et al, The impact of the composition of the bone marrow graft on engraftment and graft-versus-host disease. *Exp Hematol* 1983; **11:** 967–73.
61. Pan L, Delmonte J, Jalonen CK, Ferrara JLM, Pretreatment of donor mice with granulocyte colony-stimulating factor polarizes donor T-lymphocytes toward type-2 cytokine production and reduces severity of experimental graft-versus-host disease. *Blood* 1995; **86:** 4422–9.
62. Krenger W, Snyder KM, Byon JHC et al, Polarized type 2 alloreactive CD4+ and CD8+ donor T cells fail to induce experimental acute graft-versus-host disease. *J Immunol* 1995; **155:** 585–93.
63. Rondelli D, Raspadori D, Anasetti C et al, Alloantigen presenting capacity, T cell alloreactivity and NK function of G-CSF-mobilized peripheral blood cells. *Bone Marrow Transplant* 1998; **22:** 631–7.
64. Sugimori N, Nakao S, Yachie A et al, Administration of G-CSF to normal individuals diminishes L-selectin+ T cells in the periphal blood that respond better to alloantigen stimulation than L-selectin- T cells. *Bone Marrow Transplant* 1999; **23:** 119–24.
65. Gyger M, Stuart RK, Perreault C, Immunobiology of allogeneic peripheral blood mononuclear cells mobilized with granulocyte-colony stimulating factor. *Bone Marrow Transplant* 2000; **26:** 1–16.
66. Mielcarek M, Martin PJ, Torok-Storb B, Suppression of alloantigen-induced T-cell proliferation by CD14+ cells derived from granulocyte colony-stimulating factor-mobilized peripheral blood mononuclear cells. *Blood* 1997; **89:** 1629–34.
67. Arpinati M, Green CL, Heimfeld S et al, Granulocyte-colony stimulating factor mobilizes T helper 2-inducing dendritic cells. *Blood* 2000; **95:** 2484–90.
68. Majolino I, Saglio G, Scimè R et al, High incidence of chronic GVHD after primary allogeneic peripheral blood stem transplantation in patients with hematologic malignancies. *Bone Marrow Transplant* 1996; **17:** 555–60.
69. Sosman JA, Oettel KR, Hank JA et al, Specific recognition of human leukemic cells by allogeneic T cell lines. *Transplantation* 1989; **48:** 486–90.
70. Glass B, Uharek L, Zeis M et al, Graft-versus-leukemia activity can be predicted by natural cytotoxicity against leukemia cells. *Br J Haematol* 1996; **93:** 412–20.
71. Elmaagacli AH, Beelen DW, Opalka B et al, The risk of residual molecular and cytogenetic disease in patients with Philadelphia-chromosome positive first chronic phase chronic myelogenous leukemia is reduced after transplantation of allogeneic peripheral blood stem cells compared with bone marrow. *Blood* 1999; **94:** 384–9.
72. Beelen DW, Elmaagacli A, Peceny R et al, Prospective evaluation of the major clinical endpoints after allogenic hematopoietic stem cell transplantation: impact of the stem cell source. *Onkologie* 2000; **23**(Suppl 7): 73 (abst).
73. Bahceci E, Read EJ, Leitman S et al, CD34+ cell dose predicts relapse and survival after T-cell-depleted HLA-identical haematopoietic stem cell transplantation (HSCT) for haematological malignancies. *Br J Haematol* 2000; **108:** 408–14.
74. Giralt S, Escudier S, Kantarjian H et al, Preliminary results of treatment with filgrastim for relapse of leukemia and myelodysplasia after allogeneic bone marrow transplantation. *N Engl J Med* 1993; **329:** 757–61.
75. Glass B, Majolino I, Dreger P et al, Allogeneic peripheral blood progenitor cells for treatment

of relapse after bone marrow transplantation. *Bone Marrow Transplant* 1997; **20:** 533–41.
76. Hartung G, Uharek L, Zeis M et al, Superior antileukemic activity of murine peripheral blood progenitor cell (PBPC) grafts mobilized by G-CSF and stem cell factor (SCF) as compared to G-CSF alone. *Bone Marrow Transplant* 1998; **21**(Suppl 3): S16–20.
77. McSweeney P, Niederwieser D, Shizuru J et al, Outpatient allografting with minimally myelosuppressive, immunosuppressive conditioning of low-dose TBI and postgrafting cyclosporine and mycophenolate mofetil. *Blood* 1999; **94**(Suppl 1): 393a.
78. Giralt S, Estey E, Albitar M et al, Engraftment of allogeneic hematopoietic progenitor cells with purine analog-containing chemotherapy: harnessing graft-versus-leukemia without myeloablative therapy. *Blood* 1997; **89:** 4531–6.
79. Slavin S, Nagler A, Naparstek E et al, Nonmyeloablative stem cell transplantation and cell therapy as an alternative to conventional bone marrow transplantation with lethal cytoreduction for the treatment of malignant and nonmalignant hematologic diseases. *Blood* 1998; **91:** 756–63.
80. Childs R, Clave E, Contentin N et al, Engraftment kinetics after nonmyeloablative allogeneic peripheral blood stem cell transplantation: full donor T cell chimerism precedes alloimmune responses. *Blood* 1999; **94:** 3234–41.
81. Nagler A, Slavin S, Varadi G et al, Allogeneic peripheral blood stem cell transplantation using a fludarabine-based low intensity conditioning regimen for malignant lymphoma. *Bone Marrow Transplant* 2000; **25:** 1021–8.
82. Bornhäuser M, Thiede C, Schuler U et al, Dose-reduced conditioning for allogeneic blood stem cell transplantation: durable engraftment without antithymocyte globulin. *Bone Marrow Transplant* 2000; **26:**119–25.
83. Dreger P, Glass B, Seyfarth B et al, Reduced-intensity allogeneic stem cell transplantation as salvage treatment for patients with indolent lymphoma after failure of autologous SCT. *Bone Marrow Transplant* 2000; **26:** 1361–2.
84. Kottaridis P, Chakraverty R, Milligan DW et al, A non-myeloablative regimen for allogeneic stem cell transplantation with a low incidence of GVHD. *Bone Marrow Transplant* 2000; **25**(Suppl 1): S26 (abst).
85. Cull GM, Haynes AP, Byrne JL et al, Preliminary experience of allogeneic stem cell transplantation for lymphoproliferative disorders using BEAM–CAMPATH conditioning: an effective regimen with low procedure-related toxicity. *Br J Haematol* 2000; **108:** 754–60.
86. Müller-Ruchholtz W, Wottge HU, Müller-Hermelink HK, Bone marrow transplantation across strong histocompatibility barriers by selective elimination of lymphoid cells in bone marrow. *Transplant Proc* 1976; **8:** 537–41.
87. Marmont AM, Horowitz MM, Gale RP et al, T-cell depletion of HLA-identical transplants in leukemia. *Blood* 1991; **78:** 2120–30.
88. Cornelissen JJ, Fibbe WE, Schattenberg AV et al, A retrospective Dutch study comparing T cell-depleted allogeneic blood stem cell transplantation vs T cell-depleted allogeneic bone marrow transplantation. *Bone Marrow Transplant* 1998; **21**(Suppl 3): S66–70.
89. Dreger P, Viehmann K, Steinmann J et al, G-CSF-mobilised peripheral blood progenitor cells for allogeneic transplantation: comparison of T cell depletion strategies using different CD34+ selection systems or CAMPATH-1. *Exp Hematol* 1995; **23:** 147–54.
90. Link H, Arseniev L, Bähre O et al, Transplantation of allogeneic CD34+ blood cells. *Blood* 1996; **87:** 4903–9.
91. Bensinger WI, Buckner CD, Rowley S et al, Transplantation of allogeneic CD34+ peripheral blood stem cells in patients with advanced hematologic malignancy. *Blood* 1996; **88:** 4132–8.
92. Bensinger WI, Rowley S, Lilleby K et al, Reduction in graft-versus-host-disease (GVHD) after transplantation of CD34 selected, allogeneic peripheral blood stem cells (PBSC) in older patients with advanced hematologic malignancies. *Blood* 1996; **88**(Suppl 1): 421a.
93. Urbano-Ispizua A, Rozman C et al, Rapid engraftment without significant graft-versus-host disease after allogeneic transplantation of CD34+ selected cells from peripheral blood. *Blood* 1997; **89:** 3967–73.
94. Urbano-Ispizua A, Solano C, Brunet S et al, Allogeneic transplantation of purified CD34+ cells from peripheral blood: Spanish experience of 62 cases. Spanish Group of allo-PBT. *Bone Marrow Transplant* 1998; **21**(Suppl 3): S71–4.
95. Bensinger WI, Rowley SD, Mills B, CD34 enriched allogeneic peripheral blood stem cell used for transplantation. *Bone Marrow Transplant* 1998; **21:** S102 (abst).

96. Aversa F, Tabilio A et al, Treatment of high-risk acute leukemia with T-cell-depleted stem cells from related donors with one fully mismatched HLA haplotype. *N Engl J Med* 1998; **339:** 1186–93.
97. Fritsch G, Scharner D, Fröschl G et al, Selection of CD34-positive blood cells for allogeneic transplantation: approaches to optimize CD34-cell recovery, purity, viability, and T-cell depletion. *Onkologie* 2000; **3:** 449–56.
98. Bahceci E, Read EJ, Leitman S et al, CD34+ cell dose predicts relapse and survival after T-cell-depleted HLA-identical haematopoietic stem cell transplantation (HSCT) for haematological malignancies. *Br J Haematol* 2000; **108:** 408–14.
99. Beelen DW, Peceny R, Elmaagacli A et al, Transplantation of highly purified HLA-identical sibling donor peripheral blood CD34+ cells without prophylactic post-transplant immunosuppression in adult patients with first chronic phase chronic myeloid leukemia: results of a phase II study. *Bone Marrow Transplant* 2000; **26:** 823–9.
100. Gustafsson A, Levitsky V, Zou JZ et al, Epstein–Barr virus (EBV) load in bone marrow transplant recipients at risk to develop post-transplant lymphoproliferative disease: prophylactic infusion of EBV-specific cytotoxic T cells. *Blood* 2000; **95:** 807–14.
101. Locatelli F, Maccario R, Gerna G, Anti-cytomegalovirus T-cell clones. *N Engl J Med* 1995; **331:** 601
102. Gao L, Bellantuono I, Elsasser A et al, Selective elimination of leukemic CD34(+) progenitor cells by cytotoxic T lymphocytes specific for WT1. *Blood* 2000; **95:** 2198–203.
103. Molldrem JJ, Lee PP, Wang C et al, Evidence that specific T lymphocytes may participate in the elimination of chronic myelogenous leukemia. *Nature Med* 2000; **6:** 1018–23.

19

HLA-identical sibling transplantation

David G Savage

CONTENTS • Introduction • Background • HLA typing • Assessing the donor • Assessing the recipient • Conditioning regimens • Management of splenomegaly • Source of hematopoietic stem cells • Graft-versus-host disease prophylaxis • Results according to disease phase • Syngeneic transplantation • Prognosis • Graft-versus-leukemia effect • Minimal residual disease • Relapse after alloSCT • Treatment of relapse • General recommendations • Future developments

INTRODUCTION

Allogeneic stem cell transplantation (alloSCT) is the only curative therapy for chronic myeloid leukemia (CML) (Figure 18.1).[1–5] As discussed elsewhere in this volume, there are several therapeutic alternatives for patients who are not ideal candidates for allografting. Chemotherapy with busulfan or hydroxyurea results in median survivals of about 4 years, but hydroxyurea is less toxic and easier to administer. Interferon-α (IFN-α) provides a survival advantage relative to hydroxyurea, but complete cytogenetic responders (only 10–20% of all those treated) remain positive for leukemia-specific (*BCR/ABL*) transcripts using the reverse-transcriptase polymerase chain reaction (RT-PCR) and do eventually relapse. Preliminary studies have shown that the novel tyrosine kinase inhibitor STI571 (Glivec) has remarkable activity in the treatment of CML, but its therapeutic role remains to be defined (see Chapter 34). High-dose therapy with autologous stem cell rescue may prolong survival but does not cure patients.[5]

Allografting is the treatment of choice for young patients with a genetically HLA-identical sibling. Less straightforward issues include the upper age limit for alloSCT, the timing of the procedure during chronic phase, the role of IFN-α and autografting in older individuals, and the utility of T-cell depletion and non-myeloablative conditioning in poor-risk patients. These issues should be discussed and an overall strategy agreed at diagnosis.[6] The best treatment may be fairly clear-cut, but often the choice of therapy cannot be based on austere logic. It is important to explain the various options and to plan a provisional strategy. This plan may need modification according to later developments.

BACKGROUND

In 1969, the Seattle group began a study of bone marrow transplantation (BMT) in patients with advanced leukemia and aplastic anemia using HLA-identical siblings as donors.[7,8] The first patient received his transplant for CML in blastic phase; his donor was thought to be a matched sibling, but later refinements in HLA typing demonstrated a one-antigen mismatch. Engraftment was successful after 954 cGy of total-body irradiation (TBI). The patient recovered from acute graft-versus-host disease (GVHD), but later

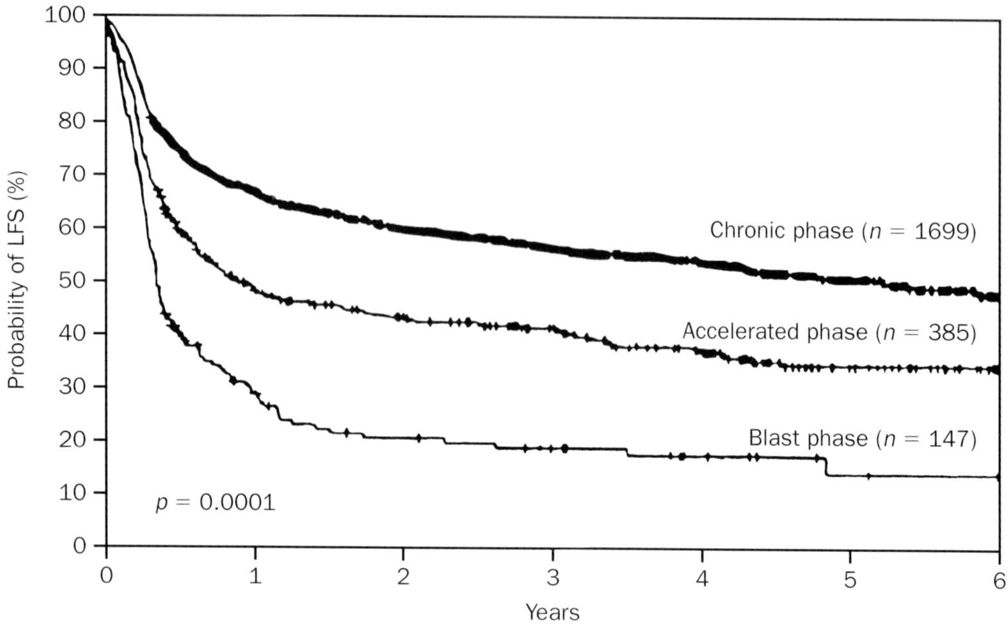

Figure 19.1 Probability of leukemia-free survival (LFS) after HLA-identical sibling bone marrow transplantation for CML in IBMTR series, 1987–1994. (From Horowitz MM, Rowlings PA, Passweg JR, Allogeneic bone marrow transplantation for CML: a report from the International Bone Marrow Transplant Registry. *Bone Marrow Transplant* 1996; **17**(Suppl 3): S5–6, with permission.)

died from an undiagnosed febrile illness, which was found at autopsy to be due to cytomegalovirus (CMV). Subsequent experience in patients with advanced hematological malignancies confirmed that engraftment of allogeneic cells was feasible after myeloablative therapy, but that the treatment was associated with significant toxicity, GVHD, opportunistic infection, and a high mortality.[8] Nevertheless, about 15% of patients undergoing alloBMT for high-risk leukemia managed to survive the procedure and remain leukemia-free. Such data provided the impetus for developing alloBMT as an important treatment for patients with leukemia, and led to investigations of its role in earlier-stage disease.

HLA TYPING

In the absence of a monozygotic twin, the risks of alloSCT are lowest in patients with an HLA-identical sibling donor.[9,10] In North America and Europe, because family sizes are generally small, most patients lack a compatible sibling. Serological typing of the A, B, and DR loci is usually sufficient to show genetic HLA identity between siblings. Because the results of serological testing are sometimes equivocal, some individuals may require high-resolution typing methods, such as PCR with sequence-specific oligonucleotide probes.[10]

ASSESSING THE DONOR

Some patients have more than one HLA-identical sibling. Donors are selected according to their general health, availability, and ability to give consent. Sisters are usually less desirable than brothers because of a greater risk of GVHD in recipients of female donor grafts;[11,12] pregnancy-related alloimmunization may account for this effect. Relapse is more common when the donor is male,[13] but this risk is probably mitigated by the efficacy of donor lymphocyte infusion (DLI) for relapse, as discussed below. The National Marrow Donor Program have reported that increasing donor age correlates with poorer outcome in recipients of unrelated allografts.[14] Similarly, greater donor age has been associated with adverse outcome in patients receiving HLA-identical sibling transplants at the Hammersmith Hospital in London (RM Szydlo, unpublished data).

If both the recipient and donor are seronegative for CMV infection, the risk of CMV disease is negligible. If the recipient is seronegative and the donor seropositive, the risk of CMV activation post transplant is about 30%.[15] The donor should be free of infection with HIV and hepatitis B and C viruses. Though desirable, ABO and Rhesus compatibility are not required.

ASSESSING THE RECIPIENT

The results of allografting using HLA-identical sibling donors seem to be improving. Transplant-related complications were fewer in the 1990s than in previous decades. Ganciclovir provides effective prophylaxis and treatment against CMV disease. The upper age limit for alloSCT for CML patients remains a matter of debate because of the increased risk of severe GVHD and other complications with increasing age. For patients with HLA-identical sibling donors, it is reasonable to offer transplantation up to the age of 60 years provided they are medically fit; the Seattle team now has an upper age limit of 65 years for conventional allografting.

There is general agreement that results achieved with patients transplanted in chronic phase are superior to those obtained in patients with more advanced disease (Figures 19.1 and 19.2). Furthermore, the results of alloSCT in chronic phase are significantly better in

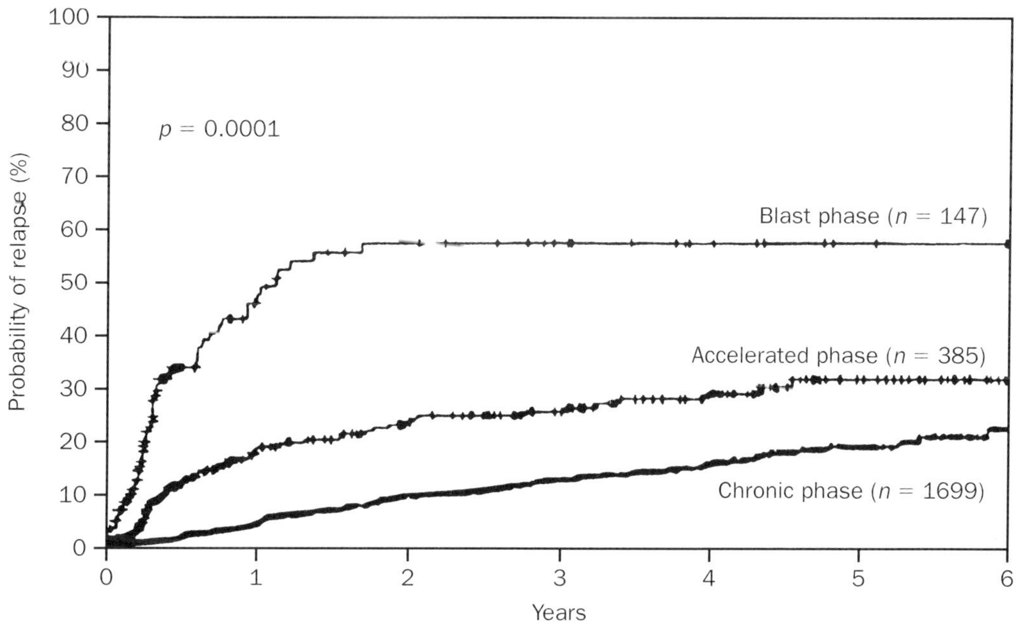

Figure 19.2 Probability of relapse after HLA-identical sibling bone marrow transplantation for CML in the IBMTR series, 1987–1994. (From Horowitz MM, Rowlings PA, Passweg JR, Allogeneic bone marrow transplantation for CML: a report from the International Bone Marrow Transplant Registry. *Bone Marrow Transplant* 1996; **17**(Suppl 3): S5–6, with permission.)

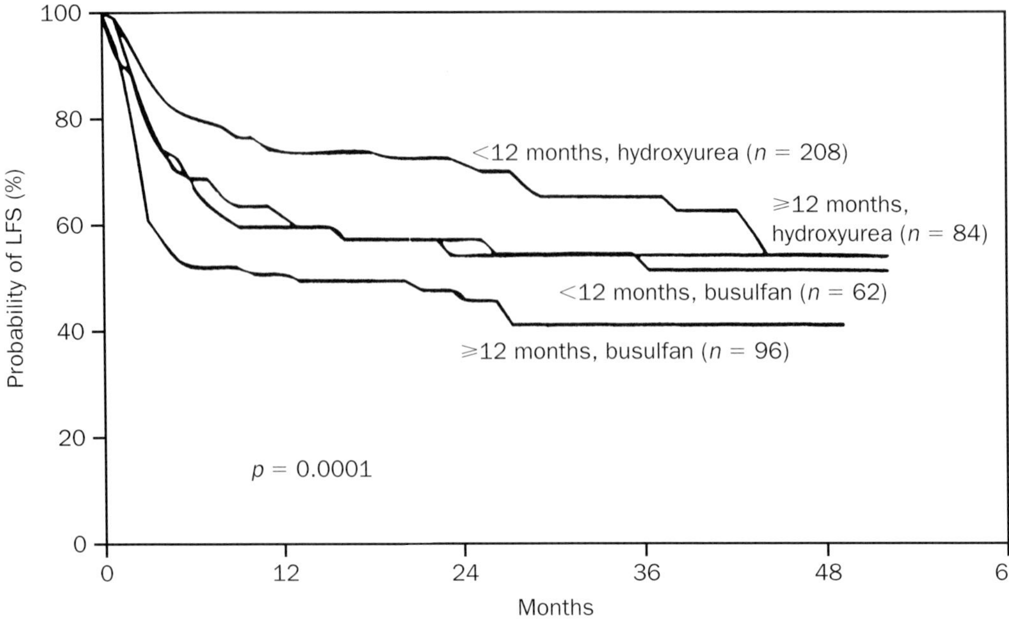

Figure 19.3 Probability of leukemia-free survival (LFS) after HLA-identical sibling BMT for CML in first chronic phase according to interval between diagnosis and transplant and type of pre-BMT treatment. (From Horowitz MM, Rowlings PA, Passweg JR, Allogeneic bone marrow transplantation for CML: a report from the International Bone Marrow Transplant Registry. *Bone Marrow Transplant* 1996; **17**(Suppl 3): S5–6, with permission.)

younger patients and if the transplant is performed early after diagnosis (Figure 19.3).[16–18] Recent reports suggest that the survival benefit of early transplantation extends into the second year following diagnosis; the results of transplant beyond the second year are inferior. The use of busulfan prior to transplant is independently associated with increased transplant-related mortality (Figure 19.3).[16,19] For patients prepared for transplant with busulfan/cyclophosphamide, the improved survival for allografts performed in chronic phase within 1 year of diagnosis only occurred in the group given prior maintenance therapy with hydroxyurea rather than with busulfan.[20] Prolonged use of IFN-α prior to alloSCT may also be associated with an adverse outcome,[21–23] but this effect appears to disappear if the drug is discontinued at least 3 months prior to the allograft (Figure 19.4).[23]

Recent analysis by the International Bone Marrow Transplant Registry (IBMTR) suggests a 30% long-term disease-free survival for patients transplanted in accelerated phase (Figure 19.1).[19] Copelan and colleagues[24] reported a striking 3-year leukemia-free survival rate of 55% in a small group of patients who received busulfan/cyclophosphamide conditioning for accelerated-phase disease, but these results have not been confirmed. The prognostic importance of the different IBMTR criteria for acceleration varies considerably,[25] but it is clear that increased numbers of blasts are associated with a poor outcome. The long-term results of alloSCT in blastic phase are poorer still (Figure 19.1). Hematological relapse post transplant is more common for advanced-phase disease, but, for unclear reasons, so also is severe acute GVHD.[25]

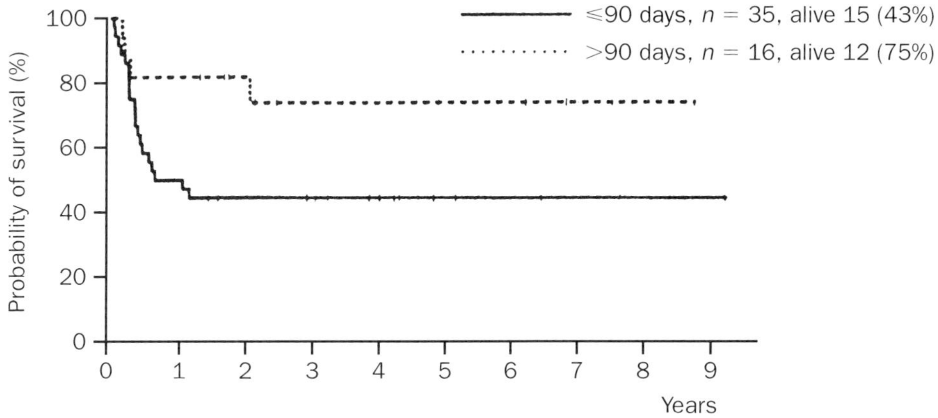

Figure 19.4 Survival after related donor BMT for CML in chronic phase according to interval of less than 90 days or more than 90 days between discontinuation of pre-transplant IFN-α and BMT. (From Hehlmann R, Hochhaus A, Kolb H-J et al, Interferon before allogeneic bone marrow transplantation in chronic myelogenous leukemia does not affect outcome adversely, provided it is discontinued at least 90 days before the procedure. *Blood* 1999; **94:** 3668–77.)

As discussed in Chapter 15, the European Group for Blood and Marrow Transplantation (EBMT) have formulated a 'risk score' that takes into account the patient's age, disease phase, duration of disease, HLA-match with the prospective donor, and patient–donor gender relationship.[26] The probability of transplant-related mortality is significantly related to pre-transplant risk score (see Figure 15.3 in Chapter 15). For example, a patient with newly diagnosed disease in chronic phase who has an HLA-identical brother may score 0, while an older patient with CML diagnosed earlier and now in transformation who only has an unrelated donor would score 6.

CONDITIONING REGIMENS

Pretransplant conditioning should be sufficiently immunosuppressive to allow engraftment of donor cells. Preparative regimens are also designed to ablate the recipient's leukemic clone. However, cure of CML is almost certainly dependent on a GVL effect as well. As reviewed in Chapter 17 and elsewhere,[5] numerous myeloablative preparative regimens have been used. The combination of cyclophosphamide (60 mg/kg/day for 2 days) and TBI has been the most popular. TBI has been administered either in a single dose or in multiple fractions. Whether fractionated treatment may be as effective as a single dose of TBI has not been formally studied in patients undergoing alloSCT for CML.

Intensification of the chemo/radiotherapy may augment antileukemic activity, but usually at the cost of greater toxicity. In a Seattle study, a dose of TBI of 1200 cGy was associated with a 36% actuarial risk of relapse at 4 years; in contrast, no relapse was observed in patients given 1575 cGy. However, overall survival was not improved for the patients receiving the higher dose, because of increased mortality from causes other than relapse.[27] Additional chemotherapy, such as busulfan, dimethylbusulfan, and anthracyclines, has provided no clear benefit.

Because of the technical demands and toxicity of TBI, many centers have employed preparative regimens that omit irradiation. The most widely used is BuCy2, which consists of busulfan (4 mg/kg/day for 4 days) combined with cyclophosphamide (120 mg/kg). BuCy2 causes a later neutrophil nadir, and may occasionally result in permanent alopecia. It should probably not be used if there has been substantial prior exposure to busulfan. An additional limitation of busulfan-based conditioning is the drug's variable pharmacokinetics. High busulfan levels may be associated with hepatic veno-occlusive disease and greater transplant-related mortality.[28] The Seattle group have suggested that BuCy2 may be less toxic and more efficacious if the oral busulfan dose is adjusted according to the busulfan plasma level.[29] Parenteral preparations of busulfan may also help to overcome the problem of erratic bioavailability.

Randomized trials performed in Seattle[30] and France[31] have compared cyclophosphamide/TBI and BuCy2 as preparative therapy for HLA-identical sibling BMT in patients with CML in chronic phase. The Seattle team reported a higher frequency of GVHD, renal dysfunction, and infection in the patients given cyclophosphamide/TBI.[30] These differences were not seen in the French study.[31] Event-free and overall survival were equivalent in patients receiving BuCy2 and cyclophosphamide/TBI in both reports. Although cyclophosphamide/TBI may be somewhat more toxic, both cyclophosphamide/TBI and BuCy2 are acceptable regimens for HLA-identical sibling alloSCT for CML in chronic phase. For advanced-phase disease, however, transplant-related mortality may be greater in patients receiving BuCy2.[32]

Novel preparative regimens

Because of the potent GVL effect of alloSCT for CML, less intensive conditioning might be feasible. At the Hammersmith Hospital, adequate immunosuppression and myeloablation have been achieved using busulfan alone before second BMT in patients relapsing after a previous allograft.[33] As discussed in Chapter 17, several groups have described exciting preliminary results of alloSCT following conditioning with non-myeloablative regimens.[34–39] With this approach, the intensity of the conditioning is lowered to reduce toxicity, but is still sufficiently immunosuppressive to allow engraftment of donor cells. Following engraftment, the procedure's success is dependent on the ability of donor-derived lymphoid cells to eradicate leukemia. The current consensus is that this procedure should not be used in standard-risk patients, but should be reserved for those who are likely to suffer severe complications with conventional alloSCT.

Because increased irradiation results in less relapse, radiation therapy that targets lymphohematopoietic organs is being developed.[40] Such treatments include ^{131}I-labeled monoclonal antibodies directed against CD33 and CD45, ^{166}Ho, an α-emitter with affinity for bone, and ^{52}Fe, which is taken up avidly by the erythroid marrow.

MANAGEMENT OF THE SPLENOMEGALY

The presence of an enlarged spleen influences survival adversely after allografting. The addition of splenic irradiation to the preparative regimen does not appear to provide any major advantage to patients receiving HLA-identical sibling transplants.[5,41] Although splenectomy might augment cytoreduction, retrospective studies have revealed no improvement in relapse rates or survival. Removal of the spleen appears to accelerate recovery of blood counts and reduce transfusion requirements in patients with marked splenomegaly, but acute GVHD and infection may be more prominent.[5]

SOURCE OF HEMATOPOIETIC STEM CELLS

Bone marrow has been the conventional source of hematopoietic stem cells in allogeneic transplantation. A blood stem cell harvest is a more convenient and less invasive approach to obtaining progenitor cells than a marrow harvest.

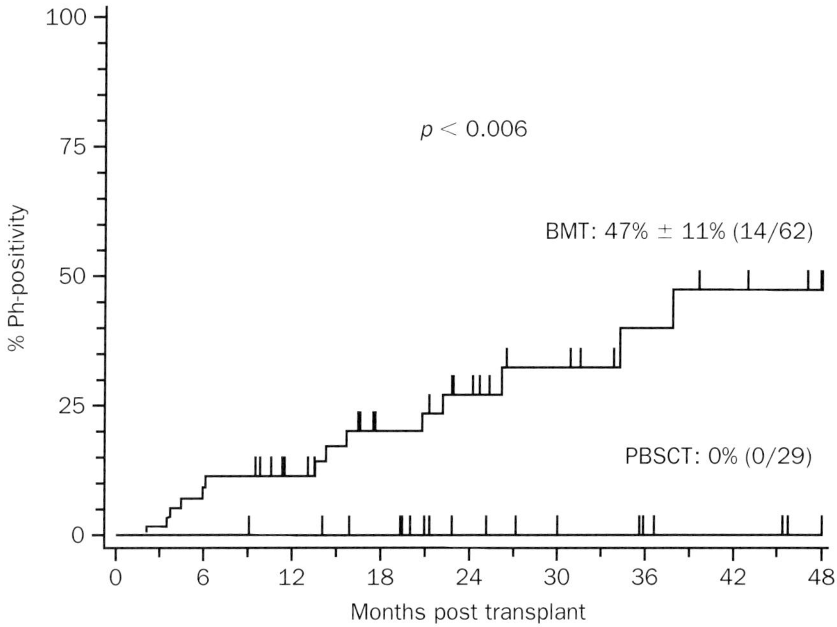

Figure 19.5 Four-year cumulative estimates of cytogenetic relapse after transplantation of allogeneic bone marrow (BMT) or peripheral blood stem cells (PBSCT) in patients with first chronic phase CML in a non-randomized study reported by the Essen group (Ph, Philadelphia chromosome). Tick marks indicate patients who survive in continuous cytogenetic remission of CML. (From Elmaagacli AH, Beelen DW, Opalka B et al, The risk of molecular and cytogenetic disease in patients with Philadelphia-chromosome positive first chronic phase chronic myelogenous leukemia is reduced after transplantation of allogeneic peripheral blood stem cells compared with bone marrow. *Blood* 1999; **94:** 384–9, with permission.)

Blood stem cells are collected by leukapheresis after treatment of the donor with recombinant human granulocyte colony-stimulating factor (G-CSF) over 5–6 days. In theory, pharmacological doses of G-CSF might perturb the donor's myelopoiesis sufficiently to cause myelodysplasia and leukemia in subsequent years, but the risk seems small.[5,42] As blood-derived transplants contain a higher number of T cells, one would anticipate more GVHD and greater GVL activity (Figure 19.5) with blood SCT.[5,43]

A multicenter randomized trial comparing allogeneic blood SCT with marrow SCT in patients with hematological malignancies has now been reported.[44] Engraftment was more rapid and survival significantly better with blood SCT. Relapse was indeed less common with blood SCT, but there has been no statistical difference in the frequency of acute or chronic GVHD. The results of other randomized studies comparing blood and marrow SCT are awaited.

GRAFT-VERSUS-HOST DISEASE PROPHYLAXIS

For the prevention of GVHD, combined cyclosporin and methotrexate therapy is preferred.[45,46] With this regimen, the frequency of severe GVHD is low, but not negligible, and the likelihood of relapse is 20–30% in the first 5 years

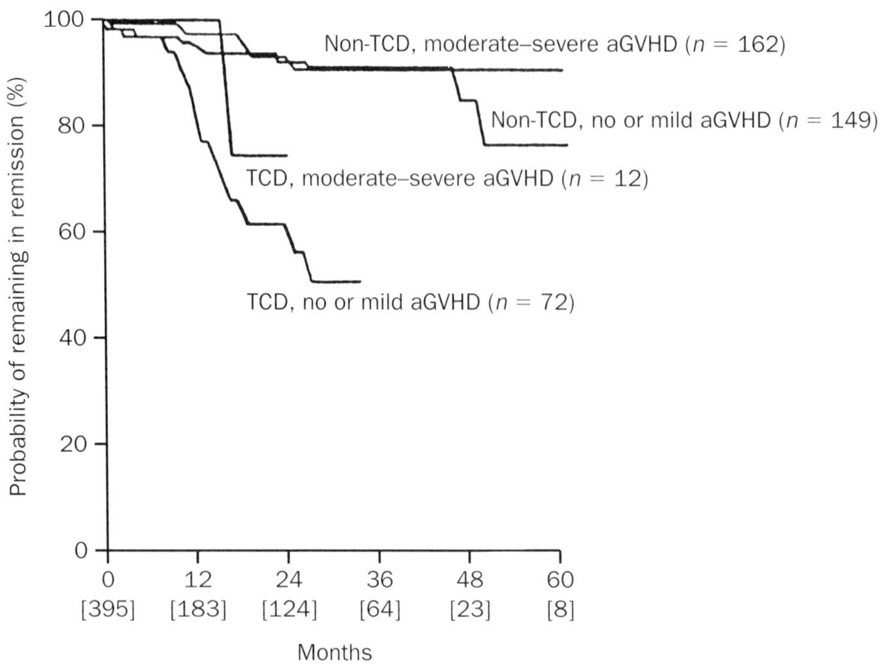

Figure 19.6 Actuarial probability of remaining in remission after T-cell-depleted (TCD) or non-T-cell-depleted (Non-TCD) HLA-identical sibling alloBMT for CML in first chronic phase according to the presence or absence of moderate to severe acute GVHD (aGVHD). Number of patients at risk are given in parentheses. (From Goldman JM, Gale RP, Horowitz MM et al, Bone marrow transplantation for chronic myelogenous leukemia in chronic phase: increased risk of relapse associated with T-cell depletion. *Ann Intern Med* 1988; **108:** 806–14.)

post alloSCT. The optimal timing and dosage of these drugs have not been established.[46]

Although GVHD is markedly reduced if the graft is depleted of T cells (Figure 19.6),[3,47–54] this also increases the risk of graft rejection and leukemic relapse. Ex vivo T-cell depletion with the monoclonal anti-CD52 antibody Campath results in an actuarial relapse rate after alloSCT in chronic phase of 60–70%. Other methods of T-cell depletion, including use of other antibodies and E-rosette formation/soybean lectin agglutination, also reduce the incidence of GVHD, but increase to varying degrees the incidence of relapse. That rejection is increased by T-cell depletion suggests that the T cells play an important role in facilitating engraftment. At most centers, T-cell depletion is reserved for patients receiving grafts from unrelated or mismatched donors. In view of the remarkable efficacy of DLI as treatment for relapse following alloSCT, however, T-cell depletion is again becoming popular as a means to minimize GVHD.[50–54]

RESULTS ACCORDING TO DISEASE PHASE

Transplant in chronic phase

Cure is possible in the majority of patients undergoing alloSCT for CML in chronic phase.[2,3,13,17,19,25] Most survivors of alloBMT have normal hematopoiesis for periods that now extend beyond 10 years. Such patients have no evidence of residual leukemia, i.e., no Philadelphia chromosome (Ph) on cytogenetic analysis or *BCR/ABL* transcripts by PCR.[55,56] In a report from the IBMTR, for 1699 patients transplanted in chronic phase between 1987 and

1994 with marrow from HLA-identical siblings, the 3-year probability of leukemia-free survival was 57% (Figure 19.1).[19] However, this figure was partially based on patients transplanted with donor marrow depleted ex vivo of T cells. As mentioned previously, T-cell depletion may impair donor hematopoietic engraftment and predispose the patient to relapse (Figure 19.6).[3,47–49] In an unpublished IBMTR analysis performed in 1992, the 5-year survival and leukemia-free survival rates were 58% and 54%, respectively, for non-T-cell-depleted transplants. The majority of hematological relapses occurred in the first 3 years following alloBMT; the overall probability of relapse at 5 years was 19%. If patients receiving T-cell-depleted marrow were excluded, the relapse rate was 13%. As discussed in Chapter 20, graft rejection, GVHD, and early death are more common in recipients of marrow from 'matched' unrelated volunteers than from HLA-identical siblings.

Transplant in advanced phase

AlloSCT results in prolonged leukemia-free survival in a substantial minority of patients in advanced phase, but the results are clearly inferior to what can be achieved in chronic phase (Figure 19.1).[1,25,47,57] GVHD,[11,25] infection, and relapse are increased. The IBMTR figures for disease-free survival rates at 3 years following BMT with HLA-identical sibling donors performed in chronic and accelerated phase are 57% and 41%, respectively (Figure 19.1).[19]

For patients undergoing alloBMT in blastic phase, the actuarial leukemia-free survival rate at 3 years is 18% in the IBMTR series (Figure 19.1).[19] Because of the abysmal prognosis of patients allografted in overt blast crisis, many centers would first administer intensive 'acute-leukemia-type' therapy and offer alloSCT to those patients able to achieve a second chronic phase.[58]

SYNGENEIC TRANSPLANTATION

In 1979, Fefer and colleagues[59] reported successful transplantation in four patients with CML in chronic phase from identical-twin donors after conditioning with cyclophosphamide, dimethylbusulfan, and a single dose of 920 cGy of TBI. Leukemic cells were

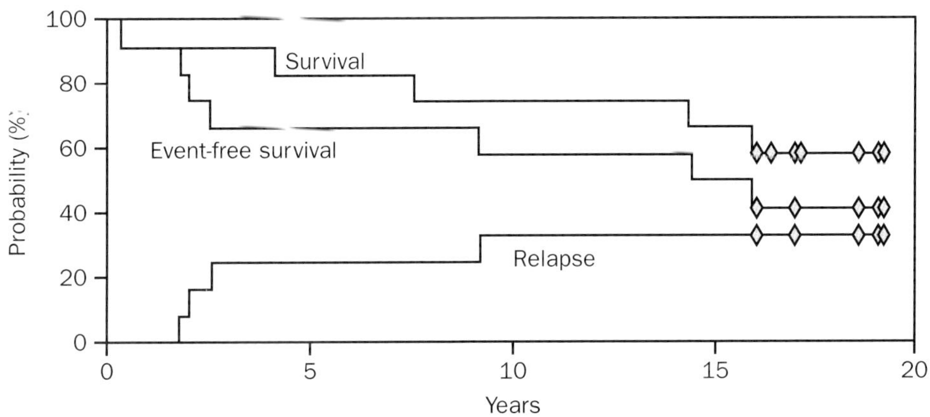

Figure 19.7 Probabilities of survival and relapse for 12 patients with CML in chronic phase transplanted from syngeneic donors before May 1981 after a regimen of cyclophosphamide, dimethylbusulfan, and TBI in Seattle. Survival and events were updated as of December 1996. (From Clift RA, Anasetti C, Allografting for chronic myeloid leukaemia. *Baillière's Clin Haematol* 1997; **10:** 319–36.)

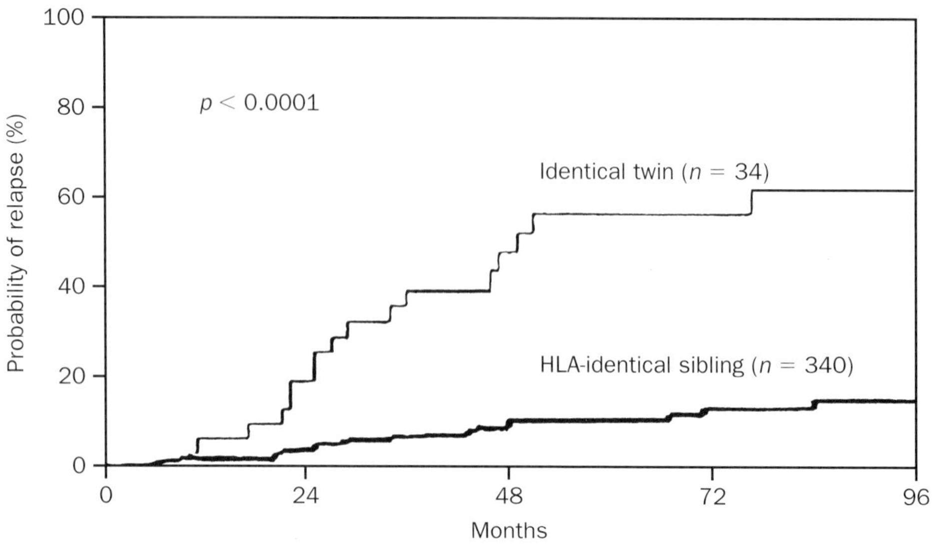

Figure 19.8 Probability of relapse after HLA-identical sibling and identical-twin transplants for CML in first chronic phase in the IBMTR series. (From Horowitz MM, Rowlings PA, Passweg JR, Allogeneic bone marrow transplantation for CML: a report from the International Bone Marrow Transplant Registry. *Bone Marrow Transplant* 1996; **17**(Suppl 3): S5–6, with permission.)

eliminated in all patients. The Seattle team and other groups extended these studies to other CML patients with identical-twin donors (Figures 19.7 and 19.8).[17,19,60,61] Because of the absence of graft rejection and GVHD with syngeneic grafts, post-transplant immunosuppressive therapy is not required, transplant-related mortality is very low (in the range of 0–10%), and overall survival is at least comparable to that of HLA-identical sibling alloSCT. The high relapse rates (Figure 19.8) are probably related to the lack of a major GVL effect. A recent report from the IBMTR suggests that relapse risk and overall outcome might be improved by infusing a relatively large dose of cells at transplant (i.e. $>3 \times 10^8$ nucleated marrow cells/kg).[60]

PROGNOSIS

Outcome of alloSCT for CML is determined by several factors, including disease phase (Figure 19.1),[12,62,63] degree of HLA mismatch,[9] and age.[1,17,19] Patients under 20 years of age have a better outcome than older patients. Results are generally inferior in patients more than 40 years of age, but survival does not differ significantly between those 41–50 years versus those 51–60 years of age. There is no clear evidence that the risk of transplant-related mortality increases as a continuum. As mentioned previously, better survival is seen if alloSCT is carried out in the first 1–2 years after diagnosis (Figure 19.3).[1,12,13,16,19] Prior busulfan therapy is an independent adverse risk factor (Figure 19.3),[16,19,20] – presumably because of the greater cumulative toxicity of this drug. In current practice, however, only rare patients have received busulfan therapy before referral for alloSCT. In patients treated with IFN-α, as already mentioned, it appears that transplant outcome is not adversely affected if the drug is discontinued at least 3 months before the allograft (Figure 19.4).[23]

GRAFT-VERSUS-LEUKEMIA EFFECT

As discussed in Chapter 23, a GVL effect plays a major role in the cure of CML after alloSCT. The greater risk of relapse seen in patients without GVHD,[12,62,63] in recipients of T-cell-depleted grafts, and in syngeneic transplants[19] all lend support to this concept. For patients who relapse following transplantation, remission has been re-induced by DLI[64] or by discontinuation of immunosuppression,[65,66] providing additional evidence for the role of GVL. Selective depletion of donor $CD8^+$ T cells has resulted in less GVHD without an increase in leukemic relapse,[67,68] suggesting that GVHD and GVL are mediated by different T-cell subsets.

MINIMAL RESIDUAL DISEASE

Patients who relapse typically do so in an orderly manner that appears to recapitulate the natural history of the original disease. Thus, a patient who has been negative on RT-PCR study of peripheral blood and also Ph-negative may become PCR-positive.[55,56,69–75] Relapses can usually be detected first at the molecular level. The number of *BCR/ABL* transcripts progressively increases (*molecular relapse*). Subsequently, Ph-positive metaphases are detected in the marrow or blood (*cytogenetic relapse*). When their level reaches 100%, the patient demonstrates a leukocytosis, splenomegaly, and other features typical of *hematological relapse* (Figure 19.9).

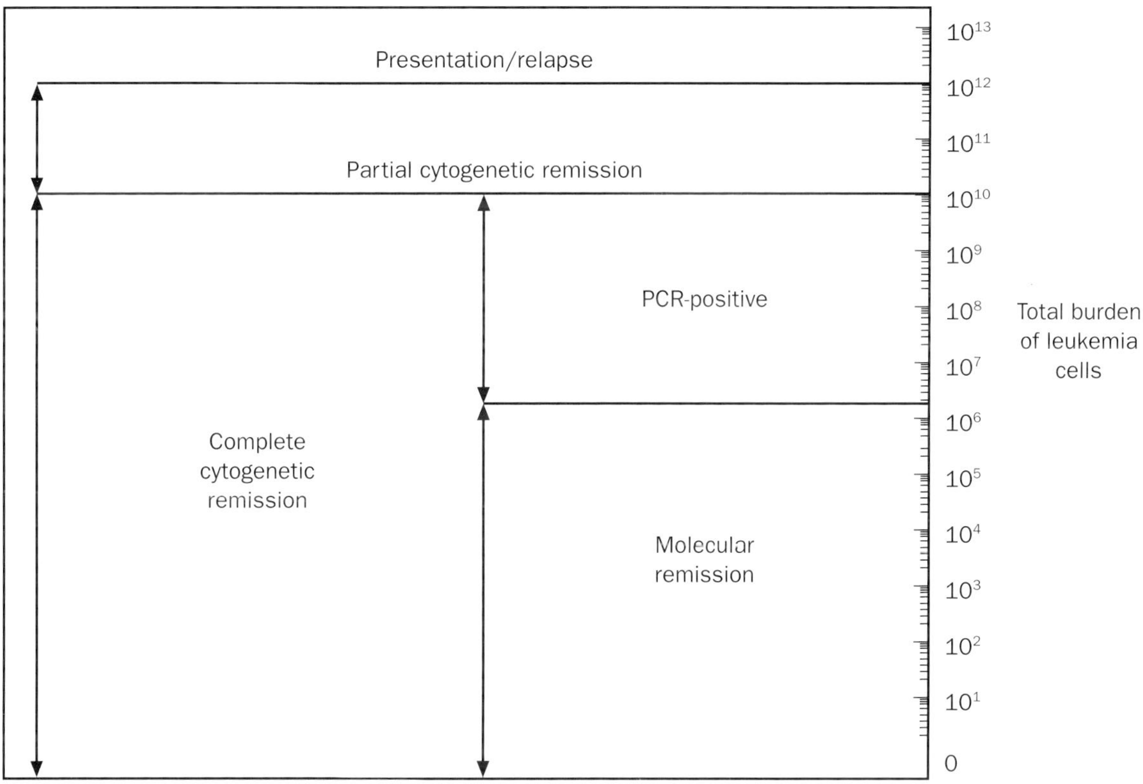

Figure 19.9 Approximate ranges of total numbers of leukemic cells at presentation, relapse and remission. Most patients in partial cytogenetic remission are also positive by Southern and Western blotting; all are positive by PCR. Most patients in complete cytogenetic remission are negative by Southern and Western blotting; however, a fraction are still PCR-positive (From Cross NCP, Assessing residual leukaemia. *Baillière's Clin Haematol* 1997; **10:** 389–403, with permission.)

These observations provide the rationale for routine use of RT-PCR to monitor *BCR/ABL* transcript numbers in patients in complete cytogenetic remission after alloSCT.[69,72,73] As discussed in Chapter 21, RNA is extracted from the buffy coat of blood or bone marrow and reverse transcribed into cDNA. Using oligonucleotide primers, a junctional region of cDNA is then amplified by two-step PCR, electrophoresed, and probed for the *BCR/ABL* rearrangement. *BCR/ABL* transcripts can be quantified using a 'competing' molecule of known concentration that co-amplifies with material from the patient.[72] As blood and marrow give equivalent results for RT-PCR measurements of *BCR/ABL* transcripts, blood alone can be used.[74] Ph-positive patients are invariably PCR-positive for *BCR/ABL* (Figure 19.9). In theory, patients might harbor a population of leukemic cells that do not express *BCR/ABL* RNA. However, RT-PCR measurements and amplification of *BCR/ABL* in genomic DNA are usually concordant.[72] The recent introduction of 'real-time' RT-PCR may make quantitative measurements of *BCR/ABL* transcripts more convenient and reliable, and allow easier standardization between laboratories.[76]

In most cases, rising numbers of *BCR/ABL* transcripts after alloSCT predict for cytogenetic and later hematological relapse.[72] Most patients will be PCR-positive at least once in the first year following transplant.[55,69] Patients destined never to relapse may have diminishing levels of *BCR/ABL* transcripts in their blood; in such cases, RT-PCR usually becomes entirely negative by the end of the first year after alloSCT. Relapse is more likely in patients who are PCR-positive after more than 1 year than in those who are persistently negative. Most 10-year survivors are PCR-negative, but occasional patients are positive without other signs of relapse.[74]

Fluorescence in situ hybridization (FISH) allows direct visualization of the Ph translocation without the risk of contamination associated with PCR. A variety of techniques have been employed, including interphase FISH, metaphase FISH, and hypermetaphase FISH, but their precise role in monitoring patients post alloSCT remains undefined.

RELAPSE AFTER alloSCT

Molecular and cytogenetic relapses

Molecular relapse can be defined as the finding of persistently high *BCR/ABL* transcript numbers or a rising number of transcripts more than 9 months after transplant.[75] A small percentage of patients in the first year after alloSCT are transiently found to have some Ph-positive metaphases in their bone marrow.[77] These Ph-positive cells commonly disappear, and many of these patients are long-term survivors. The pattern tends to be different in the cytogenetic relapse that precedes hematological relapse. At about 12–36 months after BMT, there is a progressive increase in the percentage of Ph-positive cells, usually in the absence of symptoms. Patients with rising numbers of *BCR/ABL* transcripts in blood or Ph-positive metaphases in bone marrow are candidates for treatment by DLI.[75]

Hematological relapse

Most relapses occur in the first 3 years after transplant, but some occur many years later.[74] Hematological relapse after alloBMT occurs in 10–20% of recipients of unmanipulated donor marrow, in 60–80% of those receiving marrow depleted ex vivo of T cells, and in the majority of patients transplanted in advanced phase. Although relapse usually evolves over time,[56] occasional patients present abruptly with blastic-phase disease.[78] In these patients, it is possible that a preceding relapse to chronic phase may not have been detected. A second possibility is that transformed cells present at the time of transplant persisted after BMT. Thirdly, leukemic stem cells may survive allografting and retain the ability to transform abruptly into a more primitive phenotype.

Donor cell relapse

In rare instances, leukemic relapse has been documented in donor cells.[79,80] Its mechanism is unexplained. It is most easily shown in sex-mismatched transplants, where cells with the sex chromosomes of the donor are found to contain the Ph chromosome. Residual host leukemia cells or the marrow microenvironment might interact with normal donor cells and render them leukemic.

TREATMENT OF RELAPSE

There are various approaches to the management of relapse. To unleash potential GVL effects, a reasonable initial step would be to reduce or eliminate immunosuppressive drug therapy,[65,66,81] although this may be difficult in patients with active GVHD. For patients no longer receiving cyclosporin, alternative approaches include treatment with hydroxyurea or IFN-α, or a second alloSCT.[33,81–84] As discussed in Chapter 24, however, the most effective therapy is the transfusion of lymphoid cells from the original stem cell donor.

Donor lymphocyte infusions

Transfusion of donor derived lymphocytes induces complete remission in 60–80% of patients who relapse into chronic phase and in some patients with more advanced disease.[50,51,64,84–93] Those achieving cytogenetic remission revert from PCR-positivity to PCR-negativity. Most responses are seen within 1–9 months of DLI, and are durable.[93]

The procedure is most successful when performed in the first 2 years following alloSCT for patients with molecular or cytogenetic (and not hematological) evidence of relapse.[89,90] Remissions with DLI are also more common in patients whose original transplants were T-cell-depleted, in patients with limited GVHD at DLI, and in those who develop acute and chronic GVHD following lymphocyte infusion.[88–90] However, in occasional patients, the GVHD is severe and fatal. Acute GVHD is associated with increasing patient age, donor–recipient sex mismatch,[92] and lymphocyte dose.[87] For patients relapsing following HLA-identical sibling transplantation, larger numbers of T cells must be transfused for relapse in accelerated phase than chronic phase.

Pancytopenia due to marrow aplasia occurs in about 10–20% of patients treated with DLI.[89,90] This complication is more common in those with overt hematological relapse and limited donor hematopoiesis prior to lymphocyte infusion.[90] The aplasia usually improves with transfusion of donor stem cells.[64,90]

As DLI appears to be safer and more effective if performed before the onset of hematological relapse, it may be advisable to monitor patients using PCR studies on a monthly or bimonthly basis for the 2 years following alloSCT, and thereafter at longer intervals. DLI can then be administered before hematological relapse in patients with rising numbers of *BCR/ABL* transcripts in blood or Ph-positive metaphases in marrow.[86,91] Treatment with relatively low lymphocyte doses appears to reduce the risk of GVHD and marrow aplasia,[86,87] although the optimal cell dose is not precisely defined. It is also unclear whether GVHD prophylaxis should be administered. As already mentioned, complete remissions have been observed following abrupt discontinuation of cyclosporin immunosuppression, even without DLI.[65,66,81]

In view of the efficacy of DLI, numerous groups are attempting to develop methods to maximize the GVL effect while reducing the capacity of the transfused lymphocytes to cause GVHD. One approach is to deplete the initial alloSCT of T cells, thus lessening the risk of GVHD in the early post-transplant period. After engraftment and recovery from the early toxicity of the preparative regimen, 'lymphocyte add-back' is performed to confer the GVL effect.[52] In patients who relapse following alloSCT, the MD Anderson Cancer Center group in Houston[94] have reported that DLI selectively depleted of CD8+ cells is effective treatment for relapse with a low risk of GVHD. Another approach is to begin treatment with the minimum number of lymphocytes (1×10^7 T cells/kg) thought to be effective, and then to repeat the transfusion on an escalating schedule at regular intervals until a response is seen.[87] Patients receiving escalated dose infusions have a lower incidence of GVHD than those receiving bulk dose therapy; early data suggest that the GVL effect is maintained. In an innovative approach devised in Italy,[95] relapsing patients are transfused with donor lymphocytes that have been transduced ex vivo with the herpes simplex thymidine kinase gene; those who develop unacceptable GVHD are given ganciclovir to eliminate the wayward lymphocyte population. To augment GVL, Slavin and colleagues[96] infuse interleukin-2 in conjunction with DLI.

Other treatments for relapse

Alternative approaches to relapse include administration of conventional chemotherapy or IFN-α or performance of a second alloSCT. Because of the risks associated with DLI, some centers would offer IFN-α as primary therapy to relapsing patients.[81] IFN-α in combination with DLI is an alternative approach.[64] A second alloSCT is more likely to be successful if the interval between the two transplants exceeds 2 years.[33,81–83] Because of high transplant-related mortality,[82,83] less intensive conditioning is appropriate.[33]

GENERAL RECOMMENDATIONS

Curative therapy with alloSCT should be the goal in all patients less than 60 years of age. If an HLA-identical sibling is available, alloSCT should be performed as early as feasible for younger patients. For those 40 years of age or older, one might postpone the transplant to allow a trial of IFN-α (or the new agent STI571). If the patient has a cytogenetic response, alloSCT could be postponed until there is evidence of IFN-α resistance. For those patients who become resistant to IFN-α, there should be an interval of at least 3 months between discontinuation of the drug and alloSCT.[23] Some debatable points are the upper age limit for alloSCT, the age at which an initial trial of IFN-α is appropriate, and the duration of IFN-α therapy if a cytogenetic response is not achieved within 6 months.

FUTURE DEVELOPMENTS

Although T-cell depletion is not currently used in the majority of transplant centers, the procedure might regain favor if it could eliminate the cells responsible for GVHD while leaving intact those responsible for facilitating engraftment and mediating GVL effects. The greater risk of relapse with T-cell depletion could be offset by T-cell add-back on a routine basis or at the earliest signs of relapse.[50,52–54] This approach would be enhanced by ex vivo methods to produce alloreactive, leukemia-specific donor T cells.[97] Elucidation of the mechanism of action of GVL should also lead to immunotherapeutic approaches to the management of CML that do not involve intensive conditioning regimens. In this regard, the recent introduction of allotransplantation with non-myeloablative preparative regimens[34–39] is of great interest. The results of allografting for CML in advanced phase remain unsatisfactory and highlight the need to perform alloSCT early in the course of the disease before the onset of blastic transformation.

REFERENCES

1. Thomas ED, Clift RA, Fefer A et al, Marrow transplantation for the treatment of chronic myelogenous leukemia. *Ann Intern Med* 1986; **104:** 155–63.
2. Goldman JM, Apperley JF, Jones L et al, Bone marrow transplantation for patients with chronic myeloid leukemia. *N Engl J Med* 1986; **314:** 202–7.
3. Goldman JM, Gale RP, Horowitz MM et al, Bone

marrow transplantation for chronic myelogenous leukemia in chronic phase: increased risk of relapse associated with T-cell depletion. *Ann Intern Med* 1988; **108:** 806–14.

4. Gale RP, Hehlmann R, Zhang M-J et al, Survival with bone marrow transplantation versus hydroxyurea or interferon for chronic myelogenous leukemia. *Blood* 1998; **91:** 1810–19.
5. Savage DG, Goldman JM, Chronic myelogenous leukemia. In: *High Dose Therapy: Pharmacology, Hematopoietins, Stem Cells*, 3rd edn (Armitage JO, Antman KH, eds). Baltimore: Williams & Wilkins, 1999: 705–31.
6. Silver RT, Woolf SH, Hehlmann R et al, An evidence-based analysis of the effect of busulfan, hydroxyurea, interferon, and allogeneic bone marrow transplantation in treating the chronic phase of chronic myeloid leukemia: developed for the American Society of Hematology. *Blood* 1999; **94:** 1517–36.
7. Buckner CD, Epstein RB, Rudolph RH et al, Allogeneic marrow engraftment following whole body irradiation in a patient with leukemia. *Blood* 1970; **35:** 741–50.
8. Thomas ED, A history of haemopoietic cell transplantation. *Br J Haematol* 1999; **105:** 330–9.
9. Anasetti C, Amos D, Beatty PG et al, Effect of HLA compatibility on engraftment of bone marrow transplants in patients with leukemia or lymphoma. *N Engl J Med* 1989; **320:** 197–204.
10. Charron DJ, HLA matching in unrelated donor bone marrow transplantation. *Curr Opin Hematol* 1996; **3:** 416–22.
11. Nash RA, Pepe MS, Storb R et al, Acute graft-versus-host disease: analysis of risk factors after allogeneic marrow transplantation and prophylaxis with cyclosporine and methotrexate. *Blood* 1992; **80:** 1838–45.
12. Enright H, Davies SM, DeFor T et al, Relapse after non-T-cell-depleted allogeneic bone marrow transplantation for chronic myelogenous leukemia: early transplantation, use of an unrelated donor, and chronic graft-versus-host disease are protective. *Blood* 1996; **88:** 714–20.
13. Van Rhee F, Szydlo RM, Hermans J et al, Long-term results after allogeneic bone marrow transplantation for chronic myelogenous leukemia in chronic phase: a report from the Chronic Leukaemia Working Party of the European Group for Blood and Marrow Transplantation. *Bone Marrow Transplant* 1997; **20:** 553–60.
14. Confer D, Matlack M, Kitajima D, Howe CWS, The effect of donor age on recipient outcome following unrelated donor bone marrow transplant. *Blood* 1998; **92**(Suppl 1): 686a.
15. Reusser P, Riddell SR, Meyers JD, Greenberg PD, Cytotoxic T-lymphocyte response to cytomegalovirus after human allogeneic bone marrow transplantation: pattern of recovery and correlation with cytomegalovirus infection and disease. *Blood* 1991; **78:** 1373–80.
16. Goldman JM, Szydlo R, Horowitz MM et al, Choice of pretransplant treatment and timing of transplants for chronic myelogenous leukemia in chronic phase. *Blood* 1993; **82:** 2235–8.
17. Clift RA, Anasetti C, Allografting for chronic myeloid leukaemia. *Baillière's Clin Haematol* 1997; **10:** 319–36.
18. Italian Cooperative Study Group on Chronic Myeloid Leukemia and Italian Group for Bone Marrow Transplantation, Monitoring treatment and survival in chronic myeloid leukemia. *J Clin Oncol* 1999; **17:** 1858–68.
19. Horowitz MM, Rowlings PA, Passweg JR, Allogeneic bone marrow transplantation for CML: a report from the International Bone Marrow Transplant Registry. *Bone Marrow Transplant* 1996; **17**(Suppl 3): S5–6.
20. Biggs JC, Szer J, Crilley P et al, Treatment of chronic myeloid leukemia with allogeneic bone marrow transplantation after preparation with BuCy2. *Blood* 1992; **80:** 1352–7.
21. Beelen DW, Graeven U, Elmaagacli AH et al, Prolonged administration of interferon-α in patients with chronic-phase Philadelphia chromosome-positive chronic myelogenous leukemia before allogeneic bone marrow transplantation may adversely affect transplant outcome. *Blood* 1995; **85:** 2981–90.
22. Giralt S, Szydlo RM, Goldman JM et al, Effect of short-term interferon therapy on the outcome of subsequent HLA-identical sibling transplantation for chronic myelogenous leukemia: an analysis from the International Bone Marrow Transplant Registry. *Blood* 2000; **95**: 410–15.
23. Hehlmann R, Hochhaus A, Kolb H-J et al, Interferon before allogeneic bone marrow transplantation in chronic myelogenous leukemia does not affect outcome adversely, provided it is discontinued at least 90 days before the procedure. *Blood* 1999; **94:** 3668–77.
24. Copelan EA, Grever MR, Kapoor N, Tutschka PJ, Marrow transplantation following busulfan and cyclophosphamide for chronic myelogenous

leukaemia in accelerated or blastic phase. *Br J Haematol* 1989; **71:** 487–91.

25. Savage DG, Szydlo RM, Chase A et al, Bone marrow transplantation for chronic myeloid leukaemia: the effects of differing criteria for defining chronic phase on probabilities of survival and relapse. *Br J Haematol* 1997; **99:** 30–5.
26. Gratwohl A, Hermans J, Goldman JM et al, Risk assessment for patients with chronic myeloid leukaemia before allogeneic blood or marrow transplantation. *Lancet* 1998; **352:** 1087–92.
27. Clift RA, Buckner CD, Appelbaum FR et al, Allogeneic marrow transplantation in patients with chronic myeloid leukemia in the chronic phase: a randomized trial of two irradiation regimens. *Blood* 1991; **77:** 1660–5.
28. Ljungman P, Hassan M, Békássy AN et al, High busulfan concentrations are associated with increased transplant-related mortality in allogeneic bone marrow transplant patients. *Bone Marrow Transplant* 1997; **20:** 909–13.
29. Slattery JT, Clift RA, Buckner CD et al, Marrow transplantation for chronic myeloid leukemia: the influence of plasma busulfan levels on the outcome of transplantation. *Blood* 1997; **89:** 3055–60.
30. Clift RA, Radich J, Appelbaum FR et al, Long-term follow-up of a randomized study comparing cyclophosphamide and total body irradiation with busulfan and cyclophosphamide for patients receiving allogeneic marrow transplants during chronic phase of chronic myeloid leukemia. *Blood* 1994; **84:** 2036–43.
31. Devergie A, Blaise D, Attal M et al, Allogeneic bone marrow transplantation for chronic myeloid leukemia in first chronic phase: a randomized trial of busulfan–cytoxan versus cytoxan–total body irradiation as preparative regimen: a report from the French Society of Bone Marrow Graft (SFGM). *Blood* 1995; **85:** 2263–8.
32. Ringdén O, Ruutu T, Remberger M et al, A randomized trial comparing busulfan with total body irradiation as conditioning in allogeneic marrow transplant recipients with leukemia: a report from the Nordic Bone Marrow Transplantation Group. *Blood* 1994; **83:** 2723–30.
33. Cullis JO, Schwarer AP, Hughes TP et al, Second transplants for patients with chronic myeloid leukaemia in relapse after original transplant with T-depleted donor marrow: feasibility of busulphan alone for re-conditioning. *Br J Haematol* 1992; **80:** 33–9.
34. Giralt S, Estey E, Albitar M et al, Engraftment of allogeneic haematopoietic progenitor cells with purine analog-containing chemotherapy: harnessing graft-versus-leukemia without myeloablative therapy. *Blood* 1997; **89:** 4531–6.
35. Slavin S, Nagler A, Naparstek E et al, Nonmyeloablative stem cell transplantation and cell therapy as an alternative to conventional bone marrow transplantation with lethal cytoreduction for the treatment of malignant and nonmalignant hematologic diseases. *Blood* 1998; **91:** 756–63.
36. Kelemen E, Masszi T, Reményi P et al, Reduction in the frequency of transplant-related complications in patients with chronic myeloid leukemia undergoing BMT conditioned with a new, nonmyeloablative drug combination. *Bone Marrow Transplant* 1998; **21:** 747–9.
37. Childs R, Clave E, Contentin N et al, Engraftment kinetics after nonmyeloablative allogeneic peripheral blood stem cell transplantation: full donor T-cell chimerism precedes alloimmune responses. *Blood* 1999; **94:** 3234–41.
38. Kraus A, Spitzer TR, McAfee S et al, Graft-versus-leukemia, mixed chimerism and early T-cell reconstitution in two patients with advanced stage chronic lymphocytic leukemia after bone marrow transplantation with a novel nonmyeloablative conditioning regimen. *Blood* 1999; **92**(Suppl 1): 349a.
39. McSweeney PA, Storb R, Mixed chimerism: preclinical studies and clinical applications. *Biol Blood Marrow Transplant* 1999; **5:** 192–203.
40. Corcoran MC, Press OW, Matthews DC, Appelbaum FR, Bernstein ID, The role of radioimmunotherapy in bone marrow transplantation. *Curr Opin Hematol* 1996; **3**: 438–45.
41. Gratwohl A, Hermans J, von Biezen A et al, Splenic irradiation before bone marrow transplantation. *Br J Haematol* 1996; **95:** 494–500.
42. Appelbaum FR, Choosing the source of stem cells for allogeneic transplantation: no longer a peripheral issue. *Blood* 1999; **94:** 381–3.
43. Elmaagacli AH, Beelen DW, Opalka B et al, The risk of molecular and cytogenetic disease in patients with Philadelphia-chromosome positive first chronic phase chronic myelogenous leukemia is reduced after transplantation of allogeneic peripheral blood stem cells compared with bone marrow. *Blood* 1999; **94:** 384–9.
44. Bensinger W, Martin P, Clift R et al, A prospective randomised trial of peripheral blood stem

cells or marrow for patients undergoing allogeneic transplantation for hematological malignancies. *Blood* 1999; **94**(Suppl 1): 368a.

45. Storb R, Deeg HJ, Pepe M et al, Methotrexate and cyclosporine versus cyclosporine alone for prophylaxis of graft-versus-host disease in patients given HLA-identical marrow grafts for leukemia: long-term follow-up of a controlled trial. *Blood* 1989; **73:** 1729–34.
46. Gratwohl A, Hermans J, Apperley J et al, Acute graft-versus-host disease: grade and outcome in patients with chronic myelogenous leukemia. *Blood* 1995; **86:** 813–18.
47. Apperley JF, Mauro FR, Goldman JM et al, Bone marrow transplantation for chronic myeloid leukaemia in first chronic phase: importance of a graft-versus-leukaemia effect. *Br J Haematol* 1988; **69:** 239–45.
48. Cunningham I, Castro-Malaspina H, Flomenberg N et al, Improved results of bone marrow transplantation (BMT) for chronic myelogenous leukemia using marrow depleted of T cells by soybean lectin agglutination and E-rosette depletion. In: *Progress in Bone Marrow Transplantation* (Gale RP, Champlin RE, eds). New York: Alan R Liss, 1987: 359–63.
49. Marmont AM, Horowitz MM, Gale RP et al, T-cell depletion of HLA-identical transplants in leukemia. *Blood* 1991; **78:** 2120–30.
50. Sehn LH, Alyea EP, Weller E et al, Comparative outcomes of T-cell-depleted and non-T-cell-depleted allogeneic bone marrow transplantation for chronic myelogenous leukemia: impact of donor lymphocyte infusion. *J Clin Oncol* 1999; **17:** 561–8.
51. Porter DL, Collins RH Jr, Shpilberg O et al, Long-term follow-up of patients who achieved complete remission after donor leukocyte infusions. *Biol Blood Marrow Transplant* 1999; **5:** 253–61.
52. Barrett AJ, Mavroudis D, Tisdale J et al, T cell-depleted bone marrow transplantation and delayed T cell add-back to control acute GVHD and conserve a graft-versus-leukemia effect. *Bone Marrow Transplant* 1998; **21:** 543–51.
53. Drobyski WR, Hessner MJ, Klein JP et al, T-cell depletion plus salvage immunotherapy with donor leukocyte infusions as a strategy to treat chronic-phase chronic myelogenous leukemia patients undergoing HLA-identical sibling marrow transplantation. *Blood* 1999; **94:** 434–41.
54. Cwynarski K, Craddock C, Dazzi F et al, T-cell depletion plus adoptive immunotherapy with donor lymphocyte infusions as a strategy to treat stem cell transplantation from volunteer unrelated donors. *Blood* 1999; **94**(Suppl 1): 567a.
55. Morgan GJ, Hughes T, Janssen JWG et al, Polymerase chain reaction for detection of residual leukaemia. *Lancet* 1989; **i:** 928–9.
56. Hughes TP, Morgan GJ, Martiat P, Goldman JM, Detection of residual leukemia after bone marrow transplant for chronic myeloid leukemia: role of the polymerase chain reaction in predicting relapse. *Blood* 1991; **77:** 874–8.
57. Clift RA, Buckner CD, Thomas ED et al, Marrow transplantation for patients in accelerated phase of chronic myeloid leukemia. *Blood* 1994; **84:** 4368–73.
58. Lipton JH, Messner HA, Curtis JE et al, Intensive remission induction therapy for chronic myeloid leukemia in blast phase with a goal of post-remission bone marrow transplant – a pilot study. *Eur J Haematol* 1996; **57:** 42–5.
59. Fefer A, Cheever MA, Thomas ED et al, Disappearance of Ph1-positive cells in four patients with chronic granulocytic leukemia after chemotherapy, irradiation and marrow transplantation from an identical twin. *N Engl J Med* 1979; **300:** 333–7.
60. Barrett AJ, Ringden O, Zhang M-J, Horowitz MM, Effect of nucleated marrow cell dose on relapse and survival in identical twin transplants for leukemia. *Blood* 2000; **95**: 3323–7.
61. Frassoni F, Niederweiser D, Gratwohl A et al, Long-term disease-free (PCR-negative) survival after identical twin transplant in chronic myeloid leukemia: graft-versus-tumor or reduction of leukemic burden? *Blood* 1999; **94**(Suppl 1): 641a.
62. Weiden P, Flovrnoy N, Thomas E et al, Antileukemic effects of graft-versus-host disease in human recipients of allogeneic marrow grafts. *N Engl J Med* 1979; **300:** 1068–73.
63. Sullivan KM, Weiden PL, Storb R et al, Influence of acute and chronic graft-versus-host disease on relapse and survival after bone marrow transplantation from HLA-identical siblings as treatment of acute and chronic leukemia. *Blood* 1989; **73:** 1720–8.
64. Kolb HJ, Mittermüller J, Clemm C et al, Donor leukocyte transfusions for treatment of recurrent chronic myelogenous leukemia in marrow transplant patients. *Blood* 1990; **76:** 2462–5.
65. Collins RH Jr, Rogers ZR, Bennett M et al, Hematologic relapse of chronic myelogenous leukemia following allogeneic bone marrow transplantation: apparent graft-versus-leukemia effect

following abrupt discontinuation of immunosuppression. *Bone Marrow Transplant* 1992; **10:** 391–5.
66. Suzuki R, Taji H, Iida S et al, Complete cytogenetic response with host-derived hematopoiesis induced by cyclosporin A discontinuation in a patient with relapsed chronic myelogenous leukemia after bone marrow transplantation. *Bone Marrow Transplant* 1997; **20:** 615–17.
67. Champlin R, Ho W, Gajewski J et al, Selective depletion of CD8+ T-lymphocytes for prevention of graft-versus-host disease after allogeneic bone marrow transplantation. *Blood* 1990; **76:** 418–23.
68. Alyea EP, Soiffer RJ, Canning C et al, Toxicity and efficacy of defined doses of CD41 donor lymphocytes for treatment of relapse after allogeneic bone marrow transplant. *Blood* 1998; **91:** 3671–80.
69. Negrin RS, Blume KG, The use of the polymerase chain reaction for the detection of minimal residual malignant disease. *Blood* 1991; **78:** 255–8.
70. Cross NCP, Feng L, Chase A et al, Competitive polymerase chain reaction to estimate the number of BCR–ABL transcripts in chronic myeloid leukemia patients after bone marrow transplantation. *Blood* 1993; **82:** 1929–36.
71. Radich JP, Gehly G, Gooley T et al, Polymerase chain reaction detection of the BCR–ABL fusion transcript after allogeneic marrow transplantation for chronic myeloid leukemia: results and implications in 346 patients. *Blood* 1995; **85:** 2632–8.
72. Cross NCP, Assessing residual leukaemia. *Baillière's Clin Haematol* 1997; **10:** 389–404.
73. Faderl S, Talpaz M, Kantarjian HM, Estrov Z, Should polymerase chain reaction analysis to detect minimal residual disease in patients with chronic myelogenous leukemia be used in clinical decision making? *Blood* 1999; **93:** 2755–9.
74. Van Rhee F, Lin F, Cross NC et al, Detection of residual leukaemia more than 10 years after allogeneic bone marrow transplantation. *Bone Marrow Transplant* 1994; **14:** 609–12.
75. Van Rhee F, Feng Lin, Cullis JO et al, Relapse of chronic myeloid leukemia after allogeneic bone marrow transplant: the case for giving donor leukocyte transfusions before the onset of hematologic relapse. *Blood* 1994; **83:** 3377–83.
76. Branford S, Hughes TP, Rudzki Z, Monitoring chronic myeloid leukaemia therapy by real-time quantitative PCR in blood is a reliable alternative to bone marrow cytogenetics. *Br J Haematol* 1999; **107:** 587–99.
77. Arthur CK, Apperley JF, Guo AP et al, Cytogenetic events after bone marrow transplantation for chronic myeloid leukemia in chronic phase. *Blood* 1988; **80:** 1179–86.
78. Cullis JO, Marks DI, Schwarer AP et al, Relapse into blast crisis following bone marrow transplantation for chronic phase chronic myeloid leukaemia: a report of five cases. *Br J Haematol* 1992; **81:** 378–81.
79. Marmont A, Frassoni F, Bacigalupo A et al, Recurrence of Ph9-positive leukemia in donor cells after marrow transplantation for chronic granulocytic leukemia. *N Engl J Med* 1984; **310:** 903–6.
80. McCann SR, Lawler M, Bacigalupo A, Recurrence of Philadelphia chromosome-positive leukemia in donor cells after marrow transplantation for chronic granulocytic leukemia. *Leuk Lymphoma* 1993; **10:** 419–25.
81. Elmaagacli AH, Beelen DW, Schaefer UW, A retrospective single centre study of the outcome of five different therapy approaches in 48 patients with relapse of chronic myelogenous leukemia after allogeneic bone marrow transplantation. *Bone Marrow Transplant* 1997; **20:** 1045–55.
82. Arcese W, Gratwohl A, Niederwieser D et al, Outcome for patients who relapse after allogeneic bone marrow transplantation for chronic myeloid leukemia. *Blood* 1993; **82:** 3211–19.
83. Barrett AJ, Locatelli F, Treleaven JG et al, Second transplants for leukaemic relapse after bone marrow transplantation: high early mortality but favourable effect of chronic GVHD on continued remission. *Br J Haematol* 1991; **79:** 567–74.
84. Locatelli F, The role of repeat transplantation of haemopoietic stem cells and adoptive immunotherapy in treatment of leukaemia relapsing following allogeneic transplantation. *Br J Haematol* 1998; **102:** 633–8.
85. Cullis JO, Jiang YZ, Schwarer AP et al, Donor leukocyte infusions for chronic myeloid leukemia after allogeneic bone marrow transplantation. *Blood* 1992; **79:** 1379–81.
86. Van Rhee F, Feng L, Cullis JO et al, Relapse of chronic myeloid leukemia after allogeneic bone marrow transplant: the case for giving donor leukocyte transfusions before the onset of hematologic relapse. *Blood* 1994; **83:** 3377–83.
87. Mackinnon S, Papadopoulos EB, Carabasi MH et al, Adoptive immunotherapy evaluating escalating doses of donor leukocytes for relapse of

chronic myeloid leukemia after bone marrow transplantation: separation of graft-versus-leukemia responses from graft-versus-host disease. *Blood* 1995; **86:** 1261–8.

88. Kolb HJ, Schattenberg A, Goldman JM et al, Graft-versus-leukemia effect of donor lymphocyte transfusions in marrow grafted patients. European Group for Blood and Marrow Transplantation Working Party Chronic Leukemia. *Blood* 1995; **86:** 2041–50.
89. Collins RH Jr, Shpilberg O, Drobyski WR et al, Donor leukocyte infusions in 140 patients with relapsed malignancy after allogeneic bone marrow transplantation. *J Clin Oncol* 1997; **15:** 433–44.
90. Keil F, Haas OA, Fritsch G et al, Donor leukocyte infusion for leukemic relapse after allogeneic marrow transplantation: lack of residual donor hematopoiesis predicts aplasia. *Blood* 1997; **89:** 3113–17.
91. Van Rhee F, Savage DG, Blackwell J et al, Comparison of adoptive immunotherapy for relapse of chronic myeloid leukaemia using allogeneic lymphocytes from sibling or unrelated marrow donors. *Bone Marrow Transplant* 1998; **21:** 1055–61.
92. Dazzi F, Cwynarski K, Craddock C et al, Factors influencing acute GVHD after donor lymphocyte infusion. *Blood* 1999; **94**(Suppl 1): 669a.
93. Cwynarski K, Dazzi F, Cross NCP et al, Response to donor lymphocyte infusions in patients with CML in relapse after allografting: a long-term follow-up study using RT-PCR. *Blood* 1999; **94**(Suppl 1): 669a.
94. Giralt S, Hester J, Huh Y et al, CD8-depleted donor lymphocyte infusion as treatment for relapsed chronic myelogenous leukemia after allogeneic bone marrow transplantation. *Blood* 1995; **86:** 4337–43.
95. Ciceri F, Bonini C, Marktel S et al, Long term follow-up in 30 patients receiving HSV-TK transduced donor lymphocytes after allo-BMT. *Blood* 1999; **94**(Suppl 1): 668a.
96. Slavin S, Naparstek E, Nagler A et al, Allogeneic cell therapy with donor peripheral blood cells and recombinant human interleukin-2 to treat leukemia relapse after allogeneic bone marrow transplantation. *Blood* 1996; **87:** 2195–204.
97. Falkenburg JHF, Wafelman AR, Joosten P et al, Complete remission of accelerated phase chronic myeloid leukemia after treatment with leukemia-reactive cytotoxic T lymphocytes. *Blood* 1999; **94:** 1201–8.

20

Results with alternative donors

Jane F Apperley

CONTENTS • Introduction • Transplant-related mortality • Relapse • Overall survival and disease-free survival overall • Summary

INTRODUCTION

Fifty-five percent of patients with chronic myeloid leukaemia (CML) are aged 50 years or less at diagnosis.[1] Of these, some 30% will have an HLA-identical sibling donor, and approximately two-thirds (11% of all patients) may be cured by allogeneic stem cell transplantation (SCT). Almost 90% of patients are therefore ineligible for, or do not benefit from, sibling SCT. There is an urgent need to extend the availability of SCT and to improve its outcome.

Improving the outcome of alloSCT is dependent on better patient selection, reductions in transplant-related mortality (TRM) and successful treatment of disease recurrence. Selecting the ideal patient for transplant is itself dependent on identifying patient and donor factors that affect the outcome and on developing risk assessment or prognostic scoring methods to assist patients and their physicians in making treatment choices.[2] Reductions in TRM can be achieved by modifications of conditioning regimens (see Chapter 17), the identification of more effective methods for preventing and treating graft-versus-host disease (GVHD), effective prevention and treatment of microbial infections, and the implementation of better supportive care.

All these measures to improve the outcome of SCT themselves permit the extension of alloSCT to patients who lack HLA-identical sibling donors. Alternative sources of allogeneic stem cells include HLA-antigen(s) mismatched family members, volunteer unrelated donors (VUDs), and cord blood donations.

The use of VUD stem cells and cord blood has been greatly facilitated by the establishment of large donor registries such as the National Marrow Donor Program (NMDP) in the USA and the Anthony Nolan Bone Marrow Donor Registry (ANBMDR) in the UK. The work of the registries includes recruitment, counselling, and selection of donors, followed by stem cell procurement and despatch to the appropriate transplant centre. As a result of their contribution to tissue typing potential donors, an international record of candidate donors has been established under the auspices of Bone Marrow Donors Worldwide (BMDW). Furthermore, the World Marrow Donor Association (WMDA) has been set up to provide guidance and regulations to ensure the safety of the donors and their recipients. A similar network of cord blood registries has now been established, together with international collaborative efforts to collect and analyse transplant outcome data.

The existence of unrelated and cord blood registries, together with the availability of HLA mismatched family members, results in the

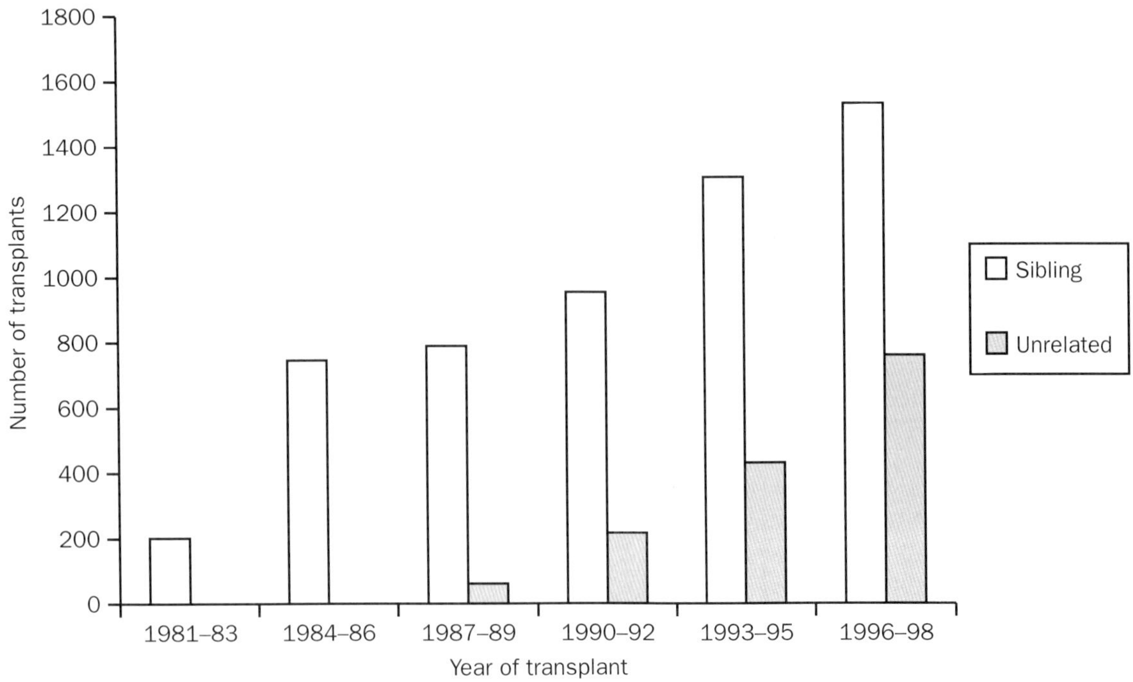

Figure 20.1 Numbers of HLA-identical sibling and volunteer unrelated donor transplants for CML per three-year period between 1981 and 1998. Data derived from the Chronic Leukaemia Registry of the EBMT.

identification of donors for up to 80% of suitable patients. The numbers of unrelated donor transplants have steadily increased over the past decade (Figure 20.1) and CML is the most frequent disease indication for the use of VUDs.

To date, the results of alternative donor transplants remain inferior to those of sibling grafts. However, awareness of the various factors affecting transplant outcome and the use of measures to overcome their harmful effects have resulted in steady improvements in transplant results (Table 20.1). In this chapter, I will discuss the various measurements of outcome and ways in which patient, donor, and procedural factors may affect these. Most of the data that will be used are derived from VUD transplants, although specific mention of family mismatched donors and cord blood will be made where appropriate.

Table 20.1 Factors that may affect the outcome of unrelated transplantation

Age
Disease status
Degree of HLA disparity
Interval from diagnosis to transplant
Recipient–donor gender combinations
Prior chemotherapy
Graft-versus-host disease prophylaxis
Conditioning regimens
Cell dose
Cytomegalovirus serostatus

TRANSPLANT-RELATED MORTALITY

Transplant-related mortality (TRM) refers to death without disease recurrence. Both transplant-related mortality and morbidity are due to a combination of adverse events following transplant, including the toxicity of the conditioning regimen, engraftment failure, GVHD, infections, and late complications such as secondary malignancies.

Conditioning regimens for conventional alloSCT include combinations of immunosuppressive and myeloablative drugs and/or total-body irradiation (TBI). Preparative regimens are the subject of Chapter 17, and will not be discussed in detail here. Briefly, any attempts to reduce the toxicity of the conditioning regimens have usually resulted in an increase in the incidence of disease recurrence, and hence no overall improvements in disease-free survival. Recently, a number of groups have been developing reduced-intensity preparative regimens where the potential for increases in the incidence of leukaemic relapse is an accepted feature of the protocol. Strategies for the prevention, pre-emptive therapy, or treatment of relapse with additional donor lymphocytes are an integral part of these protocols.[3–5]

Engraftment

Early (primary) or late (secondary) graft failures are well-recognized complications of alternative donor transplants. The graft failure rate is higher than that seen with HLA-identical siblings, and is usually attributed to the increased genetic disparity for both major and minor histocompatibility antigens.[6–9] An additional suggestion is that the graft failure rate may be increased in patients treated for CML because such patients receive relatively low amounts of chemotherapy prior to transplant, thereby increasing the risk of persistence of host alloreactive cells.[10]

A recent analysis of 1423 recipients of unrelated transplants for CML from the NMDP[11] identified a 10% incidence of primary graft failure and a further 6.6% of patients experienced late graft failure. Factors associated with problems of primary engraftment included absence of TBI in the conditioning regimen, transplant for advanced-phase disease, use of HLA-mismatched donors, and a nucleated cell dose of less than 2.1×10^8 cells/kg. Rather surprisingly, the use of T-cell depletion did not affect the incidence of graft failure. The only factor associated with an increased incidence of late graft failure was transplantation for advanced-phase disease.

Other investigations have identified donor–recipient HLA disparity as a major risk factor for problems with engraftment.[8,9,12–16] Petersdorf et al studied the role of Class I allele disparity in a group of 521 patients evaluable for engraftment after unrelated donor transplants. Of these patients, 21 (18 with CML) experienced primary graft failure. Each donor–recipient pair was case-matched with two controls for known HLA mismatch, intensity of the conditioning regimen, patient/donor demographics, and marrow cell dose. Of the pairs with graft failure, 71% were allele-mismatched for HLA-C alone, compared with 33% of control pairs, suggesting that HLA-C may act as an independent risk factor for engraftment.[9]

Previously, an increased incidence of graft failure has been associated with T-cell depletion of the donor graft.[17–19] Spencer et al described the outcome of 115 unrelated donor transplants for CML, who received ex vivo or in vivo T-cell depletion at the Hammersmith Hospital, London. The probability of graft failure at 1 year was 16%. Proportional hazards regression analysis showed an association between donor age less than 35 years and a reduced likelihood of graft failure. This was independent of the number of mononuclear cells infused.[14] Conditioning therapy at the time of transplant of these patients consisted of cyclophosphamide 120 mg/kg and 12–13.2 Gy TBI in six fractions. Since increasing the TBI dosage to 14.4 Gy, primary graft failure has not occurred (unpublished observations). The increase in intensity of the conditioning regimen has not resulted in a decrease in overall survival (Figure 20.2).

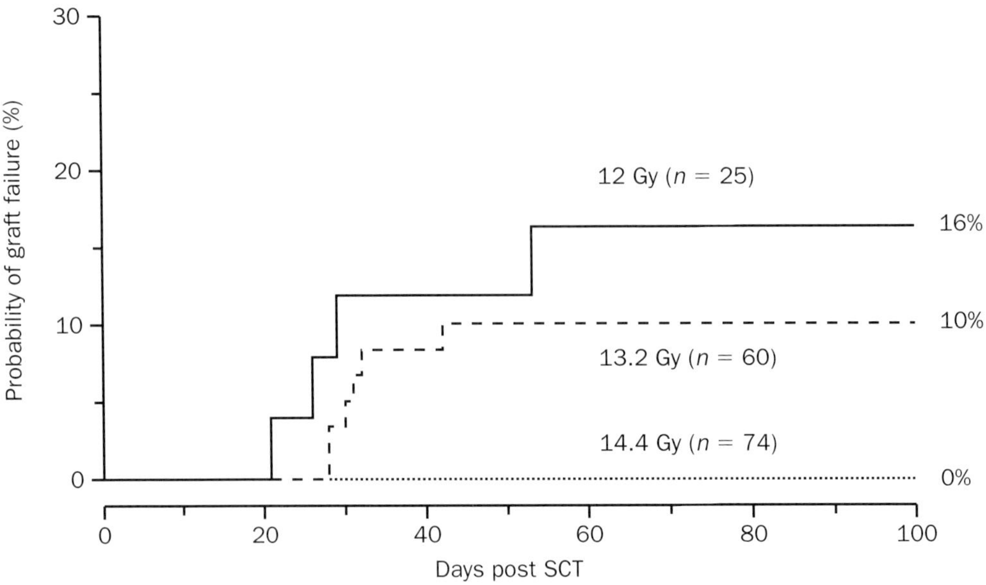

Figure 20.2 Probability of graft failure in recipients of T-cell-depleted unrelated donor transplants for CML (Hammersmith Hospital) by dose of TBI.

In summary, transplant for advanced-phase disease, the conditioning regimen, use of T-cell depletion, increasing HLA disparity, and low cell doses may all be associated with an increase in the incidence of early and late graft failure after unrelated donor transplant.

The use of cord blood in alloSCT is also associated with an increased risk of graft failure. In large part, this appears to be due to inadequate cell doses. Eurocord now recommend the use of cord blood donations only when the cell dose exceeds (1–2) × 10^7/kg. This guideline effectively limits the number of donations suitable for use in adult transplant recipients. Even when this cell dose is achieved, engraftment tends to be delayed. The adverse effects of poor graft function early after transplant may be balanced by a reduced incidence of GVHD, even when using mismatched cord blood.[20]

Graft-versus-host disease

Acute and chronic GVHD (aGVHD and cGVHD) are more common after alternative donor transplants than after HLA-identical sibling grafts. GVHD may be reduced in incidence by the use of HLA-identical donors, the avoidance of female donors for male recipients, and effective prophylaxis, including T-cell depletion.

Acute GVHD

In 1998, Hansen et al[21] reported the results of 196 patients who received unrelated donor transplants for CML in Seattle. The incidence of aGVHD grades II–IV was 77% in patients who had received cells matched for HLA-A, -B, and -DRβ1, 89% in patients with a minor mismatch at HLA-A or -B and 95% in those mismatched at HLA-DRβ1. The incidences of aGVHD grades III–IV were 35%, 37%, and 50% in those respective groups. The occurrence of GVHD was not associated with the ages of patient or donor, the interval from diagnosis to transplant, or the cell dose. Among fully matched pairs, the use of a female donor for a male patient increased the relative risk of aGVHD to

2.5.[21] Similarly high incidences of aGVHD were reported by the Seattle transplant team in 88 children who received unrelated transplants for a variety of haematological malignancies: 83% of HLA-matched and 98% of HLA-mismatched transplant recipients experienced aGVHD grades II–IV, and HLA disparity and increasing patient age (range 0.5–17 years) were associated with an increased risk of aGVHD.[22]

In the recent NMDP analysis, McGlave et al[11] reported the incidence of aGVHD as 43% by day 100. aGVHD was less frequent in patients transplanted in chronic phase, in those with an HLA-matched donor, and in recipients of T-cell-depleted grafts. Increasing recipient age and gender-mismatched donor–recipient pairs did not increase the risk of GVHD. This analysis detected a decrease in the incidence of aGVHD in more recent transplants, with occurrences of 28% in 1994–1996, 36% in 1991–1993, and 40% in 1988–1990 ($p = 0.0012$).

Other groups have suggested that the risk of aGVHD is not associated with increasing patient age, but the risk of dying of aGVHD is greater in older patients.[23,24] More recently Ringden et al[25] examined the outcome of unrelated transplants for patients over the age of 40 years, comparing 27 such patients with 69 younger patients. The incidences of aGVHD grades II–IV were 23% in patients older than 40 years and 21% in younger patients.

The use of T-cell depletion undoubtedly reduces the incidence of aGVHD. Drobyski et al[26] reported the outcome of unrelated transplant for CML from a programme using ex vivo T-cell depletion with the αβ T-cell-receptor antibody T10B9. The actuarial probability of developing aGVHD grades II–IV was 40% and of grades III–IV, 8%. No differences in the incidences of aGVHD were observed in recipients of HLA-matched or HLA-mismatched grafts.[26]

Spencer et al at the Hammersmith Hospital observed an incidence of aGVHD grades III–IV of 24% in 115 recipients of VUD marrow that had been depleted of T cells using cocktails of the Campath series of monoclonal antibodies. In this setting, the use of the functional assay for cytotoxic T-lymphocyte precursors (CTLp) proved predictive for the occurrence of GVHD. The presence of CTLp at high frequency reflects disparities at the HLA class I loci. The relative risk of aGVHD grades III–IV in patients whose donors had low CTLp frequencies was 0.28 ($p = 0.0035$). The CTLp frequency was a more useful guide to the development of aGVHD than HLA typing by serology or restriction fragment length polymorphism (RFLP).[14]

Chronic GVHD

Hansen et al[21] reported an incidence of cGVHD of 67% in 161 evaluable recipients of unrelated transplant. The degree of HLA disparity did not affect the incidence of cGVHD, which was more frequent in patients who had received grafts from women with a history of pregnancy. Similarly, the incidence of cGVHD on the NMDP analysis[11] was high at 73%, with 60% of patients experiencing extensive cGVHD.

The risk of cGVHD is also reduced in recipients of T-cell-depleted grafts, although the contrast is not as clear as with aGVHD. Drobyski et al[26] reported limited cGVHD in 29 of 35 evaluable patients, with only 4 patients experiencing extensive disease. The probability of extensive cGVHD in the Hammersmith patients was 38% at 1 year.

GVHD in family mismatched donor transplants

Limited information is available from the literature concerning the occurrence of GVHD after family mismatched transplants for CML. An extensive analysis from the IBMTR compared the outcome of alternative donor transplants for a variety of diseases with that of sibling transplants. The incidences of aGVHD grades II–IV, aGVHD grades III–IV, and cGVHD after one-antigen-mismatched related donor transplants were 44%, 27%, and 52%, respectively, while after two-antigen-mismatched related donor transplants, these incidences were 56%, 36%, and 60%. The corresponding figures for 1176 recipients in HLA-identical sibling transplants were 29%, 13%, and 42%.[27]

GVHD in recipients of cord blood transplants

Transplant of cord blood seems to result in a relatively low incidence of acute and chronic GVHD compared with the use of unrelated marrow grafts.[20,28,29] Younger patient age and recipient CMV seropositivity are associated with a reduction in the incidence and severity of aGVHD. HLA disparity does not appear to affect the occurrence of GVHD.

Role of HLA disparity in the development of GVHD

The development of more accurate methods of HLA typing using molecular technology (see Chapter 14) has increased our ability to identify more closely matched unrelated donors. However, knowledge of the complexity of modern HLA typing renders many of the earlier studies of the impact of HLA typing on transplant outcome uninterpretable.

Historically, HLA molecules were identified by allo-antisera in complement-dependent cytotoxicity assays. Analysis by genetic sequencing has revealed multiple alleles for most serologically defined specificities. In addition, there is an increasing awareness of the potential role of minor histocompatibility antigens. Most clinical centres and donor registries now use high-resolution typing of class II loci, i.e. DRβ1 and DQβ1, with PCR-based methodologies such as sequence-specific primers (SSP) and sequence-specific oligonucleotide probe hybridization (SSOPH).[30] Molecular typing of Class I loci is more complex, but is becoming more widely available through techniques such as reference strand mediated conformation analysis (RSCA).[31]

Hansen et al[21] reported the adverse effect of mismatching for HLA-DRβ1 on both the occurrences of GVHD and survival rates.[21] More recently, the Seattle transplant team have analysed the outcome of allele level matching in 300 patients with CML transplanted from unrelated donors. The risks of grade III–IV GVHD were highest for class I plus class II mismatches and for single-locus class II mismatches.[16] There was no detectable increase in the risk of aGVHD in patients mismatched with their donor or a single A1, β, or C locus allele. Earlier studies from Seattle and the European Group for Blood and Marrow Transplantation (EBMT) also reported the adverse effects of HLA-DRβ1 disparity between donors and recipients.[32,33] This effect was most profound in patients transplanted from HLA-DRβ1-disparate donors for advanced-phase disease and reported to the EBMT, where the TRM reached 94%.[33]

Petersdorf et al[34] studied 449 patient–donor pairs in an attempt to clarify the role of DQβ1. Of the 449 pairs, 335 (75%) were matched for both DRβ1 and DQβ1, and the remainder were mismatched for DRβ1 and/or DQβ1. The probability of aGVHD grades III–IV was 42% for matched transplants, 61% for single-locus DQβ1-mismatched pairs, 55% for single-locus DRβ1 mismatches, and 71% for DRβ1 and DQβ1 mismatches. The authors suggested that selection for potential unrelated donors should now include both DRβ1 and DQβ1 matching.

Sasazuki et al[15] have also reported the results of high-resolution typing for HLA-A, -B, -C, -DR, -DP, and -DQ in recipients of unrelated donor transplants from the Japan Marrow Donor Programme. They observed a harmful effect of HLA-A and HLA-C disparities on the incidence of aGVHD. Conversely, disparities for class II alleles were not associated with an increased incidence of GVHD.

Improved methods of HLA typing and consequent selection for better-matched donors may explain the reduced incidences of aGVHD seen in single-centre institutes. Nademanee et al[35] have reported a 38% incidence of aGVHD grades II–IV in patients transplanted for CML who were molecularly matched for HLA-DRβ1 and -DQβ1.

Infection

Immune reconstitution is delayed after unrelated donor transplant. This effect may be further exacerbated by the use of GVHD prophylaxis (particularly T-cell depletion) and/or immunosuppressive drugs for the treatment of aGVHD.[36]

Delays in immune recovery are associated with increased risks of fungal and viral infections. Hansen et al[21] reported improvements in the survival of unrelated transplant recipients since the introduction of prophylactic antifungal and antiviral therapy with fluconazole and ganciclovir respectively.

Cytomegalovirus (CMV) disease is a well-recognized and potentially life-threatening complication of alloSCT. However, it is only recently that the impact of CMV seropositivity in the transplant recipient has been recognized as a poor prognostic indicator. McGlave et al[11] reported an adverse effect of recipient CMV seropositivity in the outcome of more than 1400 VUD transplants for CMV. In the context of T-cell depletion, the Hammersmith group have identified cumulative risks for disease-free survival of CMV seropositivity and the presence of CTLp at high frequency in donors for T-cell-depleted unrelated transplants[37,38] (Figure 20.3).

Patients transplanted with T-cell-depleted marrow have an increased incidence of post-transplant EBV lymphoproliferative disease.[39,40] This risk may be restricted to certain methods of T-cell depletion, since this complication has not been a feature in patients receiving products depleted of T cells using the Campath series of antibodies.[41] Campath-1 recognizes the CD-52 antigen, which is expressed on the cell surface of T cells, B cells, and some monocytes. Concomitant removal of both B and T cells may maintain lymphocyte subset balance and prevent the uncontrolled proliferation of donor B cells.

RELAPSE

The cure of CML by alloSCT is attributed to a combination of the antileukaemic conditioning therapy prior to transplant and the continuous activity of all reactive donor T cells within the patient after the transplant (the graft-versus-leukaemia (GVL) effect). The incidence of the GVL effect in CML is particularly strong, and is derived from a number of sources. First,

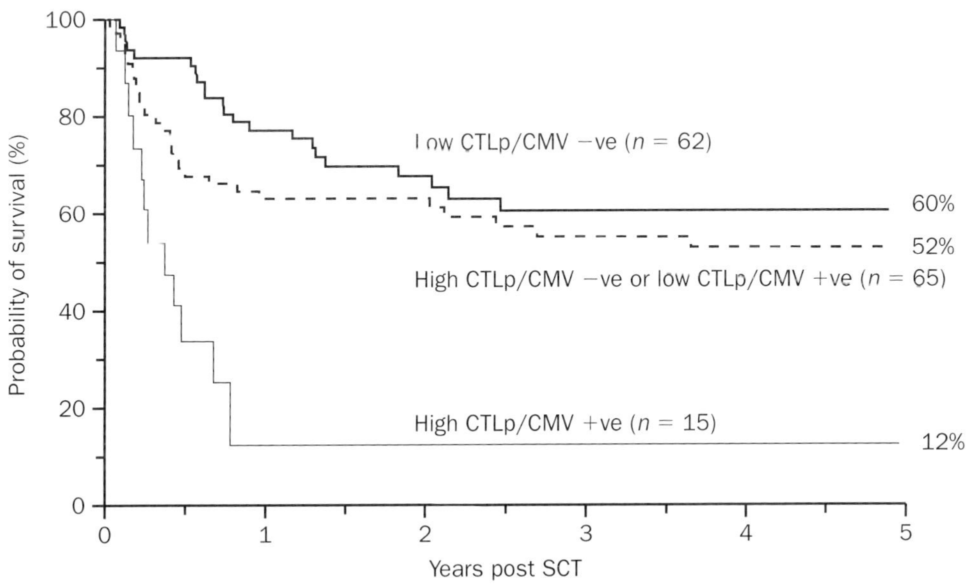

Figure 20.3 Probability of survival in recipients of T-cell-depleted unrelated donor transplants for CML in first chronic phase (Hammersmith Hospital) by combinations of CTLp frequency and CMV serostatus.

patients transplanted from syngeneic twins are at a higher risk of relapse than those transplanted from HLA-identical siblings.[42] Patients are more likely to relapse after T-cell-depleted than after T-cell-replete transplants.[43] The occurrences of non-life-threatening acute and chronic GVHD are associated with a reduced incidence of relapse. Finally, patients relapsing after transplant can be restored to remission with additional infusions of lymphocytes from the original donor.[44]

The GVL effect is a consequence of major and/or minor histocompatibility differences, and is theoretically likely to be enhanced in recipients of unrelated or family mismatched transplants. The incidence of haematological relapse after T-cell-replete HLA-identical sibling transplants is of the order of 15–20%.[45] Hansen et al[21] reported a cumulative incidence of cytogenetic and haematological relapse of 10% at 5 years post unrelated donor transplant for CML in first chronic phase, and suggested that this may reflect the increased GVL effect. McGlave et al[11] also identified a low incidence of haematological relapse of 6% for patients transplanted in first chronic phase. The incidence of relapse increased to 25% for patients transplanted in acceleration, 27% if the transplant was performed in second chronic phase, and 56% in patients treated in blast crisis. The incidence of haematological relapse was very low for chronic-phase patients who received T-cell-replete cells at 3.4% compared with 16% for recipients of T-cell-depleted stem cells. The type of conditioning regimen did not affect the incidence of relapse. In a study from Minnesota, Enright et al[46] reported an incidence of disease recurrence of 31% if the patient had not developed cGVHD, compared with 9% in patients with cGVHD.

Just as the nature of HLA typing has increased in its complexity, so too has the diagnosis of relapse. The availability of competitive and semiquantitative polymerase chain reaction (PCR) assays for the detection of *BCR/ABL* transcripts[47] has not only increased the detection of molecular relapse but has also encouraged many transplant groups to monitor their patients more frequently for evidence of disease.[48,49] The detection of rising transcript levels has become the trigger for early treatment with donor lymphocyte infusions (DLI),[49,50] since early treatment is associated with excellent response rates and a reduction in complications. This is discussed in more detail in Chapters 21 and 24.

The use of T-cell depletion is associated with an increased incidence of relapse in recipients of unrelated transplants. The risk of relapse is further increased if the transplant was performed for advanced disease.[11] Drobyski et al[51] reported the results of PCR monitoring for disease recurrence in 52 recipients of VUD transplant for CML. Twenty patients had at least one positive PCR test after transplant and 12 of these 20 had relapsed at a median of 355 days (range 97–1893 days) post grafting.

At the Hammersmith Hospital, the risk of molecular, cytogenetic, and haematological relapse in recipients of T-cell-depleted VUD transplants for CML is 49% (unpublished observations). The great majority of those patients can be restored to durable molecular remissions using DLI. This has introduced some problems in the reporting of data. The ability to restore relapsed patients to remission has led to the concept of the current leukaemia-free survival curve,[52] in which survival curves can now go up as well as down (Figure 20.4)!

The relapse risk after family mismatched transplant from CML has been reported by both the EBMT and the IBMTR.[27,53] The EBMT reported the outcome of 103 family mismatched transplant recipients treated for all stages of CML. The 2- and 5-year relapse risks for recipients of no- or one-antigen-mismatched grafts were 24% and 42%, compared with 26% and 49% if the graft was 2.3-antigen-mismatched.[53] This rather surprisingly high incidence of relapse, particularly in recipients of widely HLA-disparate grafts, was confirmed by the IBMTR, who reported 2.0 and 2.8 relative risks of relapse of CML in recipients of one-antigen- and two-antigen-mismatched related transplants compared with recipients of HLA-identical sibling transplants. These differences

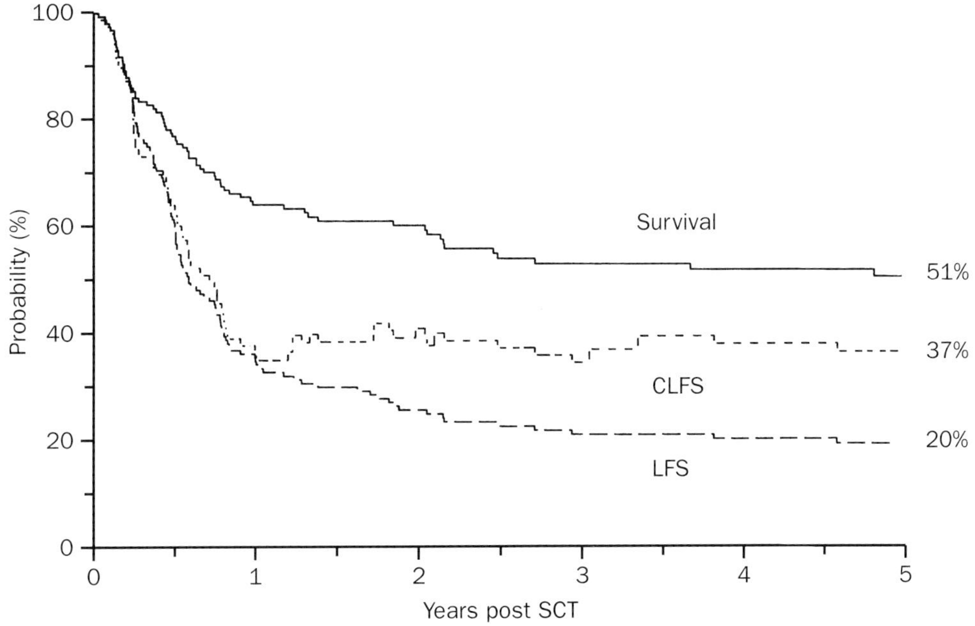

Figure 20.4 Effect of defining 'current leukaemia-free survival' (CLFS) on the outcome of T-cell-depleted unrelated donor transplants for CML in first chronic phase (Hammersmith Hospital).

persisted after stratification by disease status and after the exclusion of T-cell-depleted transplants.[27]

OVERALL SURVIVAL AND DISEASE-FREE SURVIVAL OVERALL

Overall survival (OS) and disease free survival (DFS) rates after alloSCT reflect TRM and relapse risks. Many of the factors affecting OS and DFS have therefore already been discussed. Some of these factors can be used to develop risk-assessment scores for individual patients that can assist patients and their physicians in making informed decisions regarding the nature and timing of treatment.[12] The effect of these cumulative scores on TRM and OS is shown in Figure 20.5.

Hansen et al[21] reported an OS rate for recipients of VUD transplants for CML in chronic phase of 57% at 5 years. This figure increased to 74% for patients who were 50 years or younger, were HLA-matched with their donor, and were transplanted within 12 months of diagnosis. The NMDP results confirm excellent 5-year survival rates for patients in chronic phase under the age of 35 years at transplant of 63% (age <20 years) and 67% (age 20–35 years). In their series, survival decreased in patients older than 35 years to 47%.[11] This group was also able to identify a particularly good risk group defined by age less than 35 years and transplant in first chronic phase within 12 months of diagnosis, where the DFS rate at 3 years reached 63%.

Disease phase

A number of factors have been found to have prognostic influence on OS and DFS rates in CML. The disease phase is the single most important determinant of outcome. The differences in outcome are due not only to the

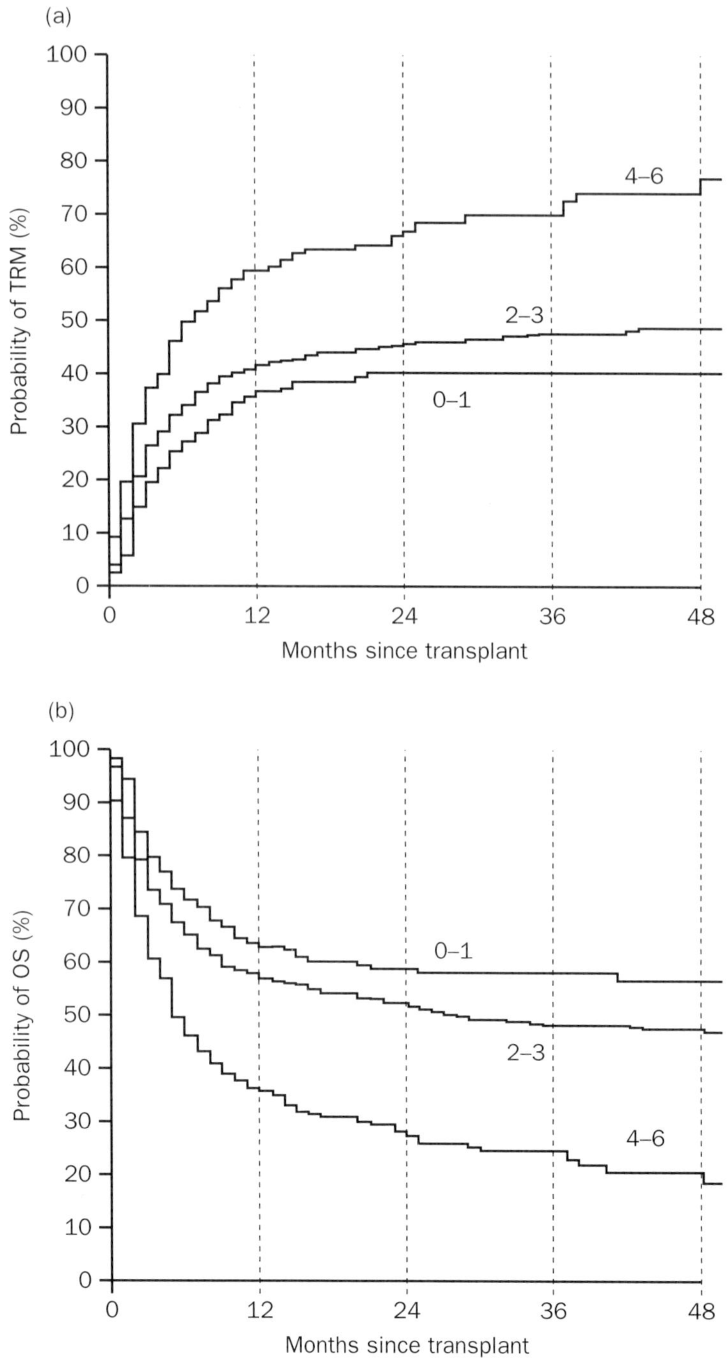

Figure 20.5 Effect of risk-assessment scores on the probabilities of transplant-related mortality (TRM) and overall survival (OS) for patients transplanted for CML from volunteer unrelated donors and reported to the Chronic Leukaemia Registry of the EBMT. Cumulative scores 0–6 obtained from known risk factors, i.e. age <20 years = 0, age 20–40 years = 1, age >40 years = 2; transplant in chronic phase = 0, in acceleration = 1, in blast crisis or subsequent chronic phase = 2; interval from diagnosis <12 months = 0, >12 months = 1; male recipient/female donor = 1, all other gender combinations = 0.

increased risk of relapse after transplant in advanced phase but also to an increase in TRM.[54,55]

Age

Increasing age has long been recognized as an adverse prognostic indicator of outcome for all forms of adult leukaemia and for all types of transplant.[2,21,54–56] The major risk for older patients is TRM.

Interval from diagnosis to treatment

Several large studies have identified decreased survival in association with increased time periods between diagnosis and transplant. The best results in HLA-identical sibling donor transplants are seen if the transplant is performed within one year of diagnosis.[55,57] Poorer outcome with later transplant is largely due to increased TRM, which is largely inexplicable, but may in part relate to the deleterious effects of prolonged treatment with conventional chemotherapy.

Until recently, the effect of delay from diagnosis to transplant in alternative donor procedures has been less clear. This must in part be due to factors such as delays in donor identification and prolonged trials of interferon-α (IFN-α), which resulted in very few patients receiving early transplants. Devergie et al[33] analysed the outcome of 366 recipients of unrelated grafts for CML. Transplant after the median duration from diagnosis to grafting of 827 days was associated with poorer outcome. Hansen et al[21] have now confirmed the adverse effect of delaying the transplant beyond 12 months from diagnosis, as have the NMDP.[11]

Gender

Several analyses have reported that the use of female donors adversely effects the outcome of HLA-identical sibling transplants, because of an increased risk of GVHD. This is clearly a complex issue. An EBMT registry study examined the effect of donor–recipient gender combinations in 1480 patients who received sibling marrow, and concluded that OS was better in female patients because of the high risk of TRM in male recipients of female cells.[58] However, a subsequent report from the same group concluded that long-term DFS was superior in recipients of female stem cells because the probability of relapse was greater with male donors.[59]

Prior chemotherapy

Recently, the Seattle transplant team reported that more than 5 months' treatment with IFN-α prior to unrelated donor transplant had a deleterious effect on overall survival.[60] These observations confirmed those of Beelen et al,[61] who showed a 22% OS rate in 27 recipients of sibling and unrelated transplants who had received more than 12 months' therapy with IFN-α, compared with 69% for patients untreated or exposed to shorter periods of treatment. In contrast, data from the IBMTR[62] did not demonstrate any adverse effect of pretreatment with IFN-α in patients undergoing sibling donor transplants. Finally, Hehlmann et al[63] have analysed the outcome of 197 patients who received sibling or unrelated transplants in the context of national studies of chemotherapy versus chemotherapy plus IFN-α. The outcome of transplant was not affected by the duration of prior therapy with IFN-α. In contrast, differences in outcome were observed depending on the duration of discontinuation of IFN-α therapy prior to alloSCT. The 5-year OS rates were 46% for 50 patients who received IFN-α within 90 days of transplant and 71% for 36 patients who discontinued therapy before this date.

Those conflicting observations reflect the difficulties of analysing two inherently different patient populations. The two groups will almost certainly differ with respect to a number of factors known to affect the outcome of transplant, namely age, phase of disease, interval from diagnosis to transplant, and time to donor identification, which may itself be a surrogate marker of increasing HLA disparity. All of these would tend to have adverse effects in patients receiving prolonged therapy with IFN-α. Paradoxically, the most appropriate reason for prolonging therapy, i.e. major or complete cytogenetic response, is not known to influence the outcome of transplant.

In summary, the harmful effects of IFN-α on survival after unrelated or related transplants are unknown. However, the possibility of such effects may be a persuasive argument for avoiding IFN-α in patients suitable for allografting. No doubt, a similar set of studies will soon emerge for the influence of prior therapy with the newly introduced tyrosine kinase inhibitor STI571.

Cell dose

Sierra et al[64] have shown that nucleated cell doses in excess of 3.65×10^8/kg are associated with improved survival in recipients of unrelated allografts. Similar results have been obtained in syngeneic and in sibling transplants.[65,66] It is often difficult to insist on high cell doses from VUDs, although collection centres should be aware of the importance of adequate harvests. The use of peripheral blood stem cells (PBSC) as an alternative to marrow may prove a simple but effective way of increasing the cell dose and reducing TRM. This is of course dependent on a lack of an increase in the incidence of acute and chronic GVHD when using PBSC. An additional benefit of PBPC may be a reduction in the incidence of disease recurrence.[67]

SUMMARY

Unrelated donor transplants for CML are feasible and effective. Improvements in the outcome of such transplants are ongoing, and will continue with increasing awareness of the effects of the various prognostic factors. The advent of more recent therapies such as STI571 may influence the use of unrelated donor transplantation over the next few years. Expectations are high that such 'designer drugs' will abrogate the need for transplant procedures. However, therapeutic trials of STI571 are likely to delay transplantation, which in itself will reduce the chances of success. Until the efficacy and durability of STI571 have been established, patients suitable for transplant with well-matched HLA-identical donors should not be denied the chance of curative therapy.

In the mean time, improvements in HLA typing for class I and II, and the identification of additional minor histocompatibility antigens, may provide additional valuable information relating to the significance of individual mismatches. In some situations, a single amino acid substitution may be capable of inducing T-cell recognition, whereas detection of serologic or molecular differences that do not induce T-cell responses may increase the potential donor pool.

REFERENCES

1. Hehlmann R, A chance of cure for every patient with chronic myeloid leukemia. *N Engl J Med* 1998; **338:** 980–2.
2. Gratwohl A, Hermans J, Goldman JM et al, Risk assessment for bone marrow transplantation in chronic myeloid leukaemia. *Lancet* 1998; **352:** 1087–92.
3. Slavin S, Nagler A, Naparstek E et al, Nonmyeloablative stem cell transplantation and cell therapy as an alternative to conventional bone marrow transplantation with lethal cytoreduction for the treatment of malignant and non-malignant diseases. *Blood* 1998; **91:** 756–63.
4. Khouri IF, Keating M, Korbling M et al, Transplant-lite: induction of graft versus malignancy using fludarabine based nonablative chemotherapy and allogeneic blood progenitor cell transplantation as treatment for lymphoid malignancies. *J Clin Oncol* 1998; **16:** 2817–24.
5. Georges GE, Storb R, Thompson JD et al, Adoptive immunotherapy in canine mixed chimeras after nonmyeloablative hematopoietic cell transplantation. *Blood* 2000; **95:** 3262–9.

6. Anasetti C, Amos D, Beatty PG et al, Effect of HLA compatibility on engraftment of bone marrow transplants in patients with leukemia or lymphoma. *N Engl J Med* 1989; **320:** 197–204.
7. Voogt PJ, Fibbe WE, Maigt WAF et al, Rejection of bone marrow graft by recipient-derived cytotoxic T-lymphocytes against minor histocompatibility antigens. *Lancet* 1990; **335:** 131–4.
8. Davies SM, Ramsay NKC, Haake RJ et al, Comparison of engraftment in recipients of matched sibling or unrelated donor marrow allografts. *Bone Marrow Transplant* 1994; **13:** 51–7.
9. Petersdorf EW, Longton GM, Anasetti C et al, Association of HLA-C disparity with graft failure after marrow transplantation from unrelated donors. *Blood* 1997; **89:** 1818–23.
10. Papadakis V, Mackinnon S, Kernan NA, Differential effect of pre-transplant cytoreduction on recovery of day 0 host circulating cells. *Bone Marrow Transplant* 1994; **14:** 623–30.
11. McGlave PB, Shu XO, Wen W et al, Unrelated donor marrow transplantation for chronic myelogenous leukemia: 9 years experience of the National Marrow Donor Program. *Blood* 2000; **95:** 2219–25.
12. Anasetti C, Beatty PG, Storb R et al, Effect of HLA incompatibility on graft versus host disease, relapse and survival after marrow transplantation for patients with leukemia or lymphoma. *Hum Immunol* 1990; **29:** 79–91.
13. Beatty PG, Anasetti C, Hansen JA et al, Marrow transplantation from unrelated donors for treatment of hematologic malignancies: effect of mismatching for one HLA locus. *Blood* 1993; **81:** 249–53.
14. Spencer A, Szydlo RM, Brookes PA et al, Bone marrow transplantation for chronic myeloid leukemia with volunteer unrelated donors using ex vivo or in vivo T-cell depletion: major prognostic impact of HLA class I identity between donor and recipient. *Blood* 1995; **86:** 3590–7.
15. Sasazuki T, Juji T, Morishima Y et al, for the Japanese Marrow Donor Program, Effect of matching of class I alleles on clinical outcome after transplantation of hematopoietic stem cells from an unrelated donor. *N Engl J Med* 1998; **339:** 1177–85.
16. Petersdorf EW, Gooley TA, Anasetti C et al, Optimizing outcome after unrelated marrow transplantation by comprehensive matching of HLA class I and II alleles in the donor and recipient. *Blood* 1998; **92:** 3515–20.
17. Kernan NA, Bordignon C, Heller G et al, Graft failure after T-cell depleted human leukocyte antigen identical marrow transplants for leukemia: I Analysis of risk factors and results of secondary transplants. *Blood* 1989; **74:** 2227–32.
18. Ash RC, Horowitz MM, Gale RP et al, Bone marrow transplantation from related donors other than HLA-identical siblings: effect of T-cell depletion. *Bone Marrow Transplant* 1991; **7:** 443–8.
19. Kernan NA, Bartsch G, Ash RC et al, Analysis of 462 transplantations from unrelated donors facilitated by the National Marrow Donor Program. *N Engl J Med* 1993; **328:** 593–602.
20. Rocha V, Wagner JE, Sobocinski KA et al, Graft versus host disease in children who have received a cord-blood or bone marrow transplant from an HLA-identical sibling. Eurocord and International Bone Marrow Transplant Registry Working Committee on Alternative Donor and Stem Cell Sources. *N Engl J Med* 2000; **342:** 1846–54.
21. Hansen JA, Gooley TA, Martin PA et al, Bone marrow transplants from unrelated donors for patients with chronic myeloid leukemia. *N Engl J Med* 1998; **338:** 962–8.
22. Balduzzi A, Gooley T, Anasetti C et al, Unrelated donor marrow transplantation in children. *Blood* 1995; **86:** 3247–56.
23. Bortin MM, Gale RP, Rimm AA, Allogeneic bone marrow transplantation for 144 patients with severe aplastic anaemia. *JAMA* 1981; **245:** 1132–9.
24. Ringden O, Nilsson B, Death by graft versus host disease associated with HLA mismatch, high recipient age, low marrow cell dose and splenectomy. *Transplantation* 1985; **40:** 39–44.
25. Ringden O, Remberger M, Mattson J et al, Transplantation with unrelated bone marrow in leukaemic patients above 40 years of age. *Bone Marrow Transplant* 1998; **21:** 43–9.
26. Drobyski WR, Ash RC, Caspar JT et al, Effect of T-depletion as graft versus host disease prophylaxis on engraftment, relapse and disease free survival in unrelated marrow transplantation for chronic myelogenous leukemia. *Blood* 1994; **83:** 1980–7.
27. Szydlo R, Goldman JM, Klein JP et al, Results of allogeneic bone marrow transplants for leukemia using donors other than HLA-identical siblings. *J Clin Oncol* 1997; **15:** 1767–77.
28. Gluckman E, Rocha V, Boyer-Chammard A et al, Outcome of cord-blood transplantation from related and unrelated donors. *N Engl J Med* 1997; **337:** 373–81.

29. Rubenstein P, Carrier C, Scaradavou A et al, Outcomes among 562 recipients of placental-blood transplants from unrelated donors. *N Engl J Med* 1998; **339:** 1565–70.
30. Heslop HE, Haemopoietic stem cell transplantation from unrelated donors. *Br J Haematol* 1999; **105:** 2–6.
31. Turner DM, Poles A, Brown J et al, HLA-A typing by reference strand mediated conformation analysis (RSCA) using a capillary based semi-automated genetic analyser. *Tissue Antigens* 1999; **54:** 400–4.
32. Petersdorf EW, Longton GM, Anasetti C et al, The significance of HLA-DRB1 matching on clinical outcome after HLA-A, B, DR identical unrelated donor marrow transplantation. *Blood* 1995; **86:** 1606–13.
33. Devergie A, Apperley JF, Labopin M et al, European results of matched unrelated donor bone marrow transplantation for chronic myeloid leukaemia: impact of HLA D class II matching. *Bone Marrow Transplant* 1997; **20:** 11–20.
34. Petersdorf EW, Longton GM, Anasetti C et al, Definition of HLA-DQ as a transplantation antigen. *Proc Natl Acad Sci USA* 1996; **93:** 15358–63.
35. Nademanee A, Schmidt GM, Parker P et al, The outcome of matched unrelated donor marrow transplantation in patients with hematologic malignancies using molecular typing for donor selection and graft versus host disease prophylaxis regimen of cyclosporine, methotrexate and prednisolone. *Blood* 1995; **86:** 1228–34.
36. Kook H, Goldman F, Padley D et al, Reconstruction of the immune system after unrelated or partially matched T-cell depleted bone marrow transplantation in children: immunophenotypic analysis and factors affecting the speed of recovery. *Blood* 1996; **88:** 1089–97.
37. Spencer A, Brookes PA, Kaminski E et al, Cytotoxic T-lymphocyte precursor frequency analyses in bone marrow transplantation with volunteer unrelated donors: value in donor selection. *Transplantation* 1995; **59:** 1302–8.
38. Craddock C, Szydlo RM, Dazzi F et al, Cytomegalovirus seropositivity adversely influences outcome after T-depleted unrelated donor transplant in patients with chronic myeloid leukaemia: the case for tailored graft-versus-host disease prophylaxis. *Br J Haematol* 2001; **112:** 228–36.
39. O'Reilly RJ, Small TN, Papadopoulos E et al, Biology and adoptive cell therapy of Epstein–Barr virus associated lymphoproliferative disorders in recipients of marrow allografts. *Immunol Rev* 1997; **157:** 195–216.
40. Aguilar LK, Rooney CM, Heslop HE, Lymphoproliferative disorders involving Epstein–Barr virus after hemopoietic stem cell transplantation. *Curr Opin Immunol* 1999; **11:** 96–101.
41. Hale G, Waldmann H, Risks of developing Epstein–Barr virus-related lymphoproliferative disorders after T-cell depleted transplants. Campath users. *Blood* 1998; **91:** 3079–83.
42. Butturini A, Gale RP, Clinical models of autotransplants in chronic myelogenous leukemia. *Leuk Lymphoma* 1993; **11**(Suppl 1): 255–7.
43. Apperley JF, Jones L, Hale G et al, Bone marrow transplantation for patients with chronic myeloid leukaemia: T-cell depletion with Campath-1 reduces the incidence of graft-versus-host disease but may increase the risk of leukaemic relapse. *Bone Marrow Transplant* 1986; **1:** 53–66.
44. Kolb HJ, Schattenberg A, Goldman JM et al, Graft-versus-leukemia effect of donor lymphocyte transfusions in marrow grafted patients. European Group for Blood and Marrow Transplantation Working Party Chronic Leukemia. *Blood* 1995; **86:** 2041–50.
45. Clift RA, Buckner CD, Thomas ED et al, Marrow transplantation for chronic myeloid leukemia: a randomised study comparing cyclophosphamide and total body irradiation with busulfan and cyclophosphamide. *Blood* 1994; **84:** 2036–43.
46. Enright H, Davies SM, DeFor T et al, Relapse after non-T-cell depleted allogeneic bone marrow transplantation for chronic myelogenous leukemia: early transplantation, use of an unrelated donor and chronic graft versus host disease are protective. *Blood* 1996; **88:** 714–20.
47. Cross NCP, Lin F, Chase A et al, Competitive polymerase chain reaction to estimate the number of BCR–ABL transcripts in chronic myeloid leukemia after bone marrow transplantation. *Blood* 1993; **82:** 1929–36.
48. Radich JP, Gehly G, Gooley T et al, Polymerase chain reaction detection of the *BCR–ABL* fusion transcript after allogeneic marrow transplantation for chronic myeloid leukaemia: results and implications in 346 patients. *Blood* 1995; **85:** 2632–8.
49. Dazzi F, Szydlo RM, Craddock C et al, Comparison of single-dose and escalating-dose

regimens of donor lymphocyte infusion for relapse after allografting for chronic myeloid leukaemia. *Blood* 2000; **95:** 67–71.

50. Mackinnon S, Papadopoulos EB, Carabasi MH et al, Adoptive immunotherapy evaluating escalating doses of donor leukocytes for relapse of chronic myeloid leukemia after bone marrow transplantation: separation of graft-versus-leukemia responses from graft-versus-host disease. *Blood* 1995; **86:** 1261–8.
51. Drobyski WR, Endean DJ, Klein JP, Hessner MJ, Detection of *BCR–ABL* RNA transcripts using the polymerase chain reaction is highly predictive for relapse in patients transplanted with unrelated marrow grafts for chronic myelogenous leukaemia. *Br J Haematol* 1997; **98:** 458–66.
52. Craddock C, Szydlo RM, Klein JP et al, Estimating leukemia free survival after allografting for chronic myeloid leukemia: a new method that takes account of patients who relapse and are restored to complete remission. *Blood* 2000; **96**: 86–90.
53. Speiser D, van Biezen A, Hermans J et al, Haploidentical related BMT in patients with chronic myeloid leukaemia. *Bone Marrow Transplant* 1997; **19:** 1197–204.
54. Goldman JM, Apperley JF, Jones L et al, Bone marrow transplantation for patients with chronic myeloid leukaemia. *N Engl J Med* 1986; **314:** 202–7.
55. Thomas ED, Clift RA, Fefer A et al, Marrow transplantation for the treatment of chronic myelogenous leukemia. *Ann Intern Med* 1986; **104:** 155–63.
56. Clift RA, Buckner CD, Storb R et al, The influence of patient age on the outcome of transplantation during chronic phase (CP) of chronic myeloid leukemia. *Blood* 1995; **86**(Suppl 1): 2457.
57. Goldman JM, Szydlo R, Horowitz MM et al, Choice of pretransplant treatment and timing of transplants for chronic myelogenous leukemia in chronic phase. *Blood* 1993; **82:** 2235–8.
58. Gratwohl A, Hermans J, Niederwieser D et al, Bone marrow transplantation for chronic myeloid leukaemia: long term results. *Bone Marrow Transplant* 1993; **12:** 509–16.
59. van Rhee F, Szydlo RM, Hermans J et al, for the EBMT Chronic Leukaemia Working Party, Long term results after allogeneic bone marrow transplantation for chronic myelogenous leukaemia. *Bone Marrow Transplant* 1997; **20:** 553–60.
60. Morton AJ, Gooley T, Hansen JA et al, Association between pretransplant interferon-α and outcome after unrelated donor marrow transplantation for chronic myelogenous leukemia in chronic phase. *Blood* 1998; **92:** 394–401.
61. Beelen DW, Graeven U, Elmaagacli AH et al, Prolonged administration of interferon-α in patients with chronic phase Philadelphia chromosome positive chronic myelogenous leukemia before allogeneic bone marrow transplantation may adversely affect transplant outcome. *Blood* 1995; **85:** 2981–90.
62. Giralt S, Szydlo R, Goldman JM et al, Effect of short-term interferon on the outcome of subsequent HLA-identical sibling bone marrow transplantation for chronic myelogenous leukemia: an analysis from the International Bone Marrow Transplant Registry. *Blood* 2000; **95:** 410–15.
63. Hehlmann R, Hochhaus A, Kolb HJ et al, Interferon-α before allogeneic bone marrow transplantation in chronic myelogenous leukemia does not affect outcome adversely, provided it is discontinued at least 90 days before the procedure. *Blood* 1999; **94:** 3668–77.
64. Sierra J, Radich J, Hansen JA et al, Marrow transplants from unrelated donors for treatment of Philadelphia chromosome positive acute leukemia. *Blood* 1997; **90:** 1410–14.
65. Lamperelli T, van Lint MT, Gualandi F et al, Bone marrow transplantation for chronic myeloid leukemia (CML) from unrelated and sibling donors: single center experience. *Bone Marrow Transplant* 1997; **20:** 1057–62.
66. Barrett AJ, Ringden O, Zhang MJ et al, Effect of nucleated marrow cell dose on relapse and survival in identical twin bone marrow transplants for leukemia. *Blood* 2000; **95:** 3323–7.
67. Elmaagacli AH, Beelen DW, Opalka B et al, The risk of residual molecular and cytogenetic disease in patients with Philadelphia-chromosome positive first chronic phase chronic myelogenous leukemia is reduced after transplantation of allogeneic peripheral blood stem cells compared with bone marrow. *Blood* 1999; **94:** 384–9.

21

Patient monitoring after allogeneic stem cell transplantation or interferon-α therapy

Andreas Hochhaus

CONTENTS • Introduction • Detection and quantification of *BCR/ABL*-positive cells • Conclusions

INTRODUCTION

Chronic myeloid leukaemia (CML) constitutes a clinical model for molecular detection and therapy surveillance of malignant disease, since this entity was the first leukaemia shown to be associated with a specific chromosomal rearrangement, the Philadelphia (Ph) translocation t(9;22)(q34;q11),[1–3] which generates two chimeric genes: *BCR/ABL*[4,5] on the derivative chromosome 22, and *ABL/BCR* on the derivative chromosome 9. *BCR/ABL* is transcribed and translated in most patients into a 210 kDa fusion protein with deregulated tyrosine kinase activity. *ABL/BCR* is expressed in about 60% of patients with CML, but probably lacks any biological function[6] (for a review, see Thijsen et al[7]).

The degree of tumour load reduction is an important prognostic factor for patients with CML on therapy.[8] Response is expressed at three levels:

(i) haematological response, defined as the normalization of the peripheral blood values and of spleen size;
(ii) cytogenetic response, defined as the proportion of residual Ph-positive metaphases;
(iii) molecular response, defined according to the method used as the proportion of the residual *BCR/ABL* gene, transcript, or protein.

The principal aim of residual disease analysis in patients with CML is to determine patient response to treatment and to enable early diagnosis of relapse.

DETECTION AND QUANTIFICATION OF *BCR/ABL*-POSITIVE CELLS

Cytogenetic analysis of bone marrow metaphases

The Ph chromosome is present in about 90% of patients with a clinical presentation consistent with CML. Between 3% and 5% of patients show a normal chromosome 22 but molecular evidence of the *BCR/ABL* translocation. At present, cytogenetic analysis usually reveals the Ph chromosome in 100% of cells analysed with standard 20–30 cell analysis. Conventional cytogenetics is still considered the 'gold standard' for evaluating this response.

Major drawbacks of cytogenetics are the requirement for bone marrow cells in mitosis, and the analysis of relatively small numbers of metaphases, resulting in significant sampling errors.[9] The major advantage of cytogenetics is the early detection of clonal evolution consistent with acceleration of the disease.[10,11]

The frequency of cytogenetic analysis can be

reduced if patients are monitored by other methods, such as quantitative Southern blot, fluorescence in situ hybridization (FISH), quantitative Western blot and quantitative reverse-transcriptase polymerase chain reaction (RT-PCR). In CML, molecular methods can be performed on peripheral blood specimens, and are therefore less invasive than conventional cytogenetic analysis of bone marrow metaphases. Furthermore, these techniques are applicable to Ph-negative, *BCR/ABL*-positive cases.

Fluorescence in situ hybridization

FISH analysis is typically performed by co-hybridization of a *BCR* and an *ABL* probe to denatured metaphase chromosomes or interphase nuclei. Probes are large genomic clones, such as cosmids or yeast artificial chromosomes (YACs), and are labelled with different fluorochromes. Dual-colour FISH using probes for *BCR* and *ABL* genes allows the specific detection of the *BCR/ABL* gene fusion in interphase and/or metaphase nuclei. Most cells exhibit four distinct signals – two of each colour corresponding to the two normal *BCR* and *ABL* alleles. CML cells are recognized by the juxtaposition of one of the *BCR* and one of the *ABL* signals.[12] FISH analysis does not depend on the presence of the typical Ph chromosome, and will detect rare *BCR* and *ABL* variant fusions.[12–15] The lineages of positive and negative cells can be determined in combination with conventional May–Grünwald staining or immunocytochemistry.[16,17]

A limitation of the interphase FISH method is the background of a variant proportion of false-positive cells, depending on the probe/detection system used.[18–21] In practice, the limit of detection of CML cells is typically 1–5%, and depends in part on which probes are used, the size of the nucleus, the precise position of the breakpoint within the *ABL* gene, and the criteria used to define co-localization.[22] The advantage of FISH over conventional cytogenetics is the analysis of a larger number of nuclei, resulting in smaller sampling errors. Therefore FISH is applicable to the quantification of residual disease in partial, minor, and non-responders to interferon-α (IFN-α)[23–25] and for determination of the *BCR/ABL* positivity of individual cell colonies,[26] of the proportion of *BCR/ABL*-positive cells in leukapheresis products[27] or in small samples, such as highly enriched cell fractions.[28]

The specificity of interphase FISH can be increased by introducing an additional probe that permits identification of both the Ph chromosome and the derivative chromosome 9 in Ph-positive cells, thus lowering the rate of false positivity.[29–32] In many cases, however, large genomic deletions around the Ph translocation breakpoints preclude the use of these techniques.[32,33]

The development of a ‘hypermetaphase FISH’ based on improved culture techniques and computerized analysis of a large number of metaphases made it possible to distinguish different levels of Ph positivity at presentation. Where readings can be obtained on 500 cells, one can reliably estimate the parameters that characterize minimal residual disease. However, hypermetaphase FISH evaluates only cycling cells, and cannot count Ph-positive cells that do not enter division.[34–36]

Southern blot analysis

Southern blotting exploits the fact that the breakpoint within the *BCR* gene falls in most cases in a limited area, the 5.8 kb major breakpoint cluster region (M-*bcr*, Figure 21.1).[4] Genomic DNA extracted from leukocytes from a patient is digested by a set of appropriate restriction enzymes (e.g. *Bgl*II, *Xba*I, *Hin*dIII, *Eco*RI, *Bam*HI), fractionated on an agarose gel, transferred to a nylon membrane, and hybridized to two labelled DNA probes derived from the 3′ and 5′ portions of the M-*bcr*. After autoradiography, a band corresponding to the unrearranged *BCR* allele is normally visible; for patients with CML, one or two additional bands may reveal the rearranged *BCR* allele

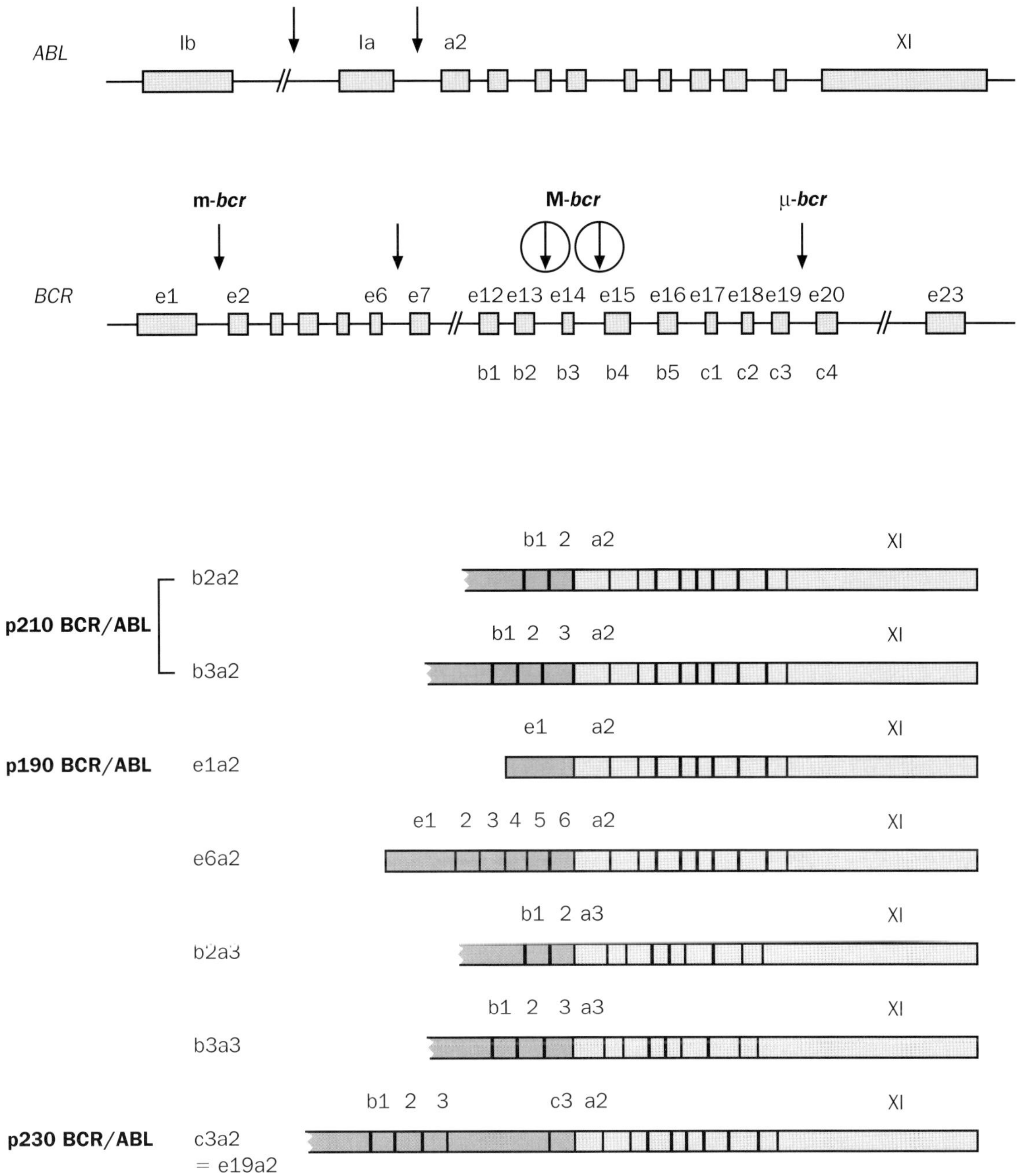

Figure 21.1
Map of the exon–intron structure of the *ABL and BCR* chromosomes and typical and atypical *BCR/ABL* mRNA variants. Arrows indicate genomic breakpoint cluster regions in the first intron of *ABL* and in introns 1, 13, 14, and 19 of *BCR*. The breakpoint cluster region in *BCR* intron 1 is designated the minor breakpoint cluster region (m-*bcr*), that in introns 13 and 14 the major breakpoint cluster region (M-*bcr*), and that in intron 19 the micro breakpoint cluster region (μ-*bcr*). Rarely, breakpoints in *BCR* intron 6 have been described.

$$BCR \text{ ratio } (\%) = \frac{2 \times R}{R + G}$$

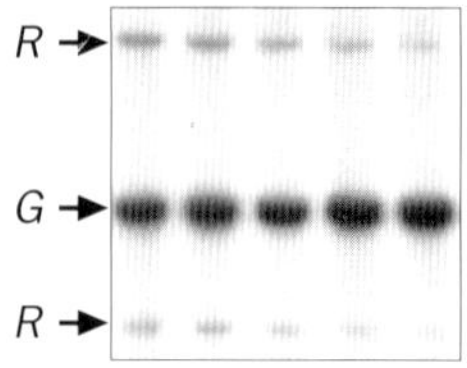

Figure 21.2
Southern blot analysis after *Bgl*II digest of genomic DNA labelled with 5' and 3' M-*bcr* probes and autoradiographed. Arrows indicate the germline band (*G*) and rearranged bands (*R*).

(Figure 21.2). Using this technique, a *BCR* rearrangement is detectable in about 98% of Ph-positive patients and in a significant proportion of Ph-negative cases.[37] For routine use, *Bgl*II and *Xba*I are sufficient, and are informative in almost all cases. However, since there are rare restriction site polymorphisms in the M-*bcr*, the finding of a rearrangement with at least two restriction enzymes is generally considered necessary to exclude a false-positive result in any new patient.[38,39] False-negative results may arise because the rearranged band is too large, too small, or coincidentally exactly the same size as the normal allele, as a result of partial deletion of *BCR* sequences on the translocated allele[40] or of rare variants that have breakpoints outside the M-*bcr*.[14,41,42] False-positive or false-negative results are, however, rare.[37]

After therapy, Southern blot analysis allows quantification of the proportion of cells with *BCR* rearrangement compared with all cells investigated. The proportion of CML cells is determined by twice the intensity of the rearranged band divided by the sum of the intensities of the rearranged plus germline bands (the *BCR* ratio). This is because each CML cell contributes signals from one normal and one rearranged chromosome 22, whereas the normal cells contribute identical signals from two normal chromosomes.[37,43] The level of disease detected in contemporaneous peripheral blood and bone marrow samples is essentially identical,[43,44] and therefore peripheral blood is usually used for analysis. Quantitative Southern blotting allows the detection and quantification of as few as 1–5% leukaemic cells.[37,44] To evaluate the response to treatment, knowledge of the initial restriction pattern and intensity of the rearranged band is mandatory. Complete cytogenetic responses are associated with disappearance of rearranged *BCR* bands in most cases.[37,45,46]

The *BCR* ratio is usually lower than the proportion of Ph-positive metaphases. The reason for this is that Southern blotting analyses a large number of dividing and resting cells, including *BCR/ABL*-negative lymphocytes, and cytogenetic analysis provides information only on a small number of dividing myeloid cells.[37,43] Empirically derived cutoff points in the *BCR* ratio were introduced in order to define molecular response groups: a *BCR* ratio of 0% was defined as complete response, and ratios of 1–24%, 25–50% and >50% were defined as partial, minor, and no molecular responses, respectively. Using these cutoff points, a major cytogenetic response could be predicted or excluded in more than 90% of cases.[37] The main advantage of Southern blotting over cytogenetics is the independence from dividing cells, which permits the use of peripheral blood instead of bone marrow.

Western blot analysis

Western blotting can be used to detect BCR/ABL proteins directly in cell extracts qualitatively and quantitatively both in bone marrow and in peripheral blood. Leukocytes are lysed in the presence of potent protease inhibitors, fractionated on a polyacrylamide gel, transferred to a nylon membrane, and probed with an anti-ABL antibody. Different types of BCR/ABL proteins (p190, p210, p230, and rare variants) can be distinguished from p145 ABL by differences in migration.[14] The limit of sensitivity is about 0.5–1%. A quantitative Western blot assay found a linear correlation between BCR/ABL : ABL protein ratios and contemporaneous conventional cytogenetics.[47,48]

Reverse-transcriptase polymerase chain reaction

In 1989, the first encouraging results were reported concerning detection of minimal residual disease by PCR in CML patients after allogeneic bone marrow transplantation.[49] However, conflicting data from a comparative multicentre study revealed serious problems with the method, with a high rate of false-positive results, and provoked an open discussion.[50,51] Over the past 10 years, PCR has been optimized and developed. Specificity has been considerably increased by the partial standardization of methodology and the introduction of rigorous precautions to avoid contamination.[52] Sensitivity has been improved by using nested primer pairs and performing two consecutive PCR steps. In view of the limited value of qualitative PCR for monitoring CML patients after therapy, quantitative *BCR/ABL* PCR assays were developed to monitor patients after stem cell transplantation[53,54] or treatment with IFN-α,[55,56] and are now in routine clinical use.

Screening for *BCR/ABL* mRNA transcripts at diagnosis

For diagnostic samples, the use of *multiplex PCR* has been suggested to detect simultaneously several kinds of *BCR/ABL* and *BCR* transcripts as internal controls in one reaction[57] by using three *BCR* and one *ABL* primers. This method allows the reliable detection of typical *BCR/ABL* transcripts, such as b2a2 or b3a2, and atypical types, such as transcripts lacking *ABL* exon a2 (b2a3 and b3a3), transcripts resulting from *BCR* breakpoints outside the M-*bcr*, such as e1a2 or e6a2,[14,15,58] or transcripts with inserts between *BCR* and *ABL* exons.[59]

Detection of minimal residual disease: 'nested' RT-PCR

Since patients with leukaemia at presentation or relapse usually have a total burden of more than 10^{12} malignant cells,[60] and cytogenetics, Western blot, and conventional FISH have a maximum sensitivity of 1%, a patient with negative results may harbour as few as zero or as many as 10^{10} residual leukaemic cells. At this point, the patient is judged to be in clinical and haematological remission, although the term 'remission' refers only to an arbitrary point of a continuum of residual leukaemic cell numbers.[61]

RT-PCR for *BCR/ABL* mRNA is by far the most sensitive assay in the context of residual disease analysis, and can detect a single leukaemic cell on a background of 10^5–10^6 normal cells. Therefore PCR is up to four orders of magnitude more sensitive than conventional methods. However, patients who have no residual disease detectable by RT-PCR may still harbour up to a million malignant cells that could contribute to subsequent relapse. The sensitivity with which residual disease can be detected will be limited by the amount of peripheral blood or bone marrow that can be analysed.

Using *nested RT-PCR* with two pairs of ('nested') primers corresponding to appropriate *BCR* and *ABL* exons employed in two rounds of amplification, residual CML cells after treatment can be specifically detected with a sensitivity of up to 1 in 10^6 cells.[62]

This qualitative method has been used for the detection of minimal residual disease after allogeneic stem cell transplantation. Most transplant centres have demonstrated that the majority of patients are PCR positive in the first 6 months after transplantation, two-thirds of patients become PCR-negative during follow-up owing to the graft-versus-leukaemia effect, persistent PCR negativity after 1 year is a marker for good prognosis, and patients who are PCR-positive more than 6 months after BMT have a great risk of relapse.[63] However, qualitative PCR cannot predict relapse in the individual patient.[53,64–66] In the majority of cases after transplantation, RT-PCR and DNA-PCR (using patient-specific primers) results are concordant, i.e. indicating that patients in remission do not generally harbour a substantial pool of CML cells that do not express *BCR/ABL* mRNA.[67]

Nested PCR is essentially useless in patients after IFN-α therapy, even in cytogenetic remission, since almost all patients remain repeatedly positive.[68]

If the RT-PCR method is pushed to the extreme, *BCR/ABL* mRNA can be detected at a very low level of 1–10 transcripts per 10^8 cells in many normal individuals, with a frequency that is age-dependent.[69,70] It has been suggested that *BCR/ABL*, and probably several other fusion genes, are being continuously formed in mitotic cells in the normal bone marrow, but only the combination of an in-frame *BCR/ABL* fusion in the correct primitive haematopoietic progenitor would have the selective advantage to become functional as an expanding clone.[71] In addition, it is possible that *BCR/ABL* alone is not sufficient to result in the expansion of myeloid cell numbers, and that other cooperating genetic events may be required.

Quantitative PCR

In view of the very limited value of qualitative PCR, several groups have developed quantitative PCR assays to estimate the amount of residual disease in positive specimens. Most groups have initially used *competitive PCR strategies* that can effectively control for variations in amplification efficiency and reaction kinetics.[53,55,72–74]

In general, nested PCR is performed using serial dilutions of a *BCR/ABL* competitor construct added to the same volume of patient's cDNA. The equivalence point at which the competitor and patient's sample bands would be of equal intensity is determined by densitometry.[53,56] In order to standardize results for both quality and quantity of blood, RNA, and cDNA, quantification of transcripts of normal housekeeping genes, such as *ABL* or glucose-6-phosphate dehydrogenase (*G6PD*), has been

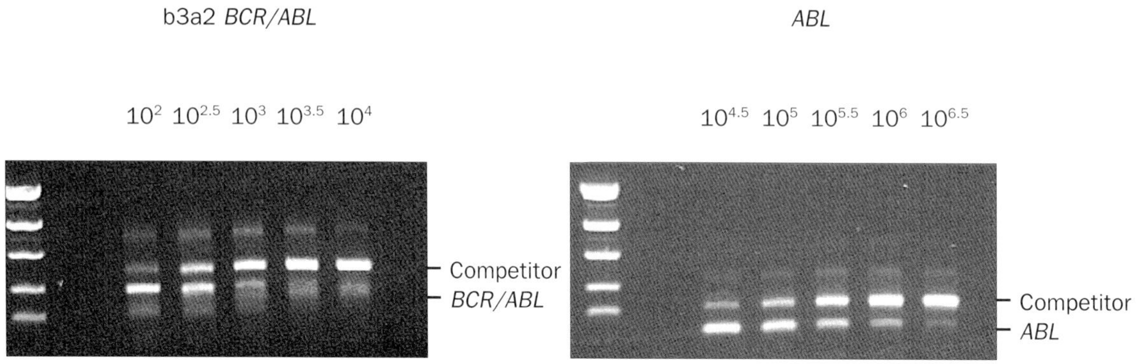

$$\text{Ratio } BCR/ABL : ABL = \frac{BCR/ABL \text{ transcripts } / \ 2.5\,\mu\text{l cDNA}}{ABL \text{ transcripts } / \ 2.5\,\mu\text{l cDNA}}$$

Figure 21.3
Quantitative competitive RT-PCR for *BCR/ABL* transcripts. Nested PCR is performed using serial dilutions of a *BCR/ABL* competitor construct added to the same volume of patient's cDNA. The equivalence point at which patient's sample and competitor bands would be of equal intensity is determined by densitometry. Total *ABL* transcripts are quantified to standardize the assay for different qualities of patient's blood, RNA, or cDNA.[56]

employed. The standardized results are expressed as the ratios of *BCR/ABL* to *ABL* or of *BCR/ABL* to *G6PD* in percent. The quantification of the transcript level of control genes is of particular importance if different RNA qualities are expected, i.e., in particular, if samples are mailed, such as in multicentre trials (Figure 21.3).

In patients after allogeneic stem cell transplantation, rising or persistently high levels of *BCR/ABL* mRNA can be detected prior to cytogenetic or haematological relapse. Low or falling *BCR/ABL* transcript levels are associated with continuous remission, while high or rising *BCR/ABL* transcript levels predict relapse (Figure 21.4).[53,54,64,75–77]

Quantitative PCR is the method of choice to determine the best time point for therapeutic interventions in the case of relapse after stem cell transplantation. Quantitative PCR data has been used to determine the optimum time point to initiate donor lymphocyte transfusions[78–80] and to monitor response.[81] Two patterns of molecular response have been described: a very rapid decline after an initial lag phase, or a more gradual decline over a period of several months.[81] The great majority of patients who respond to donor lymphocyte infusions achieve durable molecular remission (RT-PCR negativity) with a median follow-up of more than 2 years.[81]

Quantitative RT-PCR for *BCR/ABL* has been shown to be a reliable method for monitoring residual leukaemia load in mobilized peripheral blood stem cells, particularly in Ph-negative collections. Quantitative RT-PCR allows selection of the best available collections for reinfusion into patients after myeloablative therapy (autografting). A correlation has been found between low values of *BCR/ABL* : *ABL* ratios in the reinfused peripheral blood progenitor cells and the achievement of cytogenetic remission after autografting.[82]

Almost all patients are persistently positive for *BCR/ABL* transcripts following IFN-α therapy. The median ratios of complete, partial, minor and non-responders differ significantly. The results for IFN-α non-responders and patients at diagnosis are not different.[56,68] Cytogenetic response to IFN-α (complete, partial, minor/none) was compared with molecular response by introducing cutoff points for the ratio *BCR/ABL* : *ABL*. The optimum cutoff points were 2% and 14%, i.e. a complete response is associated with a ratio of up to 2%, a partial response with a ratio of 2–14%, and a minor or no response with a ratio of more than 14%.[56]

All 54 patients investigated who had achieved a complete response to IFN-α treatment had molecular evidence of residual disease during complete remission, although three

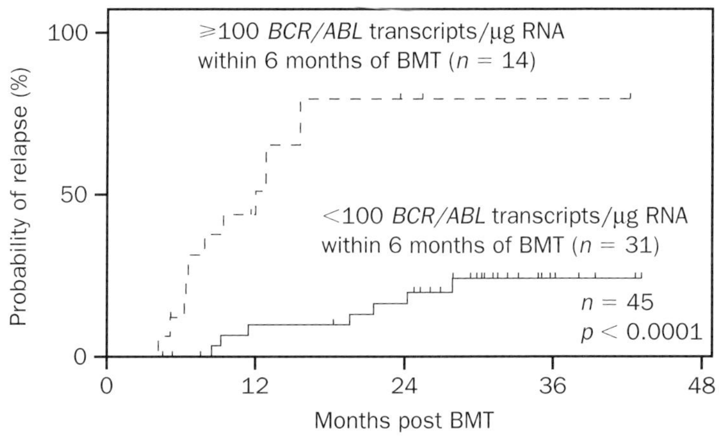

Figure 21.4
Rate of relapse in patients after allogeneic bone marrow transplantation (BMT) according to residual *BCR/ABL* transcript levels in the first 6 months after transplantation. The relapse incidence is significantly higher in patients with residual *BCR/ABL* transcripts of ≥100/µg RNA compared with patients with transcript levels of <100/µg RNA.[53]

patients were intermittently negative by RT-PCR. It should be noted that this level of sensitivity can be reached only if at least 5×10^7 cells (10–20 ml of peripheral blood) are processed and that the actual level of sensitivity for each specimen can only be determined by quantification of a control gene. The levels of residual disease in complete responders spans a range over four orders of magnitude.[68] The level of residual disease falls with time in patients who maintain their cytogenetic response to IFN-α, but molecular evidence of disease is rarely, if ever, eliminated.[83] In other series, the frequency of PCR negativity in complete cytogenetic responders is higher in a long-term follow-up using a RT-PCR strategy with a lower sensitivity (Figures 21.5 and 21.6).[84]

RT-PCR analysis of granulocyte–macrophage colony-forming units (CFU-GM) grown from bone marrow of eight complete cytogenetic responders demonstrated that residual disease resides in myeloid colony-forming cells that may have the potential to repopulate the bone marrow and contribute to relapse.[85]

Recently, novel *real-time PCR procedures* have been developed that promise to simplify existing protocols. Several procedures for quantification of *BCR/ABL* mRNA using the TaqMan system have been developed (Figure 21.7).[86–89] The assay is based on the use of the 5′ nuclease activity of *Taq* polymerase to cleave a non-extendible dual-labelled hybridization probe during the extension phase of PCR. One fluorescent dye serves as a reporter, and its emission spectrum is quenched by the second fluorescent dye. The nuclease degradation of the probe releases the quenching, resulting in an increase in fluorescent emission. The fluores-

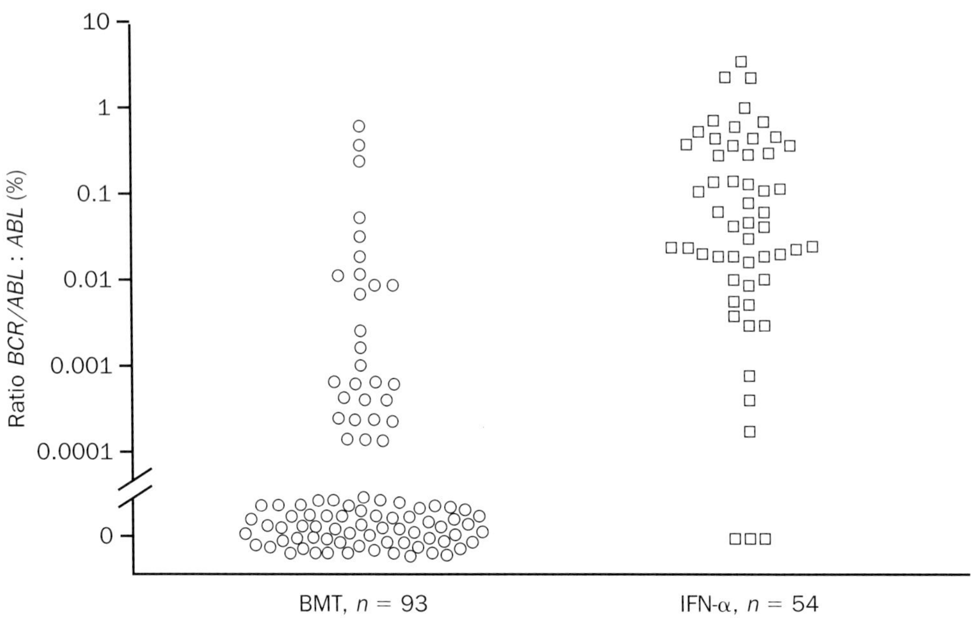

Figure 21.5
Quantitative PCR analysis for the ratio *BCR/ABL* : *ABL* in complete cytogenetic responders after allogeneic stem cell transplantation and IFN-α therapy. Two-thirds of patients after allogeneic bone marrow transplantation (BMT) are RT-PCR-negative after 6 months,[53] whereas almost all patients after IFN-α therapy are persistently RT-PCR-positive. Only 3 out of 54 patients showed transient PCR negativity.[83]

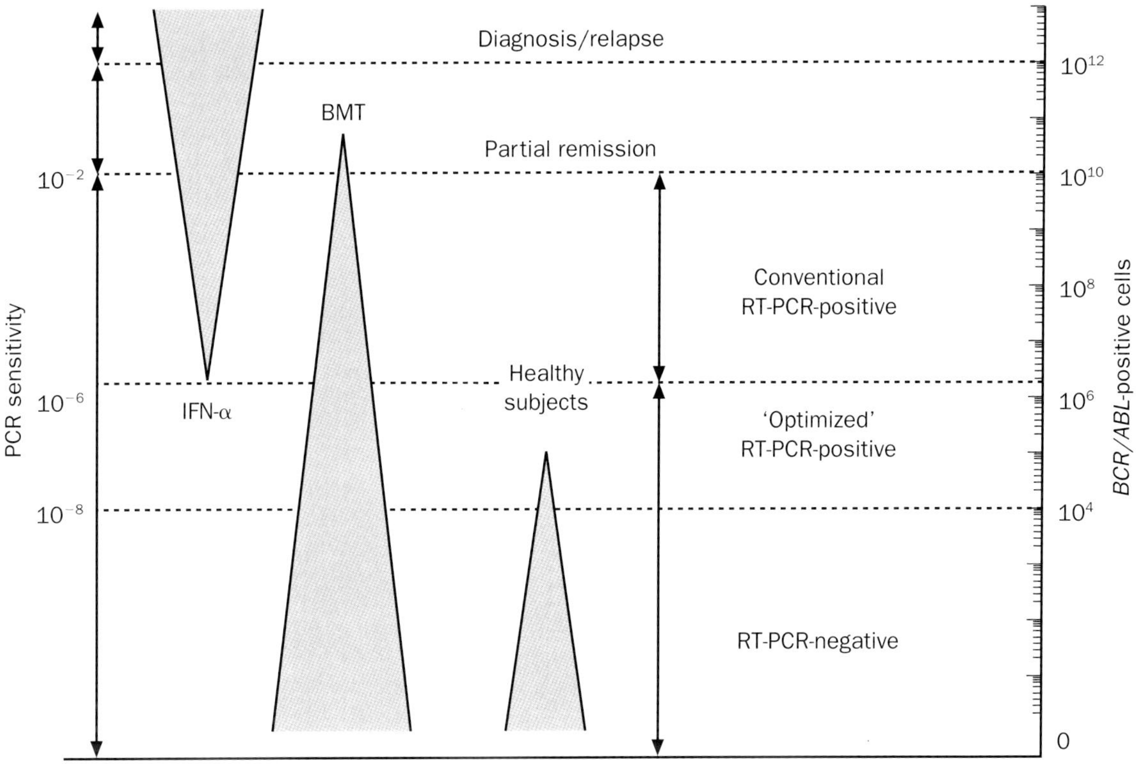

Figure 21.6
Schematic illustration of therapeutic response of CML patients on a molecular level. Almost all patients treated with IFN-α remain RT-PCR-positive;[83] the majority of patients after allogeneic stem cell transplantation (BMT) become RT-PCR-negative.[53] Healthy donors may be RT-PCR-positive for *BCR/ABL* transcripts using an optimized, very sensitive PCR strategy.[69,70]

cence is monitored by a sequence detector in real time. C_T (threshold cycle) values are calculated by determining the point at which the fluorescence exceeds a threshold limit. C_T corresponds to the number of target transcripts in the sample.[90]

An alternative real-time RT-PCR approach for detection and quantification of *BCR/ABL* fusion transcripts has been established using the LightCycler technology,[91,92] which combines rapid thermocycling with on-line fluorescence detection of PCR-product formation as it occurs. Fluorescence monitoring of PCR amplification is based on the concept of fluorescence resonance energy transfer (FRET) between two adjacent hybridization probes carrying donor and acceptor fluorophores. Excitation of a donor fluorophore (fluorescein) with an emission spectrum that overlaps the excitation spectrum of an acceptor fluorophore results in non-radioactive energy transfer to the acceptor. Once conditions are established, the amount of fluorescence resulting from the two probes is proportional to the amount of PCR product. Using amplification in glass capillaries with a low volume/surface ratio, PCR reaction times have been reduced to less than 30 minutes.

A pair of probes was designed that was complementary to *ABL* exon 3, thus enabling detection of all known *BCR/ABL* variants and also

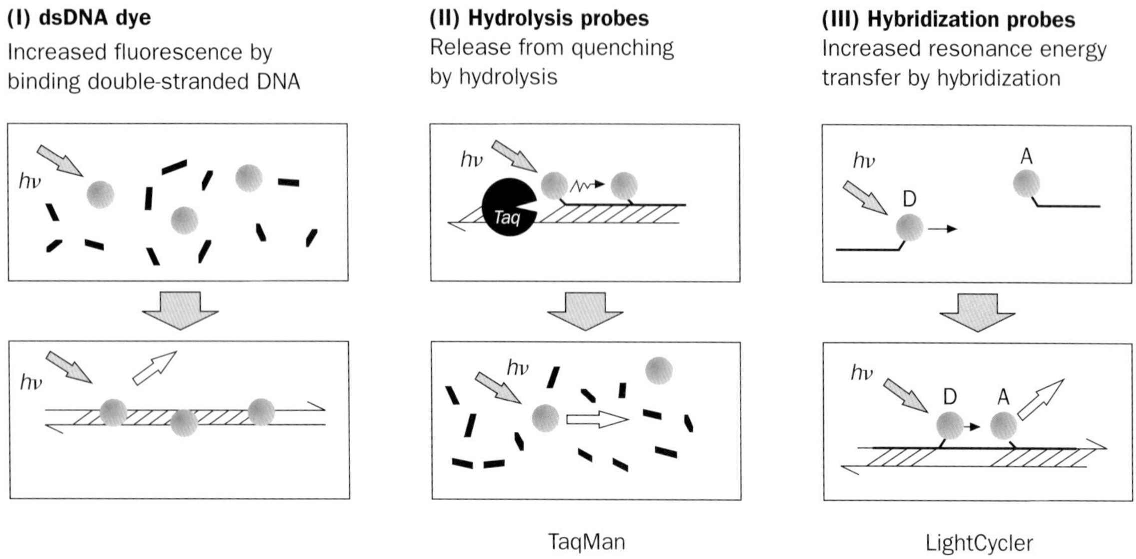

Figure 21.7
Real-time fluorescence detection of PCR products during the amplification phase (real-time PCR). Fluorescence labelling can be performed (I) by non-specific binding of an appropriate dye to double-stranded DNA (e.g. SYBR Green), (II) by hybridization of TaqMan probes carrying quencher and reporter dyes that are cleaved during elongation, or (III) by hybridization to a pair of probes labelled with a donor (D) and an acceptor (A) dye with increased fluorescence in juxtaposition (LightCycler method).

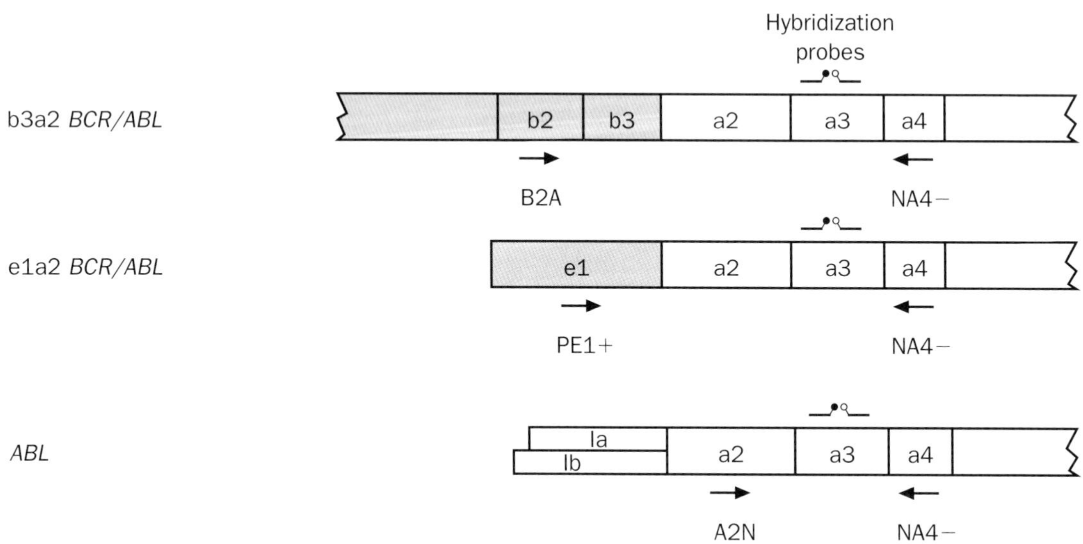

Figure 21.8
Schematic map of the amplification and detection of *BCR/ABL* and *ABL* transcripts. Specific primer pairs were used to amplify various types of *BCR/ABL* and *ABL* transcripts. The detection format was uniform, using a pair of adjacent fluorescent labelled hybridization probes to *ABL* exon 3.[93]

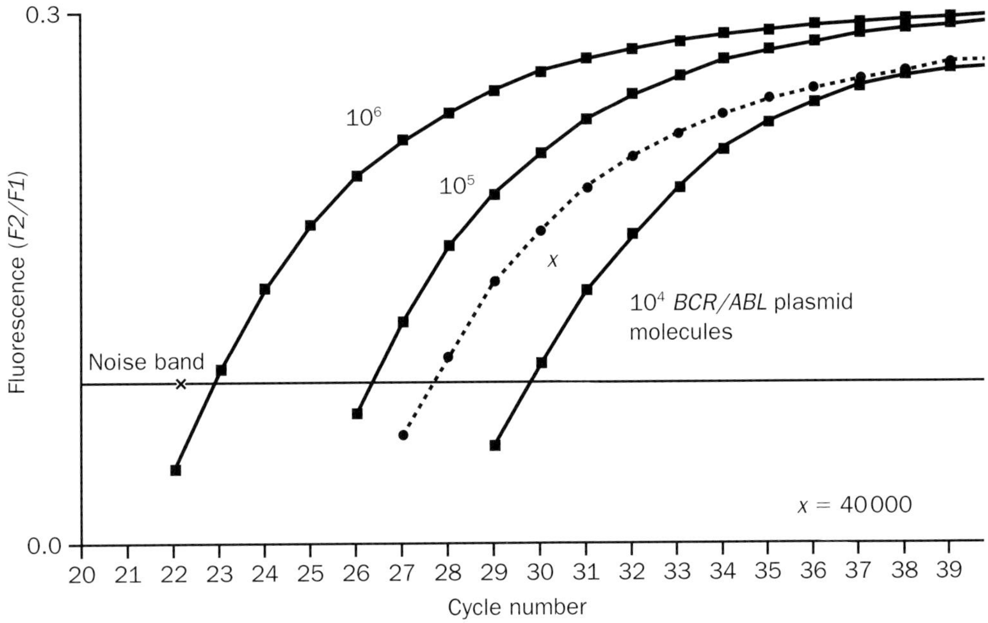

Figure 21.9
Example of real-time PCR. Three standard dilutions of plasmid pGD210 (b3a2*BCR/ABL*) were compared with a patient's sample of unknown *BCR/ABL* concentration. Each point represents the fluorescence intensity (*F2/F1*) measured after each PCR cycle. Plotting the cycle threshold of the unknown sample on the standard curve revealed that 40 000 *BCR/ABL* transcripts were present at the start of the reaction.[93]

abnormal *ABL* as an internal control (Figures 21.8 and 21.9). Conditions were established to amplify less than 10 target molecules/reaction, and to detect one CML cell in 10^5 cells from healthy donors, and one K562 cell in 10^7 HL60 cells. To determine the utility of the assay, *BCR/ABL* and *ABL* transcripts in a series of 254 samples from 120 patients with CML after therapy were quantified. The level of residual disease was expressed as the ratio of *BCR/ABL* to *ABL*. A highly significant correlation was seen between the ratios *BCR/ABL* : *ABL* determined by the LightCycler and (i) the ratios *BCR/ABL* : *ABL* obtained by nested competitive RT-PCR performed with the same cDNA samples (Figure 21.10), (ii) the proportion of Ph-positive metaphases determined by contemporaneous cytogenetics, and (iii) the *BCR* ratio determined by Southern blot analysis.[93] In CML patients, either peripheral blood or bone marrow aspirates can be processed[93,94] (Figure 21.11).

Real-time PCR approaches are reliable and sensitive methods to monitor CML patients after therapy. The major advantages of the methodology are that (i) amplification and product analysis are performed in the same reaction vessel, avoiding the risk of contamination, and (ii) the results are standardized by the quantification of housekeeping genes.

Chimerism analysis

Several alternative techniques have also been employed. They are mostly too cumbersome, inexact or underdeveloped for routine assessment of residual leukaemia. An example is *chimerism analysis*, which distinguishes between

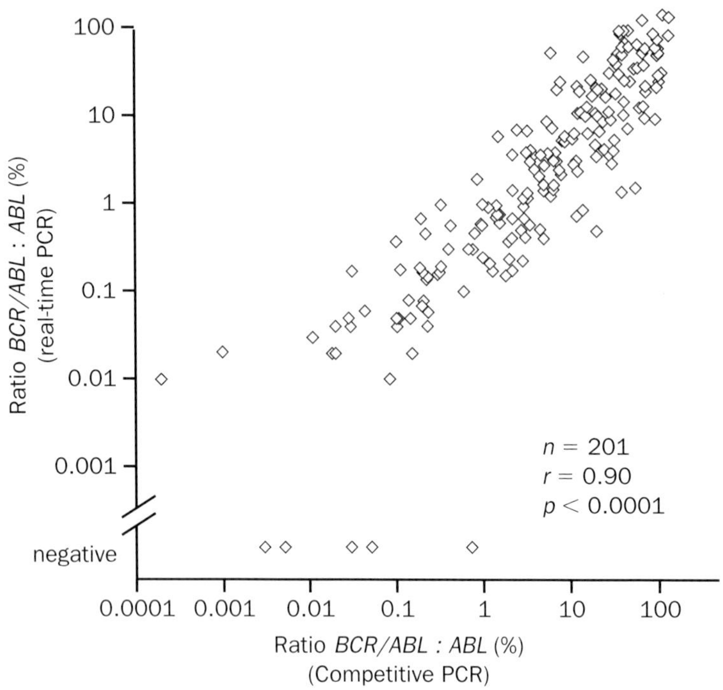

Figure 21.10
Comparison of the quantification of the ratio *BCR/ABL* : *ABL* with real-time PCR versus competitive PCR. In five samples that were positive with competitive PCR, no *BCR/ABL* transcripts were detected by real-time PCR. The ratios derived by both methods correlate with $r = 0.90$, $p < 0.0001$.[93]

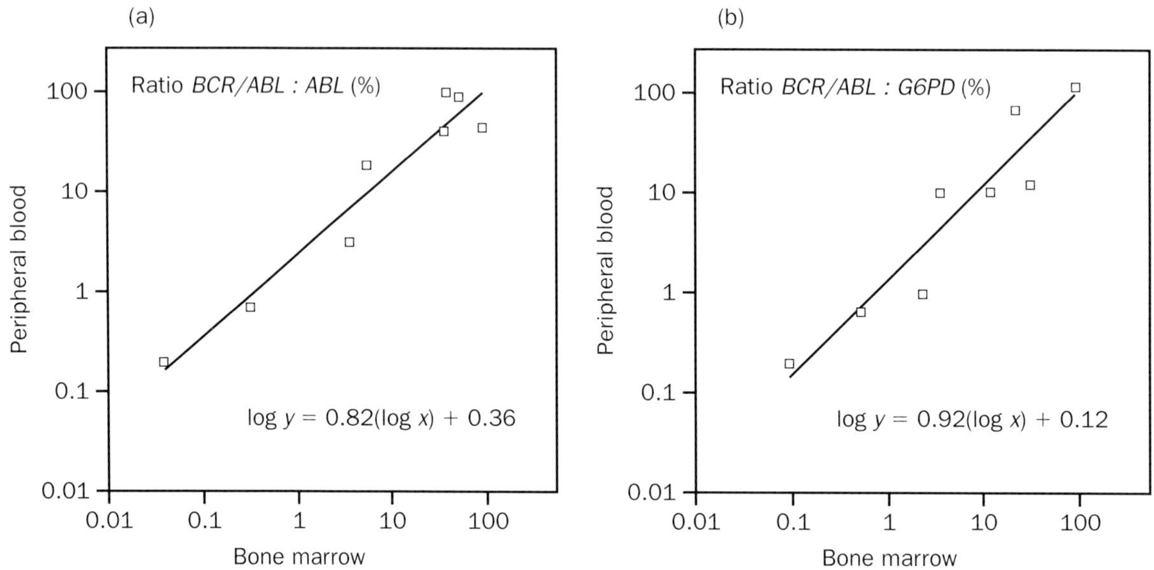

Figure 21.11
Correlations of (a) the ratio *BCR/ABL* : *ABL* and (b) the ratio *BCR/ABL* : *G6PD* obtained from eight pairs of contemporaneous peripheral blood and bone marrow samples. The coefficient of regression was $r = 0.90$ ($p = 0.0046$) for the ratio *BCR/ABL* : *ABL* and $r = 0.98$ ($p = 0.0004$) for the ratio *BCR/ABL* : *G6PD*. Therefore, in CML, the use of peripheral blood for monitoring is suggested.[93]

genomic DNA or cells from different individuals, and can be used in patients after allogeneic stem cell transplantation to calculate the proportion of host to donor cells. Typically, PCR is used to amplify polymorphic markers.[95–97] Chimerism analysis does not distinguish between malignant and normal cells, and therefore cannot be used directly to detect residual leukaemia.

CONCLUSIONS

Quantitative determination of residual disease levels after treatment for patients with CML may be achieved by various methods. However, there is a need to standardize methodologies and interpretation of results in order to reduce interlaboratory variation. The development of new real-time RT-PCR procedures offers a unique opportunity for this to be achieved. Quantitative real-time PCR will shortly become a routine and robust basis for clinical decision-making, not only in CML but also in other leukaemias with specific molecular markers.

REFERENCES

1. Nowell PC, Hungerford DA, A minute chromosome in human chronic granulocytic leukemia. *Science* 1960; **132:** 1497–501.
2. Rowley JD, A new consistent chromosome abnormality in chronic myelogenous leukaemia detected by quinacrine fluorescence and Giemsa staining. *Nature* 1973; **243:** 290–3.
3. Sawyers CL, Chronic myeloid leukemia. *N Engl J Med* 1999; **340:** 1330–40.
4. Groffen J, Stephenson JR, Heisterkamp N et al, Philadelphia chromosomal breakpoints are clustered within a limited region, bcr, on chromosome 22. *Cell* 1984; **36:** 93–9.
5. Stam K, Heisterkamp N, Grosveld G et al, Evidence of a new chimeric bcr/c-abl mRNA in patients with chronic myelocytic leukemia and the Philadelphia chromosome. *N Engl J Med* 1985; **313:** 1429–33.
6. Melo JV, Gordon DE, Cross NCP, Goldman JM, The ABL–BCR fusion gene is expressed in chronic myeloid leukemia. *Blood* 1993; **81:** 158–65.
7. Thijsen SFT, Schuurhuis GJ, van Oostveen JW, Ossenkoppele GJ, Chronic myeloid leukemia from basics to bedside. *Leukemia* 1999; **13:** 1646–74.
8. Hehlmann R, Heimpel H, Current aspects of drug therapy in Philadelphia-positive CML: correlation of tumor burden with survival. *Leuk Lymphoma* 1996; **22**(Suppl 1): 161–7.
9. Hook EB, Exclusion of chromosomal mosaicism: tables of 90%, 95%, and 99% confidence limits and comments on use. *Am J Hum Genet* 1977; **29:** 94–7.
10. Cortes J, Talpaz M, O'Brien S et al, Suppression on cytogenetic clonal evolution with interferon alfa therapy in patients with Philadelphia chromosome-positive chronic myelogenous leukemia. *J Clin Oncol* 1998; **16:** 3279–85.
11. Kantarjian HM, Dixon D, Keating MJ et al, Characteristics of accelerated disease in chronic myelogenous leukemia. *Cancer* 1988; **61:** 1441–6.
12. Tkachuk DC, Westbrook CA, Andreeff M et al, Detection of bcr–abl fusion in chronic myelogenous leukemia by in situ hybridization. *Science* 1990; **250:** 559–62.
13. Nacheva E, Holloway T, Brown K et al, Philadelphia-negative chronic myeloid leukaemia: detection by FISH of BCR–ABL fusion gene localized either to chromosome 9 or chromosome 22. *Br J Haematol* 1994; **87:** 409–12.
14. Hochhaus A, Reiter A, Skladny H et al, A novel BCR–ABL fusion gene (e6a2) in a patient with Philadelphia chromosome negative chronic myelogenous leukemia. *Blood* 1996; **88:** 2236–40.
15. Melo JV, The diversity of BCR–ABL fusion proteins and their relationship to leukemia phenotype. *Blood* 1996; **88:** 2375–84.
16. Weber-Matthiesen K, Winkemann M, Müller-Hermelink A et al, Simultaneous fluorescence immunophenotyping and interphase cytogenetics: a contribution to characterization of tumor cells. *J Histochem Cytochem* 1992; **40:** 171–5.
17. Haferlach T, Winkemann M, Nickenig C et al, Which compartments are involved in Philadelphia-chromosome positive chronic myeloid leukaemia? An answer at the single cell level by combining May–Grünwald–Giemsa staining and fluorescence in situ hybridization techniques. *Br J Haematol* 1997; **97:** 99–106.
18. Bentz M, Cabot G, Moos M et al, Detection of

chimeric BCR–ABL genes on bone marrow samples and blood smears in chronic myeloid and acute lymphoblastic leukemia by in situ hybridization. *Blood* 1994; **83:** 1922–8.

19. Garcia-Isidoro M, Tabernero MD, Garcia JL et al, Detection of the Mbcr/abl translocation in chronic myeloid leukemia by fluorescence in situ hybridization: comparison with conventional cytogenetics and implications for minimal residual disease detection. *Hum Pathol* 1997; **28:** 154–9.
20. Cuneo A, Bigoni R, Emmanuel B et al, Fluorescence in situ hybridization for the detection and monitoring of the Ph-positive clone in chronic myelogenous leukemia: comparison with metaphase banding analysis. *Leukemia* 1998; **12:** 1718–23.
21. Yanagi M, Shinjo K, Takeshita A et al, Simple and reliably sensitive diagnosis and monitoring of Philadelphia chromosome-positive cells in chronic myeloid leukemia by interphase fluorescence in situ hybridization of peripheral blood cells. *Leukemia* 1999; **13:** 542–52.
22. Chase A, Grand F, Zhang JG et al, Factors influencing the false positive and negative rates of *BCR–ABL* fluorescence in-situ hybridization. *Genes Chromosomes Cancer* 1997; **18:** 246–53.
23. Mühlmann J, Thaler J, Hilbe W et al, Fluorescence in situ hybridization (FISH) on peripheral blood smears for monitoring Philadelphia chromosome-positive chronic myeloid leukemia (CML) during interferon treatment: a new strategy for remission assessment. *Genes Chromosomes Cancer* 1998; **21:** 90–100.
24. Tchirkov A, Giollant M, Tavernier F et al, Interphase cytogenetics and competitive RT-PCR for residual disease monitoring in patients with chronic myeloid leukaemia during interferon-α therapy. *Br J Haematol* 1998; **101:** 552–7.
25. Cox Froncillo MC, Maffei L, Cantonetti M et al, FISH analysis for CML monitoring? *Ann Hematol* 1996; **73:** 113–19.
26. Verfaillie C, Bhatia R, Miller W et al, BCR/ABL-negative primitive progenitors suitable for transplantation can be selected from the marrow of most early-chronic phase but not accelerated-phase chronic myelogenous leukemia patients. *Blood* 1996; **87:** 4770–9.
27. Hess G, Reifenrath C, Friedrich-Freksa A et al, Autologous transplantation of in vivo purged PBSC in CML: comparison of FISH, cytogenetics, and PCR for detection of Philadelphia chromosome in leukapheresis products. *Cancer Genet Cytogenet* 2000; **117**: 1–8.
28. Kirk JA, Reems JA, Roecklein BA et al, Benign marrow progenitors are enriched in the CD34+/HLA-DRlo population but not in the CD34+/CD38lo population in chronic myeloid leukemia: an analysis using interphase fluorescence in situ hybridization. *Blood* 1995; **86:** 737–43.
29. Sinclair PB, Green AR, Grace C, Nacheva EP, Improved sensitivity of BCR–ABL detection: a triple-probe three-colour fluorescence in situ hybridization system. *Blood* 1997; **90:** 1395–402.
30. Buno I, Wyatt WA, Zinsmeister AR et al, A special fluorescent in situ hybridization technique to study peripheral blood and assess the effectiveness of interferon therapy in chronic myeloid leukemia. *Blood* 1998; **92:** 2315–21.
31. Dewald GW, Wyatt WA, Juneau AL et al, Highly sensitive fluorescence in situ hybridization method to detect double BCR/ABL fusion and monitor response to therapy in chronic myeloid leukemia. *Blood* 1998; **91:** 3357–65.
32. Grand F, Kulkarni S, Chase A et al, Frequent deletion of hSNF5/INI1, a component of the SWI/SNF complex, during progression of chronic myeloid leukemia. *Cancer Res* 1999; **59:** 3870–4.
33. Sinclair PB, Nacheva EP, Leversha M et al, Large deletions at the t(9;22) breakpoint are common and may identify a poor-prognosis subgroup of patients with chronic myeloid leukemia. *Blood* 2000; **95:** 738–44.
34. El Rifae W, Ruutu T, Vettentanta K et al, Minimal residual disease after allogeneic bone marrow transplantation for chronic myeloid leukaemia: a metaphase-FISH study. *Br J Haematol* 1996; **92:** 365–9.
35. Seong DC, Kantarjian HM, Ro JY et al, Hypermetaphase fluorescence in situ hybridization for quantitative monitoring of Philadelphia chromosome-positive cells in patients with chronic myelogenous leukemia during treatment. *Blood* 1995; **86:** 2343–9.
36. Seong D, Giralt S, Fischer H et al, Usefulness of detection of minimal residual disease by 'hypermetaphase' fluorescent in situ hybridization after allogeneic BMT for chronic myelogenous leukemia. *Bone Marrow Transplant* 1997; **19:** 565–70.
37. Reiter A, Skladny H, Hochhaus A et al, Molecular response of CML patients treated with interferon-α monitored by quantitative Southern blot analysis. *Br J Haematol* 1997; **97:** 86–93.

38. Fishleder AJ, Shadrach B, Tuttle C, *bcr* rearrangement: potential false positive secondary to an ECORI restriction fragment length polymorphism. *Leukemia* 1989; **3:** 746–8.
39. Grossman A, Mathew A, O'Connnell MP et al, Multiple restriction enzyme digests are required to rule out polymorphism in the molecular diagnosis of chronic myeloid leukemia. *Leukemia* 1990; **4:** 63–4.
40. Popenoe DW, Schaefer Rego K, Mears JG et al, Frequent and extensive deletion during the 9,22 translocation in CML. *Blood* 1986; **68:** 1123–8.
41. Bartram CR, Bross Bach U, Schmidt H, Waller HD, Philadelphia-positive chronic myelogenous leukemia with breakpoint 5′ of the breakpoint cluster region but within the bcr gene. *Blut* 1987; **55:** 505–11.
42. Saglio G, Guerrasio A, Rosso C et al, New type of Bcr/Abl junction in Philadelphia chromosome-positive chronic myelogenous leukemia. *Blood* 1990; **76:** 1819–24.
43. Stock W, Westbrook CA, Peterson B et al, Value of molecular monitoring during treatment of chronic myeloid leukemia: a Cancer and Leukemia Group B study. *J Clin Oncol* 1997; **15:** 26–36.
44. Verschraegen CF, Talpaz M, Hirsch Ginsberg CF et al, Quantification of the breakpoint cluster region rearrangement for clinical monitoring in Philadelphia chromosome-positive chronic myeloid leukemia. *Blood* 1995; **85:** 2705–10.
45. Steegmann JL, Requena MJ, Casado LF et al, Southern technique and cytogenetics are complementary and must be used together in the evaluation of Ph1, M-BCR positive chronic myeloid leukemia (CML) patients treated with alpha interferon (IFN-ALPHA). *Am J Hematol* 1996; **53:** 169–74.
46. Yoffe G, Blick M, Kantarjian H et al, Molecular analysis of interferon-induced suppression of Philadelphia chromosome in patients with chronic myeloid leukemia. *Blood* 1987; **69:** 961–3.
47. Guo JQ, Lian J, Glassman A et al, Comparison of *bcr–abl* protein expression and Philadelphia chromosome analyses in chronic myelogenous leukemia patients. *Am J Clin Pathol* 1996; **106:** 442–8.
48. Guo JQ, Lian JY, Xian YM et al, BCR–ABL protein expression in peripheral blood cells of chronic myelogenous leukemia patients undergoing therapy. *Blood* 1994; **83:** 3629–37.
49. Morgan GJ, Hughes T, Janssen JW et al, Polymerase chain reaction for detection of residual leukaemia. *Lancet* 1989; **i:** 928–9.
50. Hughes T, Martiat P, Morgan G et al, Significance of residual leukaemia transcripts after bone marrow transplant for CML. *Lancet* 1990; **335:** 50.
51. Hughes T, Janssen JWG, Morgan G et al, False-positive results with PCR to detect leukaemia-specific transcript. *Lancet* 1990; **335:** 1037–8.
52. Hughes T, Goldman JM, Improved results with PCR for chronic myeloid leukaemia. *Lancet* 1990; **336:** 812.
53. Cross NCP, Feng L, Chase A et al, Competitive polymerase chain reaction to estimate the number of BCR–ABL transcripts in chronic myeloid leukemia patients after bone marrow transplantation. *Blood* 1993; **82:** 1929–36.
54. Lion T, Henn T, Gaiger A et al, Early detection of relapse after bone marrow transplantation in patients with chronic myelogenous leukaemia. *Lancet* 1993; **341:** 275–6.
55. Malinge MC, Mahon FX, Delfau MH et al, Quantitative determination of the hybrid Bcr–Abl RNA in patients with chronic myelogenous leukaemia under interferon therapy. *Br J Haematol* 1992; **82:** 701–7.
56. Hochhaus A, Lin F, Reiter A et al, Quantification of residual disease in chronic myelogenous leukemia patients on interferon-α therapy by competitive polymerase chain reaction. *Blood* 1996; **87:** 1549–55.
57. Cross NCP, Melo JV, Feng L, Goldman JM, An optimized multiplex polymerase chain reaction (PCR) for detection of BCR–ABL fusion mRNAs in haematological disorders. *Leukemia* 1994; **8:** 186–9.
58. Melo JV, Myint H, Galton DA, Goldman JM, p190BCR–ABL chronic myeloid leukaemia: the missing link with chronic myelomonocytic leukaemia? *Leukemia* 1994; **8:** 208–11.
59. Rubinstein R, Purves LR, A novel BCR–ABL rearrangement in a Philadelphia chromosome-positive chronic myelogenous leukaemia variant with thrombocythaemia. *Leukemia* 1998; **12:** 230–2.
60. Clarkson B, Strife A, Linkage of proliferative and maturational abnormalities in chronic myelogenous leukemia and relevance to treatment. *Leukemia* 1993; **7:** 1683–721.
61. Morley A, Quantifying leukemia. *N Engl J Med* 1998; **339:** 627–9.
62. van Dongen JJM, MacIntyre EA, Gabert JA et al,

Standardized RT-PCR analysis of fusion gene transcripts from chromosome aberrations in acute leukemia for detection of minimal residual disease. *Leukemia* 1999; **12:** 1901–28.

63. Cross NCP, Assessing residual leukaemia. *Baillière's Clin Haematol* 1997; **10:** 389–403.
64. Cross NCP, Feng L, Zhang JG, Goldman JM, Competitive PCR to monitor residual disease after bone marrow transplantation for chronic myeloid leukaemia. In: *Molecular Diagnosis and Monitoring of Leukaemia and Lymphoma* (Borden EC, Goldman JM, Grignani F, eds). Ares-Serono Symposia Publications, Rome, 1994: 119–26.
65. Potter MN, Cross NCP, van Dongen JJ et al, Molecular evidence of minimal residual disease after treatment for leukaemia and lymphoma: an updated meeting report and review. *Leukemia* 1993; **7:** 1302–14.
66. Reiter E, Greinix HT, Keil F et al, Long-term follow-up of patients after related- and unrelated-donor bone marrow transplantation for chronic myelogenous leukemia. *Ann Hematol* 1999; **78:** 507–13.
67. Zhang JG, Lin F, Chase A et al, Comparison of genomic DNA and cDNA for detection of residual disease after treatment of chronic myeloid leukemia with allogeneic bone marrow transplantation. *Blood* 1996; **87:** 2588–93.
68. Hochhaus A, Lin F, Reiter A et al, Variable numbers of BCR–ABL transcripts persist in CML patients who achieve complete cytogenetic remission with interferon-α. *Br J Haematol* 1995; **91:** 126–31.
69. Biernaux C, Loos M, Sels A et al, Detection of major bcr–abl gene expression at a very low level in blood cells of some healthy individuals. *Blood* 1995; **88:** 3118–22.
70. Bose S, Deininger M, Gora-Tybor J et al, The presence of typical and atypical BCR–ABL fusion genes in leukocytes of normal individuals: biological significance and implications for the assessment of minimal residual disease. *Blood* 1998; **92:** 3362–7.
71. Melo JV, The molecular biology of chronic myeloid leukaemia. *Leukemia* 1996; **10:** 751–6.
72. Lion T, Izraeli S, Henn T et al, Monitoring of residual disease in chronic myelogenous leukemia by quantitative polymerase chain reaction. *Leukemia* 1992; **6:** 495–9.
73. Thompson JD, Brodsky I, Yunis JJ, Molecular quantification of residual disease in chronic myelogenous leukemia after bone marrow transplantation. *Blood* 1992; **79:** 1629–35.
74. Nagel S, Schmidt M, Thiede C et al, Quantification of Bcr–Abl transcripts in chronic myelogenous leukemia (CML) using standardized, internally controlled, competitive differential PCR (CD-PCR). *Nucleic Acids Res* 1996; **24:** 4102–3.
75. Delage R, Soiffer RJ, Dear K, Ritz J, Clinical significance of *bcr–abl* gene rearrangement detected by polymerase chain reaction after allogeneic bone marrow transplantation in chronic myelogenous leukemia. *Blood* 1991; **78:** 2759–67.
76. Lin F, van Rhee F, Goldman JM, Cross NCP, Kinetics of increasing BCR–ABL transcript numbers in chronic myeloid leukemia patients who relapse after bone marrow transplantation. *Blood* 1996; **87:** 4473–8.
77. Lin F, Kirkland MA, van Rhee F et al, Molecular analysis of transient cytogenetic relapse after allogeneic bone marrow transplantation for chronic myeloid leukaemia. *Bone Marrow Transplant* 1996; **18:** 1147–52.
78. van Rhee F, Lin F, Cullis JO et al, Relapse of chronic myeloid leukemia after allogeneic bone marrow transplant: the case for giving donor leukocyte transfusions before the onset of hematologic relapse. *Blood* 1994; **83:** 3377–83.
79. Dazzi F, Szydlo RM, Goldman JM, Donor lymphocyte infusions for relapse of chronic myeloid leukemia after allogeneic stem cell transplant: where we now stand. *Exp Hematol* 1999; **27:** 1477–86.
80. Cross NCP, Minimal residual disease in CML. *Hematol Cell Ther* 1998; **40:** 224–8.
81. Raanani P, Dazzi F, Sohal J et al, The rate and kinetics of molecular response to donor leucocyte transfusions in chronic myeloid leukaemia patients treated for relapse after allogeneic bone marrow transplantation. *Br J Haematol* 1997; **99:** 945–50.
82. Corsetti MT, Lerma E, Dejana A et al, Quantitative competitive reverse transcriptase-polymerase chain reaction for BCR–ABL on Philadelphia-negative leukaphereses allows the selection of low-contaminated peripheral blood progenitor cells for autografting in chronic myelogenous leukemia. *Leukemia* 1999; **13:** 999–1008.
83. Hochhaus A, Reiter A, Saußele S et al, for the German CML Study Group and the U.K. MRC CML Study Group, Molecular heterogeneity in complete cytogenetic responders after interferon-α therapy for chronic myeloid leukaemia:

low levels of minimal residual disease are associated with continuing remission. *Blood* 2000; **95:** 62–6.
84. Kurzrock R, Estrov Z, Kantarjian H, Talpaz M, Conversion of interferon-induced, long-term cytogenetic remissions in chronic myelogenous leukemia to polymerase chain reaction negativity. *J Clin Oncol* 1998; **16:** 1526–31.
85. Reiter A, Marley SB, Hochhaus A et al, BCR–ABL positive progenitors in chronic myeloid leukaemia patients in complete cytogenetic remission after treatment with interferon-α. *Br J Haematol* 1998; **102:** 1271–8.
86. Mensink E, van de Locht A, Schattenberg A et al, Quantitation of minimal residual disease in Philadelphia chromosome positive chronic myeloid leukaemia patients using real-time quantitative RT-PCR. *Br J Haematol* 1998; **102:** 768–74.
87. Preudhomme C, Révillion F, Merlat A et al, Detection of BCR–ABL transcripts in chronic myeloid leukemia (CML) using a 'real time' quantitative RT-PCR assay. *Leukemia* 1999; **13:** 957–64.
88. Eder M, Battner K, Kafert S et al, Monitoring of BCR–ABL expression using real-time RT-PCR in CML after bone marrow or peripheral blood stem cell transplantation. *Leukemia* 1999; **13:** 1383–9.
89. Branford S, Hughes TP, Rudzki Z, Monitoring chronic myeloid leukaemia therapy by real-time quantitative PCR in blood is a reliable alternative to bone marrow cytogenetics. *Br J Haematol* 1999; **107:** 587–99.
90. Heid CA, Stevens J, Livak KJ, Williams PM, Real time quantitative PCR. *Genome Res* 1996; **6:** 986–94.
91. Wittwer CT, Herrmann MG, Moss AA, Rasmussen RP, Continuous fluorescence monitoring of rapid cycle DNA amplification. *Biotechniques* 1997; **22:** 130–8.
92. Wittwer CT, Ririe KM, Andrew RV et al, The LightCycler™: A microvolume multisample fluorimeter with rapid temperature control. *Biotechniques* 1997; **22:** 176–81.
93. Emig M, Saussele S, Wittor H et al, Accurate and rapid analysis of residual disease in patients with CML using specific fluorescent hybridization probes for real time quantitative RT-PCR. *Leukemia* 1999; **13:** 1825–32.
94. Lin F, Goldman JM, Cross NCP, A comparison of the sensitivity of blood and bone marrow for the detection of minimal residual disease in chronic myeloid leukaemia. *Br J Haematol* 1994; **86:** 683–5.
95. Lawler M, Humphries P, McCann SR, Evaluation of mixed chimerism by in vitro amplification of dinucleotide repeat sequences using the polymerase chain reaction. *Blood* 1991; **77:** 2504–14.
96. Rapanotti MC, Arcese W, Buffolino S et al, Sequential molecular monitoring of chimerism in chronic myeloid leukemia patients receiving donor lymphocyte transfusion for relapse after bone marrow transplantation. *Bone Marrow Transplant* 1997; **19:** 703–7.
97. Gardiner N, Lawler M, O'Riordan JM et al, Monitoring of lineage-specific chimaerism allows early prediction of response following donor lymphocyte infusions for relapsed chronic myeloid leukaemia. *Bone Marrow Transplant* 1998; **21:** 711–19.

22

Recommendations for assessment and definitions of response and relapse in CML: A report from the Chronic Leukemia Working Committee of the IBMTR

Sergio A Giralt, John Goldman, Claudio Anasetti, Francisco Cervantes, Richard Champlin, Nicholas Cross, Andreas Hochhaus, John P Klein, Esperanza Papadopoulos, Kathleen Sobocinski, Daniel Weisdorf, Mary Horowitz on behalf of the Chronic Leukemia Working Committee of the IBMTR

CONTENTS • Introduction and historical perspective • Current response criteria • Relevance of monitoring for interventions to treat relapse • Impact of PCR monitoring on response assessment • Impact of monitoring strategies and effective post-transplant therapies on evaluating success of transplantation • Recommendations of the Working Group • Summary and conclusions

INTRODUCTION AND HISTORICAL PERSPECTIVE

Bennett[1] and Virchow[2] first described chronic myeloid leukemia (CML) in 1845. Early therapy (Fowler solutions or radiotherapy) produced hematologic improvement, but there were no formal attempts to quantify or qualify responses.[3–6] Formal definitions of remission and relapse were first used in acute leukemia studies during the late 1950s.[7] The introduction of busulfan in 1953[8,9] and hydroxyurea in 1966[10] and the design and conduct of trials comparing these agents with each other and with other therapies led to a need for standardized response criteria for CML.[9,11–13]

The original response criteria for CML related exclusively to clinical symptoms, peripheral blood morphology, and spleen size.[8–13] The discovery of the Philadelphia chromosome (Ph) in 1960[14] and further work elucidating its molecular abnormalities made apparent the importance of translocation of genetic material between chromosomes 9 and 22 and the resultant BCR/ABL protein in disease pathogenesis.[15]

The observation that some busulfan-treated patients who exhibited chromosome mosaicism (simultaneous presence of Ph-positive and Ph-negative cells) had prolonged survival suggested that reduction or elimination of Ph-positive cells should be a therapeutic goal.[16,17] Intensive chemotherapy sometimes produced cytogenetic responses, i.e. reduction in the percentage of Ph-positive cells among analyzed metaphases.[18–20] These responses were generally brief, however, and survival was not prolonged. The importance of obtaining complete and durable cytogenetic responses in prolonging survival was not definitely established until therapies that could reliably produce them, i.e. allogeneic transplantation and interferon-α (IFN-α), became widely available.

Allogeneic bone marrow transplantation became an established therapy for CML during the 1980s.[21–25] To date, it is the only therapy known to cure the disease in most patients treated. Cures after allografting are always associated with disappearance of Ph-positive cells as determined by conventional cytogenetic techniques. IFN-α therapy for CML was introduced in 1986.[26] It produces complete hematologic responses in 60–80% of patients, major cytogenetic responses (<35% Ph-positive metaphases) in 20–40%, and complete cytogenetic responses in 10–20%.[27–32] Retrospective analyses and randomized trials indicate that IFN-α is superior to hydroxyurea or busulfan in prolonging survival.[28–32] IFN-α is standard therapy for those CML patients who are ineligible for allogeneic transplantation.[33] The degree of cytogenetic response is the single most important factor predicting survival with IFN-α therapy, and the cytogenetic response criteria noted above and summarized in Table 22.1 are used by most investigators in the field.[28–32]

Complete cytogenetic response does not necessarily mean eradication of CML. The limit of detection of conventional cytogenetic analysis is approximately 1 in 20 cells.[34] Fluorescence in situ hybridization (FISH) techniques or 'hypermetaphase' FISH techniques increase this sensitivity to 1 in 500 cells.[34–38] Use of the polymerase chain reaction (PCR) technique to detect *BCR/ABL* transcripts allows detection of 1 in 10^4 to 1 in 10^6 Ph-positive cells.[39–48] However, the role of this very sensitive test in assessing response to treatment is still not well defined.[48–54] Some centers now use PCR testing to detect and treat CML persisting after transplantation, since effective therapies for post-transplant relapse are available. Advances in both diagnostic and therapeutic interventions make some traditional definitions of response and relapse inadequate to describe the clinical course of CML in all patients, and can lead to some confusion when comparing current results with historical outcomes or even when comparing concurrent results from diverse centers. The Chronic Leukemia Working Committee of the International Bone Marrow

Table 22.1 Hematologic and cytogenetic response criteria for CML

Hematologic response

- **Complete.** All of the following:
  WBC < 10 × 10^9/l
  Hemoglobin > 11.0 g/dl
  Platelet count < 500 × 10^9/l
  Normal differential (<1% precursor cells)
  No palpable splenomegaly

- **Partial.** Any of the following:
  WBC > 10 but < 50 × 10^9/l and 50% below pretreatment values
  Hemoglobin > 9.0 but < 11.0 g/dl
  Platelet count > 500 × 10^9/l
  Differential >1% precursor cells
  Palpable splenomegaly

Cytogenetic response

- **Complete**
  0% Ph-positive metaphases
- **Partial**
  1–35% Ph-positive metaphases
- **Minor**
  36–95% Ph-positive metaphases
- **None**
  100% Ph-positive metaphases

A minimum of 20 analyzable metaphases must be assessed for appropriate evaluation of a cytogenetic response. Response should be confirmed with repeat cytogenetic analysis within 4–12 weeks.

Transplant Registry (IBMTR) recently formed a Working Group to address these issues and propose recommendations for disease monitoring, response assessment, and definitions of relapse for CML, particularly in the transplant setting.

CURRENT RESPONSE CRITERIA

Commonly used criteria for hematologic and cytogenetic responses in CML are summarized in Table 22.1. These criteria are known to be relevant for patients receiving IFN-α therapy.[27–31] They are also frequently used in autograft studies. Hematologic response after autografting for CML correlates with survival;[55] correlation of cytogenetic response with survival is not as clear.[55–60] Allograft recipients, especially those transplanted in chronic phase, usually have complete cytogenetic and hematologic responses. Regardless of the type of therapy, the degree of cytogenetic and hematologic response can be used to determine prognosis and to allocate high-risk patients to alternative secondary treatments.

Until the advent of PCR techniques, diagnosis of relapse after allografting was relatively straightforward. Patients were followed with periodic hematologic and cytogenetic evaluations. Those with persistent leukocytosis and immature forms or extramedullary manifestations of the disease with documented Ph-positive cells were considered to have clinical relapse. Patients without hematologic or extramedullary abnormalities, but with Ph-positive cells in blood or bone marrow, usually on two or more occasions, were considered to have cytogenetic relapse.[22–25]

Most investigators agree that detection of Ph-positive cells by conventional cytogenetic techniques after allogeneic transplantation should be considered as relapse, and would propose intervention with either IFN-α or donor lymphocytes. However, up to 20% of transplant recipients have transient cytogenetic relapses, particularly if the graft was not T-cell-depleted, and a definition that depends on only one cytogenetic test would likely overestimate the true relapse rate.[61,62] Using the published literature to estimate the true relapse rate after allogeneic transplantation is made difficult by the fact that various reports use cytogenetic, hematologic, or unspecified relapse criteria (Table 22.2). The situation is further complicated by differences in frequency and intensity of post-transplant monitoring for relapse. Continued cytogenetic remission is sometimes assumed without formal cytogenetic testing if peripheral blood counts and physical examination are normal.

RELEVANCE OF MONITORING FOR INTERVENTIONS TO TREAT RELAPSE

The natural history of hematologic and cytogenetic relapse of CML after allografting was well described by Arcese et al.[61] Patients with isolated cytogenetic relapses had a median time to hematologic progression of 8 months, with a 6-year survival probability of 52%. Survival after hematologic relapse depended on the phase of the disease. Patients relapsing into chronic phase had a 6-year survival probability of 30%; none of those relapsing into accelerated or blastic phase survived 6 years. IFN-α therapy produced complete cytogenetic responses in 16% of patients with cytogenetic relapse, 14% of those with chronic-phase relapse, and 0% of those with transformed disease.[61] Other studies have confirmed these results, including the greater likelihood of a response to IFN-α when administered in cytogenetic or chronic-phase relapse.[63,64]

Since 1990, the use of donor lymphocyte infusions (DLI) to treat CML relapse has increased dramatically.[65–67] The full impact of this therapy on the natural course of CML is yet to be defined; however, long-term cytogenetic and molecular responses are frequent. Median survivals of more than 5 years are reported for patients receiving donor lymphocytes for cytogenetic or chronic-phase relapses.[65–69] Results in more advanced disease are less good. Infusion of donor lymphocytes during cytogenetic rather than hematologic

Table 22.2 Censoring events for leukemia-free survival in some representative transplant trials

Reference (year)	No. of patients	Cytogenetic	Morphologic	Comments
Thomas et al[79] (1986)	198	+	+	Cytogenetic and hematologic relapses were described separately
Goldman et al[80] (1988)	405	−	+	Registry analysis; relapse was defined using hematologic criteria
Biggs et al[81] (1992)	115	+	+	Transient cytogenetic relapse was not scored as an event
Wagner et al[82] (1992)	79	+	+	
Bacigalupo et al[83] (1993)	100	+	+	Transient cytogenetic relapse was scored as an event
McGlave et al[84] (1993)	196	−	+	Registry analysis; relapse was defined using hematologic criteria
Snyder et al[85] (1994)	94	+	+	Transient cytogenetic relapse was not considered as an event
Clift et al[86] (1994)	142	+	+	Patterns of relapse were specified
Devergie et al[87] (1995)	120	+	+	
Enright et al[88] (1996)	283	−	+	

relapse is associated with a lower incidence of cytopenia.[65,70]

Thus, current evidence suggests that both IFN-α and DLI may be effective for CMI patients relapsing after allogeneic transplantation, and that these therapies are more likely to be effective when administered early in the course of relapse. Additionally, early DLI may decrease toxicity. Therefore, periodic monitoring for CML recurrence should be routine for transplant recipients, to allow early detection and more effective intervention. Periodic monitoring after other therapies where cytogenetic response is frequent but often transient and/or incomplete, such as IFN-α and autografting, is also recommended to assess ongoing response to therapy and to allocate patients for new therapies such as STI571 or studies aimed at inhibiting or delaying disease progression.

IMPACT OF PCR MONITORING ON RESPONSE ASSESSMENT

The use of PCR to assess treatment response in CML has several problems. First, highly sensitive PCR techniques can detect the *BCR/ABL* rearrangement in a proportion of normal individuals who never develop CML.[73] Second, *BCR/ABL* can be detected by PCR in some allograft recipients for months or years without development of cytogenetic or hematologic relapse.[41–43] Third, PCR techniques vary in sensitivity from center to center, and strict attention to quality control is essential to avoid false-positive results.[53,54] Quantitative PCR techniques using nested PCR with a competitor address the first two problems by monitoring the levels, not just the presence, of *BCR/ABL* transcripts. This allows intervention at certain

Table 22.3 PCR as a predictor of CML relapse after BMT

Reference	No. of patients	PCR type/sensitivity[a]	% Relapse PCR$^+$	% Relapse PCR$^-$
Hughes et al[40]	37	Qualitative/10^5	44	0
Radich et al[41]	346	Qualitative/10^6	28	4
Miyamura et al[42]	64	Qualitative/10^6	17	9
Roth et al[43]	64	Qualitative/NS	32	0
Lee et al	20	Qualitative/NS	8	0
Mackinnon et al[71]	36	Qualitative/10^5	65	7
Lin et al[46]	98	Quantitative/10^6	72	2
Lion et al[48]	28	Quantitative/NS	100	0

[a] NS, not specified.

threshold levels or when levels are consistently increasing.[45,52–54] However, this technique is labor-intensive, has not been well standardized, and is available only in a limited number of specialized laboratories. Real-time quantitative PCR has been proposed as an easier method of *BCR/ABL* quantification. It offers a lower risk of contamination, allows greater sample throughput, and is less labor-intensive than nested PCR techniques.[74] However, only limited experience with real-time PCR monitoring is available at present.

Assessing disease activity and timing therapeutic interventions using PCR results remains controversial.[50–54] Not all groups have shown that the presence of *BCR/ABL* transcripts after allografting predicts relapse, and quantitative assays have been used in only small numbers of patients (Table 22.3). In contrast to hematologic relapse, which always portends a poor prognosis, or cytogenetic relapse, which generally progresses to hematologic relapse, the natural history of *BCR/ABL* positivity detectable only by PCR after allografting is not well known, and probably depends on various factors, including the level of positivity, donor–recipient compatibility, the type of graft, the disease stage at the time of transplantation, and concurrent or prior therapy.

IMPACT OF MONITORING STRATEGIES AND EFFECTIVE POST-TRANSPLANT THERAPIES ON EVALUATING SUCCESS OF TRANSPLANTATION

As noted above, response (and, similarly, relapse and leukemia-free survival (LFS)) may be variously defined using hematologic, cytogenetic, and/or molecular criteria. Obviously, rates of response, relapse, and LFS will differ, depending on the criteria used and the frequency with which these criteria are assessed. Approaches that assume continuing cytogenetic response beyond the date of the last formal assessment in the absence of hematologic abnormalities may also be misleading.

Regardless of the relapse criteria used, traditional LFS estimates count patients as treatment failures at the time at which relapse is first diagnosed, regardless of subsequent treatment. The efficacy of donor lymphocytes in achieving durable cytogenetic and molecular responses in 70–80% of patients treated for cytogenetic or chronic-phase relapse raises questions about this approach. First, some centers administer donor lymphocytes for molecular relapse but score treatment failures only at cytogenetic or molecular relapse. In this situation, a patient may be treated for relapse but never be reported as a relapse.[75–77] Even when treatment is given for cytogenetic or hematologic relapse, if a patient achieves a durable complete response, his or her classification as a treatment 'failure' is controversial. Recently, statistical techniques have been suggested to incorporate responses to post-relapse therapies, such as DLI, in the estimation of LFS. Such techniques may be useful, especially for evaluation of treatments such as non-myeloablative therapies, where initial establishment of donor chimerism may not lead to complete response until later, followed by planned DLI to boost the graft-versus-leukemia (GVL) effect.[78]

RECOMMENDATIONS OF THE WORKING GROUP

Recommendations for monitoring disease response, progression, and relapse after hematopoietic stem cell transplantation

The approach to assessment will depend on the availability of PCR techniques. While the use of PCR is recommended, it is recognized that such testing is not yet available in all centers.

- For patients who cannot be followed using PCR techniques, minimum disease assessment should include history and physical examination, complete blood count, and bone marrow with cytogenetic analysis every 3–6 months for the first 2 years after transplantation, every 6–12 months from years 2 to 5, and yearly thereafter.
- For patients who can be followed using PCR techniques, minimum disease assessment should include history and physical examination, complete blood count, and quantitative (preferable) or qualitative peripheral blood PCR analysis every 3–6 months for the first 2 years after transplantation, every 6–12 months from years 2 to 5, and yearly thereafter. Patients with persistently positive PCR tests or increasing levels of *BCR/ABL* transcripts should undergo bone marrow aspiration for cytogenetic analysis.

Proposed definitions for hematologic and cytogenetic response and relapse

The current response criteria used for IFN-α therapy should be also used when analyzing transplant trials. Benefits are that these criteria are well known, are used by most CML researchers, and are demonstrated to have prognostic significance. They are summarized in Table 22.1.

Relapse after a complete response should generally be defined by cytogenetic and hematologic criteria. Among patients without hematologic or extramedullary evidence of CML, relapse times should be defined by the first of two consecutive cytogenetic analyses in which more than one Ph-positive metaphase is encountered, regardless of the number of metaphases analyzed. The minimal interval between tests should be two weeks. Patients with five or more Ph-positive metaphases or with clinical evidence of CML may be scored as relapses without a second confirmatory cytogenetic test.

Proposed definitions for molecular remission and molecular relapse

No well-established criteria for molecular remission exist. Variable levels of sensitivity of PCR assays and lack of standardization make any definition difficult at present. However, molecular remission should currently imply the use of an assay with a sensitivity to allow detection of one Ph-positive cell in 10^5–10^6 cells, and the result should be confirmed by two consecutive tests done at least four weeks apart.[53] Molecular relapse is defined by the European Group of Investigators on CML (EICML) as a

10-fold or greater increase in the relative expression of the marker gene detected and confirmed by a minimum of three consecutive quantitative PCR analyses.[48,54] This definition protects against transient increases in *BCR/ABL* transcript production not related to tumor load, variability of the test, and other non-specific variations. The definition seems reasonable, but needs to be evaluated in the post-transplant setting.

Proposed recommendations for assessing survival and leukemia-free survival

Survival is and should be the most important endpoint for all CML trials. Survival times are unambiguous and allow assessment of the relative impact of diverse treatment strategies that may have different toxicities and response profiles.

Taken literally, LFS would only apply to patients achieving complete molecular remissions. Since PCR is not readily available, and nor is it adequately standardized, this definition is impractical. A practical compromise is that LFS be defined using cytogenetic criteria for relapse as defined above. It is of particular importance that time to relapse and LFS estimates should be censored at the time of the last documented negative bone marrow test (in the case of cytogenetics) or blood (if PCR is used for monitoring as described above), and not at the time of last follow-up if such testing was not performed.

Other definitions that need further study but may be useful in certain situations

Current leukemia-free survival

With DLI, it is possible to successfully induce complete cytogenetic responses in 70–80% of patients with molecular, cytogenetic, and chronic-phase relapse after allogeneic transplantation. The concept of 'current' LFS includes as non-failures patients who are alive and disease-free at the time of last follow-up, regardless of prior history. Calculating 'current LFS' requires the use of a multistate model that allows patients to move from complete response to relapse back to complete response. This type of analysis allows depiction of overall survival and disease control in one graph, and has been performed by the groups at the Hammersmith Hospital, London and the Dana-Farber Cancer Institute, Boston.[75,78]

Survival free of cytogenetic progression

Cytogenetic progression refers to patients with partial or complete cytogenetic responses who subsequently lose the response (i.e. > 35% Ph-positive metaphases) in two consecutive analyses done at least two weeks apart. Patients not achieving at least a partial response would be considered failures at the day of transplant. This concept of cytogenetic progression is important for evaluating the results of autografting and non-ablative transplant therapies, in which many patients achieve a partial but not complete cytogenetic response followed by prolonged survival with or without maintenance therapy with IFN-α or other treatment modalities.

Proposed definitions for post-transplant cellular therapy

The use of different terminologies to describe donor cells administered to treat or prevent post-transplant relapse is confusing. Terms such as 'buffy coat infusions', 'donor lymphocyte infusions', 'filgrastim-stimulated donor lymphocytes', 'cytokine-stimulated donor lymphocytes', and 'stem cell infusions or boosts' have all been used – sometimes interchangeably. Differentiation of these therapies from a second transplant with pretransplant conditioning is often arbitrary, since infusions are sometimes preceded by cytotoxic or immunosuppressive therapy. The qualitative and quantitative compositions of these products vary widely among centers and according to the indication for the therapy, i.e. relapse prevention, relapse treatment, treatment of infection, and prevention or treatment of post-transplant lymphoproliferative disease. We propose that the term 'second or subsequent transplant' be used for the infusion of any cellular product likely to contain an engrafting dose of hematopoietic stem cells (bone marrow or growth-factor-primed peripheral blood). We also propose that the term 'donor lymphocyte infusion' be restricted to the infusion of unstimulated peripheral blood.

SUMMARY AND CONCLUSIONS

Definitions of disease status and response to therapy reflect our understanding of the disease and the therapies available to treat it. Novel diagnostic and therapeutic techniques in CML necessitate the reevaluation of old standards. We are now aware that disease eradication may be an active process that can occur for many months or even years after therapy. Likewise, disease recurrence may be effectively treated with approaches that induce cytogenetic and molecular remission. These proposed guidelines and definitions should assist physicians treating CML and investigators designing trials of new agents, and should allow appropriate comparisons among treatment approaches.

REFERENCES

1. Bennett JH, Case of hypertrophy of the spleen and liver, in which death took place from suppuration of the blood. *Edinburgh Med Sci J* 1845; **64:** 413.
2. Virchow R, Weisses Blut. *Frorieps Notizen* 1845; **36:** 151.
3. Lissauer H, Zwei falle von leucaemie. *Klin Wochenschr* 1865; **2:** 403–5.
4. Ordway T, Remission in leukemia produced by radium in cases completely resistant to X-ray and benzol treatment. *Boston Med Surg J* 1917; **176:** 490–503.
5. Minot G, Buckman T, Isaacs R, Chronic myelogenous leukemia. *JAMA* 1924; **82:** 1489–94.
6. Lawrence J, Lowry-Dobson R, Low Beer B, Brown B, Chronic myelogenous leukemia. A study of 129 cases in which therapy was radioactive phosphorus. *JAMA* 1948; **136:** 672–7.
7. Bisel H, Letter to the Editor: Criteria for the evaluation of response to treatment in acute leukemia. *Blood* 1956; **11:** 676.
8. Galton DA, Chemotherapy of chronic myelocytic leukemia. *Semin Hematol* 1969; **6:** 323–43.
9. Medical Research Council's Working Party for Therapeutic Trials in Leukemia, Chronic Granulocytic Leukemia: comparison of radiotherapy and busulphan therapy. *BMJ* 1968; **i:** 201–8.
10. Kennedy B, Yarbro K, Metabolic and therapeutic effects of hydroxyurea in chronic myeloid leukemia. *JAMA* 1966; **195:** 1038–46.
11. Rundles RW, Grizzle J, Bell WN et al, Comparison of chlorambucil and myeleran in chronic lymphocytic and granulocytic leukemia. *Am J Med* 1959; **27:** 424–32.
12. Southeastern Cancer Chemotherapy Cooperative Study Group, Comparison of 6-mercaptopurine and busulfan in chronic granulocytic leukemia. *Blood* 1963; **21:** 89–100.
13. Bolin RW, Robinson WA, Sutherland J, Hamman RF, Busulfan versus hydroxyurea in long term therapy of chronic myelogenous leukemia. *Cancer* 1982; **50:** 1683–6.
14. Nowell PC, Hungerford DA, Chromosome studies on normal and leukemic human leukocytes. *J Natl Cancer Inst* 1960; **25:** 85–109.
15. Kurzrock R, Gutterman J, Talpaz M. The molecular genetics of Philadelphia positive leukemia. *N Engl J Med* 1988; **319:** 990–8.
16. Finney R, McDonald GA, Baikie AG, Douglas AS, Chronic granulocytic leukaemia with Ph^1 negative cells in bone marrow and a ten year remission after busulphan hypoplasia. *Br J Haematol* 1972; **23:** 283–8.
17. Golde DW, Bersch NL, Sparkes RS, Chromosomal mosaicism associated with prolonged remission in chronic myelogenous leukemia. *Cancer* 1976; **37:** 1849–52.
18. Canellos GP, DeVita VT, Whang-Peng J, Carbone PP, Hematologic and cytogenetic remission of blastic transformation in chronic granulocytic leukemia. *Blood* 1971; **38:** 671–9.
19. Cunningham I, Gee T, Dowling M et al, Results of treatment of Ph^1+ chronic myelogenous leukemia with an intensive treatment regimen (L-5 protocol). *Blood* 1979; **53:** 375–95.
20. Kantarjian HM, Vellekoop L, McCredie KB et al, Intensive combination chemotherapy (ROAP 10) and splenectomy in the management of chronic myelogenous leukemia. *J Clin Oncol* 1985; **3:** 192–200.

21. Thomas ED, Storb R, Clift RA et al, Bone marrow transplantation: Part I. *N Engl J Med* 1975; **292:** 832–43.
22. Goldman JM, Baughan AS, Mccarthy DM et al, Marrow transplantation for patients in the chronic phase of chronic granulocytic leukemia. *Lancet* 1982; **ii:** 623–5.
23. Fefer A, Clift RA, Thomas ED, Allogeneic marrow transplantation for chronic granulocytic leukemia. *J Natl Cancer Inst* 1986; **76:** 1269–73.
24. Speck B, Bortin MM, Champlin R et al, Allogeneic bone marrow transplantation for chronic myelogenous leukemia. *Lancet* 1984; **i:** 665–8.
25. Goldman J, Apperley J, Jones L et al, Bone marrow transplantation for chronic myeloid leukemia. *N Engl J Med* 1986; **314:** 202–7.
26. Talpaz M, Kantarjian HM, McCredie K et al, Hematologic remission and cytogenetic improvement induced by recombinant human interferon alpha in chronic myelogenous leukemia. *N Engl J Med* 1986; **314:** 1065–9.
27. Kantarjian H, O'Brien S, Anderlini P et al, Treatment of chronic myelogenous leukemia: current status and investigational options. *Blood* 1996; **87:** 3069–81.
28. Kantarjian H, Smith T, O'Brien S et al, Prolonged survival in chronic myelogenous leukemia after cytogenetic response to interferon-α therapy. *Ann Intern Med* 1995; **122:** 254–61.
29. Italian Cooperative Study Group on Chronic Myeloid Leukemia, Interferon alfa-2a as compared with conventional chemotherapy for the treatment of chronic myeloid leukemia. *N Engl J Med* 1994; **330:** 820–5.
30. Allan N, Richards S, Shepherd P, for the Medical Research Council's Working Party for Therapeutic Trials in Adult Leukaemia, Results of the Medical Research Council randomised multicentre trial of interferon alpha n 1 for chronic myeloid leukaemia: improved survival irrespective of cytogenetic response. *Lancet* 1995; **345:** 1392–7.
31. Chronic Myeloid Leukemia Trialists' Collaborative Group, Interferon alfa versus chemotherapy for chronic myeloid leukemia: a meta-analysis of seven randomized trials. *J Natl Cancer Inst* 1997; **89:** 1616–20.
32. Guilhot F, Chastang C, Michallet M et al, Interferon alfa-2b combined with cytarabine versus interferon alone in chronic myelogenous leukemia. *N Engl J Med* 1997; **337:** 223–9.
33. Silver RT, Woolf SH, Hehlmann R et al, An evidence-based analysis of the effect of busulfan, hydroxyurea, interferon, and allogeneic bone marrow transplantation in treating the chronic phase of chronic myeloid leukemia: developed for the American Society of Hematology. *Blood* 1999; **94:** 1517–36.
34. O'Brien S, Thall P, Siciliano M, Cytogenetics of chronic myelogeneous leukemia. *Baillière's Clin Haematol* 1997; **10:** 259–76.
35. Lichter P, Ledbetter S, Ledbetter D, Ward D, Fluorescence in situ hybridization with Alu and Li polymerase chain reaction probes for the rapid characterization of human chromosomes in hybrid cell lines. *Proc Natl Acad Sci USA* 1990; **87:** 6634–8.
36. Liu P, Siciliano M, Seong D et al, Dual Alu PCR primers and conditions for isolation of human chromosome painting probes from hybrid cells. *Cancer Genet Cytogenet* 1993; **65:** 93–9.
37. Seong D, Kantarjian H, Ro J et al, Hypermetaphase FISH for quantitative monitoring of Philadelphia-positive cells in chronic myelogenous leukemia patients during treatment. *Blood* 1995; **86:** 2343–9.
38. Seong D, Giralt S, Fischer H et al, Usefulness of detection of minimal residual disease by hypermetaphase fluorescent in situ hybridization after allogeneic BMT for chronic myelogenous leukemia. *Bone Marrow Transplant* 1997; **19:** 565–70.
39. Sklar J, Polymerase chain reaction: the molecular microscope of residual disease. *J Clin Oncol* 1991; **9:** 1521.
40. Hughes T, Morgan G, Martiat P, Goldman J, Detection of residual leukemia after bone marrow transplant for chronic myeloid leukemia: role of polymerase chain reaction in predicting relapse. *Blood* 1991; **77:** 874–8.
41. Radich J, Gehly G, Gooley T et al, Polymerase chain reaction detection of the BCR–ABL fusion transcript after allogeneic marrow transplantation for chronic myeloid leukemia: results and implications in 346 patients. *Blood* 1995; **85:** 2632–8.
42. Miyamura K, Taharo T, Tanimoto M et al, Long persistent bcr–abl positive transcript detected by polymerase chain reaction after marrow transplant for chronic myelogenous leukemia without clinical relapse: a study of 64 patients. *Blood* 1993; **81:** 1089–93.
43. Roth M, Antin J, Ash R et al, Prognostic significance of Philadelphia chromosome-positive cells

detected by the polymerase chain reaction after bone marrow transplant for chronic myelogenous leukemia. *Blood* 1992; **79:** 276–82.
44. Hochhaus A, Lin F, Reiter A et al, Quantification of residual disease in chronic myelogenous leukemia patients on interferon-α therapy by competitive polymerase chain reaction. *Blood* 1996; **87:** 1549–55.
45. Cross N, Lin F, Chase A et al, Competitive polymerase chain reaction to estimate the number of BCR–ABL transcripts in chronic myeloid leukemia patients after bone marrow transplantation. *Blood* 1993; **82:** 1929–36.
46. Lin F, van Rhee F, Goldman J, Cross N, Kinetics of increasing BCR–ABL transcript numbers in chronic myeloid leukemia patients who relapse after bone marrow transplantation. *Blood* 1996; **87:** 4473–8.
47. Raanani P, Dazzi F, Sohal J et al, The rate and kinetics of molecular response to donor leukocyte transfusions in chronic myeloid leukaemia patients treated for relapse after allogeneic bone marrow transplantation. *Br J Haematol* 1997; **99:** 945–50.
48. Lion T, Clinical implications of qualitative and quantitative polymerase chain reaction analysis in the monitoring of patients with chronic myelogenous leukemia. The European Investigators on Chronic Myeloid Leukemia Group. *Bone Marrow Transplant* 1994; **14:** 505.
49. Cross N, Minimal residual disease in CML. *Hematol Cell Ther* 1998; **40:** 224.
50. Faderl S, Talpaz M, Kantarjian H, Estrov Z, Should polymerase chain reaction analysis to detect minimal residual disease in patients with chronic myelogenous leukemia be used in clinical decision making? *Blood* 1999; **93:** 2755–9.
51. Moravcova J, Nadvornikova S, Lukasova M, Klamova H, Letter to the Editor: Polymerase chain reaction analysis should be used as a basis for clinical decision making in patients with chronic myelogenous leukemia. *Blood* 1999; **94:** 3609–10.
52. Goldman J, Kaeda J, Cross N et al, Letter to the Editor: Clinical decision making in chronic myeloid leukemia based on polymerase chain reaction analysis of minimal residual disease. *Blood* 1999; **94:** 1484–5.
53. Cross N, Assessing residual leukaemia. *Baillière's Clin Haematol* 1997; **10:** 389–403.
54. Lion T, Bartram C, Talpaz M et al, Debate Round Table. Monitoring of residual disease in chronic myelogenous leukemia. Methodological approaches and clinical aspects. *Leukemia* 1996; **10:** 896–906.
55. Pigneux A, Faberes C, Boiron JM et al, Autologous stem cell transplantation in chronic myeloid leukemia: a single center experience. *Bone Marrow Transplant* 1999; **24:** 265–70.
56. Boiron JM, Cahn JY, Meloni G et al, Chronic myeloid leukemia in first chronic phase not responding to interferon: outcome and prognostic factors after autologous transplantation. *Bone Marrow Transplant* 1999; **24:** 259–64.
57. Carella A, Lerma E, Corsetti M et al, Autografting with Philadelphia chromosome-negative mobilized hematopoietic progenitor cells in chronic myelogenous leukemia. *Blood* 1999; **93:** 1534–9.
58. Khouri IF, Kantarjian HM, Talpaz M et al, Results with high-dose chemotherapy and unpurged autologous stem cell transplantation in 73 patients with chronic myelogenous leukemia: the MD Anderson experience. *Bone Marrow Transplant* 1996; **17:** 775–9.
59. Hoyle C, Gray R, Goldman J, Autografting for patients with CML in chronic phase: an update. *Br J Haematol* 1994; **86:** 76–81.
60. McGlave PB, De Fabritiis P, Deisseroth A et al, Autologous transplants for chronic myelogenous leukaemia: results from eight transplant groups. *Lancet* 1994; **343:** 1486–8.
61. Arcese W, Goldman J, D'Arcangelo E et al, Outcome for patients who relapse after allogeneic bone marrow transplantation for chronic myeloid leukemia. *Blood* 1993; **82:** 3211–19.
62. Arthur C, Apperley J, Guo A et al, Cytogenetic events after bone marrow transplantation for chronic myeloid leukemia in chronic phase. *Blood* 1988; **71:** 1179–86.
63. Higano CS, Chielens D, Raskind W et al, Use of alpha-2a-interferon to treat cytogenetic relapse of chronic myeloid leukemia after marrow transplantation. *Blood* 1997; **90:** 2549–54.
64. Steegmann JL, Casado LF, Tomas JF et al, Interferon alpha for chronic myeloid leukemia relapsing after allogeneic bone marrow transplantation. *Bone Marrow Transplant* 1999; **23:** 483–7.
65. Kolb H, Schattenberg A, Goldman J et al, Graft-versus-leukemia effect of donor lymphocyte transfusions in marrow grafted patients. *Blood* 1995; **86:** 2041–50.
66. Collins R, Shpilberg O, Drobyski W et al, Donor

leukocyte infusions in 140 patients with relapsed malignancy after allogeneic bone marrow transplantation. *J Clin Oncol* 1997; **15:** 433–44.

67. Guglielmi C, Arcese W, Hermans J et al, Risk assessment in patients with Ph+ chronic myelogenous leukemia at first relapse after allogeneic stem cell transplant: an EBMT retrospective analysis. *Blood* 2000; **95:** 3328–34.
68. Shimoni A, Anderlini P, Andersson B et al, CD8-depleted donor lymphocytes (DLI) for the treatment of CML relapse after allogeneic transplant: long term follow up and factors predicting outcome. *Blood* 1999; **94**(Suppl 1)**:** 160a.
69. Porter DL, Collins RH, Shpilberg O et al, Long-term follow-up of patients who achieved complete remission after donor leukocyte infusions. *BBMT* 1999; **5:** 253–61.
70. Van Rhee F, Lin F, Cullis J et al, Relapse of chronic myeloid leukemia after allogeneic bone marrow transplant: the case for giving donor leukocyte transfusions before the onset of hematologic relapse. *Blood* 1994; **83:** 3377–83.
71. Mackinnon S, Papadopoulos EB, Carabasi MH et al, Adoptive immunotherapy evaluating escalating doses of donor leukocytes for relapse of chronic myeloid leukemia after bone marrow transplantation: separation of graft-versus-leukemia responses from graft-versus-host disease. *Blood* 1995; **86:** 1261–8.
72. Dazzi F, Szydlo RM, Craddock C et al, Comparison of single-dose and escalating-dose regimens of donor lymphocyte infusion for relapse after allografting for chronic myeloid leukemia. *Blood* 2000; **95:** 67–71.
73. Biernaux C, Loos M, Sels A et al, Detection of major bcr–abl gene expression at a very low level in blood cells of some healthy individuals. *Blood* 1995; **86:** 3118–122.
74. Branford S, Hughes TP, Rudzki Z, Monitoring chronic myeloid leukaemia therapy by real-time quantitative PCR in blood is a reliable alternative to bone marrow cytogenetics. *Br J Haematol* 1999; **107:** 587–99.
75. Sehn L, Alyea E, Weller E et al, Comparative outcomes of T-cell depleted and non T-cell depleted allogeneic bone marrow transplantation for chronic myelogenous leukemia: impact of donor lymphocyte infusion. *J Clin Oncol* 1999; **17:** 561–8.
76. Drobyski WR, Hessner MJ, Klein JP et al, T-cell depletion plus salvage immunotherapy with donor leukocyte infusions as a strategy to treat chronic phase chronic myelogenous leukemia patients undergoing HLA-identical sibling marrow transplantation. *Blood* 1999; **94:** 434–41.
77. Giralt S, Gajewski J, Khouri I et al, Induction of graft-vs-leukemia as primary treatment of chronic myelogenous leukemia. *Blood* 1997; **90**(Suppl 1)**:** 418a.
78. Craddock C, Szydlo R, Klein JP et al, Estimating leukemia free survival after allografting for chronic myeloid leukemia: a new method that takes into account patients who relapse and are restored to complete remission. *Blood* 2000; **96:** 86–90.
79. Thomas ED, Clift R, Fefer A et al, Marrow transplantation for the treatment of chronic myelogenous leukemia. *Ann Intern Med* 1986; **104:** 155–63.
80. Goldman J, Gale R, Horowitz M et al, Bone marrow transplantation for chronic myelogenous leukemia in chronic phase. Increased risk of relapse associated with T-cell depletion. *Ann Intern Med* 1988; **108:** 806–14.
81. Biggs J, Szer J, Crilley P et al, Treatment of chronic myeloid leukemia with allogeneic bone marrow transplantation after preparation with BuCy2. *Blood* 1992; **80:** 1352–7.
82. Wagner J, Zahurak M, Piantadosi S et al, Bone marrow transplantation of chronic myelogenous leukemia in chronic phase: evaluation of risks and benefits. *J Clin Oncol* 1992; **10:** 779–89.
83. Bacigalupo A, Gualandi F, Vam Lint M et al, Multivariate analysis of risk factors for survival and relapse in chronic granulocytic leukemia following allogeneic marrow transplantation: impact of disease related variables (Sokal score). *Bone Marrow Transplant* 1993; **12:** 443–8.
84. McGlave P, Bartsch G, Anasetti C et al, Unrelated donor marrow transplantation therapy for chronic myelogenous leukemia: initial experience of the National Marrow Donor Program. *Blood* 1993; **81:** 543–50.
85. Snyder D, Negrin R, O'Donnell M et al, Fractionated total-body irradiation and high dose etoposide as a preparatory regimen for bone marrow transplantation for 94 patients with chronic myelogenous leukemia in chronic phase. *Blood* 1994; **84:** 1672–9.
86. Clift R, Buckner C, Thomas E et al, Marrow transplantation for chronic myeloid leukemia: a randomized study comparing cyclophosphamide and total body irradiation with busulfan–cyclophosphamide. *Blood* 1994; **84:** 2036–43.
87. Devergie A, Blaise D, Attal M et al, Allogeneic

bone marrow transplantation for chronic myeloid leukemia in first chronic phase: a randomized trial of busulfan–cytoxan versus total body irradiation as preparative regimen: a report from the French Society of Bone Marrow Graft (SFGM). *Blood* 1995; **85:** 2263–8.

88. Enright H, Davies S, DeFor T et al, Relapse after non-T-cell-depleted allogeneic bone marrow transplantation for chronic myelogenous leukemia: early transplantation use of an unrelated donor, and chronic graft-versus-host disease are protective. *Blood* 1996; **88:** 714–20.

23

Basis of GVL

John M Barrett

CONTENTS • Introduction • Clinical basis of GVL in CML • Immunological mechanisms in GVL • Optimizing the GVL response after allogeneic SCT • Separating GVH and GVL • Amplifying GVL responses • Conclusions

INTRODUCTION

The idea that allogeneic immunity conferred by bone marrow transplantation (BMT) could exert an antileukemic effect has its origins in experiments in mice by Barnes and Loutit[1] in 1956, who showed that allogeneic BMT prolonged survival from a lethal experimental leukemia at the same time as causing graft-versus-host disease (GVHD). Clinical investigators, however, have been slow to appreciate the potential of this so-called graft-versus-leukemia (GVL) effect. Only in the last decade have concerted attempts to characterize and optimize GVL been made. The study of GVL reactions in chronic myeloid leukemia (CML) is particularly rewarding, since, of all leukemias, CML is the most susceptible to control and eradication by alloimmune processes. Furthermore, the study of GVL in CML has been greatly facilitated by our ability to quantitate residual disease using the polymerase chain reaction (PCR) to detect *BCR/ABL* mRNA.[2,3] In this chapter, the clinical features of GVL in CML are summarized, cellular mechanisms are outlined, and current and future immunotherapeutic applications are discussed.

CLINICAL BASIS OF GVL IN CML

Historical background

The first clear evidence that alloimmune effects could impact on leukemic relapse after BMT came from observations by the Seattle group that patients developing either acute[4] or chronic[5] GVHD had a lower risk of leukemic relapse. At the time, it seemed that clinically significant GVHD was an inevitable accompaniment of GVL, thereby rendering it unsafe to manipulate the antileukemic effect of the graft. This perception changed in 1990 with the publication by the International Bone Marrow Transplant Registry (IBMTR) of a large analysis of relapse in allogeneic marrow transplants for leukemia.[6] The study conclusively identified a powerful effect of donor lymphocytes on disease relapse, as evidence by the much higher relapse rate in recipients of T-cell-depleted transplants. The effect of T-cell depletion on relapse was especially noticeable in CML. Of particular interest was the finding of a GVL effect independent of GVHD, evident because even T-cell-replete transplants not developing GVHD had a relapse rate nearly sevenfold lower than T-cell-depleted transplants. In CML, GVL was shown to be related to an alloimmune effect, since identical-twin transplants had a higher relapse rate than T-cell-replete transplants from HLA-identical siblings.[6,7] In the same years as the IBMTR report, dramatic proof of a therapeutic role of lymphocytes in GVL came from studies by Kolb and colleagues[8] in Munich showing that donor lymphocyte infusions (DLI) could induce durable remission in patients relapsing with CML after allogenic marrow transplantation. Following these important observations, much has been accomplished in clinical practice, characterizing the features of the GVL effect and the factors affecting it. In the laboratory, the cellular mechanisms underlying the GVL response have been defined, thereby laying the foundations for therapeutic strategies to enhance the effect and separate it from GVHD.

Factors affecting the GVL reaction

The factors determining the effectiveness of the GVL response in eliminating CML are listed in Table 23.1 and discussed below.

Histocompatibility antigen disparity

Since histocompatibility differences drive GVHD, it is not surprising that, in general, the GVL effect is also greater the more disparate the match between donor and recipient. There is evidence for a GVL effect from both major histocompatibility complex (MHC) and minor histocompatibility antigen (mHA) differences. In a comparative study, Japanese CML recipients of HLA-identical sibling marrow had less GVHD and more prolonged persistence of minimal residual disease than a cohort of patients transplanted in the UK.[9] This suggested that greater antigenic disparity in the genetically

Table 23.1 Factors determining the antileukemic potential of the GVL effect

Antigenic disparity

Decreasing GVL effect:

- mismatched family donors > molecularly matched unrelated donors > HLA-identical siblings–diverse racial origins > HLA identical siblings–genetically homogeneous populations > identical-twin donors

Disease stage

Decreasing GVL effect:

- chronic phase > accelerated phase > blastic phase
- molecularly detectable disease > karyotypic relapse > hematological relapse

T-lymphocyte dose

Decreasing GVL effect:

- DLI > T-replete transplants > T-cell-depleted transplants

Stem cell dose

- $CD34^+$ cell doses greater than 3×10^6/kg
- peripheral blood transplants > bone marrow

Immunosuppression

- Cyclosporin, methotrexate

Factors leading to mixed lymphocyte chimerism

- Low-intensity preparative regimens
- T-cell depletion

diverse European cohort resulted in a more powerful GVL effect from mHA. Evidence for MHC differences causing more GVL is less clear, but several studies suggest that relapse rates are lower in recipients of unrelated donor marrow and mismatched related marrow donors.[10,11]

Disease status

A major factor determining the efficacy of the GVL effect is the disease status – CML in chronic phase is much more susceptible to GVL than CML in accelerated phase, which in turn is more susceptible than CML in blast crisis.[6,12,13]

Donor alloreactivity

The use of immunosuppressives to prevent GVHD is closely linked to a weakening of the GVL response. Cyclosporin exerts a powerful inhibitory effect on GVL, and several case reports attest to the favorable impact of cyclosporin withdrawal on relapsed or persisting leukemia.[14,15]

T-cell depletion

This has a major impact on donor alloreactivity. Both GVHD and GVL are diminished by T-cell depletion, resulting in high relapse rates in CML transplant recipients.[15,16] The more intense the T-cell depletion, the greater is the relapse risk.

Mixed chimerism

Persisting mixed donor–host lymphoid chimerism is a powerful risk factor for relapse in CML.[17–19] Mixed chimerism is encountered when host T cells persist after transplant – either when the preparative regimen is of low immunosuppressive potential or when the recovery of the donor immune system is diminished by T-cell depletion of the graft.[20] To minimize graft rejection, full donor lymphoid chimerism without immunosuppression is required. This can be achieved with additional transfusions of lymphocytes at transplant.[21] Unfortunately, this strategy has been abandoned because it induced severe GVHD.

GVL and DLI

Many factors affecting the relapse rate after BMT also determine success of DLI. The antileukemic effect of DLI is greatest in the absence of immunosuppression, and when it induces full donor lymphoid chimerism.[22] As with transplantation, the occurrence of GVHD results in a much higher probability of leukemic response.[23] Considerable experience with DLI has demonstrated a correlation of lymphocyte dose with probability of remission. The consensus is that a $CD3^+$ T-cell dose of 10^7/kg is the threshold for an optimum GVL effect that maintains the risk of GVHD at a minimum.[24] GVL is enhanced by interferon (IFN)-α[25] and interleukin (IL)-2.[26,27] Experience with DLI has helped to define the time required for a functional GVL response. Molecular remission in CML is achieved between 3 and 12 months after DLI. In unrelated donor transplants, the effect is generally more rapid, but the range is still wide.[28]

Lymphocytes and GVL

Several investigators have studied the GVL response after BMT for CML by measuring the frequency of leukemia-reactive helper or cytotoxic T-lymphocyte precursors (HTLP/CTLP).[29–32] Using a limiting-dilution assay to detect leukemia-specific cytotoxic T cells, we found a higher frequency of CTLP in patients remaining in sustained remission, and a rise in CTLP frequency following DLI in patients who achieved a remission.[31,32] After BMT, we also observed a correlation of high natural killer (NK) and lymphokine-activated killer (LAK) cell function with sustained remission and a similar rise in NK and LAK cell activity after DLI.[32,33] These findings implicate both T cells and NK cells in the GVL response. Leukemia-reactive T cells have also been detected by analysis of T-cell receptor (TCR) Vβ subsets. After transplant, oligoclonal expansions of TCR Vβ families are frequently encountered, with particular expansions coinciding with leukemic remission after DLI.[34] These studies provide strong, albeit indirect, proof of a leukemia-specific T-cell response.

IMMUNOLOGICAL MECHANISMS IN GVL

Basis of the alloresponse

The GVH reaction serves as the basis for our understanding of the GVL response, which can be regarded as a special form of the GVH reaction. The basis of the GVH response is the initiation of an alloreaction through the stimulation of donor T cells by either host or donor antigen-presenting cells (APC) (reviewed by Lord and Lechler[35]). The central molecular event is the interaction of the responder TCR complex ($CD3^+$ TCR) with antigenic peptides aligned within the antigen-presenting groove of MHC class I or II molecules. To succeed in triggering T-cell proliferation and subsequently an effector T-cell response, a second co-stimulatory signal from B7-1 and B7-2 molecules on the APC surface to the CD28 molecule on the T cell is necessary.[36] In the absence of the second signal, T-cell anergy results. In its presence, expansion of the T-cell clone bearing the selected TCR follows in both $CD4^+$ and $CD8^+$ T cells. The expansion is driven by IL-2 and IL-12, modulated by IL-4 and IL-10 and controlled by $CD4^+$ helper T cells and feedback to the APC via CD40 and its ligand on the T cell. Both $CD4^+$ and $CD8^+$ T cells have effector/cytotoxic function.[37] This involves direct killing of host target cells bearing the appropriate MHC molecule via Fas ligand on the killer cell interacting with Fas on the target cell surface. Death of the target follows by activation of caspase and subsequent apoptosis. Cytotoxic T lymphocytes (CTL) also kill targets directly through a calcium-dependent mechanism involving membrane damage by perforin, causing cell lysis, and damage to the target by a package of proteases called granzymes (released from the granules of large granular lymphocytes). Granzymes kill by direct damage to membranes and by caspase activation leading to apoptosis. On this framework, a picture of GVL mechanisms in CML has been constructed.

Induction of the immune response

CML is unique among myeloid malignancies in generating a complete hierarchy of functioning leukocytes, including monocytes, dendritic cells (DC), and B-lymphocyte APC. Unlike many other malignancies, which evade the immune response by a variety of mechanisms to avoid antigen presentation, CML cells have an intact antigen-presenting ability. Both monocytes and DC from CML can process and present exogenous antigens, as well as internally processed self-antigens presented through MHC class I molecules.[38–40] It is possible that the unique sensitivity of CML to control by alloimmune lymphocytes resides in this property. However, in the context of allogeneic BMT, the uniqueness of the antigen-presenting capacity of the malignancy may have less importance, because tumor antigen recognition is also established through malignant cell antigen presentation by donor-derived APC.[41]

Recognition of CML by the responding donor T cell

This implies the presentation of antigens to the donor through MHC molecules. The nature of these antigens is considered in detail in the next section. The next step in the process of the GVL response is the provision of an adequate co-stimulatory signal. This is mediated by B7-1 and B7-2 interaction with CD28 and CD40/CD40 ligand interaction through 'professional APC' of either recipient or donor origin. Subsequently, clonal expansion of leukemia-reacting T cells follows, involving both $CD4^+$ and $CD8^+$ T cells. We have recently gained an insight into the early expansion of recipient reactive donor T cells using the Spectratyping technique to study clonal expansions within TCR Vβ families. Within 14 days, cultures of donor T cells exposed to patient's leukemic or non-leukemic cells exhibit leukemia-restricted skewing of particular TCR Vβ families. In six of eight donor–recipient pairs studied, these clonally expanded leukemia-restricted patterns of TCR Vβ families were also identifiable after allogeneic BMT.[42]

Effector function

To be a target for immune attack by T cells, a malignant cell must ideally express both class I and II MHC molecules, present antigen, and be susceptible to destruction by perforin and granzymes or by apoptosis. Studies with CML cells indicate that they express functional Fas molecules on their surface and that cytotoxic T cells can kill CML by apoptosis.[38] CTL probably also kill CML cells by perforin-mediated lysis. The cytotoxicity of CTL to CML extends to early progenitor cells – CTL inhibit granulocyte–macrophage colony growth (CFU-GM), and can inhibit induction of leukemia in a severe combined immunodeficient (SCID) mouse model, indicating that the progenitors required for leukemogenesis are also successfully inhibited.[43] Other factors that exert an antileukemic effect on CML are the cytokines produced by effector cells – we showed that CML CFU-GM inhibition by leukemia-specific T-cell clones was achieved both by a cell-contact-mediated killing and by cytokine production by the clone – in particular tumor-necrosis factor (TNF)-α and IFN-γ.[44] It is also likely that other effector cells, such as NK cells and macrophages, are involved in the effector phase of the GVL response, but multicellular mechanisms have not been well studied in vitro.[45]

Tumor escape

Despite the near-perfect immune susceptibility of CML, it is abundantly clear from the high relapse rate of advanced CML that, given time, the leukemia is also adept at escaping from immune regulation.[46] The ability to escape from immune attack may depend upon the rate of proliferation of the leukemic stem cell, which could outstrip the pace of T-cell clonal expansion to control the process. Alternatively, the leukemia may use several classical pathways of downregulation of key surface molecules such as MHC, adhesion molecules, and co-stimulatory molecules to evade immune recognition and destruction.[47] We studied a series of patients relapsing with leukemia after BMT, and found a diversity of surface molecular changes that could facilitate immune escape. Furthermore, relapsed leukemic cells were found to be less susceptible than the pretransplant leukemia to lysis by CTL, or, in one case, by NK cells.[48] Figure 23.1 illustrates our current view of CML antigenicity and the role of alloimmune lymphocytes in GVL.

Leukemia antigens

The prerequisite for an alloimmune T-cell response to CML is the interaction between donor lymphocytes with antigens on the leukemia cell. As discussed above, antigen presentation is necessary at both the initiation and the effector phase of the alloresponse. Antigens presented by leukemic cells can be classified as shown in Table 23.2.

Minor histocompatibility antigens

mHA are defined as alleleic variants of cellular proteins presented through MHC class I and II molecules to donor lymphocytes lacking the precise polymorphism of the stimulator.[49] It is clear from mouse genetic studies that many hundreds of mHA exist.[50] Minor antigens can be derived from any region of the cell – known examples include proteins with close homology to known cytoskeletal proteins. So far only a few protein sequences of mHA have been defined. It can be assumed that GVL responses are mediated through mHA, some of which show tissue-restriction and, therefore, possibly GVL-restricted behavior.

Myeloid-specific antigens

Evidence that at least some mHA are restricted to myeloid lineages comes from in vitro experiments where donor T-cell clones, generated against recipient CML, exhibit tissue-restricted cytotoxicity against myeloid but not lymphoid cells.[51,52] In a search for myeloid-specific proteins that could be used to induce CML-restricted alloresponses, we studied well-characterized differentiation antigens restricted to

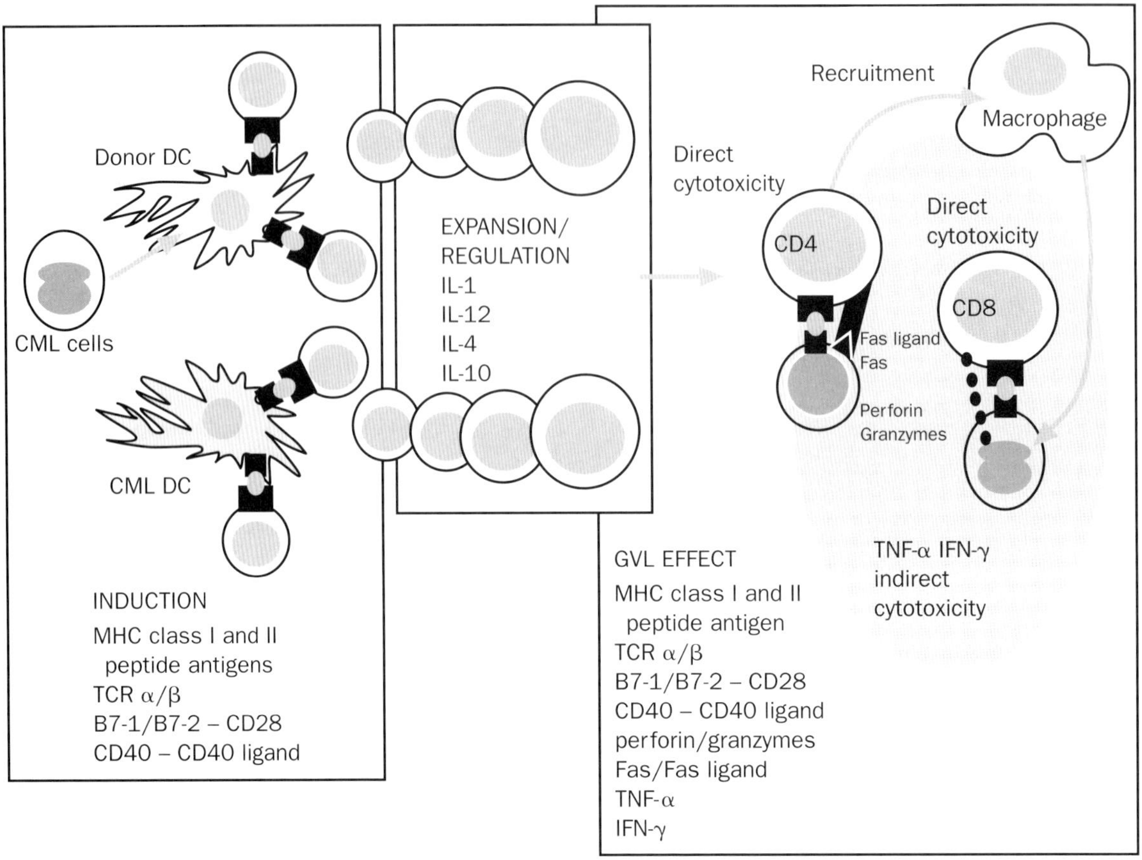

Figure 23.1 Cellular mechanisms and key molecules regulating GVL in CML. *Induction* of donor T-cell responses requires presentation of antigens on leukemia cells to CD4$^+$ and CD8$^+$ cells of the donor by CML dendritic cells (DC), or indirectly via donor DC. The critical steps involved in this process are presentation of peptide antigens by MHC class I and II molecules together with co-stimulation via B7-1/B7-2 interaction with CD28 on the T cell and (for professional APC such as DC) CD40 with CD40 ligand on the T cell. *Expansion* of the immune response generates CD4$^+$ and CD8$^+$ antigen-specific T cells. The cytokines IL-2 and IL-12 promote T-cell proliferation; IL-10 and IL-4 control the balance between Th1 and Th2 cells, modifying the effector behavior – Th1 cells in favor of cytotoxic responses and Th2 cells in favor of humoral responses (not shown). *GVL effect* is mediated by both CD4$^+$ and CD8$^+$ T cells, with possible involvement of other non-specific effectors, such as macrophages. CML cells, including progenitors, are killed directly by perforin and granzyme release inducing cytoplasmic damage and apoptosis, and by Fas-ligand interaction with Fas on the target surface inducing apoptosis (both CD4$^+$ and CD8$^+$ cells use these pathways). Cytokines such as TNF-α and IFN-α also suppress CML by inhibiting cell proliferation and inducing apoptosis.

cells of the myeloid lineage. We used two strategies to identify potential myeloid-restricted antigens: (1) examination of known protein sequences for peptide motifs predicted to bind to common HLA class I antigens; (2) DNA sequencing of known proteins for polymorphisms in a series of marrow cell donors and their recipients. We found peptide sequences in

Table 23.2 Potential antigenic targets for immune responses to CML

Antigen category	Refs
Minor histocompatibility antigens	
Ubiquitously represented: H-Y, HA-1, . . . , HA-7	48
Defined myeloid-restricted antigens	
CD33, CD45	37, 53–56
Primary granule protein proteinase-3, peptides PR-1, PR-7	
Undefined myeloid-restricted antigens	50, 51
BCR/ABL fusion protein (b2a2, b3a2)	59

the primary granule protein, proteinase-3, that bound to HLA-A2. Peptide-loaded APC were used to generate CTL in normal HLA-A2 donors. The CTL were peptide-specific and HLA-A2-restricted, and were cytotoxic to CML cells and their CFU-GM progenitors, but not to normal CFU-GM.[53,54] It was subsequently shown that the PR-1 proteinase-3 peptide could be eluted from MHC molecules of CML cells, confirming that the peptide represents a naturally processed antigen.[55] This discriminatory property of the CTL for the leukemia resided in the much greater cytoplasmic expression of proteinase-3 in the leukemic cells.[54] We also found alleleic variants in proteinase-3[56] and in CD33[57] that could induce alloresponses in donor–recipient pairs disparate for the two alleles.

BCR/ABL fusion protein

The possibility that the novel peptide sequence spanning the breakpoint of the BCR/ABL fusion protein might be presented as an antigen has received much attention as the ideal leukemia-specific target in CML cells.[58,59] BCR/ABL protein expression is unique to CML and essential for the leukemic phenotype, and has only three common variant sequences (b2a2, b3a2, and e1a2). Thus a strategy to induce CTL against BCR/ABL would have universal applicability in all CML patients. Critical to this approach is whether the relevant peptides are naturally presented in sufficient amounts through MHC molecules, whether T cells recognize and respond to the peptide sequences, and whether BCR/ABL-specific T cells can be identified in the blood of patients in remission after allogeneic BMT. So far, there has been no success in eluting BCR/ABL peptides from CML cells.[55] Many investigators have succeeded in generating BCR/ABL or ABL peptide-specific $CD4^+$ and $CD8^+$ T cells.[60,61] However, evidence that such T cells can recognize and kill CML cells specifically is not convincing. Pawelec et al[65] describe recognition by BCR/ABL-specific $CD4^+$ T cells of CML. Oettel et al[66] raised CTL against Philadelphia chromosome (Ph)-positive CML cells, but found that they were also cytotoxic to Ph-negative cells from the same individual. Similarly, ten Bosch et al[67] found that BCR/ABL peptide-specific CTL recognized but did not kill CML targets. It is possible that the amount of BCR/ABL expression via class I and II is not high enough to reproducibly induce damage by CTL. Alternatively, it may be that only T cells with low affinity for BCR/ABL have been generated. Further experience with BCR/ABL vaccines may clarify the ability of normal individuals to generate T-cell responses and identify the target susceptibility of BCR/ABL-positive CML cells.[68]

OPTIMIZING THE GVL RESPONSE AFTER ALLOGENEIC SCT

Stem cell dose

The high yields of progenitor cells obtained with granulocyte colony-stimulating factor (G-CSF)-stimulated peripheral blood stem cell transplantation (PBSCT) have facilitated the study of the effect of $CD34^+$ cell dose on transplant outcome. Several studies have identified a beneficial effect of stem cell dose following allogeneic transplants. In a series of 78 recipients of BMT or PBSCT, we found lower transplant-related mortality and lower relapse rates in recipients of high $CD34^+$ cell doses. Patients with CML in chronic phase had a significantly lower relapse rate if the transplant contained more than 2×10^6 $CD34^+$ cells.[69] These observations suggest that $CD34^+$ dose, independently of $CD3^+$ dose, can affect the relapse risk. Even in transplants from identical twins, a high nucleated cell dose appears to protect against relapse.[70] A possible explanation is that higher stem cell doses result in more rapid reconstitution of APC, with a concomitant improvement in antigen processing of recipient leukemia antigens.

Optimizing DLI

In the decade since the first use of DLI to treat relapsed CML after BMT, much progress has been made in determining the kinetics of the response, the effect of immune activation by cytokines and immune suppression by cyclosporin, the optimum lymphocyte dose required to achieve an effect, and the timing of the DLI in relation to the progression of the relapse. Careful sequential dose studies carried out by the Memorial Sloan–Kettering group identified a $CD3^+$ cell dose of 1×10^7/kg as usually sufficient to achieve a response of relapsed CML within 3 months.[24] The Hammersmith Hospital group compared the use of DLI at the first sign of molecular relapse with DLI given to treat hematological relapse, and concluded that early treatment yielded the highest probability of complete response.[71] It was also clear from large multicenter studies that CML relapsing in accelerated phase or in blast crisis had a much lower chance of responding to DLI.[23] Several investigators have used DLI in conjunction with IFN-α.[25] Although there are no controlled studies, it appears that addition of IFN-α may increase the number of remissions. Despite some benefit of reduced GVHD incidence and severity achieved by judicious dosing of DLI, GVHD still remains a major complication of the procedure, especially when unrelated donors are used.[23] Two studies have evaluated the effect of selected $CD4^+$ donor lymphocytes on disease control and GVHD. The results indicate a favorable effect of selected DLI on GVHD, with comparable antileukemic effects to those seen with unmanipulated lymphocytes.[72,73]

Non-myeloablative stem cell transplants (NMT)

The observation that patients with CML achieve durable remissions when given donor lymphocytes alone to treat leukemia relapsing after BMT is the basis for the use of low-intensity non-myeloablative transplants (NMT) to treat CML. We treated two patients with chronic-phase CML with a PBSCT regimen consisting of cyclophosphamide and fludarabine.[74] Both patients achieved a molecular remission within 100 days following transplant. The GVL effect was the main mechanism involved in disease eradication, because, after the low-dose preparative regimen and the transplant, the CML persisted until full donor T-cell reconstitution was established. The ease of leukemia suppression after NMT strongly supports a central role for the GVL effect in the cure of CML after allogeneic BMT.

SEPARATING GVH AND GVL

Prophylaxis or pre-emptive treatment of relapse after T-cell depletion

One of the continuing challenges in allogeneic BMT is the separation of the beneficial GVL effect from the unwanted GVH response. That the two can be separated is no longer a contentious issue – current thinking is that malignant cells exhibit a variety of antigens restricted to cells of that lineage, as well as tumor-specific antigens.[49] Thus, at a clonal level, it should be possible to find CTL that show a high degree of specificity for the malignant cell without reactivity to other tissues. However, without full knowledge of the target antigens on malignant cells, clinically applicable approaches to separating GVHD from GVL are currently imperfect. Several clinical strategies have been used to prevent GVHD while conserving the GVL effect. Drobyski et al[75] performed T-cell-depleted transplants for CML and monitored patients for relapse. Those patients developing molecular relapse were given DLI. GVHD was reduced by sparing patients who did not require donor lymphocytes to remain in remission and, in those who required DLI, by diminished severity of GVHD associated with the delayed lymphocyte add-back. To prevent relapse while minimizing GVHD, Naparstek et al[76] employed pre-emptive add-back of increasing doses of donor T cells at monthly intervals following T-cell-depleted BMT, and reported low relapse rates and controllable GVHD. An alternative strategy adopted by our group was to give a planned add-back of 1×10^7 CD3 cells on day 45 following a T-cell-depleted transplant.[77] About half of the patients with CML were negative for BCR/ABL by PCR by day 100. Those who still had detectable disease received a further transfusion of 5×10^7 $CD3^+$ cells/kg, and cyclosporin was discontinued. This approach reduced the incidence and severity of GVHD and conferred an antileukemic effect comparable to T-cell-replete transplants.

CD8 depletion

The demonstration of CML-specific cytotoxicity from $CD4^+$ cells justifies the use of CD4-subset selected transfusions. In HLA-matched individuals, the removal of $CD8^+$ cells reduces or prevents GVHD. Several groups have reported effective GVL reactivity against CML using $CD8^+$-depleted T cells to prevent CML relapse.[78,79]

Suicide genes

Another way to control GVHD while permitting the GVL effect is to insert a 'suicide gene' into donor T cells given with the SCT. T cells transfected with the herpes simplex virus (HSV) thymidine kinase (Tk) gene die on exposure to ganciclovir. After transplantation with these genetically modified lymphocytes, GVHD can be aborted with ganciclovir treatment.[80–82] However, there are concerns that genetically manipulated T cells lose their function. The strategy has also been criticized for its lack of selectivity – the abrogation of donor immune cells by ganciclovir treatment leaves the patient with impaired immune function and defective GVL reactivity. Furthermore, incomplete transfection with the HSV-Tk gene could lead to the selection of ganciclovir-resistant strains with unwanted alloreactivity.

Selective depletion

To overcome the problem of non-specific immune depletion, several approaches to selective depletion of donor anti-host reactivity are under investigation. The principle is to induce donor lymphocytes before administration with lymphocytes from the patient. Alloactivated donor cells expressing CD25 or CD69 activation markers can be eliminated by an immunotoxin directed against the activation marker, or removed using magnetic beads coated with the relevant antibody.[51,83–85] Selective depletion has been shown in vitro and in an animal model to remove GVHD-reacting T cells while conserving immunity to third-party cells, Epstein–Barr virus (EBV)-transformed B cells, and, importantly, recipient's CML cells.[84–86] This technique has yet to be fully evaluated in clinical trials.

TCR Vβ selection

Analysis of T-cell clones induced against CML in vitro reveals three common patterns of alloreactivity: leukemia-specific cells recognizing leukemia but not phytohemagglutinin (PHA)-stimulated blasts from the patient, PHA-blast-specific clones, and clones recognizing both cell types. In one donor–recipient pair, we examined the TCR Vβ subtype of 18 of 78 T-cell clones generated against the patient's CML. We found a marked restriction in Vβ family usage, with only one dominant clonotype with leukemia-specific reactivity.[87] This observation suggested that the antigens inducing leukemia-specific responses are immunodominant and few in number. We subsequently showed that short-term culture of donor lymphocytes with HLA-identical sibling leukemia or normal cells reveals oligoclonal expansions within specific Vβ T-cell families, detectable within two weeks of culture. We found the same oligoclonal expansions of donor T cells in the blood following PBSCT.[42] The ability to predict what appear to be biologically relevant expansions of specific TCR Vβ subsets presents us with the opportunity to use antibody-coated magnetic beads to select for DLI T cells of the relevant (GVL-reacting) TCR Vβ family. The approach is clinically attractive because of its relative simplicity. However, more studies are needed to determine whether in vitro expansion of TCR Vβ T-cell subsets is a reliable predictor of in vivo antileukemic capability.

AMPLIFYING GVL RESPONSES

The techniques described so far only result at best in the conservation but not the amplification of GVL reactivity. Augmentation of GVL reactivity requires the generation of large numbers of CTL with leukemia specificity. This could be achieved by adoptive transfer of in vitro expanded CTL, or by the use of vaccines to enhance either the donor's or the recipient's generation of leukemia-specific CTL.

Adoptive transfer of leukemia-specific CTL

After considerable effort and with much technical expertise, it was recently shown by Falkenburg et al[88] in Leiden that donor CTL expanded in vitro against recipient's leukemia induced remission in CML patients relapsing with leukemia after transplantation. Impressively, both patients treated were refractory to the standard DLI approach using unmanipulated lymphocytes, while only small numbers of leukemia-specific CTL were needed to achieve remission.[88] While these experiments demonstrate the proof of principle that in-vitro-generated leukemia-specific CTL are effective in vivo, the variability in the ability to generate such CTL in every donor–recipient pair and the technical competence required for prolonged T-cell culture limit the more general application of the technique. In future, with the identification of specific antigens, the generation of leukemia-specific CTL should be easier to achieve and more reproducible, thus facilitating clinical application.

Vaccines

In contrast to the complexity of adoptive transfer of leukemia-specific T cells, vaccination has the attraction of simplicity and ease of clinical application. Clinical trials using BCR/ABL fusion proteins are underway in the autologous setting, which could be readily adapted to allogeneic transplantation by vaccination of either the patient or the donor.[67] Vaccination of CML patients with PR-1 peptide of proteinase-3 is also under investigation (J Molldrem, personal communication). Ultimately, both ex vivo and in vivo approaches to boosting the GVL response could be combined to maximize the effect.

CONCLUSIONS

CML remains one of the best leukemia models that we have to further the study of alloimmune events. Through in vivo analysis of minimal residual disease, T-cell chimerism, and specific reactivity, we have learned much about the kinetics of the immune response. From in vitro studies, facilitated by the ability to grow CML in culture, the basis of the GVL response has been characterized. Now we are on the threshold of delivering highly targeted and effective immunotherapy to patients with CML undergoing BMT. A continuing concern is whether immune escape will limit the success of these techniques. As immunotherapy begins to be more widely applied, we will inevitably have to learn more about the mechanisms resulting in failure of GVL to eradicate disease. In the future, understanding tumor escape and developing ways to modify malignant cells to be better immune targets will be crucial to the success of this approach.

REFERENCES

1. Barnes DWH, Loutit JF, Treatment of murine leukemia with X-rays and homologous bone marrow. *BMJ* 1956; **2:** 626–7.
2. Radich JP, Gehly G, Gooley T et al, Polymerase chain reaction detection of the BCR–ABL fusion transcript after allogeneic marrow transplantation for chronic myeloid leukemia: results and implications in 346. *Leukemia* 1994; **8:** 735–9.
3. Costello RT, Kirk J, Gabert J, Value of PCR analysis for long term survivors after allogeneic bone marrow transplant for chronic myelogenous leukemia: a comparative study. *Biol Blood Marrow Transplant* 1995; **1:** 24–31.
4. Weiden PL, Fluornoy N, Thomas D, Antileukemic effects of graft versus host disease in human recipients of allogeneic marrow grafts. *N Engl J Med* 1969; **300:** 1068–72.
5. Sullivan K, Storb R, Buckner C et al, Graft versus host disease as adoptive immunotherapy in patients with advanced hematologic malignancies. *N Engl J Med* 1989; **320:** 828–34.
6. Horowitz MM, Gale RP, Sondel PM et al, Graft-versus-leukemia reactions after bone marrow transplantation. *Blood* 1990; **75:** 555–62.
7. Gale RP, Horowitz MM, Ash RC et al, Identical twin bone marrow transplants for leukemia. *Ann Intern Med* 1994; **12:** 646–52.
8. Kolb H-J, Mitmuller J, Clemm Ch et al, Donor leukocyte transfusions for treatment of recurrent chronic myelogenous leukemia in marrow transplant patients. *Blood* 1990; **76:** 2462–5.
9. Miyamura K, Barrett AJ, Kodera Y, Saito H, Minimal residual disease after bone marrow transplantation for chronic myelogenous leukemia and implications for graft-versus-leukemia effect: a review of recent results. *Bone Marrow Transplant* 1994; **14:** 201–10.
10. Hessner M, Endean D, Casper J et al, Use of unrelated marrow grafts compensates for reduced graft-versus-leukemia reactivity after T-cell-depleted allogeneic marrow transplantation for chronic myelogenous leukemia. *Blood* 1995; **86:** 3987–96.
11. Henslee-Downey PJ, Abhyankar SH, Parrish PRS et al, Use of partially mismatched related donors extends access to allogeneic marrow transplant. *Blood* 1997; **89:** 3864–72.
12. Clift RA, Buckner CD, Thomas ED et al, Marrow transplantation for patients in accelerated phase of chronic myeloid leukaemia. *Blood* 1994; **84:** 4368–73.
13. Frassoni F, Martinelli G, Saglio G et al, bcr/abl chimeric transcript in patients in remission after marrow transplantation for chronic myeloid leukemia: higher frequency of detection and slower clearance in patients grafted in advanced disease as compared to patients grafted in chronic phase. *Blood* 1995; **85:** 2632–8.
14. Higano CS, Brixey M, Bryant EM et al, Durable complete remission of acute non-lymphoblastic leukaemia associated with discontinuation of immunosuppression following relapse after allogeneic bone marrow transplantation. A case report of a probable graft-versus-leukaemia effect. *Transplantation* 1990; **50:** 175–7.

15. Collins RH, Rogers ZR, Bennett M et al, Hematologic relapse of chronic myelogenous leukemia following allogeneic bone marrow transplantation: apparent graft-versus-leukemia effect following abrupt discontinuation of immunosuppression. *Bone Marrow Transplant* 1992; **10:** 391–5.
16. Apperley JF, Jones L, Hale G, Goldman JM, Bone marrow transplantation for chronic myeloid leukaemia: T cell depletion with Campath-1 reduces the incidence of acute graft-versus-host disease but may increase the risk of leukaemic relapse. *Bone Marrow Transplant* 1986; **1:** 53–66.
17. Champlin RE, Passweg JR, Zhang M-J et al, T-cell depletion of bone marrow transplants for leukemia from donors other than HLA-identical siblings: advantages of T-cell antibodies with narrow specificities. *Blood* 2000; **95:** 3996–4003.
18. Mckinnon S, Barnett L, Heller G, O'Reilly RJ, Minimal residual disease is more common in patients who have mixed T-cell chimerism after bone marrow transplantation for chronic myelogenous leukemia. *Blood* 1994; **83:** 3409–16.
19. Kogler G, Hernandez A, Heyll A et al, Qualitative assessment of mixed chimerism after allogeneic bone marrow transplantation with regard to leukemic relapse. *Cancer Detect Prev* 1996; **20:** 601–9.
20. Roux E, Helg C, Dumont-Girard F et al, Analysis of T-cell repopulation after allogeneic bone marrow transplantation: significant differences between recipients of T-cell depleted and unmanipulated grafts. *Blood* 1996; **87:** 3984–92.
21. Sullivan KM, Weiden PL, Storb R et al, Influence of acute and chronic graft-versus-host disease after relapse and survival after bone marrow transplantation from HLA identical siblings as treatment of acute and chronic leukemia. *Blood* 1989; **73:** 1720–8.
22. Gardiner N, Lawler M, O'Riordan JM et al, Monitoring of lineage-specific chimaerism allows early prediction of response following donor lymphocyte infusions for relapsed chronic myeloid leukaemia. *Bone Marrow Transplant* 1998; **21:** 711–19.
23. Kolb HJ, Schattenberg A, Goldman JM et al, Graft-versus-leukemia effect of donor lymphocyte transfusions in marrow grafted patients. *Blood* 1995; **86:** 2041–50.
24. Mackinnon S, Papadopoulos E, Carabasi M et al, Adoptive immunotherapy evaluating escalating doses of donor leukocytes for relapse of chronic myeloid leukemia after bone marrow transplantation: separation of graft-versus-leukemia responses from graft-versus-host disease. *Blood* 1995; **86:** 1261–8.
25. Higano CS, Chielens D, Raskind W et al, Use of α-2a-interferon to treat cytogenetic relapse of chronic myeloid leukemia after marrow transplantation. *Blood* 1997; **90:** 2549–54.
26. Giralt S, O'Brien S, Talpaz M et al, Interferon-α and interleukin-2 as treatment for leukemia relapse after allogeneic bone marrow transplantation. *Cytokines Mol Ther* 1995; **1:** 115–22.
27. Slavin S, Naparstek E, Nagler A et al, Allogeneic cell therapy with donor peripheral blood cells and recombinant human interleukin-2 to treat leukemia relapse after allogeneic bone marrow transplantation. *Blood* 1996; **87:** 2195–204.
28. van Rhee F, Savage D, Blackwell J et al, Adoptive immunotherapy for relapse of chronic myeloid leukemia after allogeneic bone marrow transplant: equal efficacy of lymphocytes from sibling and matched unrelated donors. *Bone Marrow Transplant* 1998; **21:** 1055–61.
29. Salomo M, Steinmann J, Glass B et al, Leukemia-specific allogeneic donor T cells: quantification by limiting dilution assay. *Bone Marrow Transplant* 1995; **15:** 179–86.
30. Hoffmann T, Theobald M, Bunjes D et al, Frequency of bone marrow T cells responding to HLA-identical non-leukemic and leukemic stimulator cells. *Bone Marrow Transplant* 1993; **12:** 1–8.
31. Jiang YZ, Kanfer E, Macdonald D et al, Graft-versus-leukemia following allogeneic bone marrow transplantation: emergence of cytotoxic T lymphocytes reacting to host leukemia cells. *Bone Marrow Transplant* 1991; **8:** 253–8.
32. Jiang YZ, Cullis J, Kanfer E et al, T cell and NK cell mediated graft-versus-leukemia reactivity following donor buffy coat transfusion to treat relapse after marrow transplantation for chronic myeloid leukemia. *Bone Marrow Transplant* 1993; **11:** 133–8.
33. Jiang YZ, Barrett AJ, Goldman JM, Mavroudis DA, Evidence for natural killer cell modulation of a graft-versus-graft-versus-leukaemia effect without graft-versus-host disease following allogeneic bone marrow transplantation. *Ann Hematol* 1997; **74:** 1–6.
34. Claret EJ, Alyea EP, Orsini E et al, Characterization of T cell repertoire in patients with graft-versus-leukemia after donor lymphocyte infusion. *J Clin Invest* 1997; **100:** 855–66.

35. Lord GM, Lechler RI, The immune response to alloantigens. In: *Tumor Alloimmunotherapy* (Barrett AJ, Jiang YZ, eds). New York: Marcel Dekker, 2000: 13–38.
36. Matulonis UA, Dosiou CD, Lamont C et al, Role of B7.1 in mediating an immune response to myeloid leukaemia cells. *Blood* 1995; **85:** 2507–15.
37. Jiang YZ, Mavroudis D, Dermime S et al, Alloreactive CD4+ T lymphocytes can exert cytotoxicity to chronic myeloid leukaemia cells processing and presenting exogenous antigen. *Br J Haematol* 1996; **93:** 606–12.
38. Barrett AJ, Mechanisms of the graft-vs-leukaemia reaction. *Stem Cells* 1997; **15:** 248–58.
39. Choudhury A, Gajewski JL, Liang JL et al, Use of leukemic dendritic cells for the generation of antileukemic cellular cytotoxicity against Philadelphia-chromosome positive chronic myelogenous leukemia. *Blood* 1997; **89:** 1133–42.
40. Jiang YZ, Mavroudis D, Dermime S et al, Alloreactive CD4+ T lymphocytes can exert cytotoxicity to chronic myeloid leukaemia cells processing and presenting exogenous antigen. *Br J Haematol* 1996; **93:** 606–12.
41. Auchincloss H Jr, Sultan H, Antigen processing and presentation in transplantation. *Curr Opin Immunol* 1996; **8:** 681–7.
42. Epperson D, Margolis DA, McOlash LM et al, In vitro T cell receptor Vβ repertoire analysis can identify which T cells mediate graft vs. leukemia (GVL) and graft vs. host (GVH) responses after HLA-matched sibling bone marrow transplantation *Blood* 1999; **94**:(Suppl 1a) 325a.
43. Warren EH, Greenberg PD, Riddell SR, Cytotoxic T-lymphocyte-defined human minor histocompatibility antigens with a restricted tissue distribution. *Blood* 1998; **91:** 2197–207.
44. Jiang YZ, Barrett AJ, Cellular and cytokine mediated effects of CD4-positive lymphocyte lines generated in vitro against chronic myelogenous leukemia. *Exp Hematol* 1995; **23:** 1167–72.
45. Albi N, Ruggeri L, Aversa F et al, Natural killer cell function and antileukemic activity of a large population of CD3+/CD8+ T cells expressing NK receptors for major histocompatibility complex class I after 'three-loci' HLA-incompatible bone marrow transplantation. *Blood* 1996; **87:** 3993–4000.
46. Sondel PM, Hank JA, Molanda J et al, Relapse of host leukaemic lymphoblasts following engraftment by an HLA-mismatched marrow transplant: mechanisms of escape from the 'graft versus leukaemia' effect. *Exp Hematol* 1985; **13:** 782–90.
47. Delain M, Tiberghien P, Racadot E et al, Variability of the alloreactive T-cell response to human leukemic blasts. *Leukemia* 1994; **8:** 642–7.
48. Dermime S, Hensel N, Jiang YZ et al, Does immune escape from a graft-versus-leukemia effect play a role in the relapse of myelogenous leukemias following allogeneic bone marrow transplantation? *Bone Marrow Transplant* 1997; **19:** 989–99.
49. Goulmy E, Human minor histocompatibility antigens: new concepts for marrow transplantation and adoptive immunotherapy. *Immunol Rev* 1997; **157:** 125–40.
50. Perreault C, Decary F, Brochu S et al, Minor histocompatibility antigens. *Blood* 1990; **76:** 1269–77.
51. Datta AR, Barrett AJ, Jiang YZ et al, Distinct T cell populations distinguish chronic myeloid leukemia cells from lymphocytes in the same individual: a model for separating GVHD from GVL reactions. *Bone Marrow Transplant* 1994; **14:** 517–24.
52. van Lochem E, de Gast B, Goulmy E, In vitro separation of host specific graft-versus-host and graft-versus-leukemia cytotoxic T cell activities. *Bone Marrow Transplant* 1992; **10:** 181–3.
53. Molldrem J, Dermime S, Parker K et al, Targeted T cell therapy for human leukemia: cytotoxic T lymphocytes specific for a peptide derived from proteinase 3 preferentially lyse human myeloid leukemia cells. *Blood* 1996; **88:** 2450–7.
54. Molldrem JJ, Clave E, Jiang YZ et al, Cytotoxic T lymphocytes specific for a nonpolymorphic proteinase 3 peptide preferentially inhibit chronic myeloid leukemia colony-forming units. *Blood* 1997; **90:** 2529–34.
55. Papadopoulos KP, Suciu-Foca N, Harris PE et al, Naturally processed tissue- and differentiation stage-specific autologous peptides bound by HLA class I and II molecules of chronic myeloid leukemia blasts. *Blood* 1997; **90:** 4938–46.
56. Clave E, Molldrem J, Hensel N et al, Donor–recipient polymorphism of the proteinase 3 gene in bone marrow transplantation. *J Immunother* 1999; **22:** 1–6.
57. Raptis A, Clave E, Mavroudis D et al, Polymorphism in CD33 and CD34 genes: a source of minor histocompatibility antigens on hematopoietic stem cells? *Br J Haematol* 1998; **102:** 1323–30.
58. Barrett AJ, Jiang YZ, Immune responses to

chronic myeloid leukaemia. *Bone Marrow Transplant* 1992; **9:** 305–11.
59. Cheever MA, Disis ML, Bernhard H et al, Immunity to oncogenic proteins. *Immunol Rev* 1995; **145:** 33–59.
60. Chen W, Peace DJ, Rovira DK et al, T-cell immunity to the joining region of p210BCR–ABL protein. *Proc Natl Acad Sci USA* 1992; **89:** 1468–75.
61. Bocchia M, Wentworth PA, Southwood S et al, Specific binding of leukemia oncogene fusion proteins peptides to HLA class I molecules. *Blood* 1995; **85:** 2680–4.
62. Smit WM, Rijnbeek M, van Bergen CAM et al, Generation of dendritic cells expressing bcr–abl from CD34-positive chronic myeloid leukemia cells. *Hum Immunol* 1997; **53:** 216–23.
63. Buzyn A, Ostankovich M, Zerbib A et al, Peptides derived from the whole sequence of BCR–ABL bind to several class I molecules allowing specific induction of human cytotoxic T lymphocytes. *Eur J Immunol* 1997; **27:** 2066–72.
64. Bocchia M, Korontsvit T, Xu Q et al, Specific human cellular immunity to bcr/abl oncogene-derived peptides. *Blood* 1996; **87:** 3587–92.
65. Pawelec G, Max H, Halder T et al, BCR/ABL leukemia oncogene fusion peptides selectively bind to certain HLA-DR alleles and can be recognized by T cells found at low frequency in the repertoire of normal donors. *Blood* 1996; **88:** 2118–24.
66. Oettel K, Wesly O, Albertini M et al, Allogeneic T cell clones able to selectively destroy Philadelphia chromosome-bearing human leukemia lines can also recognize Ph− cells from the same patient. *Blood* 1994; **83:** 3390–402.
67. ten Bosch GJA, Joosten AM, Kessler JH et al, Recognition of BCR–ABL positive leukemic blasts by human CD4+ T cells elicited by primary in vitro immunization with a BCR–ABL breakpoint peptide. *Blood* 1996; **88:** 3522–30.
68. Caron PC, Scheinberg DA, The biological therapy of acute and chronic leukemia. *Cancer Invest* 1997; **15:** 342–52.
69. Bahçeci E, Read EJ, Leitman S et al, CD34+ cell dose predicts relapse and survival following T cell depleted HLA-identical hematopoietic stem cell transplantation for hematologic malignancies. *Br J Haematol* 2000; **108**: 408–15.
70. Barrett AJ, Ringden O, Zhang M-J et al, Effect of nucleated marrow cell dose on relapse and survival in identical twin transplants for leukemia. *Blood* 2000; **95**: 3323–7.
71. van Rhee F, Feng L, Cullis JO et al, Relapse of chronic myeloid leukemia after allogeneic bone marrow transplantation: the case for giving donor leukocyte transfusions before the onset of hematologic relapse. *Blood* 1994; **83:** 3377–83.
72. Giralt S, Hester J, Huh Y et al, CD8+-depleted donor lymphocyte infusion as treatment for relapsed chronic myelogenous leukemia after allogeneic bone marrow transplantation: graft vs. leukemia without graft vs. host disease. *Blood* 1995; **86:** 4337–43.
73. Alyea EP, Soiffer RJ, Canning C et al, Toxicity and efficacy of defined doses of CD4(+) donor lymphocytes for treatment of relapse after allogeneic bone marrow transplant. *Blood* 1998; **91:** 3671–80.
74. Childs R, Epperson D, Bahçeci E et al, Molecular remission of chronic myeloid leukaemia following a non-myeloablative allogeneic peripheral blood stem cell transplant: in vivo and in vitro evidence for a graft-versus-leukaemia effect. *Br J Haematol* 1999; **107:** 396–400.
75. Drobyski WR, Hessner MJ, Klein JP et al, T-cell depletion plus salvage immunotherapy with donor leukocyte infusions as a strategy to treat chronic-phase myelogenous leukemia patients undergoing HLA-identical sibling marrow transplantation. *Blood* 1999; **94:** 434–41.
76. Naparstek E, Or R, Nagler A et al, T-cell depleted allogeneic bone marrow transplantation for acute leukemia using Campath-1 antibodies and post-transplant administration of donor's peripheral blood lymphocytes for prevention of relapse. *Br J Haematol* 1995; **89:** 506–15.
77. Barrett J, Mavroudis D, Tisdale J et al, T-cell depleted bone marrow transplantation followed by delayed T-cell add-back to prevent severe acute GVHD. *Bone Marrow Transplant* 1998; **21:** 543–21.
78. Champlin R, Ho W, Gajewski J et al, Selective depletion of CD8+ T lymphocytes for prevention of graft-versus-host disease after allogeneic bone marrow transplantation. *Blood* 1990; **76:** 418–23.
79. Nimer SD, Giorgi J, Gajewski JL et al, Selective depletion of CD8+ cells for prevention of graft-versus-host disease after bone marrow transplantation. *Blood* 1994; **57:** 82–7.
80. Bonini C, Verzeletti S, Servida P et al, HSV-TK gene transfer into donor lymphocytes for control of allogeneic graft-versus-leukemia. *Science* 1997; **276:** 1719–23.

81. Tiberghien P, Reynolds CW, Keller J et al, Ganciclovir treatment of herpes simplex thymidine kinase-transduced primary T lymphocytes: an approach for specific in vivo donor T-cell depletion after bone marrow transplantation? *Blood* 1994; **84:** 1333–40.
82. Gallot G, Hallet M, Gaschet J et al, Human HLA-specific T-cell clones with stable expression of a suicide gene: a possible tool to drive and control a graft-versus-host-graft-versus-leukemia reaction? *Blood* 1996; **88:** 1098–103.
83. Rencher SD, Houston JA, Lockey TD et al, Eliminating graft-versus-host potential T cell immunotherapeutic populations. *Bone Marrow Transplant* 1996; **18:** 415–20.
84. Mavroudis DA, Jiang YZ, Hensel N et al, Specific depletion of alloreactivity against haplotype mismatched related individuals: a new approach to graft-versus-host disease prophylaxis in haploidentical bone marrow transplantation. *Bone Marrow Transplant* 1996; **17:** 793–9.
85. Mavroudis DA, Dermime S, Molldrem JJ et al, Specific depletion of alloreactive T cells in HLA-identical siblings – a method for separating graft-vs-host and graft-vs-leukaemia reactions. *Br J Haematol* 1998; **101:** 565–70.
86. Cavazzana-Calvo M, Stephan JL, Sarnacki S et al, Attenuation of graft-versus-host disease and graft rejection by ex-vivo immunotoxin elimination of alloreactive T cells in an H-2 haplotype disparate mouse combination. *Blood* 1994; **83:** 288–98.
87. Jiang YZ, Mavroudis D, Hensel N, Barrett AJ, Preferential usage of T cell receptor (TCR) Vβ by allogeneic T cells recognising myeloid leukemia cells: implications for separating GVL from GVHD. *Bone Marrow Transplant* 1997; **19:** 899–903.
88. Falkenburg JH, Wafelman AR, Joosten P et al, Complete remission of accelerated phase chronic myeloid leukemia by treatment with leukemia-reactive cytotoxic T lymphocytes. *Blood* 1999; **94:** 1201–8.

24

Donor lymphocyte infusions

Francesco Dazzi, Hans J Stauss

CONTENTS • Relapse of CML after allogeneic SCT: the immunologic scenario • Therapeutic options for CML at relapse: is DLI the most rational option? • Use of DLI for CML • How to tackle GVHD • Time to treat: 'the sooner the better'? • Association of DLI with other treatments • Potential targets of DLI • New trends in the immunotherapy of CML • Conclusions

RELAPSE OF CML AFTER ALLOGENEIC SCT: THE IMMUNOLOGIC SCENARIO

Allogeneic stem cell transplantation (SCT) is the only approach capable of curing chronic myeloid leukaemia (CML).[1,2] However, a proportion of patients can relapse. The actuarial probability of relapse is very low for patients allografted in chronic phase with unmanipulated marrow cells and with the use of cyclosporin alone as prophylaxis for graft-versus-host disease (GVHD). However, the incidence of relapse becomes much higher when the transplant is performed in patients in advanced phase[3] and when the GVHD prophylaxis is more intensive.[4] In particular, the observation that the use of T-cell-depleted stem cells significantly increases the incidence of relapse provided *prima facie* evidence that allogeneic T cells play a pivotal role in eradicating leukaemic cells and/or maintaining remission.[4,5]

Allogeneic SCT allows donor allogeneic haematopoiesis to be established in the recipient. This event implies that recipient T cells reacting against donor cells are deleted or anergized so that donor cells are recognized as self (transplantation tolerance). Furthermore, disappearance of GHVD correlates with the deletion of anti-recipient donor T cells,[6,7] so that, in the case of relapse, some of the recipient leukaemic cells cannot be recognized by the donor T-cell repertoire. However, this chimeric condition provides the opportunity to exploit lymphocytes from the original donor once again, without any immunosuppressive regimen, to kill leukaemic cells.

THERAPEUTIC OPTIONS FOR CML AT RELAPSE: IS DLI THE MOST RATIONAL OPTION?

The identification of molecular markers specific for CML has allowed investigators to develop laboratory assays that are now of fundamental importance in monitoring disease and for diagnosing relapse after transplant. In general, relapse of CML after allogeneic SCT can be recognized first as a result of a progressive rise in the numbers of *BCR/ABL* transcripts on reverse-transcriptase polymerase chain reaction (RT-PCR) in the blood (molecular relapse).[8] Subsequently, Philadelphia chromosome (Ph)-positive metaphases can be identified in the marrow (cytogenetic relapse), and eventually patients show features of haematologic relapse.

Haematologic relapse can be subclassified into chronic, accelerated, and blastic phase, in accordance with the standard criteria.[9]

Occasionally, molecular or cytogenetic relapses are reversible, but such 'transient' relapses are rare.[8] Therefore, when relapse is detected, a treatment to restore remission is mandatory. Therapeutic options for patients in relapse were initially limited either to a second transplant or to the use of interferon-α (IFN-α). However, the former is associated with significant mortality,[10] whereas the latter can restore remission only in a minority of cases.[11] The graft-versus-leukaemia (GVL) effect exerted by donor T lymphocytes plays a major role in the control or eradication of leukaemia. However, the concomitant administration of immunosuppressive treatment to prevent GVHD, and in selected cases the low number of T cells administered at the time of transplant, can potentially limit the efficacy of the transplant procedure and favour the reappearance of leukaemia.

Therefore Kolb and colleagues[12] proposed the infusion of lymphocytes from the original stem cell donor to restore remission in patients with CML in relapse after allografting. This proved to be possible. Donor lymphocyte infusions (DLI) have since been widely employed to treat relapses of all types of leukaemia after allogeneic SCT. Their ability to react against cells of recipient origin has also been used to reverse defective bone marrow engraftment due to graft rejection. Furthermore, the state of selective tolerance induced in the recipient by the transplantation of donor cells allows donor T cells to be utilized to reconstitute immune deficiency, and to cure viral diseases that may complicate transplantation.

USE OF DLI FOR CML

Efficacy

Whereas the existence of a graft-versus-tumour effect in solid malignancies is still a matter of debate, adoptive immunotherapy is a clinical reality in the treatment of haematologic malignancies in relapses after allografting. However, the results vary amongst the different types of tumours.

The studies conducted with DLI in patients with CML have clearly demonstrated that this leukaemia is exquisitely sensitive to immune recognition and that DLI should be considered as the first-choice option to treat patients in relapse after allografting. Table 24.1 illustrates the response rates reported by the most representative studies.[13–23] DLI results in complete remission in a high percentage of patients, although the figures vary significantly. These differences might be explained by the heterogeneity of the patients treated.

Factors for response

It has been clearly demonstrated that an important factor predicting response to DLI is the disease stage at the time of DLI. In fact, patients who are treated when the disease is detected only by molecular or cytogenetic analysis respond better than those whose disease is in frank haematologic relapse.[13,14,17,18,23] Furthermore, among patients with haematologic relapse, those in chronic phase fare better than those with disease in accelerated or blastic phase. However, some groups have reported excellent results also in patients with disease in advanced phase.[15,21] It has been suggested that the stage of disease at the time of transplantation may be as important as the stage of disease at the time of DLI in determining response to DLI,[17] but it is not known which of the two factors is more relevant.

The tumour burden – as measured by the disease stage – is not the only factor affecting the outcome of the DLI treatment. The interval between transplant and DLI has been observed to influence the response to DLI. In fact, it appears that response rates are higher if this interval is shorter than 2 years.[14] However, it has also been shown that patients who relapse less than 9 months after allografting are less likely to respond to DLI than patients who relapse relatively late after allografting.[24] This

Table 24.1 Responsiveness of chronic myeloid leukaemia to DLI in the most representative studies

Ref	Responder/Total no. of patients[a]			
	Molecular/ cytogenetic relapse	Haematologic relapse (CP)	Haematologic relapse (AP)	Total (%)
13	11/11 (100)	8/14 (57)	1/5 (20)	20/30 (66)
14	3/3 (100)	25/34 (73)	5/18 (27)	33/42 (78)
15	–	–	6/8 (75)	–
16	–	NS	NS	26/39 (66)
17	14/17 (82)	39/53 (73)	1/14 (7)	54/84 (64)
18	8/8 (100)	9/10 (90)	2/4 (50)	19/22 (86)
19	6	12	NS	10/18 (55)
20	15/19 (79)		0/5 (0)	15/24 (62)
21	–	9/9 (100)	4/5 (80)	13/14 (93)
22	NS	NS	NS	19/23 (82)
23	16	23	9	67–91%[b]

[a] Percentages in parentheses. CP, chronic phase; AP, advanced phase; NS, not specified.
[b] Probability of cytogenetic response.

contradiction might be explained by the fact that the interval from transplant to DLI comprises the interval from transplant to diagnosis of relapse plus the interval from relapse to initiation of DLI. Despite the apparent discrepancy, both findings may suggest that the tumour burden at the time of relapse correlates with the probability of response.[13] Alternatively, they may reflect different tempos of disease in different patients, with those whose disease progresses relatively rapidly to haematologic relapse being relatively resistant to remission induction by DLI.

The type of donor cells used for DLI does not seem to correlate with response. A recent report has shown that the overall probability of achieving remission does not differ significantly between patients receiving leukocytes from HLA-matched volunteer unrelated donors (VUD) and patients transfused with cells from HLA-identical siblings (SIB).[25] This apparently contrasts with the observation that patients receiving a T-cell-depleted transplant respond better to DLI than those receiving a T-cell-replete allograft.[17] In fact, in the cited study, the VUD and SIB groups received a T-cell-depleted and T-cell-replete transplant respectively. The role of T-cell depletion has not been confirmed by others.[14]

In conclusion, the amount of disease and its kinetics remain the major factors influencing response to DLI. An important issue that remains to be addressed is whether advanced disease is refractory to the effect of DLI because leukaemic cells are intrinsically resistant to the effector T cells, as is widely documented for other tumours. Alternatively, an unfavourable ratio between donor T cells and recipient leukaemic cells could account for treatment failure.

Toxicity

The most frequent complication of DLI is acute and chronic GVHD. The overall incidence varies between 41%[17] and 60%,[14] and is similar for both acute and chronic GVHD. The incidence of acute GVHD is higher in patients receiving cells from HLA-matched unrelated donors than in those receiving cells from siblings. GVHD is closely correlated with disease response. Notably, one study has reported that only 8% of the patients who did not develop GVHD had responded to DLI.[26] Despite this association, there is evidence that complete remissions can be attained with minimal or no GVHD, and no difference in the GVL effect has been demonstrated when using VUD or SIB donor cells.[25] These findings support the concept that biological GVH/GVL does not necessarily produce the disease (clinical GVHD).[17,18]

DLI can also produce as a side-effect a pancytopenia of variable intensity, which, in some cases, is irreversible and requires the infusion of donor stem cells. This event is related to the donor anti-recipient immune response, which kills host stem cells and thus causes bone marrow failure. However, pancytopenia does not correlate with GVHD. Aplasia occurs almost exclusively in patients who were treated in florid chronic phase or in advanced disease where donor haematopoiesis is low or absent. In fact, a correlation has been found between bone marrow failure and lack of residual donor haematopoiesis.[27] The lack of donor haematopoiesis is also more important as a predictor of aplasia than the assessment of BCR/ABL-positive haematopoiesis.

Administration regimen

Donor lymphocytes were initially administered in single 'bulk' doses containing variable numbers of CD3+ T cells (bulk dose regimen, BDR) depending on the collection. This regimen is still in use, and is associated with a high incidence of acute and chronic GVHD as described before. In order to circumvent this problem, the Memorial Sloan-Kettering transplant group proposed to transfuse donor cells in multiple aliquots by escalating the cell dose until a remission was achieved (escalating dose regimen, EDR).[18] This approach was based on the observation that a proportion of responders do not experience GVHD, thus suggesting that the GVL effect can be separated from GVHD. Using this regimen, they noticed that a substantial GVL effect could be achieved with relatively small doses of lymphocytes and that the incidence and severity of GVHD could be minimized. The obvious conclusion was that the chance of developing GVHD post DLI is correlated with the use of high cell doses. A recent study from the Hammersmith transplant group has compared the response rate and the incidence of GVHD in patients treated with DLI according to an EDR or a BDR. They confirmed that the GVL effect is similar with the two administration regimens, but the incidence and severity of GVHD is much reduced using EDR. Interestingly, they found that the incidence of acute and chronic GVHD associated with EDR is low – not because the final cell dose is small, but because lymphocytes are administered over a period of months.[23] A possible explanation for these findings is that the initial low dose or doses of donor cells that are insufficient for a GVL effect are 'anergized' by recipient tissues and thereby reduce the capacity of the subsequent higher dose or doses to produce GVHD.[28] The hypothesis of a cell population with a suppressor function capable of downregulating GVHD has been postulated also in a preclinical model of bone marrow transplantation.[29] Alternatively, the EDR protocol might produce less GVHD because the high cell doses are infused late after transplant. In this regard, delayed administration of donor splenocytes in a murine model of allogeneic bone marrow transplantation greatly reduces the incidence and severity of GVHD.[30] Notably, four studies have adopted the EDR protocol, with different intervals between infusions;[18,19–21,23] regardless of the cell dose administered, the lowest incidence of GVHD was observed in the study where DLI were given at a longer interval.[23]

Effective cell dose

The course of CML is characterized by three different phases with different disease activity and variable tumour burden. Identification of the minimal effective cell dose (ECD) required to achieve remission in each phase would be desirable. Since responsiveness to DLI correlates with the disease phase at the time of treatment, it would be sensible to believe that the ECD is also correlated with the leukaemic cell number. In vivo studies conducted in animal models have shown that the balance between recipient leukaemic cells and donor effector cells[31,32] is probably the main factor in determining the efficacy of the antileukaemic response after bone marrow transplant. A preliminary study from the Hammersmith transplant group does not seem to support this view. Although they found that there is a dose–response effect, the ECD does not correlate with disease stage and thus with the leukaemic burden. However, the ECD is lower for VUD than for SIB recipients. Therefore the multiple non-MHC mismatches, which are more extensive in donor–recipient pairs when a VUD is used, may play a major role in determining the efficacy of donor lymphocytes and influencing the ECD.[33]

Durability of response

Although DLI are highly effective in restoring remission in patients who relapse after allogeneic SCT for CML, the durability of these remissions is not yet known. The very few data generated so far are inconclusive, since the definition of remission has not been consistent and therefore the final outcome for patients achieving different levels of remission can be significantly different. Porter and colleagues[16] recently reported a long-term follow-up (median time 40 months) of 39 patients with relapsed CML treated with DLI. Only 13% of the patients achieving a cytogenetic remission subsequently relapsed. A more recent report[24] has assessed the long-term outcome of 66 consecutive patients receiving DLI for CML in relapse after allografting. The probability of attaining molecular remission was 68% at 3 years post DLI. For the majority of patients (70%) who achieved molecular remission, its duration exceeded the duration of remission after the original transplant procedure. Whether these remissions are durable because the disease has been eradicated or because of the continuous immune surveillance by donor T cells on leukaemia remains to be elucidated. Studies conducted using gene-marked donor T-cell lines to treat post-transplant viral diseases have shown that donor T cells can be detected at least 18 months after infusion, and can be recruited again in the case of viral reactivation.[34] It has been observed that some patients may respond only transiently to DLI,[33] thus suggesting either that donor lymphocytes can be effective only for a limited period of time or that donor T lymphocytes are anergized by the tumour cells.[35]

HOW TO TACKLE GVHD

GVHD is a potentially threatening complication of DLI. Multiple efforts have been made in order to prevent or minimize this problem. A very simple and convenient solution has been to administer donor cells in escalating doses, thus avoiding unnecessary high cell doses potentially associated with GVHD. The merits and demerits of such an approach have been discussed above.

Other strategies are based on the in vitro manipulation of donor lymphocytes prior to infusion into patients. Data from both mice and humans[36,37] have suggested that CD8+ cytotoxic/suppressor T lymphocytes contain most of the effector T cells responsible for GVHD but not for GVL. The Houston group has pursued this hypothesis and used CD8-depleted DLI. These in vitro selected lymphocytes seem to reduce the risk of GVHD without affecting GVL activity.[20,38]

An alternative method to deplete potentially harmful cells has been developed independently by two groups.[39–41] Donor alloreactive

T cells are specifically activated in vitro by recipient cells and selectively depleted using an antibody specific for the α-chain of the interleukin-2 (IL-2) receptor (CD25), which is expressed by activated T cells. $CD25^+$ cells are then removed either by virtue of a toxin bound to the antibody[39,41] or by immunomagnetic separation.[40] In vitro functional studies have shown that this technique efficiently removes alloreactive cells, while preserving antileukaemic and antiviral cytotoxic responses.[41] Based on the same principle, a group from Boston has developed a similar approach in clinical bone marrow transplantation. They showed that donor T cells can be specifically anergized in vitro to recipient mononuclear cells by CTLA-4-Ig, an inhibitor of B7-CD28-mediated co-stimulation. This ex vivo procedure was performed on donor bone marrow preparation prior to infusion in 12 transplants mismatched for one HLA haplotype. All 11 evaluable patients engrafted, and only 3 had GVHD.[42]

A very elegant procedure has also been proposed, which involves the use of a suicide gene. Suicide genes code for enzymes that render cells sensitive to otherwise non-toxic compounds. The thymidine kinase encoded by the herpes simplex virus type 1 (HSV-Tk) converts ganciclovir into a metabolite that inhibits DNA elongation.[43] This event, which does not occur in normal cells, leads to cell death. This approach has been exploited to control the DLI-induced GVHD by transducing the HSV-Tk gene into donor T lymphocytes prior to infusion into the patient.[44,45] However, this technique is not free of problems. In fact, in some cases, a strong immune response has been detected against transduced lymphocytes, and the procedure does not apparently work in chronic GVHD.[46] Furthermore, ganciclovir cannot discriminate between the lymphocytes that mediate GVHD and the lymphocytes mediating GVL, thus potentially jeopardizing the therapeutic effect of DLI. Therefore this fascinating approach warrants further study to assess its true efficacy.

A very elegant approach has also been proposed based on blockade of MHC molecules with analogue peptides. Although conducted exclusively in murine models, these studies have shown the effectiveness of synthetic peptides in blocking MHC on antigen-presenting cells, and in preventing T-cell activation and GVHD.[47,48]

TIME TO TREAT: 'THE SOONER THE BETTER'?

We have mentioned above that molecular and cytogenetic relapses are more responsive to DLI than to haematologic relapse.[13] Therefore it seems reasonable to treat patients as soon as relapse has been recognized at the molecular level. However, there is still no consensus as to whether one should treat a patient in molecular relapse, because in some – though rare – cases, molecular relapses are only transient. The numbers of *BCR/ABL* transcripts assessed by sequential RT-PCR analysis at frequent intervals after transplant can guide a therapeutic decision.[8,49]

The use of techniques aimed at reducing the incidence of GVHD after allogeneic SCT is associated with a significantly higher relapse rate. Similarly, patients transplanted after non-myeloablative conditioning regimens are more likely to relapse than those receiving conventional preparation regimens. In these cases, the proposal to use prophylactic DLI treatment even before the molecular detection of relapse may deserve attention,[50] although a proper clinical trial is required to substantiate such a hypothesis.

ASSOCIATION OF DLI WITH OTHER TREATMENTS

Antiproliferative drugs

Patients who are treated in haematologic relapse often present with high white cell counts. It is conceivable that high numbers of proliferating leukaemic cells hinder the ability of donor T cells to be primed. Antiproliferative drugs capable of debulking the tumour burden might enhance the efficacy of DLI and/or reduce the cell dose required to achieve remission. However, the utility of such a complementary approach has to be demonstrated, and the intensity of the regimen is still a matter of debate. Furthermore, it is likely that drugs inhibiting cell cycling in general can also inhibit antigen-induced T-cell proliferation,[51] thus jeopardizing the GVL effect.

Steroids

Another situation that sometimes complicates the treatment of patients with DLI is when relapse is accompanied by immune haemolytic anaemia (IHA). The pathogenesis of IHA is unknown in most cases, but it can be related to the immune response of donor cells against the emerging recipient erythropoiesis or, alternatively, to the immune response of recipient cells against residual donor red cells. This hypothesis is consistent with the fact that response to DLI – which coincides with restoration of donor haematopoiesis – also cures the haemolysis. However, in some cases, the haemolysis is so severe as to require the use of steroids. It is unknown to what extent steroids affect donor lymphocytes and whether there is a dose that can be used safely.

Immune modulators

In theory, IL-2 might expand donor T cells infused with DLI and primed by the allogeneic leukaemic cells, enhance natural cell immunity amongst donor lymphocytes, and increase the survival of T cells infused in vivo.[52] It has been suggested that IL-2 could be a suitable adjuvant to circumvent DLI failures[53] in patients who are refractory to the DLI treatment or who respond only partially and/or transiently. It appears that its efficacy could be confined to patients with a very limited tumour burden.[54]

Some centres administer DLI with IFN-α since this molecule is supposed to enhance the immune response.[55] However, multivariate analyses of large groups of CML patients have failed to identify any difference in response rate,[14,17] as initially suggested by others.[12]

POTENTIAL TARGETS OF DLI

The specificity of donor T lymphocytes that recognize and eliminate leukaemic cells has remained elusive. Elimination of leukaemic cells is often associated with attack on normal cells in the skin, gut, liver, and bone marrow, resulting in GVHD and bone marrow aplasia. However, the notion that the clinical effects of DLI are mediated by distinct T-cell clones is supported by the observation that the elimination of leukaemic cells is not always associated with GVHD and/or bone marrow aplasia. Similarly, the linked occurrence of GVL and GVHD in most patients treated by DLI may reflect the simultaneous activity of two discrete donor T-cell populations with distinct specificities: T-cell clones specific for leukaemia antigens and T-cell clones specific for antigens of normal cells. Alternatively, the same population of donor T-cell clones specific for shared antigens expressed in leukaemic and normal cells may mediate both GVL and GVHD.

The GVL effect is exclusively a GVH effect

In the majority of cases, the stem cell allograft is matched for the MHC of the recipient. Therefore GVH and graft rejection are caused by disparities at the level of transplantation antigens that are not encoded by the MHC, namely the minor histocompatibility H antigens. Minor H antigens are polymorphic (generally bi-allelic) cell-derived self-peptides that are inherited independently of MHC. They are presented on the cell surface by MHC molecules[56] and are recognized by alloreactive T cells. That these molecules play a major role in allogeneic SCT has been suggested by the fact that mismatches for minor H antigens between donor and recipient have been found to correlate with GVHD.[57–60]

The reactivity of donor T cells against minor antigens on recipient tissues also supports the notion that minor H antigens may be the major target of the GVL effect. Although this would argue against the possibility of separating GVH from GVL, some minor H antigens appear to exhibit a restricted tissue distribution.[61–64] The minor H antigens HA-1 and HA-2 appear to be expressed exclusively on haematopoietic cells. HA-1- and HA-2-specific cytotoxic T lymphocytes have recently been generated using synthetic peptides that efficiently lyse leukaemic cells but not skin fibroblasts. They might be used to treat leukaemia relapses after allogeneic bone marrow transplantation with low risk of GVHD.[64,65] However, it is unclear why these 'leukaemia-specific' mHA have been found to induce high levels of specific T cells in patients developing acute GVHD.[66]

Evidence for leukaemia-specific immune response

Numerous attempts have been made to identify leukaemia-specific antigens. Although no evidence of such specificity has been provided, the bulk of studies have led investigators to focus on a restricted number of targets.

The CML-specific Ph chromosomal translocation leads to the formation of a fusion peptide that is unique to the leukaemic cells. For a long time, the BCR/ABL fusion protein has been considered as an ideal target for CML-specific T-cell responses, because sequences covering the fusion region of BCR/ABL are only present in leukaemic but not in normal cells. It has been demonstrated that some synthetic peptides spanning the BCR/ABL fusion region are capable of binding to HLA-A3, -A11, and -B8 molecules[67,68] and can induce a specific T-cell response.[69–72] A very recent multicentre case–control study comparing patients with CML with unaffected individuals may support the view that presentation of BCR/ABL breakpoint peptides in these HLA molecules can induce a protective immune response.[73] In fact, the results have indicated that HLA-B8, especially when co-expressed with HLA-A3, is associated with a diminished incidence of CML. Similar results have suggested positive and negative associations between certain HLA-DRB1 alleles and CML.[74] However, restrictions in the natural antigen processing pathways are likely to limit the usefulness of BCR/ABL fusion peptides. In order to serve as targets for cytotoxic and helper T lymphocytes, it is essential that the MHC class I and class II antigen processing pathways produce relevant fusion peptides and that these peptides can bind efficiently to the groove of HLA class I and class II molecules. Failure to produce relevant peptide epitopes and lack of efficient binding to HLA molecules are likely to confine T-cell responses to a limited number of patients expressing HLA alleles that are particular suitable for the high-affinity binding of BCR/ABL fusion peptides produced by natural processing.

Along this line, another interesting strategy to generate leukaemia-specific T cells has come from the use of dendritic cells. These are the most potent antigen-presenting cells for initiation of primary immune responses, and have been used as adjuvants for cancer vaccines.[75] CML dendritic cells belong to the leukaemic clone, and as such they are potentially capable of presenting endogenously derived tumour peptides. In fact, dendritic cells generated from the peripheral blood cells of CML patients can stimulate autologous T cells to mount a leukaemia-specific immune response. These T cells exhibit vigorous proliferative and cytotoxic activity against CML cells but low reactivity to allogeneic normal cells.[76] Although promising, this observation has not been confirmed by others.

NEW TRENDS IN THE IMMUNOTHERAPY OF CML

Taken together, the manifestations of GVHD and/or GVL are probably determined by the relative prevalence of donor T-lymphocyte clones with three distinct specificities. T-cell clones specific for antigens of normal cells will cause GVHD, and clones specific for antigens shared between normal and leukaemic cells will cause GVHD and GVL. To further improve the existing immunotherapy of CML, it is essential to dissociate GVL and GVHD by defining the specificity of infused T lymphocytes. The challenge is to identify leukaemia-associated antigens suitable to direct T-cell responses selectively against CML cells without causing damage to normal cells.

The notion that proteins encoded by mutated genes are not commonly recognized by tumour-specific cytotoxic T lymphocytes (CTL) is supported by studies in melanoma patients. It has been shown that peptide epitopes derived from mutated genes can trigger melanoma-specific CTL responses in individual patients.[77] However, these responses are frequently case reports, and they are not commonly detected in a large number of melanoma patients. In contrast, CTL responses against differentiation antigens that are expressed at high levels in melanoma cells are commonly detected in most melanoma patients.[78] Patients expressing different HLA alleles present different peptide epitopes from the same differentiation antigen. Thus immune responses against these antigens are not limited to a specific peptide epitope containing a particular mutation. Consequently, CTL responses are much less confined by restrictions of natural antigen processing pathways and by HLA binding preferences. This hypothesis has been exploited to raise CML-specific CTL against a peptide derived from the primary granule enzyme proteinase-3.[79] These CTL showed HLA-restricted colony inhibition of CML cells – which overexpress proteinase-3 – but were ineffective on normal haematopoietic cells.

Whether haematopoietic differentiation antigens that are expressed at elevated levels in leukaemia can serve as targets for leukaemia-specific CTL responses is currently being explored. In contrast to melanocyte-specific differentiation antigens that are expressed only in a limited number of normal melanocytes, haematopoietic-specific antigens are more widely expressed in cells of the haematopoietic lineage. Thus most haematopoietic differentiation antigens are probably accessible to developing T cells, leading to the establishment of T-cell tolerance by deletion in the thymus or by post-thymic tolerance mechanisms in the periphery. However, based on the observation that tolerance is self MHC-restricted, an approach to circumvent CTL tolerance has recently been developed. It has been shown that responder lymphocytes from healthy donors can be immunized in vitro to generate CTL responses against selected peptide epitopes derived from normal cellular proteins presented in the context of allogeneic MHC molecules.[80–82] Such allo-restricted CTL can selectively kill tumour cells expressing elevated levels of a chosen cellular protein, but not normal cells with physiologic levels of protein expression. Therefore the allo-restricted CTL approach is ideally suited to: (i) identify CTL-recognized peptide epitopes in haematopoietic differentiation antigens; (ii) test whether the CTL selectively kill leukaemic cells expressing elevated levels of the antigen; (iii) explore whether the identified epitopes can be used to activate autologous, leukaemia-specific CTL responses.

The Wilms' tumour antigen 1 (WT1) has been used to explore these points. WT1 is a transcription factor that is expressed in several embryonic tissues and is involved in normal development and differentiation. Targeted deletion of WT1 in knockout mice is embryonically lethal because of a failure to develop normal kidneys. After birth, WT1 is switched off in most tissues, except for some cells of mesenchymal origin, including renal podocytes, testicular Sertoli cells, and ovarian granulosa cells. Interestingly, WT1 is also expressed in $CD34^+$ haematopoietic stem cells.[83] Differentiation of haematopoietic stem cells is associated with WT1 downregulation.[84] Consequently, mature white and red blood cells do not express this molecule. Studies in leukaemia patients suffering from acute myeloid or lymphoblastic leukaemia or from blast-crisis CML have demonstrated elevated levels of WT1 expression.[85] Furthermore, it has been shown that WT1 is selectively overexpressed in $CD34^+$ progenitor cells of CML patients but not in mature

$CD34^-$ mononuclear cells. Thus WT1 is an ideal target antigen to direct CTL responses selectively against $CD34^+$ leukaemic progenitor cells. There is good evidence that the $CD34^+$ cell population contains the leukaemic stem cells, and that immunologic responses against $CD34^+$ cells are associated with remission in CML patients treated with DLI.

Evidence that the leukaemic stem cells are $CD34^+$ comes from transfer experiments into SCID/NOD mice, showing that the leukaemia-initiating cells are present in purified $CD34^+$ populations isolated from CML patients.[86,87] The evidence that immune responses against $CD34^+$ cells are beneficial stems from a study of CML patients who relapsed after allogeneic bone marrow transplantation and were treated by DLI. It was shown that CTL responses against $CD34^+$ cells were associated with remission, while CTL responses against more mature $CD34^-$ mononuclear cells were not associated with a favourable clinical response.[88] However, the antigens that might direct CTL responses against leukaemic $CD34^+$ progenitor cells have not been identified in this study.

Using the allo-restricted CTL approach, it was possible to identify CTL epitopes in the WT1 protein. The CTL were generated against peptide epitopes presented by the HLA-A0201 class I molecule, an allele that is expressed by nearly 50% of Caucasian individuals. Two distinct HLA-A0201-presented peptide epitopes from the WT1 protein were identified as CTL target epitopes. CTL specific for these epitopes killed leukaemic cell lines expressing WT1, but not control cells that did not express this protein.

Preclinical in vitro experimentation has yielded exciting results.[89] CTL specific for WT1 epitopes were found to kill $CD34^+$ stem cell populations isolated from CML patients. As expected, $CD34^+$ cells from HLA-A0201-negative patients were not recognized. The most promising observation was made when WT1-specific CTL were tested against normal $CD34^+$ cells from healthy HLA-A0201-positive adult donors or from cord blood. No killing of normal haematopoietic progenitor cells was detectable. Colony-forming assays with $CD34^+$ cells from CML patients revealed that the CTL eliminated between 80% and 100% of clonogenic progenitors of the erythrocyte, monocyte, and granulocyte lineages. The clonogenic progenitors of normal $CD34^+$ cells were not affected by WT1-specific CTL.

These results show that WT1 can serve as target for CTL with exquisite specificity for leukaemic $CD34^+$ progenitors. This suggests that adoptive transfer of these CTL would selectively eliminate leukaemic progenitors without causing damage to normal progenitors or mature cells of the haematopoietic lineage. Furthermore, since WT1 is only expressed at low levels in a relatively small number of cells in other tissues (e.g. renal podocytes, testicular Sertoli cells, and ovarian granulosa cells), it is unlikely that adoptive therapy with WT1-specific CTL would cause damage to these tissues or trigger GVHD. This prediction was tested in a murine model. Infusion of WT1-specific CTL into partially myeloablated recipients did not cause GVHD or kidney damage. Importantly, the CTL infusion did not interfere with haematopoietic recovery, indicating that the functional activity of haematopoietic stem cells was unaffected. These in vivo experiments suggest that WT1-specific CTL may be able to mount a highly selective attack against leukaemic progenitor cells, resulting in strong GVL without GVHD.[89]

It is not yet known whether CTL specific for the identified HLA-A0201 epitopes of WT1 are present in the autologous T-cell repertoire. Since WT1 is switched off in the majority of cells in postnatal life, it is likely that autologous CTL are not deleted during thymic T-cell selection or rendered tolerant in the periphery. A recent study demonstrated lack of tolerance to a WT1-derived peptide epitope presented in the context of HLA-A24 class I molecules.[90] It was possible to isolate WT1-specific CTL by in vitro stimulation of T lymphocytes from HLA-A24-positive normal donors. Whether such CTL are present in leukaemia patients, and whether they can be activated, has not yet been explored.

Adoptive therapy with WT1-specific CTL remains an attractive treatment option, particularly if autologous CTL responses are ineffective. Murine experiments have demonstrated that the infusion of allo-restricted CTL from MHC-mismatched donors is feasible.[80] The experiments involved CTL specific for a peptide epitope of the MDM2 protein that is frequently overexpressed in tumours but also expressed at low levels in normal tissues. When given at the time of bone marrow transplantation, the CTL were detectable for at least 14 weeks post injection. They maintained their peptide-specific killing activity, and did not cause GVHD.

CONCLUSIONS

The efficacy of DLI in restoring remission in patients with CML in relapse after allografting has paved the way to exploring new approaches of adoptive immunotherapy in order to minimize the risk of GVHD. Different methodologies have successfully been proposed to eliminate alloreactive donor T cells, but the major challenge is to generate leukaemia-specific T cells. The results derived from preclinical models suggest that allo-restricted CTL specific for HLA-A0201-presented WT1 peptides is safe and may mediate lasting protection against leukaemic relapse. Future experiments will show whether further peptide epitopes can also be extended to patients with other malignancies expressing WT1.

REFERENCES

1. Clift R, Anasetti C, Allografting for chronic myeloid leukemia. *Baillière's Clin Haematol* 1997; **10:** 319-36.
2. Hansen JA, Gooley TA, Martin PJ et al, Bone marrow transplants from unrelated donors for patients with chronic myeloid leukemia. *N Engl J Med* 1998; **338:** 962–8.
3. Gratwohl A, Hermans J, Goldman JM et al, Risk assessment for patients with chronic myeloid leukaemia before allogeneic blood or marrow transplantation. Chronic Leukemia Working Party of the European Group for Blood and Marrow Transplantation. *Lancet* 1998; **352:** 1087–92.
4. Goldman JM, Gale RP, Horowitz MM et al, Bone marrow transplantation for chronic myelogenous leukemia in chronic phase. Increased risk for relapse associated with T-cell depletion. *Ann Intern Med* 1988; **108:** 806–14.
5. Fefer A, Sullivan KM, Weiden P et al, Graft versus leukemia effect in man: the relapse rate of acute leukemia is lower after allogeneic than after syngeneic marrow transplantation. *Prog Clin Biol Res* 1987; **244:** 401–8.
6. Irschick EU, Hladik F, Niederwieser D et al, Studies on the mechanism of tolerance or graft-versus-host disease in allogeneic bone marrow recipients at the level of cytotoxic T-cell precursor frequencies. *Blood* 1992; **79:** 1622–8.
7. Nierle T, Bunjes D, Arnold R et al, Quantitative assessment of posttransplant host-specific interleukin-2-secreting T-helper cell precursors in patients with and without acute graft-versus-host disease after allogeneic HLA-identical sibling bone marrow transplantation. *Blood* 1993; **81:** 841–8.
8. Lin F, van Rhee F, Goldman JM, Cross NC, Kinetics of increasing BCR–ABL transcript numbers in chronic myeloid leukemia patients who relapse after bone marrow transplantation. *Blood* 1996; **87:** 4473–8.
9. Clift R, Goldman J, Gratwohl A, Horowitz M, Proposals for standardized reporting of results of bone marrow transplantation for leukaemia. *Bone Marrow Transplant* 1989; **4:** 445–8.
10. Arcese W, Goldman JM, D'Arcangelo E et al, Outcome for patients who relapse after allogeneic bone marrow transplantation for chronic myeloid leukemia. Chronic Leukemia Working Party. European Bone Marrow Transplantation Group. *Blood* 1993; **82:** 3211–19
11. Higano CS, Chielens D, Raskind W et al, Use of alpha-2a-interferon to treat cytogenetic relapse of chronic myeloid leukemia after marrow transplantation. *Blood* 1997; **90:** 2549–54.
12. Kolb HJ, Mittermuller J, Clemm C et al, Donor leukocyte transfusions for treatment of recurrent chronic myelogenous leukemia in marrow transplant patients. *Blood* 1990; **76:** 2462–5.
13. van Rhee F, Lin F, Cullis JO et al, Relapse of chronic myeloid leukemia after allogeneic bone marrow transplant: the case for giving donor

leukocyte transfusions before the onset of hematologic relapse. *Blood* 1994; **83:** 3377–83.

14. Collins RH Jr, Shpilberg O, Drobyski WR et al, Donor leukocyte infusions in 140 patients with relapsed malignancy after allogeneic bone marrow transplantation. *J Clin Oncol* 1997; **15:** 433–44.
15. Drobyski WR, Keever CA, Roth MS et al, Salvage immunotherapy using donor leukocyte infusions as treatment for relapsed chronic myelogenous leukemia after allogeneic bone marrow transplantation: efficacy and toxicity of a defined T cell dose. *Blood* 1993; **82:** 2310–18.
16. Porter DL, Collins RH Jr, Shpilberg O et al, Long-term follow-up of patients who achieved complete remission after donor leukocyte infusions. *Biol Blood Marrow Transplant* 1999; **5:** 253–61.
17. Kolb HJ, Schattenberg A, Goldman JM et al, Graft-versus-leukemia effect of donor lymphocyte transfusions in marrow grafted patients. European Group for Blood and Marrow Transplantation Working Party Chronic Leukemia. *Blood* 1995; **86:** 2041–50.
18. Mackinnon S, Papadopoulos EB, Carabasi MH et al, Adoptive immunotherapy evaluating escalating doses of donor leukocytes for relapse of chronic myeloid leukemia after bone marrow transplantation: separation of graft-versus-leukemia responses from graft-versus-host disease. *Blood* 1995; **86:** 1261–8.
19. Bacigalupo A, Soracco M, Vassallo F et al, Donor lymphocyte infusions (DLI) in patients with chronic myeloid leukemia following allogeneic bone marrow transplantation. *Bone Marrow Transplant* 1997; **19:** 927–32.
20. Alyea EP, Soiffer RJ, Canning C et al, Toxicity and efficacy of defined doses of CD4+ donor lymphocytes for treatment of relapse after allogeneic bone marrow transplant. *Blood* 1998; **91:** 3671–80.
21. Verdonck LF, Petersen EJ, Lokhorst HM et al, Donor leukocyte infusions for recurrent hematologic malignancies after allogeneic bone marrow transplantation: impact of infused and residual donor T cells. *Bone Marrow Transplant* 1998; **22:** 1057–63.
22. Sehn LH, Alyea EP, Weller E et al, Comparative outcomes of T-cell-depleted and non-T-cell-depleted allogeneic bone marrow transplantation for chronic myelogenous leukemia: impact of donor lymphocyte infusion. *J Clin Oncol* 1999; **17:** 561–8.
23. Dazzi F, Szydlo RM, Craddock C et al, Comparison of single-dose and escalating-dose regimens of donor lymphocyte infusion for relapse after allografting for chronic myeloid leukemia. *Blood* 2000; **95:** 67–71.
24. Dazzi F, Szydlo RM, Craddock C et al, Durability of responses following donor lymphocyte infusions for patients who relapse after allogeneic stem cell transplantation for chronic myeloid leukemia. *Blood* 2000; **96**: 2712–16.
25. van Rhee F, Savage D, Blackwell J et al, Adoptive immunotherapy for relapse of chronic myeloid leukemia after allogeneic bone marrow transplant: equal efficacy of lymphocytes from sibling and matched unrelated donors. *Bone Marrow Transplant* 1998; **21:** 1055–61.
26. Mackinnon S, Papadopoulos EB, Carabasi MH et al, Adoptive immunotherapy using donor leukocytes following bone marrow transplantation for chronic myeloid leukemia: Is T cell dose important in determining biological response? *Bone Marrow Transplant* 1995; **15:** 591–4.
27. Keil F, Haas OA, Fritsch G et al, Donor leukocyte infusion for leukemic relapse after allogeneic marrow transplantation: lack of residual donor hematopoiesis predicts aplasia. *Blood* 1997; **89:** 3113–17.
28. Lombardi G, Sidhu S, Batchelor R, Lechler RI, Anergic T cells as suppressor cells in vitro. *Science* 1994; **264:** 1587–9.
29. van Bekkum DW, Kinwel-Bohre EPM, Risk of donor lymphocyte infusions following allogeneic bone marrow transplantation. *Exp Hematol* 1987; **25:** 478–80.
30. Johnson BD, Truitt RL, Delayed infusion of immunocompetent donor cells after bone marrow transplantation breaks graft-host tolerance allows for persistent antileukemic reactivity without severe graft-versus-host disease. *Blood* 1995; **85:** 3302–12.
31. Aizawa S, Kamisaku H, Sado T, Possible induction of graft-versus-leukemia effect against a leukemia refractory to antileukemia response in ordinary MHC-compatible, allogeneic bone marrow transplantation. *Transplantation* 1998; **65:** 893–8.
32. Zeis M, Uharek L, Glass B et al, Eradication of residual disease by administration of leukemia-specific T cells after experimental allogeneic bone marrow transplantation. *Exp Hematol* 1998; **26:** 1068–73.
33. Dazzi F, Raanani P, van Rhee F et al, Responses

to donor lymphocyte infusion (DLI) in CML patients in relapse after BMT may be partial and transient: further evidence for a dose–response effect. *Blood* 1997; **90:** 518 (abst).

34. Heslop HE, Ng CY, Li C et al, Long-term restoration of immunity against Epstein–Barr virus infection by adoptive transfer of gene-modified virus-specific T lymphocytes. *Nature Med* 1996; **2:** 551–5.
35. Antonia SJ, Extermann M, Flavell RA, Immunologic nonresponsiveness to tumors. *Crit Rev Oncog* 1998; **9:** 35–41.
36. Nimer SD, Giorgi J, Gajewski JL et al, Selective depletion of CD8$^+$ cells for prevention of graft-versus-host disease after bone marrow transplantation. A randomized controlled trial. *Transplantation* 1994; **57:** 82–7.
37. Korngold R, Sprent J, T cell subsets and graft-versus-host disease. *Transplantation* 1987; **44:** 335–9.
38. Giralt S, Hester J, Huh Y et al, CD8-depleted donor lymphocyte infusion as treatment for relapsed chronic myelogenous leukemia after allogeneic bone marrow transplantation. *Blood* 1995; **86:** 4337–43.
39. Mavroudis DA, Dermime S, Molldrem J et al, Specific depletion of alloreactive T cells in HLA-identical siblings: a method for separating graft-versus-host and graft-versus-leukaemia reactions. *Br J Haematol* 1998; **101:** 565–70.
40. Garderet L, Snell V, Przepiorka D et al, Effective depletion of alloreactive lymphocytes from peripheral blood mononuclear cell preparations. *Transplantation* 1999; **67:** 124–30.
41. Montagna D, Yvon E, Calcaterra V et al, Depletion of alloreactive T cells by a specific anti-interleukin-2 receptor p55 chain immunotoxin does not impair in vitro antileukemia and antiviral activity. *Blood* 1999; **93:** 3550–7.
42. Guinan EC, Boussiotis VA, Neuberg D et al, Transplantation of anergic histoincompatible bone marrow allografts. *N Engl J Med* 1999; **340:** 1704–14.
43. St Clair MH, Richards CA, Spector T et al, 3'-Azido-3'-deoxythymidine triphosphate as an inhibitor and substrate of purified human immunodeficiency virus reverse transcriptase. *Antimicrob Agents Chemother* 1987; **31:** 1972–7.
44. Tiberghien P, Reynolds CW, Keller J et al, Ganciclovir treatment of herpes simplex thymidine kinase-transduced primary T lymphocytes: an approach for specific in vivo donor T-cell depletion after bone marrow transplantation? *Blood* 1994; **84:** 1333–41.
45. Bonini C, Ferrari G, Verzeletti S et al, HSV-TK gene transfer into donor lymphocytes for control of allogeneic graft-versus-leukemia. *Science* 1997; **276:** 1719–24.
46. Verzeletti S, Bonini C, Marktel S et al, Herpes simplex virus thymidine kinase gene transfer for controlled graft-versus-host disease and graft-versus-leukemia: clinical follow-up and improved new vectors. *Hum Gene Ther* 1998; **9:** 2243–51.
47. Schlegel PG, Aharoni R, Smilek DE et al, Prevention of graft-versus-host disease by peptides binding to class II major histocompatibility complex molecules. *Blood* 1994; **84:** 2802–10.
48. Schlegel PG, Aharoni R, Chen Y et al, A synthetic random basic copolymer with promiscuous binding to class II major histocompatibility complex molecules inhibits T-cell proliferative responses to major and minor histocompatibility antigens in vitro and confers the capacity to prevent murine graft-versus-host disease in vivo. *Proc Natl Acad Sci USA* 1996; **93:** 5061–6 [Erratum 93: 8796].
49. Olavarria E, Kaeda J, Carnicero F et al, Early detection of BCR–ABL transcripts by RT-PCR predicts outcome after allogeneic stem cell transplantation for chronic myeloid leukemia. *Blood* 1999; **94:** 632 (abst).
50. Barrett AJ, Mavroudis D, Tisdale J et al, T cell-depleted bone marrow transplantation and delayed T cell add-back to control acute GVHD and conserve a graft-versus-leukemia effect. *Bone Marrow Transplant* 1998; **21:** 543–51.
51. Pierson BA, Miller JS, CD56+bright and CD56+dim natural killer cells in patients with chronic myelogenous leukemia progressively decrease in number, respond less to stimuli that recruit clonogenic natural killer cells, and exhibit decreased proliferation on a per cell basis. *Blood* 1996; **88:** 2279–87.
52. Cheever MA, Chen W, Therapy with cultured T cells: principles revisited. *Immunol Rev* 1997; **157:** 177–94.
53. Slavin S, Naparstek E, Nagler A et al, Allogeneic cell therapy with donor peripheral blood cells and recombinant human interleukin-2 to treat leukemia relapse after allogeneic bone marrow transplantation. *Blood* 1996; **87:** 2195–204.
54. Dazzi F, Kaeda J, Kanfer E et al, Interleukin-2 may induce complete remission in patients who

respond only partially to donor lymphocyte infusion (DLI) for relapse following allogeneic bone marrow transplantation. *Br J Haematol* 1998; **102:** 287 (abst).

55. Oka T, Sastry KJ, Nehete P et al, Evidence for specific immune response against p210 BCR–ABL in long term remission CML patients treated with interferon. *Leukemia* 1998; **12:** 155–63.
56. Wallny HJ, Rammensee HG, Identification of classical minor histocompatibility antigen as cell-derived peptide. *Nature* 1990; **343:** 275–8.
57. den Haan JM, Meadows LM, Wang W et al, The minor histocompatibility antigen HA-1: a diallelic gene with a single amino acid polymorphism. *Science* 1998; **279:** 1054–7.
58. den Haan JM, Bontrop RE, Pool J et al, Conservation of minor histocompatibility antigens between human and non-human primates. *Eur J Immunol* 1996; **26:** 2680–5.
59. Goulmy E, Schipper R, Pool J et al, Mismatches of minor histocompatibility antigens between HLA-identical donors and recipients and the development of graft-versus-host disease after bone marrow transplantation. *N Engl J Med* 1996; **334:** 281–5.
60. den Haan JM, Sherman NE, Blokland E et al, Identification of a graft versus host disease-associated human minor histocompatibility antigen. *Science* 1995; **268:** 1476–80.
61. Dolstra H, Fredrix H, Preijers F et al, Recognition of a B cell leukemia-associated minor histocompatibility antigen by CTL. *J Immunol* 1997; **158:** 560–5.
62. de Bueger M, Bakker A, van Rood JJ et al, Tissue distribution of human minor histocompatibility antigens. Ubiquitous versus restricted tissue distribution indicates heterogeneity among human cytotoxic T lymphocyte-defined non-MHC antigens. *J Immunol* 1992; **149:** 1788–94.
63. Warren EH, Greenberg PD, Riddell SR, Cytotoxic T-lymphocyte-defined human minor histocompatibility antigens with a restricted tissue distribution. *Blood* 1998; **91:** 2197–207.
64. Dolstra H, Fredrix H, Maas F et al, A human minor histocompatibility antigen specific for B cell acute lymphoblastic leukemia. *J Exp Med* 1999; **189:** 301–8.
65. Mutis T, Verdijk R, Schrama E, Esendam B, Brand A, Goulmy E, Feasibility of immunotherapy of relapsed leukemia with ex vivo-generated cytotoxic T lymphocytes specific for hematopoietic system-restricted minor histocompatibility antigens. *Blood* 1999; **93:** 2336–41.
66. Mutis T, Gillespie G, Schrama E et al, Tetrameric HLA class I-minor histocompatibility antigen peptide complexes demonstrate minor histocompatibility antigen-specific cytotoxic T lymphocytes in patients with graft-versus-host disease. *Nature Med* 1999; **5:** 839–42.
67. Cullis JO, Barrett AJ, Goldman JM, Lechler RI, Binding of BCR/ABL junctional peptides to major histocompatibility complex (MHC) class I molecules: studies in antigen-processing defective cell lines. *Leukemia* 1994; **8:** 165–70.
68. Bocchia M, Wentworth PA, Southwood S et al, Specific binding of leukemia oncogene fusion protein peptides to HLA class I molecules. *Blood* 1995; **85:** 2680–4.
69. Bocchia M, Korontsvit T, Xu Q et al, Specific human cellular immunity to bcr–abl oncogene-derived peptides. *Blood* 1996; **87:** 3587–92.
70. Bosch GJ, Joosten AM, Kessler JH et al, Recognition of BCR–ABL positive leukemic blasts by human $CD4^+$ T cells elicited by primary in vitro immunization with a BCR–ABL breakpoint peptide. *Blood* 1996; **88:** 3522–7.
71. Pawelec G, Max H, Halder T et al, BCR/ABL leukemia oncogene fusion peptides selectively bind to certain HLA-DR alleles and can be recognized by T cells found at low frequency in the repertoire of normal donors. *Blood* 1996; **88:** 2118–24.
72. Buzyn A, Ostankovitch M, Zerbib A et al, Peptides derived from the whole sequence of BCR–ABL bind to several class I molecules allowing specific induction of human cytotoxic T lymphocytes. *Eur J Immunol* 1997; **27:** 2066–72.
73. Posthuma EF, Falkenburg JH, Apperley JF et al, HLA-B8 and HLA-A3 coexpressed with HLA-B8 are associated with a reduced risk of the development of chronic myeloid leukemia. The Chronic Leukemia Working Party of the EBMT. *Blood* 1999; **93:** 3863–5.
74. Yasukawa M, Ohminami H, Kojima K et al, Analysis of HLA-DRB1 alleles in Japanese patients with chronic myelogenous leukemia. *Am J Hematol* 2000; **63:** 99–101.
75. Celluzzi CM, Mayordomo JI, Storkus WJ et al, Peptide-pulsed dendritic cells induce antigen-specific CTL-mediated protective tumor immunity. *J Exp Med* 1996; **183:** 283–7.
76. Choudhury A, Gajewski JL, Liang JC et al, Use of leukemic dendritic cells for the generation of antileukemic cellular cytotoxicity against

Philadelphia chromosome-positive chronic myelogenous leukemia. *Blood* 1997; **89:** 1133–42.
77. Chiari R, Foury F, De Plaen E et al, Two antigens recognized by autologous cytolytic T lymphocytes on a melanoma result from a single point mutation in an essential housekeeping gene. *Cancer Res* 1999; **59:** 5785–92.
78. Boon T, Coulie PG, Van den EB, Tumor antigens recognized by T cells. *Immunol Today* 1997; **18:** 267–8.
79. Molldrem JJ, Clave E, Jiang YZ et al, Cytotoxic T lymphocytes specific for a nonpolymorphic proteinase 3 peptide preferentially inhibit chronic myeloid leukemia colony-forming units. *Blood* 1997; **90:** 2529–34.
80. Sadovnikova E, Stauss HJ, Peptide-specific cytotoxic T lymphocytes restricted by nonself major histocompatibility complex class I molecules: reagents for tumor immunotherapy. *Proc Natl Acad Sci USA* 1996; **93**: 13114–18.
81. Sadovnikova E, Jopling LA, Soo KS, Stauss HJ, Generation of human tumor-reactive cytotoxic T cells against peptides presented by non-self HLA class I molecules. *Eur J Immunol* 1998; **28:** 193–200.
82. Stauss HJ, Immunotherapy with CTLs restricted by nonself MHC. *Immunol Today* 1999; **20:** 180–3.
83. Baird PN, Simmons PJ, Expression of the Wilms' tumor gene (WT1) in normal hemopoiesis. *Exp Hematol* 1997; **25:** 312–20.
84. Inoue K, Tamaki H, Ogawa H et al, Wilms' tumor gene (WT1) competes with differentiation-inducing signal in hematopoietic progenitor cells. *Blood* 1998; **91:** 2969–76.
85. Inoue K, Ogawa H, Sonoda Y et al, Aberrant overexpression of the Wilms tumor gene (WT1) in human leukemia. *Blood* 1997; **89:** 1405–12.
86. Dazzi F, Capelli D, Hasserjian R et al, The kinetics and extent of engraftment of chronic myelogenous leukemia cells in non-obese diabetic/severe combined immunodeficiency mice reflect the phase of the donor's disease: an in vivo model of chronic myelogenous leukemia biology. *Blood* 1998; **92:** 1390–6.
87. Wang JC, Lapidot T, Cashman JD et al, High level engraftment of NOD/SCID mice by primitive normal and leukemic hematopoietic cells from patients with chronic myeloid leukemia in chronic phase. *Blood* 1998; **91:** 2406–14.
88. Smit WM, Rijnbeek M, van Bergen CA et al, T cells recognizing leukemic CD34+ progenitor cells mediate the antileukemic effect of donor lymphocyte infusions for relapsed chronic myeloid leukemia after allogeneic stem cell transplantation. *Proc Natl Acad Sci USA* 1998; **95:** 10152–7.
89. Gao L, Bellantuono I, Elsässer A et al, Selective elimination of leukemic $CD34^+$ progenitor cells by cytotoxic T lymphocytes specific for WT1. *Blood* 2000; **95**: 2198–203.
90. Ohminami H, Yasukawa M, Fujita S, HLA class I-restricted lysis of leukemia cells by a CD8(+) cytotoxic T-lymphocyte clone specific for WT1 peptide. *Blood* 2000; **95:** 286–93.

25

Late complications, including late relapse

Gérard Socié, Rochelle E Curtis, John P Klein

CONTENTS • Introduction • Long-term outcome and late relapses after alloSCT • Secondary malignancies after alloSCT • Non-malignant complications after alloSCT

INTRODUCTION

Since its introduction in the early 1970s, allogeneic stem cell transplantation (alloSCT) for chronic myeloid leukemia (CML) has gained wide acceptance.[1] It is generally considered as the only form of therapy with the capacity to cure CML.[2] The efficacy of alloSCT in the treatment of chronic-phase CML has been evaluated in a number of observational studies and several retrospective studies (for reviews, see Goldman,[3,4] Clift et al,[5] and Gratwohl et al[6]). Projected actuarial 3-year to 5-year survival rates in these studies are in the 50–60% range, with slightly lower probabilities of disease-free survival. The prospect of cure in this disease came from projected survival curves that appear to plateau (or taper more slowly) after 3–7 years.[7] However, while SCT was introduced nearly 30 years ago, it is of note that only a few published studies have reported data with a median follow-up of more than 40 months.

During the last decade, new approaches such as the combined use of cyclosporin and methotrexate,[8] or the use of ganciclovir to treat cytomegalovirus (CMV) infection have reduced early treatment-related mortality and improved the general outcome following alloSCT. Furthermore, in CML, the impact of the conditioning regimen on transplant outcomes has been prospectively tested in three randomized studies.[9–11] In the short term, the association of busulfan with cyclophosphamide seemed to be as efficacious as the association of cyclophosphamide with total-body irradiation (TBI). Since some late effects of alloSCT have clearly been linked with the use of TBI,[12] the long-term follow-up of such randomized trials would be of obvious clinical importance. All these changes in the practice of alloSCT may have a strong impact on the incidence and risk factors of late events occurring after transplantation, but, when reporting these data, few studies have restricted the study population to patients transplanted for CML. Thus, we would like to remind the reader that when summarizing the long-term outcome of transplantation in CML in this chapter, we have to deal with a limited number of sets of reported data, in which patients with CML are often mixed with those transplanted for other diseases. As a consequence, what could be considered to be true for the overall population (risk factor or incidence rate) for any complication may not strictly be applied when considering complications in the setting of transplantation for CML.

In this chapter, we will summarize the long-term outcome and causes of late death, the incidence and risk factors of secondary malignancies, and the incidence and risk factors of non-malignant complications following alloSCT for CML.

LONG-TERM OUTCOME AND LATE RELAPSES AFTER alloSCT

The IBMTR survey

We recently reported the long-term survival and the analysis of late death in a cohort of 6691 patients who survived more than 2 years and were free of their original disease.[13] Among these patients, roughly a third (2146) were transplanted for CML. For the purpose of this chapter, we have analyzed these 2146 CML patients in greater detail. Their characteristics are summarized in Table 25.1. They were transplanted from January 1980 to December 1993, and were disease-free (i.e. without hematological relapse) for at least 2 years after transplantation. Data on these patients had been reported to the International Bone Marrow Transplant Registry (IBMTR) by 221 transplantation centers worldwide. Less than 4% of the population were lost to follow-up within 2 years after SCT. Thus this cohort represents the largest population of long-term survivors studied today. The median duration of follow-up was 80 months. In this analysis, patients who died as a result of a relapse after transplantation were considered to have died of their original disease, even if this was not recorded as the proximate cause of death. Similarly, patients who died of active chronic graft-versus-host disease (GVHD) were considered to have died of this complication even if other complications (e.g. infection or bleeding) were considered as the proximate cause of death. Deaths due to infection included only those among patients without GVHD.

Among the 2146 patients with CML who were free of their primary disease 2 years after transplantation, the probability of surviving for 5 more years was 88%, the probability of relapse 5 years later was 11%, and the probability of relapse-related death was 6%. The primary causes of death are summarized in Table 25.2. As previously reported, recurrent leukemia was the most frequent cause of late death after transplantation for CML (47% of the cases who died after 2 years), with chronic GVHD being the second most frequent cause (36%). However, it is of note that the primary causes of death were strongly influenced by whether or not a T-cell-depleted graft was used. Of the 283 patients who received a T-cell-depleted transplant, 50 (17.7%) died more than 2 years after transplant, as compared with 188 out of 1863 (10%) of those who received a T-cell-replete graft. Relapse accounted for 80% of the causes of late death in patients who received a T-cell-depleted graft, and 36% in those who received a non-T-cell-depleted one.

We then calculated estimates of relative mortality as described by Andersen et al,[14] taking into account differences among patients with regard to age, gender, race, and nationality. Relative mortality with respect to a transplant recipient is the relative risk of dying at a given time post transplantation as compared with a person of similar age, sex, and nationality in the general population. Relative mortalities with 95% confidence intervals that included 1.0 were not considered to indicate significant differences from the rates in a normal population. Among patients who underwent transplantation for CML, the relative mortality rate was 11.2 (95% confidence interval (CI) 8.2–14.1) 5 years after transplantation, and 19.1 (95% CI 8.8–29.4) 10 years after transplantation, as previously described. However, the analysis of the relative mortalities in patients who received a T-cell-depleted transplant or a non-T-cell-depleted graft again disclosed major differences (Figure 25.1).

Finally, multivariate analyses of late death were performed. As shown in Table 25.3, patients who received a T-cell-depleted transplant had a higher risk of transplant-related death than those whose grafts were not T-cell-depleted; patients with active chronic GVHD or previous acute GVHD had higher risks of death not due to relapse.

Table 25.1 Characteristics of 2146 recipients of allogeneic bone marrow transplants who were disease-free 2 years after transplantation for CML

Variable[a]		
Age (in years) median (range)	34	(1–62)
Gender (%):		
Male	1221	(57%)
Female	925	(43%)
Karnofsky score before SCT <90, *n* (%)	228	(11%)
Disease stage before SCT, *n* (%):		
First chronic phase	1716	(80%)
Second chronic phase or accelerated phase	361	(17%)
Blast phase	65	(3%)
Time from diagnosis to SCT (in months), median (range)	12	(1–201)
Type of donor, *n* (%):		
Matched sibling	1812	(84%)
Identical twin	32	(1%)
Mismatched related	104	(5%)
Unrelated	188	(9%)
Prophylaxis against GVHD, *n* (%)		
MTX + CSA ± other drugs	1199	(56%)
MTX ± other drugs (not CSA)	134	(6%)
CSA ± other drugs (not MTX)	493	(23%)
T-cell depletion ± drugs	283	(13%)
Other methods or none	35	(2%)
Year of transplantation, *n* (%):		
1980–1983	151	(7%)
1984–1987	614	(29%)
1988–1990	759	(35%)
1991–1993	622	(29%)
Acute GVHD grade ⩾II, *n* (%)	586	(27%)
Chronic GVHD, *n* (%):		
None before 2 years	1034	(48%)
Resolved by 2 years	393	(18%)
Active by 2 years	716	(33%)

[a] *n*, number; MTX, methotrexate; CSA, cyclosporin.

Table 25.2 Primary causes of death among 2146 recipients of allogeneic bone marrow transplants who were disease-free 2 years after transplantation for CMT[a]

Cause of death	Non-TCD graft: late death 188 patients	TCD graft: late death 50 patients	Total: 2146 patients; late death 248 patients
Relapse	68 (36%)	40 (80%)	108 (45%)
GVHD	75 (40%)	6 (12%)	81 (34%)
Infection without GVHD	12 (6%)	2 (4%)	14 (6%)
New cancer	8 (4%)	0 (0%)	8 (3%)
Organ failure	9 (4%)	1 (2%)	10 (4%)
Other	16 (7%)	1 (2%)	17 (7%)
Unknown	10 (5%)	0 (0%)	10 (4%)

[a] Percentages are rounded and may not add to 100%. Other causes of death included: hemorrhage, interstitial pneumonia, and miscellaneous causes.
TCD, T-cell-depleted.

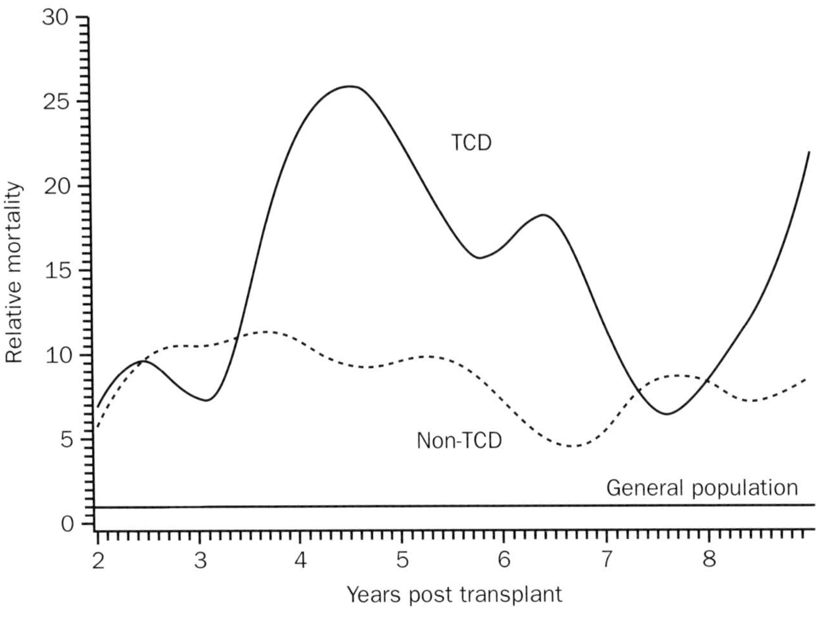

Figure 25.1 Mortality relative to the general population among 2146 recipients of allogeneic bone marrow transplants who were disease-free 2 years after transplantation for CML. TCD, T-cell-depleted.

Long-term follow-up of randomized studies comparing busulfan and cyclophosphamide with cyclophosphamide and TBI as pretransplant conditioning regimen

Two main conditioning regimens are currently used before transplantation for CML: the association of cyclophosphamide (Cy) and total-body irradiation (TBI)[15] and the association of busulfan (Bu) with Cy.[16,17] In the early 1990s, three randomized studies compared the outcome of patients with CML who underwent allogeneic SCT either after Cy–TBI or after Bu–Cy.[9–11] Among these trials, the French trial

Table 25.3 Relative risk (RR) of late death among 2146 recipients of allogeneic bone marrow transplants who were disease-free 2 years after transplantation for CML

Variable	Death from any cause			Death not related to relapse			Death related to relapse		
	RR	95% CI	*p*	RR	95% CI	*p*	RR	95% CI	*p*
Disease phase:									
Chronic	1.0		0.002	1.0		0.12	1.0		0.004
Accelerated	1.4	1.0–2.0		1.1	0.7–1.7		1.9	1.3–3.0	
Blast	2.2	1.3–3.7		2.0	1.0–3.9		2.3	1.0–5.8	
T-cell depletion	1.9	1.4–2.6	<0.001	0.7	0.4–1.4	0.34	3.3	2.2–5.0	<0.001
Previous acute GVHD	1.4	1.1–1.9	0.009	2.0	1.4–2.9	<0.001	0.9	0.5–1.4	0.56
Chronic GVHD at 2 years:									
None	1.0		<0.001	1.0		<0.001	1.0		0.09
Resolved	0.7	0.5–1.1		0.9	0.4–1.9		0.7	0.4–1.2	
Active	1.78	1.3–2.4		4.2	2.7–6.6		0.6	0.4–1.0	

and the Seattle group trial included only patients with CML in first chronic phase,[9,10] while the Nordic group trial included not only CML patients at various stages of their disease but also other diagnoses.[11] At present, these trials have more than 7 years' median follow-up. Olle Ringden and co-workers from the Nordic group recently updated their results, showing an increased risk of chronic GVHD, obstructive bronchiolitis, and alopecia in patients who received Bu–Cy as compared with those who were given Cy–TBI, irrespective of the primary diagnoses.[18] In this study, 30 patients with CML received Bu–Cy and 27 Cy–TBI. The updated analysis with 7 years' follow-up in patients with CML in first chronic phase receiving Cy–TBI (24 patients) or Bu–CY (22 patients) did not show any differences in the two arms (Figure 25.2; Olle Ringden, personal communication, November 1999). Similarly, Clift and co-workers from the Seattle group recently updated their results on 69 patients who received Bu–Cy and 73 who were given Cy–TBI. All patients were transplanted in first chronic phase and none had T-cell-depleted grafts. With a median duration of follow-up of more than 7 years, no difference in leukemia-free survival was observed in the two groups (RA Clift, personal communication, August 1999). However, as shown in Figure 25.3, this large study demonstrates that late relapses do occur in patients transplanted for CML (the latest being observed 8 years after transplantation). Furthermore, what is clearly illustrated by these two studies is the apparent equivalence of the two conditioning regimens with regard to disease control. It would thus be of clinical importance to determine the quality of life and the incidences of late malignancies and non-malignant late effects in patients assigned to the two types of conditioning. Such a study is in progress. It will compare in the long term patients who have been enrolled in these two trials, and will update the results of the French trial (by Socié et al).

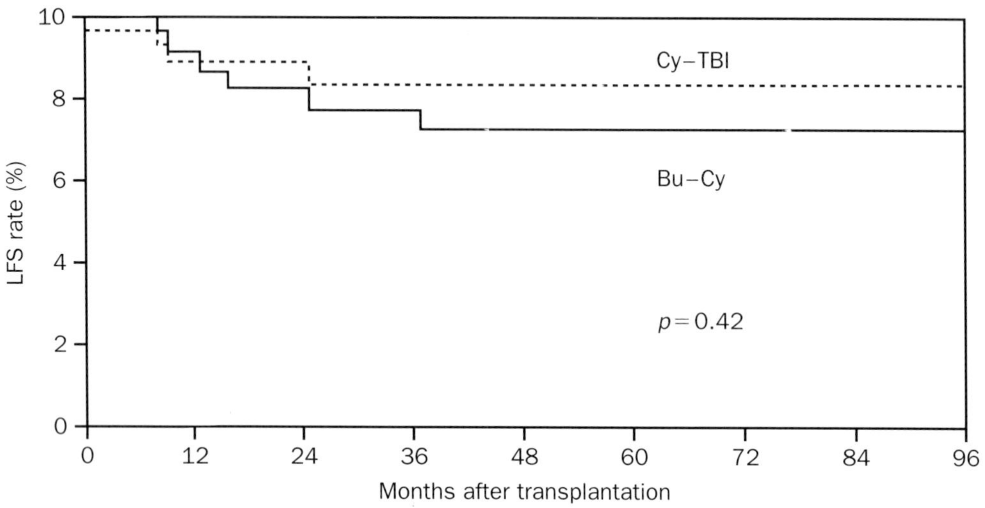

Figure 25.2 Kaplan–Meier estimates of leukemia-free survival (LFS) for 46 patients conditioned for HLA-identical marrow transplantation with the busulfan–cyclophosphamide (Bu–Cy) and cyclophosphamide plus total-body irradiation (CY–TBI) regimens. Updated results from the Nordic Bone Marrow Transplantation Group.

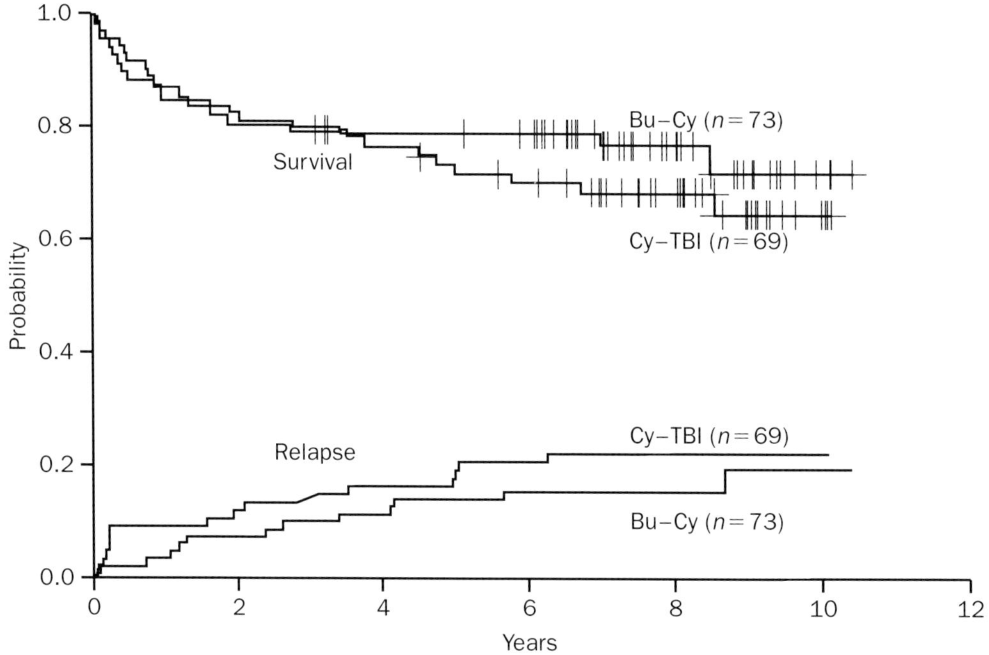

Figure 25.3 Kaplan–Meier estimates of survival and cumulative incidence of relapse for patients conditioned for HLA-identical marrow transplantation with the Bu–Cy or Cy–TBI regimens. Updated results from the Fred Hutchinson Cancer Research Center.

Long-term follow-up after transplantation: literature data with emphasis on late relapses

Most aspects of alloSCT for CML are covered in the other chapters in this volume. However, when we looked for series reported in the literature in which the median follow-up was longer than 3 years (as 'long-term' could be defined), it turned out that only a few data were available.

One of the most useful reports in this regard is the one published by Van Rhee and co-workers on behalf of the European Group for Blood and Marrow Transplantation (EBMT).[19] In this study, data on 373 patients transplanted in first chronic phase of CML using unmanipulated marrow cells from HLA-identical sibling donors were reported. The median follow-up of surviving patients was 7 years. The probabilities of survival and leukemia-free survival at 8 years were 54% and 47%, respectively. Twenty-seven patients died more than 2 years after transplant. Leukemia relapse accounted for more than 40% of these late deaths. Relapse of CML occurred in 40 patients. In a further 7 cases, a transient cytogenetic relapse was observed. Twenty-four patients experienced relapse 2 years after SCT. The latest documented relapse was at 6.5 years. The probabilities of relapses at 2 and 8 years after SCT were 10% (95% CI 7–15) and 18.9% (95% CI 14–25). Late relapses (later than 2 years) were less frequent in patients who developed chronic GVHD (relative risk 0.21) and in patients with female donors (relative risk 0.18). Finally, 67 patients in hematological remission were studied for residual disease by two-step reverse-transcriptase polymerase chain reaction (RT-PCR) for *BCR/ABL* mRNA, and 61 (91%) tested negative. These results closely match those of other cooperative groups and of single-center studies (Table 25.4).

Long-term outcome and comparisons with sibling transplants are still lacking for unrelated transplants. However, it should be noted that reported relapse rates following unrelated SCT for CML seem to be relatively low, especially in patients who received unmanipulated grafts Hansen et al[20,21] for the Seattle group reported an analysis on 196 patients transplanted for CML from an unrelated donor. The median follow-up was over 5 years. Fifteen patients relapsed, yielding a 10% cumulative incidence rate at 5 years. Devergie et al[22] for the EBMT reported a relapse rate as low as 2% in patients transplanted while in chronic phase, from an HLA-DRB1-matched donor, using a non-T-cell-depleted graft. Finally, in a study involving 283 patients by the Minneapolis group,[23] the relapse rate among recipients from unrelated donors (106 patients) was significantly lower (relative risk 0.22) than that in recipients from related donors (177 patients). Patients who underwent SCT from related donors had a median follow-up of 60 months, but those with unrelated donors have only been followed for a median of 20 months.[23]

Finally, studies comparing the outcome of grafted patients with that of non-grafted patients who were treated with interferon-α (IFN-α) have not reported the impact of late relapses in grafted patients.[24,25] This point should be kept in mind, because patients who relapse after transplant may have prolonged survival following donor leukocyte infusion (DLI).

Long-term follow-up after transplantation: concluding remarks

Some data reported here deserve additional comments. First, it is now clear that long-term molecular cure can be achieved after alloSCT in up to 50–60% of patients, provided that they are transplanted in chronic phase. It is therefore important to pay attention to parameters that influence the long-term outcome of these patients, with the aim of reducing both relapse-related and non-relapse-related deaths. Second, data reported in this section, in particular those of the IBMTR survey, are retrospective analyses of patients transplanted some years ago. With the advent of cellular therapy, it may again become possible to use T-cell depletion in

Table 25.4 Long-term follow-up studies of alloSCT for chronic-phase CML

Authors	No. of patients	Conditioning[a]	GVHD prophylaxis[b]	Median follow-up (months)	Relapse rate (%)	OS rate (%)	DFS rate (%)
Van Rhee et al[19]	373	Cy–TBI	CSA ± PDN ± MTX	84	19	54	47
Clift and Anasetti[71]	351	Cy–TBI	CSA + MTX	NR[c]	20	70	60
Devergie et al[72]	170	Cy–TBI	CSA + MTX/TCD	44	19	56	46
Beelen et al[73]	135	Cy–TBI	CSA + MTX	59	17	59	49
Aschan et al[74]	42	Cy–TBI	CSA + MTX/TCD	60–65	NR[c]	38–54	NR[c]
Galimberti et al[75]	34	Bu–Cy	CSA + MTX + PDN	43	0	71	71

[a] Cy, cyclophosphamide; TBI, total-body irradiation; Bu, busulfan.
[b] CSA, cyclosporin; PDN, prednisone; MTX, methotrexate; TCD, T-cell depletion.
[c] Not reported.

patients with high risks of transplant-related mortality (i.e. older patients). In this regard, it is interesting to note that excellent results have recently been reported by the Milwaukee group using T-cell depletion and DLI in patients who eventually relapsed.[26]

SECONDARY MALIGNANCIES AFTER alloSCT

Few studies have assessed the risks of second malignancies among long-term survivors of SCT[27–32] (for a review, see Deeg and Socie[33]). While classically the problem of secondary malignancy has been subdivided into lymphoproliferative disorders, secondary leukemia, and solid cancers, it is mainly the third of these that may arise as late events following SCT. To the best of our knowledge, no cases of secondary leukemia (i.e. leukemia developing in donor cells) have been reported after SCT for CML.

Lymphoproliferative disorders are mainly B-cell malignancies of donor origin occurring mostly during the first year after SCT. In the largest series, involving 18 014 patients, 4770 (26.5%) patients had CML.[34] There was no increased risk per se in CML patients. Risk factors included transplantation from an unrelated or from an HLA-mismatched related donor (relative risk 4.1), T-cell depletion of the graft (relative risk 12.7), grade II–IV acute GVHD (relative risk 1.9), and the use of anti-thymocyte globulin (ATG) (relative risk 6.4) or anti-CD3 (relative risk 43.2) antibody to treat acute GVHD. It is clear that most of these risk factors apply to patients with CML, especially with the growing use of unrelated donors in such patients. In this survey, two additional points deserve comment. First, for the first time, it was clearly demonstrated that the risk of lymphoproliferative disorders in recipients of T-cell-depleted grafts varied greatly with the method used for T-cell depletion (with the highest risk being associated with methods targeting only T cells and/or natural killer (NK) cells and the lowest with the use of Campath-1). Second, this study demonstrated that late-occurring (beyond a year) lymphoproliferative disorders do exist. These late disorders closely resemble non-Hodgkin's lymphoma. None of the above risk factors emerged, and only chronic GVHD was significantly linked with these late lymphomas.

None of the reports on second solid cancers specifically restricted the study population to patients who underwent SCT for CML. The largest study on solid cancers involved 19 229 patients who were transplanted at the Fred Hutchinson Cancer Research Center or reported to the IBMTR.[35] In this cohort, 4885 patients (25.4%) underwent alloSCT for CML. For the purpose of this chapter, data on patients with CML were re-analyzed. Sixteen solid tumors occurred in these 4885 patients, and of these 16 tumors, 14 were invasive. The projected 10-year incidence of invasive solid cancer using Kaplan–Meier estimates was 0.7% (95% CI 0.3–1.1%). The different tumor types and the times between transplant and the occurrence of the cancer are summarized in Table 25.5. We then calculated the observed incidence of invasive cancer in CML patients and compared it with that in the general population, matched for age, gender, and year of diagnosis of cancer. Overall, the observed-to-expected ratio was 1.2 (95% CI 0.6–2). This ratio means that there is a slight but not statistically significant increased incidence of solid cancers in patients transplanted for CML. However, when looking at age at transplantation, there was a significant 9.7 excess risk in patients transplanted before 30 years of age but not in patients older than this (Table 25.6).

NON-MALIGNANT COMPLICATIONS AFTER alloSCT

A number of late complications have already been described, but few data on risk factors for these long-term effects of SCT are available. Besides long-term complications, evaluation of the quality of life (QOL) of cured patients is of obvious importance.[36,37] Our goal is not only to cure the patients of their original disease but also to help them to return to work or school

Table 25.5 Solid cancers developing in 16 patients among 4885 recipients transplanted for CML

No. of tumors	Tumor type	Location	Latency (years)
4	Adenocarcinoma	Breast	0.3, 2.9, 4.2, and 4.1
2	Papillary carcinoma	Thyroid	0.2 and 2.8
2	In situ epidermoid carcinoma	Uterine cervix	1.2 and 3.4
2	Rhabdomyosarcoma	Temporalis muscle, tight	0.7 and 2.7
2	Malignant melanoma	Skin	1.0 and 2.0
1	Malignant fibrous histiocytoma	Liver	1.4
1	Chondrosarcoma	Scapula	15.3
1	Epidermoid carcinoma	Skin	2.2
1	Astrocytoma	Spinal chord	3.2

Table 25.6 Ratio of observed (O) to expected (E) cases and absolute excess risk of new invasive solid cancers according to age at transplantation in patients with CML

Age at transplantation							
Less than 30 years				More than 30 years			
O	E	O : E	Excess risk	O	E	O : E	Excess risk
6	1.4	4.3 ($p < 0.05$)	9.7	8	10.5	0.8	−4.1

and to be able to lead a social life as close as possible to the 'normal' general population. The major goal in assessing late complications after SCT is not only to analyze late complications and QOL of transplanted patients but also to compare them with those of non-transplanted patients. In fact, while some of the late complications might be more frequent after SCT (such as radiation- or steroid-induced cataracts), other late complications have also been described in non-transplanted patients with CML (for a review, see Silver et al[7]). In this section, we will cover only the main non-malignant complications, and will focus on the few data that are available after SCT for CML.

Thyroid abnormalities

Thyroid dysfunction has been recognized as one of the potential late effects of the intensive treatment for obtaining cancer survival. Irradiation and busulfan seem to be the leading causes of thyroid disorders after SCT.[38–42] The most frequent thyroid disorder found in these patients is frank or subclinical primary hypothyroidism (compensated hypothyroidism). Hypothyroidism is a relatively early complication in patients after SCT, but it can also manifest years after transplant. None of the reported series dealing with hypothyroidism after alloSCT looked specifically for this complication in patients transplanted for CML. Boulad and co-workers[40] reported that in a large series involving 150 patients who were alive and disease-free 1 year after transplantation, 3 out of 36 patients with CML (8%) developed hypothyroidism. In a cohort of 86 patients from Genoa who underwent SCT during childhood (A Cohen et al, unpublished data), 9 (10%) developed frank hypothyroidism (5 received fractionated TBI; 4 received busulfan), 0.5–6 years after transplant (median 1 year); 22 patients (25%) developed subclinical hypothyroidism (18 fractionated TBI; 4 chemotherapy only), 0.5–7 years after transplant (median 3 years). In a series of 77 patients who underwent SCT without the use of TBI, 26 patients had CML (34%).[42] Peripheral thyroid insufficiency was observed in 4 out of these 26 patients (14%), who received Bu–Cy as conditioning regimen (G Socié, unpublished data). Thus, when treating patients with CML, physicians must be aware of this relatively frequent complication, even in the absence of TBI. Regular measurement of thyroid-stimulating hormone (TSH), and free T3 and free T4 thyroid hormones allows early detection of peripheral thyroid insufficiency. Treatment with L-thyroxine is indicated in those cases of frank primary hypothyroidism with high basal TSH concentration and low free thyroid hormone levels. There is a debate on whether or not to treat patients with subclinical hypothyroidism.[43] On the one hand, treatment might induce early osteoporosis in patients who are already at risk of developing osteoporosis due to sex-hormone deficiency. Furthermore, the majority of cases with subclinical hypothyroidism after SCT were found to be mild, compensated, and resolved spontaneously. On the other hand, treatment with L-thyroxine will cause a decrease in TSH levels, which, although not proven, has been incriminated as a contributory factor in thyroid carcinogenesis.[43,44] Thus, treatment of subclinical hypothyroidism should be carefully discussed with an endocrinologist.

Ophthalmologic complications

Cataracts

Cataract formation has been recognized in SCT recipients as one of the first and most frequently occurring late complications of TBI.[45,50] Single-dose TBI of 10 Gy or more causes cataracts in nearly 100% of patients. Fractionation of TBI was first thought to reduce the incidence of this complication; however, it is now clear that fractionated TBI only delays the appearance of cataracts and consequently will probably lead to a high probability of cataracts requiring surgery on the long-term follow-up. In addition to TBI fractionation, TBI dose rate (high dose rate) is an additional risk factor for the development of cataracts. In patients who underwent SCT following irradiation-free conditioning regimens, steroids (given for GVHD prophylaxis and/or treatment) emerge as significant risk factors. Finally, it is not clear at present whether Bu–Cy per se (i.e. in the absence of steroids given for GVHD) will lead to a significant incidence of cataracts. In a series from the Fred Hutchinson Cancer Research Center studying, in the long term, the incidence of and risk factors for developing cataracts in adult patients who received either single-dose or fractionated TBI, 131 patients had CML (the total population studied comprised 492 patients).[47] In patients with CML, the 10-year probability of cataracts was 35% in those who were given fractionated TBI (121 patients) and 42% in patients receiving single-dose TBI (10 patients). In addition to TBI, steroid therapy for GVHD was an independent risk factor. Both in this study from Seattle and in another one from the Basel group,[50,51] single-dose TBI lead to more severe cataracts. Steroid use was a risk factor in both studies. Long-term outcome analysis of patients randomized to receive either Bu–Cy or Cy–TBI from the Nordic group[18] demonstrated that cataract risk was higher in the TBI group (31%) than in the Bu–Cy group (10%, $p = 0.007$) (data according to primary disease unknown). Thus there should be a systematical search for cataracts in patients transplanted for CML, irrespective of the conditioning regimen used, and surgical treatment discussed when visual acuity is lowered.

Late-onset keratoconjunctivitis sicca syndrome

This complication occurs in nearly 25% of the patients. It is clearly associated with chronic GVHD, older age, and female gender. Adequate treatment can avoid severe corneal defects.[52]

Avascular necrosis of bone

Among late complications, avascular necrosis of bone has been reported, but few studies have included enough patients to allow analysis of the risk factors.[53,56] In a multicenter retrospective study of 4388 patients, 77 developed avascular necrosis, leading to a 4.3% projected incidence at 5 years. Symptoms developed 2–132 months after transplantation. In these 77 patients, a mean of 1.87 joints per patient were affected (range 1–7). The hip joint was the most often affected (88% of patients), and 48% of the patients required joint replacement. All but 2 patients received steroids for acute and/or chronic GVHD over a mean period of 15 months. In multivariate logistic regression analysis, five factors were significantly associated with an increased risk for developing avascular necrosis: chronic GVHD (odds ratio (OR) = 3.52), acute GVHD (OR = 3.73), age over 16 years (OR = 5.81), aplastic anemia (OR = 3.90), and acute leukemia (OR = 1.72).[55] Although patients with CML seemed to have a lower risk of avascular necrosis than patients with either aplastic anemia or acute leukemia, the incidence of this complication in patients with CML was far from negligible. In fact, among 970 patients with CML, 18 developed avascular necrosis, leading to 5-year incidence of 4%.

Fertility

Gonadal failure is an almost-inevitable consequence of high-dose chemotherapy and radiotherapy, and recovery is rare. Over the last two decades, the outcome for patients undergoing high-dose therapy has continued to improve. The inability to parent children, and for women the immediate onset of menopause, are factors that further impair the quality of life of patients with CML, and which must now be addressed. For women, there are a number of risk factors for the development of ovarian failure, including the nature, dose, and duration of treatment. However, the most important factor is the age at the time of transplant, with the incidence of irreversible ovarian failure increasing with increasing age. Furthermore, women who initially recover menses, and even those who subsequently bear children, are more likely to enter menopause at an earlier age than the normal female population. For men, the age at treatment is less important than for women. In contrast, the underlying disease, the type of drug, the total dose, and the duration of administration all affect the likelihood of permanent azoospermia. For both sexes, alkylating agents are more likely to induce infertility than cytotoxics of other drug classes, although the gonadal consequences of modern high-dose combination regimens is virtually unknown (including Bu–Cy).[57]

Within the Late Effects Working Party of the EBMT, there has recently been a survey of the outcome of conceptions from men and women previously treated by transplantation. Information was provided by 199 of 229 European SCT teams. Of these, 71 teams were aware of a total of 261 conceptions, in 199 patients. Although the patients were heterogeneous with respect to underlying disease, treatment prior to transplant, conditioning regimens, and type of transplant, some general conclusions can be drawn. First, parenting a child after transplant is a rare event (as illustrated by numerous case reports in the literature);[58–69] second, the interval from transplant to first conception was longer in patients receiving allografts than in those receiving autografts, reflecting both an increased time to gonadal recovery and the younger age at transplant. Third, female patients transplanted for hematological malignancies may require assisted conception and appear to experience more complications, including a higher rate of spontaneous abortion. Babies born to these patients are more likely to be born prematurely and to be of low birth weight. Fourth, at present, the children born to such patients do not appear to be at increased risk of congenital malformations and are developing normally. Similar results have been reported from the Seattle transplant team.[70]

Despite these encouraging results, the majority of patients undergoing high-dose therapy will experience at least temporary gonadal failure. For most women, ovarian damage results in immediate menopause, with its troublesome symptoms and loss of sexual interest, and, in the longer term, an enhanced risk of osteoporosis and arterial vascular disease. An immediate and relatively easily satisfied requirement post therapy is therefore adequate hormone replacement therapy (HRT). The goal of HRT must be to find a combination of hormones that suits each individual, thereby controlling symptoms, protecting against future complications, and ensuring compliance with therapy.

The restoration of fertility is more difficult, and at present relies upon semen and embryo cryopreservation prior to treatment. In the future, ovarian, oocyte, and testicular freezing may become a real possibility (for a review, see Apperley and Reddy[57]). Fertilization can now be achieved in vitro by techniques of micromanipulation, thus requiring only a single sperm. It therefore follows that all male patients should be offered semen cryopreservation even if their sperm quality is poor. If a woman has a partner who has agreed to the procedure then cryopreservation of her own fertilized oocytes can be undertaken. Ovarian hyperstimulation is essential for the collection of several oocytes, and the time required for this may not be available in women who require immediate treatment for their underlying disease. For women with chronic illnesses such as CML, this technique may be possible. The ability to collect and fertilize good-quality oocytes is dependent on adequate ovarian function at the time of hyperstimulation. Increasing age and gonadal dysfunction due to prior exposure to chemotherapy will undoubtedly diminish the chances of successful collection cycles. For patients in whom embryo/semen cryopreservation is not practical, there remain three other possibilities to parent a child after transplant. First, following therapy and recovery, patients can receive donated ova or sperm, or donated embryos from an unrelated couple. Second, they could arrange for a surrogate to produce a live infant, and finally, according to local legal requirements, they may be able to adopt an infant.

Finally, one point should be stressed for patients with CML. In the EBMT survey on conception following SCT, three women requiring embryo transfer relapsed post SCT, and all three had CML. It is thus tempting to speculate that relapse in these patients reflected a disturbance of the graft-versus-leukemia effect consequent to pregnancy. However, in this survey, six further female patients with CML conceived and none relapsed with a median follow-up time of more than 3 years post conception. We cannot therefore recommend exclusion of patients with CML from assisted conception programs. We would, however, recommend the following for patients with CML: first, there should be a delay of 2 years after SCT, and patients should be *BCR/ABL*-negative before embarking on pregnancy; second, there should be close molecular monitoring of these patients during and after pregnancy.

ACKNOWLEDGEMENTS

This work was supported by Public Health Service grants (R01-CA54706-07) from the US National Cancer Institute (JPK), and by Contracts CP-51027 and CP-51028 from the US National Cancer Institute (REC).

REFERENCES

1. Thomas ED, A history of haemopoietic cell transplantation. *Br J Haematol* 1999; **105:** 330–9.
2. Gratwohl A, Hermans J, Goldman JM et al, Risk assessment for patients with chronic myeloid leukaemia before allogeneic blood or marrow transplantation. *Lancet* 1998; **352:** 1087–92.
3. Goldman JM, Management of chronic myeloid leukaemia. *Blood Rev* 1994; **8:** 21–9.
4. Goldman JM, The treatment of chronic myeloid leukaemia – much still to be achieved. *J Intern Med* 1994; **235:** 289–91.
5. Clift RA, Appelbaum FR, Thomas ED, Bone marrow transplantation for chronic myelogenous leukemia – Reply. *Blood* 1994; **83:** 2752–3.
6. Gratwohl A, Hermans J, Allogeneic bone marrow transplantation for chronic myeloid leukemia. *Bone Marrow Transplant* 1996; **17:** S7–9.
7. Silver RT, Woolf SH, Hehlmann R et al, An evidence-based analysis of the effect of busulfan, hydroxyurea, interferon, and allogeneic bone marrow transplantation in treating the chronic phase of chronic myeloid leukemia: developed for the American Society of Hematology. *Blood* 1999; **94:** 1517–36.
8. Storb R, Deeg HJ, Pepe M et al, Methotrexate and cyclosporine versus cyclosporine alone for prophylaxis of graft-versus-host disease in patients given HLA-identical marrow grafts for leukemia: long-term follow-up of a controlled trial. *Blood* 1989; **73:** 1729–34.
9. Clift RA, Buckner CD, Thomas ED et al, Marrow transplantation for chronic myeloid leukemia: a randomized study comparing cyclophosphamide and total body irradiation with busulfan and cyclophosphamide. *Blood* 1994; **84:** 2036–43.
10. Devergie A, Blaise D, Attal M et al, Allogeneic bone marrow transplantation for chronic myeloid leukemia in first chronic phase: a randomized trial of busulfan–cytoxan versus cytoxan–total body irradiation as preparative regimen: a report from the French Society of Bone Marrow Graft (SFGM). *Blood* 1995; **85:** 2263–8.
11. Ringden O, Ruutu T, Remberger M et al, A randomized trial comparing busulfan vs total body irradiation in allogeneic marrow transplant recipients with hematological malignancies. *Transplant Proc* 1994; **26:** 1831–2.
12. Socie G, Kolb HJ, Ljungman P, Malignant disease after allogeneic bone marrow transplantation: the case for assessment of risk factors. *Br J Haematol* 1992; **80:** 427–30.
13. Socie G, Stone JV, Wingard JR et al, Long-term survival and late deaths after allogeneic bone marrow transplantation. *N Engl J Med* 1999; **341:** 14–21.
14. Andersen PK, Horowitz MM, Klein JP et al, Modelling covariate adjusted mortality relative to a standard population. *Stat Med* 1999; **18:** 1529–40.
15. Clift RA, Appelbaum FR, Thomas ED, Treatment of chronic myeloid leukemia by marrow transplantation. *Blood* 1993; **82:** 1954–6.
16. Santos GW, The development of busulfan cyclophosphamide preparative regimens. *Semin Oncol* 1993; **20:** 12–16.
17. Tutschka PJ, Use of busulfan containing chemotherapy for conditioning patients with leukemia for bone marrow allografting. *Bone Marrow Transplant* 1993; **12:** 34–6.
18. Ringden O, Remberger M, Ruutu T et al, Increased risk of chronic graft-versus-host disease, obstructive bronchiolitis, and alopecia with busulfan versus total body irradiation: long-term results of a randomized trial in allogeneic marrow recipients with leukemia. *Blood* 1999; **93:** 2196–201.
19. Van Rhee F, Szydlo RM, Hermans J et al, Long-term results after allogeneic bone marrow transplantation for chronic myelogenous leukemia in chronic phase: a report from the Chronic Leukemia Working Party of the European Group for Blood and Marrow Transplantation. *Bone Marrow Transplant* 1997; **20:** 553–60.
20. Hansen JA, Petersdorf E, Martin PJ, Anasetti C, Hematopoietic stem cell transplants from unrelated donors. *Immunol Rev* 1997; **157:** 141–50.
21. Hansen JA, Gooley TA, Martin PJ et al, Bone marrow transplants from unrelated donors for patients with chronic myeloid leukemia. *N Engl J Med* 1998; **338:** 962–8.
22. Devergie A, Apperley JF, Labopin M et al, European results of matched unrelated donor bone marrow transplantation for chronic myeloid leukemia. Impact of HLA class II matching. *Bone Marrow Transplant* 1997; **20:** 11–19.
23. Enright H, Davies SM, Defor T et al, Relapse after non-T-cell-depleted allogeneic bone marrow transplantation for chronic myelogenous leukemia: early transplantation use of an unrelated donor, and chronic graft-versus-host disease are protective. *Blood* 1996; **88:** 714–20.
24. Baccarani M, Monitoring treatment and survival

in chronic myeloid leukemia. *J Clin Oncol* 1999; **17:** 1858–68.
25. Gale RP, Hehlmann R, Zhang MJ et al, Survival with bone marrow transplantation versus hydroxyurea or interferon for chronic myelogenous leukemia. *Blood* 1998; **91:** 1810–19.
26. Drobyski WR, Hessner MJ, Klein JP et al, T-cell depletion plus salvage immunotherapy with donor leukocyte infusions as a strategy to treat chronic-phase chronic myelogenous leukemia patients undergoing HLA-identical sibling marrow transplantation. *Blood* 1999; **94:** 434–41.
27. Witherspoon RP, Deeg HJ, Storb R, Secondary malignancies after marrow transplantation for leukemia or aplastic anemia. *Transplantation* 1994; **57:** 1413–18.
28. Witherspoon RP, Fisher L, Schoch G et al, Secondary cancers after bone marrow transplantation for leukemia or aplastic anemia. *N Engl J Med* 1989; **321:** 784–9.
29. Deeg HJ, Socie G, Schoch G et al, Malignancies after marrow transplantation for aplastic anemia and Fanconi anemia: a joint Seattle and Paris analysis of results in 700 patients. *Blood* 1996; **87:** 386–92.
30. Lowsky R, Lipton J, Fyles G et al, Secondary malignancies after bone marrow transplantation in adults. *J Clin Oncol* 1994; **12:** 2187–92.
31. Socie G, Henryamar M, Bacigalupo A et al, Malignant tumors occurring after treatment of aplastic anemia. *N Engl J Med* 1993; **329:** 1152–7.
32. Bhatia S, Ramsay NKC, Steinbuch M et al, Malignant neoplasms following bone marrow transplantation. *Blood* 1996; **87:** 3633–9.
33. Deeg HJ, Socie G, Malignancies after hematopoietic stem cell transplantation: many questions, some answers. *Blood* 1998; **91:** 1833–44.
34. Curtis RE, Travis LB, Rowlings PA et al, Risk of lymphoproliferative disorders after bone marrow transplantation: a multi-institutional study. *Blood* 1999; **94:** 2208–16.
35. Curtis RE, Rowlings PA, Deeg HJ et al, Solid cancers after bone marrow transplantation. *N Engl J Med* 1997; **336:** 897–904.
36. Duell T, van Lint MT, Ljungman P et al, Health and functional status of long-term survivors of bone marrow transplantation. *Ann Intern Med* 1997; **126:** 184–92.
37. Wingard JR, Functional ability and quality of life of patients after allogeneic bone marrow transplantation. *Bone Marrow Transplant* 1994; **14:** S29–33.
38. Alfiar FZ, Colwill R, Lipton JH et al, Abnormal thyroid stimulating hormone (TSH) levels in adults following allogeneic bone marrow transplants. *Bone Marrow Transplant* 1997; **19:** 1019–22.
39. Bakker B, Massa GG, vanRijn AM et al, Effects of total-body irradiation on growth, thyroid and pituitary gland in rhesus monkeys. *Radiother Oncol* 1999; **51:** 187–92.
40. Boulad F, Bromley M, Black P et al, Thyroid dysfunction following bone marrow transplantation using hyperfractionated radiation. *Bone Marrow Transplant* 1995; **15:** 71–6.
41. Kauppila M, Koskinen P, Irjala K et al, Long-term effects of allogeneic bone marrow transplantation (BMT) on pituitary, gonad, thyroid and adrenal function in adults. *Bone Marrow Transplant* 1998; **22:** 331–7.
42. Toubert ME, Socie G, Gluckman E et al, Short- and long-term follow-up of thyroid dysfunction after allogeneic bone marrow transplantation without the use of preparative total body irradiation. *Br J Haematol* 1997; **98:** 453–7.
43. Cohen A, Rovelli R, Zecca S et al, Endocrine late effects in children who underwent bone marrow transplantation: review. *Bone Marrow Transplant* 1998; **21:** S64–7.
44. Uderzo C, Vanlint MT, Rovelli A et al, Papillary thyroid carcinoma after total body irradiation. *Arch Dis Child* 1994; **71:** 256–8.
45. Belkacemi Y, Ozsahin M, Pene F et al, Cataractogenesis after total body irradiation. *Int J Radiat Oncol Biol Phys* 1996; **35:** 53–60.
46. Belkacemi Y, Labopin M, Vernant JP et al, Cataracts after total body irradiation and bone marrow transplantation in patients with acute leukemia in complete remission: A study of the European Group for Blood and Marrow Transplantation. *Int J Radiat Oncol Biol Phys* 1998; **41:** 659–68.
47. Benyunes MC, Sullivan KM, Deeg HJ et al, Cataracts after bone marrow transplantation: long-term follow-up of adults treated with fractionated total body irradiation. *Int J Radiat Oncol Biol Phys* 1995; **32:** 661–70.
48. Fife K, Milan S, Westbrook K et al, Risk factors for requiring cataract surgery following total body irradiation. *Radiother Oncol* 1994; **33:** 93–8.
49. Hamon MD, Gale RF, Macdonald ID et al, Incidence of cataracts after single fraction total body irradiation – the role of steroids and graft versus host disease. *Bone Marrow Transplant*

1993; **12:** 233–6.
50. Tichelli A, Gratwohl A, Egger T et al, Cataract formation after bone marrow transplantation. *Ann Intern Med* 1993; **119:** 1175–80.
51. Tichelli A, Late ocular complications after bone marrow transplantation. *Nouv Rev Fr Hematol* 1994; **36:** S79–82.
52. Tichelli A, Duell T, Weiss M et al, Late-onset keratoconjunctivitis sicca syndrome after bone marrow transplantation: Incidence and risk factors. *Bone Marrow Transplant* 1996; **17:** 1105–11.
53. Bizot P, Witvoet J, Sedel L, Avascular necrosis of the femoral head after allogenic bone-marrow transplantation – a retrospective study of 27 consecutive THAs with a minimal two-year follow-up. *J Bone Joint Surg [Br]* 1996; **78B:** 878–83.
54. Fink JC, Leisenring WM, Sullivan KM et al, Avascular necrosis following bone marrow transplantation: a case–control study. *Bone* 1998; **22:** 67–71.
55. Socie G, Cahn JY, Carmelo J et al, Avascular necrosis of bone after allogeneic bone marrow transplantation: analysis of risk factors for 4388 patients by the Société Française de Greffe de Moelle (SFGM). *Br J Haematol* 1997; **97:** 865–70.
56. Wiesmann A, Pereira P, Bohm P et al, Avascular necrosis of bone following allogeneic stem cell transplantation: MR screening and therapeutic options. *Bone Marrow Transplant* 1998; **22:** 565–9.
57. Apperley JF, Reddy N, Mechanism and management of treatment-related gonadal failure in recipients of high dose chemoradiotherapy. *Blood Rev* 1995; **9:** 93–116.
58. Arcese W, Iori AP, Pregnancy and secondary cancer after allogeneic bone marrow transplantation. *Bone Marrow Transplant* 1999; **23:** 752.
59. Atkinson HG, Apperley JF, Dawson K et al, Successful pregnancy after allogeneic bone marrow transplantation for chronic myeloid leukaemia. *Lancet* 1994; **344:** 199.
60. Borgnapignatti C, Marradi P, Rugolotto S, Marcolongo A, Successful pregnancy after bone marrow transplantation for thalassaemia. *Bone Marrow Transplant* 1996; **18:** 235–6.
61. Delmer A, Rio B, Bauduer F et al, Pregnancy during myelosuppressive treatment for chronic myelogenous leukaemia. *Br J Haematol* 1992; **82:** 783–4.
62. Gulati SC, Vanpoznak C, Pregnancy after bone marrow transplantation. *J Clin Oncol* 1998; **16:** 1978–85.
63. Lipton JH, Derzko C, Fyles G et al, Pregnancy after BMT – 3 case reports. *Bone Marrow Transplant* 1993; **11:** 415–18.
64. Lipton JH, Virro M, Solow H, Successful pregnancy after allogeneic bone marrow transplant with embryos isolated before transplant. *J Clin Oncol* 1997; **15:** 3347–9.
65. Maruta A, Matsuzaki M, Miyashita H et al, Successful pregnancy after allogeneic bone marrow transplantation following conditioning with total body irradiation. *Bone Marrow Transplant* 1995; **15:** 637–8.
66. Milpied N, Moreau P, Cuillere JC et al, Successful pregnancy after allogeneic bone marrow transplantation following conditioning including a 10-Gy single exposure total body irradiation. *Bone Marrow Transplant* 1996; **17:** 467.
67. Nicholson HS, Byrne J, Fertility and pregnancy after treatment for cancer during childhood or adolescence. *Cancer* 1993; **71:** 3392–9.
68. Rio B, Leturkonirsch H, Ajchenbaumcymbalista F et al, Full-term pregnancy with embryos from donated oocytes in a 36-year-old woman allografted for chronic myeloid leukemia. *Bone Marrow Transplant* 1994; **13:** 487–8.
69. Wang WS, Tzeng CH, Hsieh RK et al, Successful pregnancy following very high-dose total body irradiation (1575 cGy) and bone marrow transplantation in a woman with acute myeloid leukemia. *Bone Marrow Transplant* 1998; **21:** 415–17.
70. Sanders JE, Hawley J, Levy W et al, Pregnancies following high-dose cyclophosphamide with or without high-dose busulfan or total-body irradiation and bone marrow transplantation. *Blood* 1996; **87:** 3045–52.
71. Clift RA, Anasetti C, Allografting for chronic myeloid leukemia. *Baillière's Clin Haematol* 1997; **10:** 319–36.
72. Devergie A, Reiffers J, Vernant JP et al, Long-term follow-up after marrow transplantation for chronic myelogenous leukemia: factors associated with relapse. *Bone Marrow Transplant* 1990; **5:** 379–86.
73. Beelen DW, Graeven U, Elmaagacli AH et al, Prolonged administration of interferon-alpha in patients with chronic-phase Philadelphia chromosome-positive chronic myelogenous leukemia before allogeneic bone marrow transplantation may adversely affect transplant outcome. *Blood* 1995; **85:** 2981–90.
74. Aschan J, Ringden O, Sundberg B et al, Increased

risk of relapse in patients with chronic myelogenous leukemia given T-cell depleted marrow compared to methotrexate combined with cyclosporin or monotherapy for the prevention of graft-versus-host disease. *Eur J Haematol* 1993; **50:** 269–74.

75. Galimberti M, Polchi P, Lucarelli G et al, Allogeneic marrow transplantation in patients with chronic myeloid leukemia in chronic phase following preparation with busulfan and cyclophosphamide. *Bone Marrow Transplant* 1994; **13:** 197–201.

Part 4

Autografting in chronic myeloid leukaemia

26

Autografting with unmanipulated stem cells: The European experience

Arnaud Pigneux, Eduardo Olavarria, François X Mahon, Josy Reiffers

CONTENTS • Introduction • Autografting in chronic phase: rationale • Choice of progenitor cells • Autografting in chronic phase: results • Autografting in chronic phase: the EBMT survey • Toxicity and post-SCT therapy • Final considerations

INTRODUCTION

Autologous stem cell transplantation (ASCT) was first attempted for patients with CML in transformation in order to restore a second chronic phase. In 1978, Buckner et al[1] used bone marrow harvested during the chronic phase to rescue haematopoiesis after a supralethal myeloablative conditioning regimen including total-body irradiation (TBI). Subsequently, Goldman et al[2] reported that peripheral blood progenitor cells collected at diagnosis could be used efficiently to reconstitute haematopoiesis after similar conditioning. The results of ASCT for CML in transformation have been extensively reviewed,[3–7] and can be summarized as follows:

- Haematopoietic recovery is faster after peripheral blood than bone marrow stem cell transplantation.
- Following ASCT, some patients exhibit a 'cytogenetic conversion' due to the re-emergence of Philadelphia (Ph)-negative cells, and they seem to have prolonged survival.
- Unsurprisingly, the survival of patients transplanted in accelerated phase is longer than that of those transplanted in blast crisis.
- Patients who have received a 'double' transplant seem to have a longer survival than those undergoing a single transplant.
- Patients treated with interferon-α (IFN-α) after transplant survive longer than others.
- A second chronic phase is obtained in most cases, but its duration is usually short, since most patients develop a recurrent blast crisis within 6–9 months due to the clone implicated in the first transformation.

Thus, in most patients with advanced disease, restoring a prolonged second chronic phase has not proved possible, and so ASCT has progressively been abandoned for patients with CML in transformation. However, a double ASCT followed by IFN-α may be beneficial for patients in accelerated phase without a suitable donor. As has been shown in Bordeaux, there is a survival advantage for patients who received a double autograft (a 3-year survival rate of 47% ± 22%), and for those treated with IFN-α after transplant.[7]

AUTOGRAFTING IN CHRONIC PHASE: RATIONALE

Autografting in chronic phase is now becoming increasingly used, since some preliminary results suggest that ASCT could increase the proportion of patients with a cytogenetic response, and thus prolong survival.[8] It is well known that the reinfused material contributes to the reappearance of the disease.[9] The rationale for autografting in chronic phase is based on the reduction of the tumour burden and the number of leukaemic cells at risk of developing a second genetic event responsible for the blastic transformation.[10,11] This, in turn, would delay the emergence of a blastic phase and prolong survival. A second possibility is the 'setting back the clock' effect, by which the cells that have already mutated will be eradicated and new, fresh, non-transformed cells will replace them after the transplant.[12] Thirdly, there is the possibility of reverting IFN-α resistance so that IFN-α can achieve a cytogenetic response when used after autografting in patients previously resistant to it. More recently, the group in Genoa has shown the feasibility of collecting Ph-negative stem cells after in vivo purging with chemotherapy (mini-ICE). These 'normal' Ph-negative cells can be used in an autografting procedure, and most patients recover with Ph-negative haemopoiesis.[13,14]

CHOICE OF PROGENITOR CELLS

Although in the early years most stem cell transplants were performed with bone marrow material, the vast majority of autologous transplants today are done with peripheral blood stem cells (PBSC). The advantages of PBSC include more convenient and easier collection, increased numbers of stem cells collected, the possibility of multiple collections, and the option of collecting stem cells after different therapies. The possibility of manipulation of PBSC (either in vitro or in vivo) is discussed in Chapter 28. Several attempts have been made to collect stem cells following treatment with IFN-α in patients with some degree of cytogenetic response.[15–18] It is now accepted that totally or partially Ph-negative PBSC can be collected after IFN-α and used unmanipulated for autografting. The use of bone marrow cells is technically more difficult.[19,20] Although no survival advantage was seen in early studies,[21,22] it has recently been shown that bone marrow cells may carry a higher mortality risk and therefore a worse survival after ASCT.[23] In a recent report, Ph-negative PBSC have been collected after ASCT, thus allowing for sequential transplants.[24]

AUTOGRAFTING IN CHRONIC PHASE: RESULTS

No prospective study has compared ASCT with IFN-α or other treatment modalities, so it remains unknown whether ASCT can prolong survival in CML, and if so in which category of patients. The results of ASCT are still very difficult to interpret, since most of the studies performed were pilot studies or phase II trials, with a small number of patients included and a short follow-up (shorter in many cases than the usual median survival of CML!). Moreover, in most series, the indications for ASCT were unclear, although most patients seem to have been transplanted for poor prognostic factors such as resistance to IFN-α treatment. Many single-centre and multicentre studies have now been published, and their main results are summarized in Table 26.1. They are very difficult to compare, given the wide heterogeneity in the characteristics of patients (inclusion criteria) and transplants (conditioning regimens, source of stem cells, and treatment administered after ASCT). Despite this heterogeneity, the overall results look similar.

Three main single-centre studies have been reported in Europe. Meloni et al[25] reported 34 patients who were transplanted in chronic phase after melphalan (L-PAM, 60 mg/m^2) and busulfan (4 mg/kg/day × 4 days). Twenty-two treated in the early phase of the disease were transplanted with PBSC within 12 months of diagnosis (group A). Twelve other patients pretreated and responding to IFN-α had marrow (10 cases) or PBSC collection (2 cases) after a median of 5 months from discontinuation of IFN-α (group B). All patients engrafted, and

Table 26.1 Summary of results of ASCT for CML in chronic phase in Europe using unmanipulated stem cells

Number of patients	Source of stem cells[a]	Cytogenetic conversion	Outcome	Ref
34	Unmanipulated PBSC (24); unmanipulated MSC (10)	18/32 patients	10-year survival rate of 55%	25 (updated 2000)
21	Unmanipulated PBSC	11/17 patients	5-year survival rate of 56%	26
20	Unmanipulated PBSC	13/20 patients	5-year survival rate of 75% ± 42%	7
20	Unmanipulated PBSC	14/20 patients	5-year survival rate of 59% ± 22%	27 (updated 2000)
23	Unmanipulated PBSC/MSC	14/23 patients	3-year survival rate of 67% ± 23%	28
316	Unmanipulated PBSC	70/207 patients	5-year survival rate of 71%	23

[a]PBSC, peripheral blood stem cells; MSC, marrow stem cells.

only one patient died early from interstitial pneumonitis. Thirty transplanted patients showing complete haematological reconstitution received low-dose IFN-α treatment (1×10^6 IU/m^2) as maintenance therapy. At the time of first analysis, 19 patients in group A and all in group B were in chronic phase after median times from transplant of 13 and 1.5 months respectively. At 2 months from transplant, 18 of the 32 patients evaluated had a reduction of Ph-positive metaphases greater than 50% (11 among the 22 group A patients and 7 among the 12 group B patients). A recent update of these patients, using the European Group for Bone Marrow Transplantation (EBMT) database, shows 15 patients still alive after more than 8 years of (median) follow-up. Three of them remain in complete cytogenetic remission. The 8-year probability of survival is just over 50% for the entire group. In London (Hammersmith Hospital), 21 patients were treated with high-dose chemotherapy (busulfan, 4 mg/kg/day × 4 days combined with melphalan (13) or with cyclophosphamide (4) or alone (1)) or with cyclophosphamide and TBI (3), followed by the reinfusion of unmanipulated PBSC. One patient failed to engraft and died 4 months post transplant. Of the 17 patients studied during the first year post transplant, 11 had a cytogenetic conversion and seemed to have prolonged survival.[26] The 5-year survival rate after transplantation was 56%. The survival of these 21 patients was compared with that of 636 age-matched controls in the UK Medical Research Council's (MRC) database who had been treated with conventional chemotherapy (without IFN-α) over the same period. Autografted patients had a significantly longer survival at 5 years than chemotherapy patients (56% versus 28%). In Bordeaux, 20 patients with poor-prognosis CML (6 with initial Sokal index > 1.2 and 14 with no response to IFN-α) were transplanted with PBSC collected at diagnosis before any treatment and without any mobilization, after a conditioning regimen consisting of busulfan (4 mg/kg/day × 4 days) and melphalan (140 mg/m^2).[7] All 20 of these patients received IFN-α post ASCT. Thirteen patients achieved a cytogenetic response, of which 5 were major and 8 minor remissions. For the 6 patients transplanted with a Sokal index > 1.2, one partial and one minor cytogenetic response were observed, and for the 14 patients resistant to IFN-α, 4 major cytogenetic responses (one complete) and 7 minor responses were obtained. No patient died before haematopoietic reconstitution. The 5-year survival rate was 75% ± 42%, which is similar to that of the London and Rome series. A trend for better survival was observed in patients achieving a major cytogenetic response.

These European results are similar to those reported in USA by the Houston group.[29] They transplanted 22 patients who were either resistant to IFN-α or unable to tolerate it. The preparative regimens used were CBV (cyclophosphamide 1.5 g/m^2/day × 4 days, carmustine (BCNU) 300 mg/m^2, etoposide (VP-16) 125 mg/m^2 every 12 hours daily × 3 days) or Cy/VP-16/TBI (cyclophosphamide 60 mg/kg/day × 2 days, etoposide 125 mg/m^2 every 12 hours × 3 days, fractionated TBI of 10.2 Gy). One patient died early and two had graft failure. Eighteen patients achieved a complete haematological response, and five of these a partial or complete cytogenetic response. Three of the 18 patients received IFN-α maintenance therapy after ASCT. The median survival of these 22 patients was 34 months (from transplantation).

AUTOGRAFTING IN CHRONIC PHASE: THE EBMT SURVEY

Not surprisingly, the results of the retrospective analysis of multicentre studies correspond to those of single-centre studies. In a recent survey of the EBMT database, 581 patients with CML in chronic phase have been reported to undergo an ASCT for the first time.[23] The median follow-up at the time of analysis was 18 months. The median age at SCT was 44 years. The interval between diagnosis and SCT was 20 months. Most patients were transplanted after more than 12 months in chronic phase, and the majority had been treated with IFN-α before SCT. Sixty-seven percent of IFN-α-treated patients were refractory at the chromosomal level, and one-third were classified as having high-risk disease. The transplant procedure was performed using peripheral blood cells alone in more than 70% of cases. Most centres used busulfan alone or in combination with cyclophosphamide or melphalan in the preparative conditioning, although 60 patients received TBI. There has been an increase in the numbers of autografts performed with mobilized stem cells in recent years, with nearly 100 cases reported in this survey between 1994 and 1998. The overall transplant mortality rate was low (4.6%), and seemed to be greater in transplants done with bone marrow stem cells and/or TBI. It was less than 1% for patients transplanted soon after diagnosis. The overall survival rate was 65% at 5 years from transplant, with more than 50% of all patients remaining in chronic phase at 5 years. The use of IFN-α post autograft was beneficial, with more than 80% of patients treated with IFN-α after SCT surviving at 3 years, compared with 55% if they were not given IFN-α post SCT. Patients transplanted within 6 months from diagnosis and treated with IFN-α after haematological recovery had an extremely good prognosis, with more than 85% alive at 5 years from diagnosis.

McGlave et al[28] reported the results observed in 200 patients transplanted in eight major transplant centres (four from Europe). Of these 200 patients, 44 received purged stem cells. One hundred and twenty patients received unmanipulated peripheral blood or bone marrow stem cells while in chronic phase; their 5-year survival rate was 58% with a median follow-up of 30 months. Transplant-related mortality was influenced by age at the time of transplantation, so that 17% of patients over 40 years old died during the first year after SCT, compared with 1 out of 63 patients younger than 40 years. The source of stem cells (blood versus marrow) and the use of ex vivo cell treatment did not influence survival.

TOXICITY AND POST-SCT THERAPY

ASCT performed during chronic phase has a low toxicity (the transplant-related mortality does not exceed 5% in most series). The mortality seems higher in patients transplanted with bone marrow cells and receiving TBI.[23] Most centres now use chemotherapy only (such as busulfan with cyclophosphamide or with melphalan, or even busulfan alone), with similar results and a reduced toxicity.[30] Haematopoietic reconstitution using peripheral blood stem cells is usually rapid (less than 15 days), and the 5-year survival rate from transplantation varies between 50% and 70%. These results compare favourably with those after allogeneic SCT. However, unlike the latter, almost all patients have persistent disease after ASCT.

Thus, ASCT is not a curative treatment for CML, but could restore IFN-α sensitivity and prolong survival. In the EBMT retrospective analysis of transplantation for CML in chronic phase resistant to IFN-α, some patients were restored to IFN-α sensitivity after ASCT: one-third of 41 IFN-α-resistant patients achieved complete cytogenetic response after ASCT and IFN-α after a median of 2 years of treatment with IFN-α.[31] The best results were obtained for patients with the lowest tumour mass at diagnosis. These findings suggest that IFN-α following transplantation may be beneficial either in maintaining a complete cytogenetic response obtained after transplant or in decreasing the percentage of Ph-positive cells in patients who did not respond immediately after transplant. In a report from Bordeaux, encouraging results were found for 14 IFN-α-resistant patients: with no toxic deaths, a 5-year survival rate of 100%, and 11 patients obtaining cytogenetic responses, of which 4 were major.[7] In the recent EBMT survey, there is a suggestion that patients previously resistant or refractory to IFN-α could obtain a cytogenetic remission after autograft and more importantly maintain the cytogenetic response when IFN-α is used after SCT. Fifteen percent of IFN-α refractory patients could expect to achieve complete cytogenetic remission and 20% a major response.[23]

While ASCT might be able to prolong survival, it is important to know which category of patients with CML in chronic phase could benefit from ASCT. For patients responding to IFN-α,[32–34] especially those who achieve a major (≥65% Ph-negative cells) or complete cytogenetic response, the probability of surviving at 5 years is 90%. For these patients, it would be very difficult to demonstrate a survival advantage for ASCT. As most of these IFN-α-responding patients do not have a high Sokal index, it could be that ASCT is indicated only for patients with high-risk CML. In France, such ASCT was performed in 20 CML patients with a Sokal index > 1.2.[27] They were given busulfan and melphalan, and were then reinfused with blood stem cells. Of these patients, 16 received IFN-α after ASCT and 3 achieved a major cytogenetic response. The results have been recently updated: 8 of the 20 patients are still alive 56–166 months after transplant. In the EBMT survey, 52 patients (high-risk disease) were autografted early after diagnosis (27 patients) or in late chronic phase (25 patients), with a trend to a better survival for patients autografted early (72% versus 39% survival at 5 years).

The use of immunomodulator agents after ASCT has been explored with limited success. Growth factors such as granulocyte–macrophage colony-stimulating factor (GM-CSF) may selectively favour the proliferation of Ph-negative cells, and this has been used in combination with hydroxyurea after autografting with unmanipulated peripheral blood progenitor cells (PBSC)[35] or with PBSC incubated in vitro with GM-CSF.[36] A small group of 17 patients received the immunomodulator roquinimex following autologous bone marrow transplantation and cytogenetic responses were seen in all patients, occasionally developing over time, suggesting an immune-mediated and not a post-SCT transient effect.[37] Most of the current evidence suggests that IFN-α post SCT is beneficial. In one case report, a case of post-autograft graft-versus-host disease was described after re-treatment with IFN-α.[38]

FINAL CONSIDERATIONS

The use of autografting remains controversial for patients who have an HLA-identical sibling or unrelated donor.[22,39,40] Transplant-related mortality remains high for allografts (15–20% for sibling and 25–40% for unrelated).[41] It has been suggested that allogeneic SCT should be reserved for patients who are younger and that a trial of IFN-α (with or without ASCT) could be offered to older patients.[42] Others suggest that a trial of IFN could be attempted in most cases.[43]

For many years, ASCT has been performed using either unmodified bone marrow harvested during chronic phase or peripheral blood cells collected at diagnosis before treatment. In 1978, Goldman et al[2] first reported that very high numbers of granulocyte–macrophage colony-forming units (CFU-GM) were present in the blood of CML patients at diagnosis and could easily be collected by leukapheresis. Other investigators have subsequently confirmed this. For example, in Bordeaux, 1103 leukaphereses were performed in 212 CML patients, at diagnosis and before any treatment. The median number of nucleated cells and CFU-GM collected per leukapheresis were $2.7\ (0.9–12.8) \times 10^8$/kg and $31.2\ (0–1255.2) \times 10^4$/kg respectively. The median number of CFU-GM collected by a single leukapheresis was 17.5×10^4/kg, and was higher than that usually obtained from marrow harvest. Not surprisingly, the cell yield (CFU-GM) was correlated not only with the initial white blood cell count ($r \leqslant 0.24$, $p < 0.001$) but also with the platelet count ($r = 0.12$, $p = 0.0001$) and the Sokal index ($r = 0.2$, $p = 0.005$).[44] When transplanted, these cells engraft very quickly in about 15 days, which is more rapidly than observed after autologous bone marrow transplantation for patients with CML.[45] It has now been reported that both peripheral blood and bone marrow in early chronic phase contain some Ph-negative progenitors.[46–49] These normal progenitors are able to engraft, and are probably responsible for the cytogenetic conversions that are regularly seen after ASCT, since they have a proliferative advantage (when transplanted) over leukaemic Ph-positive progenitor cells.[3,50,51] Thus, as peripheral blood seems to be equivalent to bone marrow for observing cytogenetic conversion and to contain more progenitors (leading to more rapid engraftment) than bone marrow, most autologous transplants are now performed with PBSC.

In summary, retrospective and single-centre trials have shown that autologous SCT in CML could prolong survival if performed in chronic phase. Unfortunately, no randomized trial has been conducted to compare outcome after autografting with IFN-α-based therapy. Results from the French and Italian groups showed that similar results can be obtained with a combination of IFN-α and cytarabine (cytosine arabinoside, Ara-C). It is therefore of the utmost importance that such a comparison be made. Several national groups (SFGM, GETH, German CML III Study group, MRC, and ECOG) have initiated randomized trials comparing different forms of autografting with IFN-α. More recently, the EBMT has launched a multicentre, multinational study comparing autografting with IFN-α. This trial is going to include the French, Spanish, and British initiatives, and will be analysed together with the second randomization of the German CML III-A trial in a meta-analysis. So, a very important question is being addressed here: Does the addition of autografting early in the course of the disease improve the response to IFN-α-based therapy in newly diagnosed CML? Autografting has been performed in Europe for more than 20 years, and we still do not know the exact role that it should play in the management of CML. Many questions will be left unanswered: What is the best way of doing an autograft? Is mobilization necessary? Does the use of mainly Ph-negative stem cells influence outcome? But at least we shall be ready to ask these and other relevant questions regarding the use of autografting in combination with the newly developed tyrosine kinase inhibitors such as STI571 in the near future.

REFERENCES

1. Buckner CD, Stewart P, Clift RA et al, Treatment of blastic transformation of chronic granulocytic leukaemia by chemotherapy, total body irradiation and infusion of cryopreserved autologous marrow. *Exp Hematol* 1978; **6:** 96–109.
2. Goldman JM, Th'ng KH, Park DS et al, Collection, cryopreservation and subsequent viability of haemopoietic stem cells intended for treatment of chronic granulocytic leukaemia in blast-cell transformation. *Br J Haematol* 1978; **40:** 185–95.
3. Haines ME, Goldman JM, Worsley AM et al, Chemotherapy and autografting for chronic granulocytic leukaemia in transformation: probable prolongation of survival in some patients. *Br J Haematol* 1984; **58:** 711–21.
4. Butturini A, Keating A, Goldman J, Gale RP, Autotransplants in chronic myelogenous leukaemia: strategies and results. *Lancet* 1990; **335:** 1255–8.
5. Reiffers J, Trouette R, Marit G et al, Autologous blood stem cell transplantation for chronic granulocytic leukaemia in transformation: a report of 47 cases. *Br J Haematol* 1991; **77:** 339–45.
6. Reiffers J, Mahon FX, Boiron JM et al, Autografting in chronic myeloid leukaemia: an overview. *Leukaemia* 1996; **10:** 385–8.
7. Pigneux A, Faberes C, Boiron JM et al, Autologous stem cell transplantation in chronic myeloid leukemia: a single center experience. *Bone Marrow Transplant* 1999; **24:** 265–70.
8. Hehlmann R, Hochhaus A, Berger U, Reiter A, Current trends in the management of chronic myelogenous leukemia. *Ann Hematol* 2000; **79:** 345–54.
9. Deisseroth AB, Zu Z, Claxton D et al, Genetic marking shows that Ph+ cells present in autologous transplants of chronic myelogenous leukemia (CML) contribute to relapse after autologous bone marrow in CML. *Blood* 1994; **83:** 3068–76.
10. Daley GQ, Rationalizing autotransplant strategies for chronic myeloid leukemia. *Leuk Lymphoma* 1996; **21:** 353–8.
11. Bhatia R, Forman SJ, Autologous transplantation for the treatment of chronic myelogenous leukemia. *Hematol Oncol Clin North Am* 1998; **12:** 151–72.
12. Miller JS, Innovative therapy for chronic myelogenous leukemia. *Hematol Oncol Clin North Am* 1998; **12:** 173–206.
13. Carella AM, Frassoni F, ICE, mini-ICE or high-dose hydroxyurea to mobilize Philadelphia [Ph]-negative PBPC in chronic myelogenous leukaemia. *Br J Haematol* 1996; **95:** 213–14.
14. Carella AM, Lerma E, Corsetti MT et al, Autografting with Philadelphia chromosome negative mobilized hematopoietic progenitor cells in chronic myelogenous leukemia. *Blood* 1999; **83:** 1534–9.
15. Reiffers J, Taylor K, Gluckman E et al, Collection of Ph-negative progenitor cells with granulocyte-colony stimulating factor in patients with chronic myeloid leukaemia who respond to recombinant alpha-interferon. *Br J Haematol* 1998; **102:** 639–46.
16. Archimbaud E, Michallet M, Philip I et al, Granulocyte colony-stimulating factor given in addition to interferon-alpha to mobilize peripheral blood stem cells for autologous transplantation in chronic myeloid leukaemia. *Br J Haematol* 1997; **99:** 678–84.
17. Olavarria E, Parker S, Craddock C et al, Collection of Ph-negative progenitor cells from interferon responsive patients with chronic myeloid leukemia: effect of granulocyte-colony-

stimulating factor mobilization. *Haematologica* 2000; **85:** 647–52.
18. Russo D, Martinelli G, Montefusco V et al, Collection of Ph-negative progenitor cells from Ph+ CML patients in complete cytogenetic remission after long-term interferon-alpha therapy. *Haematologica* 1999; **84:** 953–5.
19. Meloni G, Russo D, Baccarani M et al, A prospective study of alpha-interferon and autologous bone marrow transplantation in chronic myeloid leukemia. The Italian Co-operative Study Group on Chronic Myeloid Leukemia. *Haematologica* 1999; **84:** 707–15.
20. The Italian Cooperative Study Group on Chronic Myeloid Leukaemia, Karyotype conversion by Interferon as preparative treatment for autologous BMT in Ph positive CML. *Leuk Lymphoma* 1993; **11**(Suppl 1): 277–80.
21. Reiffers J, Goldman J, Meloni G et al, on behalf of the Chronic Leukaemia Working Party of the EBMT, Autologous stem cell transplantation in chronic myelogenous leukaemia: a retrospective analysis of the European Group for Bone Marrow Transplantation. *Bone Marrow Transplant* 1994; **14:** 407–10.
22. Goldman JM, Treatment of chronic myeloid leukaemia: some topical questions. *Baillière's Clin Haematol* 1997; **10:** 405–21.
23. Olavarria E, Mandelli F, Goldman J et al, The role of autologous stem cell transplantation in the management of chronic myeloid leukaemia: the EBMT experience. *Bone Marrow Transplant* 2000; **25**(Suppl 1): S76.
24. Spencer A, Granter N, Fagan K et al, Collection and analysis of peripheral blood mononuclear cells during haemopoietic recovery following PBSCT for CML: autografting as an in vivo purging manoeuvre? *Bone Marrow Transplant* 1998; **21:** 101–3.
25. Meloni G, De Fabritiis P, Alimena F et al, Autologous bone marrow transplantation or peripheral blood stem cell transplantation for patients with chronic myelogenous leukaemia in chronic phase. *Bone Marrow Transplant* 1990; **4**(Suppl 4): 92–4.
26. Hoyle C, Gray R, Goldman J, Autografting for patients with CML in chronic phase: an update. *Br J Haematol* 1994; **86:** 76–81.
27. Reiffers J, Cahn JY, Montastruc M et al, Peripheral blood stem cell transplantation followed by recombinant alpha interferon for chronic myelogenous leukemia in chronic phase: preliminary results. *Stem Cells* 1993; **11:** 23–4.
28. McGlave PB, De Fabritis P, Deisseroth J et al, Autologous transplants for chronic myelogenous leukaemia: results from eight transplant groups. *Lancet* 1994; **343:** 1486–8.
29. Khouri IF, Kantarjian H, Talpaz M et al, Results with high-dose chemotherapy and unpurged autologous stem cell transplantation in 73 patients with chronic myelogenous leukaemia: the MD Anderson experience. *Bone Marrow Transplant* 1996; **17:** 775–9.
30. Olavarria E, Kanfer E, Szydlo R et al, High-dose busulphan alone as cytoreduction before allogeneic or autologous stem cell transplantation for chronic myeloid leukaemia: a single-centre experience. *Br J Haematol* 2000; **108:** 769–77.
31. Boiron JM, Cahn JY, Meloni G et al, Chronic myeloid leukaemia in first chronic phase not responding to α-interferon: outcome and prognostic factors after autologous transplantation. *Bone Marrow Transplant* 1999; **24:** 259–64.
32. Kantarjian HM, Smith TL, O'Brien S et al, Prolonged survival in chronic myelogenous leukaemia following cytogenetic response to alpha interferon therapy. *Ann Intern Med* 1995; **122:** 254–61.
33. Mahon FX, Faberes C, Pueyo S et al, Response at three months is a good predictive factor for newly diagnosed chronic myeloid leukemia patients treated by recombinant alpha interferon. *Blood* 1998; **92:** 4059–65.
34. The Italian Cooperative Study Group on Chronic Myeloid Leukaemia, Interferon alpha-2a as compared with conventional chemotherapy for the treatment of chronic myeloid leukaemia. *N Engl J Med* 1994; **330:** 820–5.
35. Carlo-Stella C, Regazzi E, Andrizzi C et al, Use of granulocyte–macrophage colony-stimulating factor (GM-CSF) in combination with hydroxyurea as post-transplant therapy in chronic myelogenous leukemia patients autografted with unmanipulated hematopoietic cells. *Haematologica* 1997; **82:** 291–6.
36. Gladstone DE, Bedi A, Miller CB et al, Philadelphia chromosome-negative engraftment after autologous transplantation with granulocyte–macrophage colony-stimulating factor for chronic myeloid leukemia. *Biol Blood Marrow Transplant* 1999; **5:** 394–9.
37. Rowe JM, Rapoport AP, Ryan DH et al, Treatment of chronic myelogenous leukemia with autologous bone marrow transplantation

followed by Roquinimex. *Bone Marrow Transplant* 1999; **24:** 1057–63.

38. Rainey MG, Harrison P, Hows JM et al, Spontaneous graft-versus-host disease following autologous peripheral blood progenitor cell transplantation in chronic myeloid leukaemia. *Bone Marrow Transplant* 1996; **17:** 1077–9.
39. O'Brien SG, Autografting for chronic myeloid leukaemia. *Baillière's Clin Haematol* 1997; **10:** 369–88.
40. Carella AM, Frassoni F, Negrin RS, Autografting in chronic myelogenous leukemia: new questions. *Leukemia* 1995; **9:** 365–9.
41. Silver RT, Woolf SH, Helhmann R et al, An evidence-based analysis of the effect of busulfan, hydroxyurea, interferon, and allogeneic bone marrow transplantation in treating the chronic phase of chronic myeloid leukemia: developed for the American Society of Hematology. *Blood* 1999; **94**(Suppl 1): 1517–36.
42. Enright H, McGlave P, Bone marrow transplantation for chronic myelogenous leukemia. *Curr Opin Oncol* 1998; **10:** 100–7.
43. Kantarjian HM, Giles FJ, O'Brien SG et al, Therapeutic choices in younger patients with chronic myelogenous leukemia. *Cancer* 2000; **83:** 1647–58.
44. Bouzgarrou R, Reiffers J, Cellules souches circulantes et LMC: modalités de prélèvement, congélation, décongélation, reconstitution hématologique après greffe. Réunion du Groupe Hémobiologie du FAG, 22 Octobre 1991.
45. Reiffers J, Autologous transplantation in chronic myelogenous leukaemia. *Rev Fr Transfus Immunohematol* 1985; **28:** 509–20.
46. Coulombel L, Kalousek DK, Eaves CJ et al, Long-term marrow culture reveals chromosomally normal hematopoietic progenitor cells in patients with Philadelphia chromosome positive chronic myelogenous leukaemia. *N Engl J Med* 1983; **308:** 1493–8.
47. Jazwieck B, Mahon FX, Pigneux A et al, 5-Fluorouracil-resistant CD34+ cell population from peripheral blood of chronic myelogenous leukemia patients contains BCR–ABL negative progenitor cells. *Exp Hematol* 1995; **23:** 1509–14.
48. Kirk JA, Reems JA, Roecklein BA et al, Benign marrow progenitors are enriched in CD34+/HLA-DR^{lo} population but not in the CD34+/38^{lo} population in chronic myeloid leukaemia: an analysis using interphase fluorescence in situ hybridization. *Blood* 1995; **86:** 737–43.
49. Petzer AL, Eaves CJ, Lansdorp PM et al, Characterization of primitive subpopulation of normal and leukemic cells in the blood of patients with newly diagnosed. *Blood* 1996; **88:** 2162–71.
50. Brito-Babapulle F, Bowcock SJ, Marcus RE et al, Autografting for patients with chronic myeloid leukaemia in chronic phase: peripheral blood stem cells may have a finite capacity for maintaining haematopoiesis. *Br J Haematol* 1989; **73:** 76–81.
51. Reiffers J, Goldman JM, Meloni G et al, Autologous stem cell transplantation (ASCT) for chronic myeloid leukemia (CML) in chronic phase: a report of the European Blood and Marrow Transplant (EBMT) Group. *Bone Marrow Transplant* 1996; **17**(Suppl 1): S3 (Abst 56).

27

Autografting with cultured marrow

Michael J Barnett, Connie J Eaves, Allen C Eaves

CONTENTS • **Introduction** • **Long-term culture of hematopoietic cells** • **Vancouver studies** • **Manchester study** • **Discussion**

INTRODUCTION

The intent of this chapter is to review the use of a culture-based strategy to prepare autografts for patients with chronic myeloid leukemia (CML). As with other in vitro techniques, the goal is to minimize the content of leukemic stem cells in the autograft while retaining sufficient Philadelphia chromosome (Ph)-negative stem cells to enable prompt restoration of blood cell formation.

Intensive therapy

Intensive ('myeloablative') therapy followed by transplantation of marrow from a suitable donor results in long-term leukemia-free survival for a significant proportion of patients who are able to undergo this treatment.[1] Considerations of age and histocompatibility do however, limit the use of allogeneic bone marrow transplantation (BMT) to only a minority of patients.[2] Although it is now appreciated that the graft-versus-leukemia (GVL) effect makes a significant contribution to eradication of CML after allogeneic BMT,[3] experience with syngeneic BMT for patients with chronic-phase disease suggests that ablative therapy alone has the capacity to eradicate the leukemic clone.[4]

Residual normal stem cells

Both laboratory[5–7] and clinical[8–10] evidence support the persistence of Ph-negative hematopoietic stem cells in many patients. Various markers of clonality have been used to show that at least some of these cells do not belong to the leukemic clone and are presumably normal.[11–13] It is likely, therefore, that residual normal stem cells represent a quantitatively useful reservoir from a therapeutic standpoint (Figure 27.1), particularly early in the course of the disease.[14–16]

The constraints on the applicability of allogeneic BMT and the results of syngeneic BMT (arguably the perfect autograft), together with the availability of normal stem cells in many patients, offer a rationale for intensive therapy with autografting in CML.

Transplantation of leukemic stem cells

Past experience with unirradiated granulocyte transfusions from donors with CML,[17–19] as well as recent studies using immunodeficient mice[6,7]

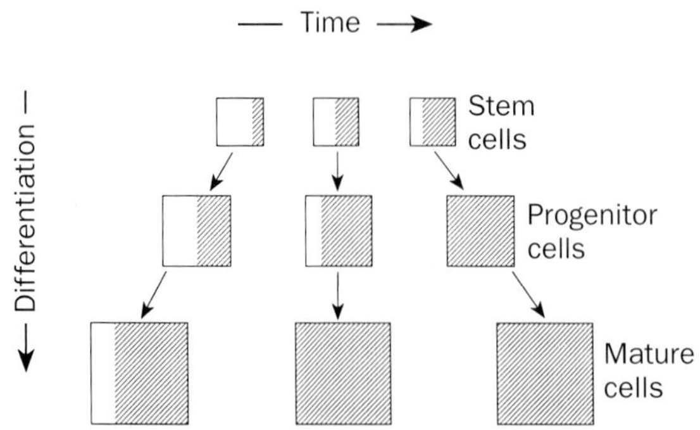

Figure 27.1
Diagram of leukemic (hatched) and normal (open) cell compartments in CML over time and during the process of differentiation. Reproduced, with permission, from Barnett MJ, Eaves CJ, Chronic myeloid leukemia. In: *Leukemia*, 6th edn (Henderson ES, Lister TA, Greaves MF, eds). Orlando, FL: WB Saunders, 1996.

or analyses of patients transplanted with genetically marked autologous cells,[20] have provided evidence that the CML clone can be transplanted. Thus, although of lesser concern than the bulk of disease residing in the patient, contamination of the autograft with leukemic stem cells is an important consideration in the development of autograft-based protocols.

LONG-TERM CULTURE OF HEMATOPOIETIC CELLS

Background

When high concentrations of marrow cells are placed in liquid culture containing serum and other supplements, but not exogeneously provided growth factors, near input levels of primitive hematopoietic cells can be maintained for approximately two weeks.[21] This so-called long-term culture (LTC) system was first developed for murine marrow in the mid 1970s,[22] and then applied to human cells a few years later.[23–25] In LTC, stromal cells have a key supportive function,[26,27] although details of the mechanisms involved remain to be determined. Nevertheless, the ability of the system to support hematopoiesis for prolonged periods of time has been exploited as the basis of a cell culture assay for a primitive progenitor cell, the long-term culture-initiating cell (LTC-IC).[28,29]

In the early 1980s, studies conducted in Vancouver demonstrated a 'switch' to normal hematopoiesis in LTC initiated with marrow from patients with either acute myeloid leukemia (AML)[30] or CML,[5] thereby suggesting a therapeutic role for the LTC system in the autograft setting. Later studies in CML have demonstrated that this differential behavior of normal and leukemic cells in LTC is due in part to unexpectedly high concentrations of normal, relative to leukemic, LTC-IC in the marrow, as well as to the intrinsically compromised self-renewal of leukemic LTC-IC.[31,32] Typically, Ph-negative LTC-IC are maintained at input levels for the first 10 days in culture, whereas Ph-positive LTC-IC decrease 30-fold under the same conditions (Figure 27.2).

Large-scale culture of cells for autografting

The group at the Christie Hospital in Manchester was the first to exploit the LTC system clinically. In 1986, Chang and colleagues[33] reported the case of a patient with AML in relapse autografted with marrow cells that had been cultured under conditions previously found to enable the establishment of LTC from a single inoculum of unseparated marrow. After marrow harvest, 2.1×10^{10} nucleated cells were cultured for 10 days in plastic flasks and, during the interval, the patient received myeloablative therapy (cyclophosphamide and total-body irradiation (TBI)). At the end of this time, 6.7×10^9 cells, i.e. 1.35×10^8 cells/kg, comprising both adherent and non-adherent fractions of the culture were collected and infused. The patient recovered with normal hematopoiesis (by morphological and karyotypic examination), although a prolonged period of time elapsed before recovery of neutrophil and platelet counts.

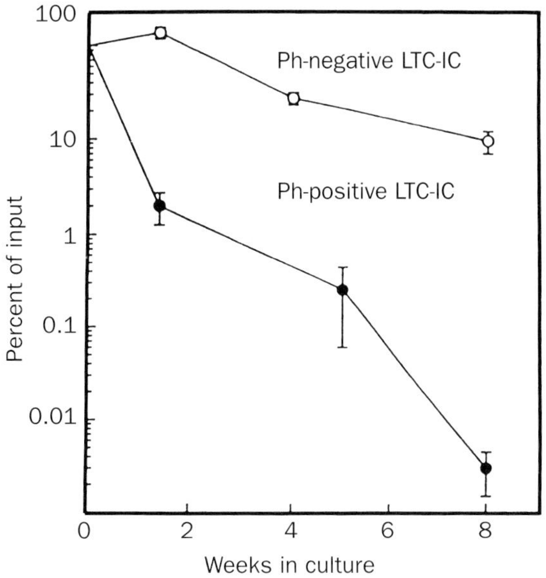

Figure 27.2
Differential maintenance of Ph-negative and Ph-positive LTC-IC under long-term culture conditions. Reproduced, with permission, from Barnett MJ, Eaves CJ, Chronic myeloid leukemia. In: *Leukemia*, 6th edn (Henderson ES, Lister TA, Greaves MF, eds). Orlando, FL: WB Saunders, 1996.

In 1987, we began a pilot study to evaluate the feasibility of using cultured marrow autografts to support intensive treatment of patients with CML. Influenced by our own laboratory findings as well as the preliminary clinical experience of the Manchester group,[34] we adopted a protocol that also employed a 10-day culture period.[35] The methodology used in Vancouver involved dispensing aliquots of 2×10^8 nucleated cells from a buffy coat preparation into approximately 100 separate 175 cm^2 tissue culture flasks, each containing 60 ml of LTC medium (to give a final cell concentration of approximately 3×10^6/ml). The flasks were then incubated at 37°C for the first 3 days and subsequently at 33°C for the remaining 7 days. After this period in culture, the adherent cells were suspended by trypsinization and combined with the non-adherent cells for infusion.

VANCOUVER STUDIES

Study 1

For the first Vancouver study, patient entry was restricted to those with disease in morphological chronic phase (although not necessarily the first) and the Ph detectable on routine cytogenetic analysis, who were no older than 60 years and ineligible for allogeneic BMT. Such patients were further selected according to the results of a laboratory test on a preliminary marrow sample. The latter required that after 10 days in culture, the concentration of Ph-negative LTC-IC be 2% or more of that present in a comparable specimen of normal marrow and that the concentration of Ph-positive LTC-IC be below the limit of detectability (usually <1 per 2×10^7 initial marrow cells). The rationale for this 'screening' test was to increase the likelihood of identifying patients in whom a subsequently harvested and similarly treated marrow would be likely to contain sufficient primitive normal hematopoietic cells to allow engraftment and might also have had its content of leukemic stem cells significantly reduced.

The intensive treatment was either a busulfan-based or TBI-based regimen, on completion of which patients were given an infusion of autologous marrow cells that had been cultured for 10 days. Patients in whom complete cytogenetic remission was achieved post autograft were followed off therapy until Ph-positive metaphases reappeared in marrow samples.

Between 1987 and 1993, 100 patients were identified as eligible for this study before their marrow was tested in culture, and in 40 of them (40%) the laboratory selection criteria were met. In this 6-year period, 26 of these 40 patients (Table 27.1) were treated with intensive therapy and then autografted with cultured marrow. The results of this first study were published in 1994,[36] and are now presented with the addition of 4 similarly selected patients and a further 6 years of follow-up.

Hematological recovery occurred in 20 of the 26 patients, with median times to 0.5×10^9/l neutrophils and 20×10^9/l platelets of 26

Table 27.1 Vancouver studies: details of patients at autografting

	Study 1	Study 2
Period of study	1987–1993	1994–1998
Number of patients	26	27
Disease status,[a] CP1 : AP : ≥CP2	20 : 3 : 3	25 : 2 : 0
Median age (years)	42 (range 22–59)	49 (range 23–60)
Prior interferon-α	6	10
Median interval from diagnosis (months)	12 (range 5–64)	15 (range 5–61)

[a]CP1, first chronic phase; AP, accelerated phase; CP2, second chronic phase.

(range 11–52) and 46 (range 16–337) days post autograft, respectively. Both neutrophil ($p < 0.0001$) and platelet ($p = 0.032$) recoveries were significantly faster in patients who had undergone splenectomy prior to autografting. No correlation was found between the speed of neutrophil or platelet recovery and the number of nucleated cells, clonogenic cells, or LTC-IC infused. In 5 patients (none of whom had undergone splenectomy), satisfactory neutrophil recovery was not achieved during the first 6 weeks after autografting (Table 27.2). All of these patients then received an infusion of unmanipulated marrow or peripheral blood cells that had been kept frozen in reserve. In all 5, this was followed by recovery of the neutrophil count, but, in spite of this, 2 died soon thereafter because of therapy-related toxicity (TRT). There was no correlation between graft failure and the size of the spleen, marrow fibrosis, and number of nucleated cells, clonogenic cells or LTC-IC infused.

Table 27.2 Vancouver studies: details of recovering hematopoiesis

	Study 1		Study 2
	Spleen	No spleen	No spleen
Number of patients[a]	17	6	27
Number of graft failures	5	0	1
Median time to neutrophils ≥ 0.5×10^9/l (days)	30 (range 19–52)	15 (range 11–18)	21 (range 12–57)
Median time to platelets ≥ 20×10^9/l (days)	50 (range 31–337)	45 (range 16–62)	27 (range 15–256)
Cytogenetic remission[b]	100%	83%	77%

[a]Excludes 3 patients from study 1 who were autografted in ≥second chronic phase.
[b]Percentage of patients with ≥66% Ph-negative cells in marrow on recovery.

Overall, 4 of the 26 patients died of TRT. One patient (unique patient number (UPN) 857) developed a post-transplant lymphoproliferative disorder about 30 days after autografting that later resolved.[37]

Marrow samples from 14 of the 20 patients who had satisfactory hematological recovery after infusion of cultured marrow achieved a complete cytogenetic remission (100% Ph-negative metaphases) 4–6 weeks after autografting, and in 5 of the other 6, a partial cytogenetic remission (66–99% Ph-negative metaphases) was achieved. In all but 1 (who died in remission) of the 14 patients in whom a complete cytogenetic remission was achieved initially, Ph-positive cells became detectable 4–36 (median 12) months post autograft. Nine of these 13 patients were subsequently treated with interferon-α (IFN-α), 3–5 × 10^6 units, 3 days per week, and 6 were returned to a complete cytogenetic remission.

All 3 of the patients who were treated after development of blastic-phase disease died post autograft: 1 of TRT and 2 of recurrent blastic phase. Of the other 23 patients, 3 died of TRT, 9 of transformed disease, 1 (who refused treatment) of uncontrolled chronic-phase disease, and 1 (at 6 years post autograft) of sepsis related to dialysis for chronic renal failure. Nine patients remain alive 7–11.5 (median 10) years after autografting: 5 in cytogenetic remission and 4 in chronic phase (Figure 27.3). Details of the 5 patients who continue in cytogenetic remission are shown in Table 27.3; hematopoiesis is 100% Ph-negative in 4 (2 of whom have no disease detectable by reverse-transcriptase polymerase chain reaction (RT-PCR) analysis of *BCR/ABL* transcripts) and 96% Ph-negative in 1. One of the patients (UPN 857) who continues in chronic phase has developed a squamous cell carcinoma of the tongue 6.5 years post autograft.

Study 2

For the second study, based on experience from the first, the protocol was modified to include elective splenectomy pre autograft (to avoid graft failure and ensure consistently faster hematological recovery) and the administration of low-dose IFN-α early post autograft (to reduce the likelihood of regrowth of the leukemic clone). In addition, selection of patients on the basis of laboratory criteria was abandoned.

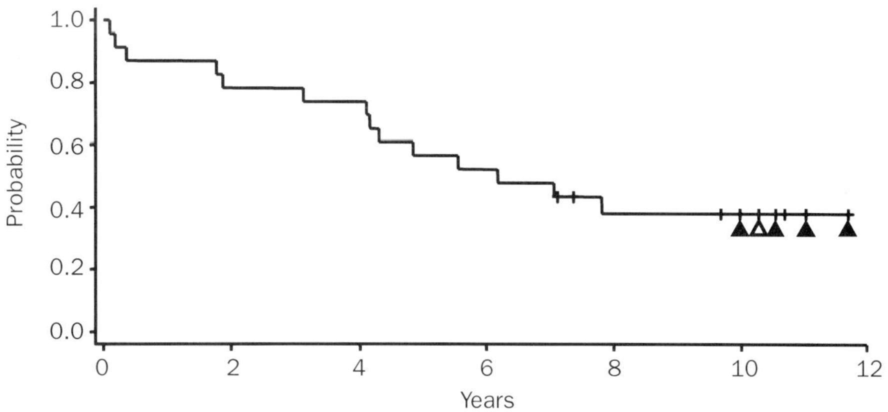

Figure 27.3
Survival after autografting in 23 patients with CML who were treated in either chronic phase (20 patients) or accelerated phase (3 patients) in the first Vancouver study. Patients who remain in complete (▲) or partial (△) cytogenetic remission are indicated.

Table 27.3 Vancouver studies: details of patients from Study 1 who remain in cytogenetic remission

UPN[a]	Diagnosis	Autografting		
	Sokal index[b]	Age	Prior treatment[c]	Interval from diagnosis (months)
208	0.67	44	Hu	64
365	0.57	22	Hu	15
399	0.48	27	Hu	6
409	0.68	53	Hu	6
448	0.61	33	Hu	17

[a]Unique patient number.
[b]Low risk, <0.8; intermediate risk, 0.8–1.2; high risk, >1.2.[63]
[c]Hu, hydroxyurea.

As in the first study, eligibility for the second required patients to have CML in morphological chronic phase (but only the first) with the Ph (a cytogenetic abnormality in addition to the Ph was acceptable), and be no more than 60 years old. In an attempt to improve patient accrual, a Canadian network was formed, including BMT centers in Edmonton, Winnipeg, Ottawa, Montreal, and Halifax. Patients were referred to Vancouver for collection, manipulation, and storage of the autograft, but underwent intensive therapy and autografting at their local center. The intensive therapy was a busulfan-based regimen, and, as in the first study, the autograft was of marrow cells that had been grown in culture for 10 days. After hematological recovery had been achieved, patients received IFN-α 1–3 × 10^6 units/m^2, 3 days per week as maintenance.

Between 1994 and 1998, 27 patients were treated (Table 27.1). Hematological recovery occurred in all except 1 who died of graft failure (Table 27.2). There were no other deaths due to TRT.

In 22 of 26 patients, a marrow sample was evaluated cytogenetically at the time of hematological recovery after infusion of cultured marrow. Cytogenetic remission was achieved in 17 (10 complete and 7 partial) of these 22 patients. The relationship between LTC-IC content of the autograft and subsequent achievement of cytogenetic remission is shown in Table 27.4.

Five patients have died of transformed disease. Twenty-one patients remain alive 1.5–6 (median 3.5) years after autografting: 7 in cytogenetic remission, 5 in hematological remission, 7 in chronic phase, and 2 in accelerated phase (Figure 27.4). The 7 patients in cytogenetic remission (5 complete and 2 partial) continue to receive IFN-α.

MANCHESTER STUDY

The Manchester group has also conducted a pilot study of the use of cultured marrow autografts in CML.[38] In order to determine eligibility for the study, marrow was assessed in LTC, and the laboratory selection criteria were met in 40% of patients tested. Nine patients aged 9–48 (median 38) years, 7–42 (median 15) months from diagnosis, including 4 who had received prior IFN-α, were autografted in first chronic phase.

The details of recovering hematopoiesis are

Table 27.4 Vancouver studies: achievement of cytogenetic remission in Study 2 according to LTC-IC content of the autograft

LTC-IC in autograft[a] Ph-negative : Ph-positive	Ph-negative metaphases in marrow on recovery from autografting		
	100% (n = 10)	76–98%[b] (n = 6)	0–19%[c] (n = 5)
>10 : 1	8	3	1
1–10 : 1	2	0	1
<1 : 1	0	3	3

[a]Median numbers of LTC-IC infused per kg body weight: Ph-negative, 2.73×10^3 (range 0–2.71×10^4); Ph-positive, 7 (range 0–1.57×10^5).
[b]Excludes 1 patient in whom partial cytogenetic remission was achieved but for whom LTC-IC data were not available.
[c]Includes 1 patient in whom a marrow sample could not be obtained but in whom metaphases from the blood were 0% Ph-negative.

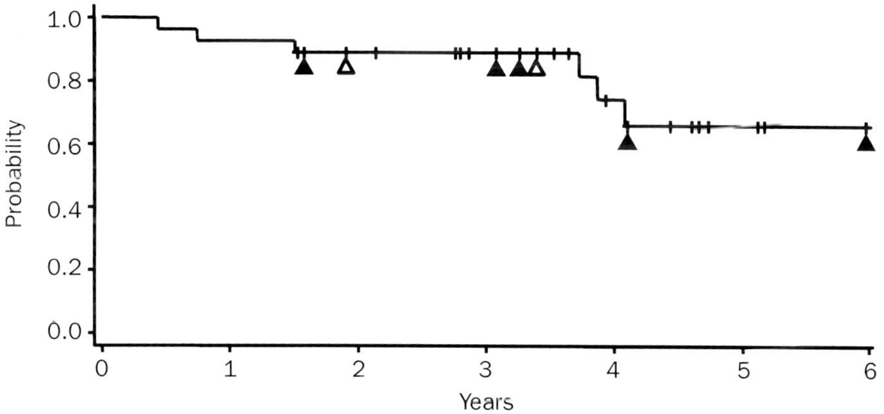

Figure 27.4
Survival after autografting in 27 patients with CML who were treated in the second Vancouver study. Patients who remain in complete (▲) or partial (△) cytogenetic remission are indicated.

shown in Table 27.5. Two patients died of graft failure and 1 died at 16 months post autograft as a consequence of prolonged thrombocytopenia. Complete cytogenetic remission lasted 6–12 months before Ph-positive cells recurred, at which time IFN-α was started. Two patients died after unrelated-donor BMT carried out for chronic-phase disease. At the time of the report, 4 patients remained alive 40–87 months after autografting: 2 in complete cytogenetic remission on IFN-α, 1 in hematological remission on IFN-α, and 1 in chronic phase.

Table 27.5 Manchester study: details of recovering hematopoiesis

Number of patients[a]	9
Number of graft failures	2
Median time to neutrophils $\geq 0.5 \times 10^9$/l (days)	26 (range 15–39)
Median time to platelets $\geq 20 \times 10^9$/l (days)	95 (range 54–252)
Cytogenetic remission[b]	100%

[a]None had undergone splenectomy.
[b]Percentage of patients with ≥66% Ph-negative cells in marrow on recovery.

DISCUSSION

In view of their keen interest in the LTC system, it is understandable that the Vancouver and Manchester groups have pursued cell culture as a means to prepare autografts for patients with CML. The reluctance of others to adopt this strategy may have a number of explanations. First, the results of some preclinical studies that evaluated growth of CML marrow in LTC were less supportive of clinical application, perhaps related to assessment of samples from patients relatively late in the course of the disease.[39,40] Second, the methodology for large-scale culture has, quite correctly, been considered laborious, and – undeservedly – a mystique has been attached to it. Third, early clinical experience elsewhere suggested that graft failure might be a complication of autografting with cultured marrow.[41] Fourth, leukapheresis of the blood during hematopoietic recovery after combination chemotherapy, developed by the Genoa group, provided a more convenient method to collect Ph-negative progenitors.[42,43]

These reservations notwithstanding, the pilot studies conducted in Vancouver[36] and in Manchester[38] have established the feasibility of this approach to prepare autografts in CML. These results and those from the second Vancouver study will be discussed in terms of the achievement of two goals: that of the autograft, i.e. the prompt restoration of Ph-negative hematopoiesis; and that of the treatment, i.e. the achievement of long-term leukemia-free and overall survival. Finally, possible future directions will be outlined.

The autograft

Cytogenetic remission was achieved in the majority of patients who had satisfactory hematological recovery after infusion of the cultured marrow autograft (Tables 27.2 and 27.5). Furthermore, this recovery with predominantly Ph-negative cells was within a time frame consistent with an origin from hematopoietic progenitors in the autograft. This is in contrast to the situation after autografting with unmanipulated blood[44] or marrow[45] cells, when recovery with Ph-positive cells is the norm. Although in both pilot studies, patients were selected according to the marrow content of primitive normal cells (i.e. Ph-negative LTC-IC), this was not the case in the second Vancouver study, in which a cytogenetic remission rate of about 75% was still achieved. It is of interest to note that this latter result is similar to that reported by the Genoa group in patients autografted with mobilized Ph-negative progenitors collected from the blood.[46]

The genotype of the regenerating cells post autograft correlated with the predominant genotype of LTC-IC that infused (Table 27.4). This observation is in accord with results from other studies that show that achievement of cytogenetic remission after autografting in CML depends on the content (i.e. Ph-positive versus Ph-negative cells) of the graft.[47–49] In turn, it seems likely that the composition of the graft is influenced more by the 'biology of the disease', as assessed for example by the Sokal prognostic index,[50] than the methodology employed for its collection.

In the combined Vancouver and Manchester experience, 10% of patients died after a prolonged period of cytopenia. This is of particular concern, since it is likely that such deaths could have been avoided had satisfactory neutrophil and platelet counts been achieved earlier. It was not possible to predict this outcome from the hematopoietic progenitor content of the autograft. Indeed, in the Vancouver pilot study, the only factor found to correlate with graft failure and speed of hematological recovery was whether or not patients had previously undergone splenectomy (thus confirming an earlier observation[51]). In order to address these concerns, patients in the second Vancouver study underwent elective splenectomy pre autograft, and perhaps some may have gained benefit from this maneuver in terms of avoidance of graft failure and faster restoration of counts (Table 27.2). Nevertheless, it should be noted that the time to both neutrophil and platelet recovery in this study was still significantly slower than that reported for blood-derived autografts.[46]

In summary, the use of cultured marrow cells as an autograft results in the restoration of Ph-negative hematopoiesis in the majority of patients with CML, but hematological recovery is relatively slow and primary (but not late) graft failure occurs not infrequently.

The treatment

The basic rationale for subjecting patients with CML to intensive therapy supported by autografting in first chronic phase is that a reduction in the target population of leukemic stem cells available for secondary mutational events will delay the emergence of a blastic-phase subclone and thereby prolong survival. In this regard, the achievement of unmaintained cytogenetic remissions for a significant length of time (typically about 12 months, but in one patient for 3 years[52]) in both pilot studies is perhaps relevant. In any event, the fact that Ph-positive cells subsequently became detectable should come as no surprise given the experience with syngeneic transplants[53] and evidence that the GVL effect makes an important contribution to the prevention of disease recurrence after allogeneic BMT.[3]

In the pilot studies, low-dose IFN-α was effective in reducing the recurrent Ph-positive population in over half of the patients so treated. In addition, it was well tolerated. It therefore seemed reasonable to use IFN-α as maintenance therapy in the second Vancouver study, and the 7 patients who remain in cytogenetic remission continue to receive this agent.

Although a significant number of patients in these studies continue free of blastic phase, some in cytogenetic remission, many years post autograft, these results have to be reviewed with circumspection, since it is likely that many belonged to a 'good-prognosis' subgroup.[54] For example, the 5 patients in the first Vancouver study who remain in cytogenetic remission now more than 10 years post autograft all had a low Sokal prognostic index at diagnosis and had only received hydroxyurea as prior treatment (Table 27.3), thus raising the possibility that they may have fared just as well with IFN-α in full dose as primary therapy.[55] On the other hand, it would be difficult not to conclude that these patients had gained significant benefit from the actual treatment received. A similar argument can be made about certain patients treated on other autograft studies;[56] however, the value of this treatment in CML will only be known upon completion of randomized controlled trials currently underway in Europe.

In summary, this treatment has resulted in prolonged leukemia-free (i.e. Ph-negative) and overall survival for a significant minority of patients with CML, although the contribution of disease-related variables confounds an assessment of efficacy in comparison to other therapies.

Future directions

A number of new avenues of clinical research in this area are possible. First, both in vivo[57] and in vitro[58] strategies may be employed to improve the quality of the autograft. Second, the recent demonstration that CML progenitors are dependent upon autocrine production of interleukin-3 and granulocyte colony-stimulating factor[59] suggests that interference with this pathway may have clinically useful application in autografting. Third, and perhaps the most promising, new immunological,[60] genetic[61] and molecular[62] treatments could be used after autografting in order to maintain cytogenetic remission.

In the next 5–10 years, it should become apparent whether these and other approaches can be incorporated with autografting to produce an improved treatment for patients with CML.

ACKNOWLEDGEMENTS

The Vancouver studies described in this chapter were supported in part by grants from the British Columbia Health Research Foundation and the National Cancer Institute of Canada, with funds from the Canadian Cancer Society and Schering Canada. Significant contributions to these studies were made by numerous individuals from the technical staff of the Terry Fox Laboratory, and the medical and nursing staff at the British Columbia Cancer Agency and Vancouver General Hospital, as well as staff from BMT centers in Edmonton, Winnipeg, Ottawa, Montreal, and Halifax. The efforts of Giovanna Cameron (collation of laboratory data), Daphne Brockington (management of clinical data), and Shawna Lumer (preparation of manuscript) are much appreciated.

REFERENCES

1. van Rhee F, Lin F, Cross NCP et al, Detection of residual leukaemia more than 10 years after allogeneic bone marrow transplantation for chronic myelogenous leukaemia. *Bone Marrow Transplant* 1994; **14:** 609–12.
2. Barnett MJ, Eaves AC, Phillips GL, An overview of bone marrow transplantation for chronic myeloid leukemia. *Can Med Assoc J* 1990; **143:** 187–93.
3. Horowitz MM, Gale RP, Sondel PM et al, Graft-versus-leukemia reactions after bone marrow transplantation. *Blood* 1990; **75:** 555–62.
4. Fefer A, Radich J, Pavletic Z et al, Syngeneic bone marrow transplantation (BMT) for chronic myelogenous leukemia in chronic phase: update of the original 14 Seattle patients, including PCR results. *Blood* 1994; **84**(Suppl 1): 252a.
5. Coulombel L, Kalousek DK, Eaves CJ et al, Long-term marrow culture reveals chromosomally normal hematopoietic progenitor cells in patients with Philadelphia chromosome-positive chronic myelogenous leukemia. *N Engl J Med* 1983; **308:** 1493–8.
6. Wang JCY, Lapidot T, Cashman JD et al, High level engraftment of NOD/SCID mice by primitive normal and leukemic hematopoietic cells from patients with chronic myeloid leukemia in chronic phase. *Blood* 1998; **91:** 2406–14.
7. Holyoake T, Jiang X, Eaves C, Eaves A, Isolation of a highly quiescent subpopulation of primitive leukemic cells in chronic myeloid leukemia. *Blood* 1999; **94:** 2056–64.
8. Goto T, Nishikori M, Arlin Z et al, Growth characteristics of leukemic and normal hematopoietic cells in Ph^1+ chronic myelogenous leukemia and effects of intensive treatment. *Blood* 1982; **59:** 793–808.
9. Kantarjian HM, Vellekoop L, McCredie KB et al, Intensive combination chemotherapy (ROAP 10) and splenectomy in the management of chronic myelogenous leukemia. *J Clin Oncol* 1985; **3:** 192–200.
10. Talpaz M, Kantarjian H, Kurzrock R et al, Interferon-alpha produces sustained cytogenetic responses in chronic myelogenous leukemia. Philadelphia chromosome-positive patients. *Ann Intern Med* 1991; **114:** 532–8.
11. Dube ID, Arlin ZA, Kalousek DK et al, Nonclonal hemopoietic progenitor cells detected in long-term marrow cultures from a Turner syndrome mosaic with chronic myeloid leukemia. *Blood* 1984; **64:** 1284–7.
12. Hogge DE, Coulombel L, Kalousek DK et al, Nonclonal hemopoietic progenitors in a G6PD

heterozygote with chronic myelogenous leukemia revealed after long-term marrow culture. *Am J Hematol* 1987; **24:** 389–94.
13. Turhan AG, Humphries RK, Eaves CJ et al, Detection of breakpoint cluster region-negative and nonclonal hematopoiesis in vitro and in vivo after transplantation of cells selected in cultures of chronic myeloid leukemia marrow. *Blood* 1990; **76:** 2404–10.
14. Petzer AL, Eaves CJ, Lansdorp PM et al, Characterization of primitive subpopulations of normal and leukemic cells present in the blood of patients with newly diagnosed as well as established chronic myeloid leukemia. *Blood* 1996; **88:** 2162–71.
15. Verfaillie CM, Bhatia R, Miller W et al, BCR/ABL-negative primitive progenitors suitable for transplantation can be selected from the marrow of most early-chronic phase but not accelerated-phase chronic myelogenous leukemia patients. *Blood* 1996; **87:** 4770–9.
16. Frassoni F, Podesta M, Piaggio G et al, Normal primitive haemopoietic progenitors are more frequent than their leukaemic counterpart in newly diagnosed patients with chronic myeloid leukaemia but rapidly decline with time. *Br J Haematol* 1999; **104:** 538–45.
17. Levin RH, Whang J, Tjio JH et al, Persistent mitosis of transfused homologous leukocytes in children receiving antileukemic therapy. *Science* 1963; **142:** 1305–11.
18. Graw RGJ, Buckner CD, Whang-Peng J et al, Complication of bone-marrow transplantation. Graft-versus-host disease resulting from chronic-myelogenous-leukaemia leucocyte transfusions. *Lancet* 1970; **ii:** 338–41.
19. Lowenthal RM, Grossman L, Goldman JM et al, Granulocyte transfusions in treatment of infections in patients with acute leukaemia and aplastic anaemia. *Lancet* 1975; **i:** 353–8.
20. Deisseroth AB, Zu Z, Claxton D et al, Genetic marking shows that Ph^+ cells present in autologous transplants of chronic myelogenous leukemia (CML) contribute to relapse after autologous bone marrow in CML. *Blood* 1994; **83:** 3068–76.
21. Eaves CJ, Cashman JD, Eaves AC, Methodology of long-term culture of human hemopoietic cells. *J Tissue Cult Meth* 1991; **13:** 55–62.
22. Dexter TM, Allen TD, Lajtha LG, Conditions controlling the proliferation of haemopoietic stem cells in vitro. *J Cell Physiol* 1977; **91:** 335–44.
23. Gartner S, Kaplan HS, Long-term culture of human bone marrow cells. *Proc Natl Acad Sci USA* 1980; **77:** 4756–9.
24. Greenberg HM, Newburger PE, Parker LM et al, Human granulocytes generated in continuous bone marrow culture are physiologically normal. *Blood* 1981; **58:** 724–32.
25. Coulombel L, Eaves AC, Eaves CJ, Enzymatic treatment of long-term human marrow cultures reveals the preferential location of primitive hemopoietic progenitors in the adherent layer. *Blood* 1983; **62:** 291–7.
26. Eaves AC, Cashman JD, Gaboury LA et al, Unregulated proliferation of primitive chronic myeloid leukemia progenitors in the presence of normal marrow adherent cells. *Proc Natl Acad Sci USA* 1986; **83:** 5306–10.
27. Verfaillie CM, Direct contact between human primitive hematopoietic progenitors and bone marrow stroma is not required for long-term in vitro hematopoiesis. *Blood* 1992; **79:** 2821–6.
28. Sutherland HJ, Eaves CJ, Eaves AC et al, Characterization and partial purification of human marrow cells capable of initiating long-term hematopoiesis in vitro. *Blood* 1989; **74:** 1563–70.
29. Sutherland HJ, Lansdorp PM, Henkelman DH et al, Functional characterization of individual human hematopoietic stem cells cultured at limiting dilution on supportive marrow stromal layers. *Proc Natl Acad Sci USA* 1990; **87:** 3584–8.
30. Coulombel L, Eaves C, Kalousek D et al, Long-term marrow culture of cells from patients with acute myelogenous leukemia. Selection in favor of normal phenotypes in some but not all cases. *J Clin Invest* 1985; **75:** 961–9.
31. Udomsakdi C, Eaves CJ, Swolin B et al, Rapid decline of chronic myeloid leukemic cells in long-term culture due to a defect at the leukemic stem cell level. *Proc Natl Acad Sci USA* 1992; **89:** 6192–6.
32. Eaves CJ, Cashman JD, Zoumbos NC et al, Biological strategies for the selective manipulation of normal and leukemic stem cells. *Stem Cells* 1993; **11**(Suppl 3): 109–21.
33. Chang J, Coutinho L, Morgenstern G et al, Reconstitution of haemopoietic system with autologous marrow taken during relapse of acute myeloblastic leukaemia and grown in long-term culture. *Lancet* 1986; **i:** 294–5.
34. Chang J, Morgenstern GR, Coutinho LH et al, The use of bone marrow cells grown in long-

term culture for autologous bone marrow transplantation in acute myeloid leukaemia: an update. *Bone Marrow Transplant* 1989; **4:** 5–9.
35. Barnett MJ, Eaves CJ, Phillips GL et al, Successful autografting in chronic myeloid leukaemia after maintenance of marrow in culture. *Bone Marrow Transplant* 1989; **4:** 345–51.
36. Barnett MJ, Eaves CJ, Phillips GL et al, Autografting with cultured marrow in chronic myeloid leukemia: results of a pilot study. *Blood* 1994; **84:** 724–32.
37. Shepherd JD, Gascoyne RD, Barnett MJ et al, Polyclonal Epstein–Barr virus-associated lymphoproliferative disorder following autografting for chronic myeloid leukemia. *Bone Marrow Transplant* 1995; **15:** 639–41.
38. Coutinho LH, Chang J, Brereton ML et al, Autografting in Philadelphia (Ph)+ chronic myeloid leukaemia using cultured marrow: an update of a pilot study. *Bone Marrow Transplant* 1997; **19:** 969–76.
39. Santucci MA, Zaccaria A, Testoni N et al, Long-term culture of chronic myeloid leukemia (CML) bone marrow cells. *Haematologica* 1991; **76:** 357–62.
40. Brandwein JM, Dube ID, Laraya P, Keating A, Maintenance of Philadelphia-chromosome-positive progenitors in long-term marrow cultures from patients with advanced chronic myeloid leukemia. *Leukemia* 1992; **6:** 556–61.
41. Stoppa AM, Maraninchi D, Lafage M et al, Liquid culture and cryopreservation of marrow cells of leukaemic patients prior to autologous bone marrow transplantation. *Br J Haematol* 1989; **72:** 519–23.
42. Carella AM, Gaozza E, Raffo MR et al, Therapy of acute phase chronic myelogenous leukemia with intensive chemotherapy, blood cell autotransplant and cyclosporine A. *Leukemia* 1991; **5:** 517–21.
43. Carella AM, Podesta M, Frassoni F et al, Collection of 'normal' blood repopulating cells during early hematopoietic recovery after intensive conventional chemotherapy in chronic myelogenous leukemia. *Bone Marrow Transplant* 1993; **12:** 267–71.
44. Brito-Babapulle F, Bowcock SJ, Marcus RE et al, Autografting for patients with chronic myeloid leukaemia in chronic phase: peripheral blood stem cells may have a finite capacity for maintaining haemopoiesis. *Br J Haematol* 1989; **73:** 76–81.
45. Kantarjian HM, Talpaz M, LeMaistre CF et al, Intensive combination chemotherapy and autologous bone marrow transplantation leads to the reappearance of Philadelphia chromosome-negative cells in chronic myelogenous leukemia. *Cancer* 1991; **67:** 2959–65.
46. Carella AM, Lerma E, Corsetti MT et al, Autografting with Philadelphia chromosome-negative mobilized hematopoietic progenitor cells in chronic myelogenous leukemia. *Blood* 1999; **93:** 1534–9.
47. Talpaz M, Kantarjian H, Liang J et al, Percentage of Philadelphia chromosome (Ph)-negative and Ph-positive cells found after autologous transplantation for chronic myelogenous leukemia depends on percentage of diploid cells induced by conventional-dose chemotherapy before collection of autologous cells. *Blood* 1995; **85:** 3257–63.
48. Verfaillie CM, Bhatia R, Steinbuch M et al, Comparative analysis of autografting in chronic myelogenous leukemia: effects of priming regimen and marrow or blood origin of stem cells. *Blood* 1998; **92:** 1820–31.
49. Corsetti MT, Lerma E, Dejana A et al, Cytogenetic response to autografting in chronic myelogenous leukemia correlates with the amount of BCR–ABL positive cells in the graft. *Exp Hematol* 2000; **28:** 104–11.
50. Hughes TP, Grigg A, Szer J et al, Mobilization of predominantly Philadelphia chromosome-negative blood progenitors using cyclophosphamide and rHUG-CSF in early chronic-phase chronic myeloid leukemia: correlation with Sokal prognostic index and haematological control. *Br J Haematol* 1997; **96:** 635–40.
51. Goldman JM, Johnson SA, Islam A et al, Haematological reconstitution after autografting for chronic granulocytic leukaemia in transformation: the influence of previous splenectomy. *Br J Haematol* 1980; **45:** 223–31.
52. Brummendorf TH, Holyoake TL, Rufer N et al, Prognostic implications of differences in telomere length between normal and malignant cells from patients with chronic myeloid leukemia measured by flow cytometry. *Blood* 2000; **95:** 1883–90.
53. Gale RP, Horowitz MM, Ash RC et al, Identical-twin bone marrow transplants for leukemia. *Ann Intern Med* 1994; **120:** 646–52.
54. Cervantes F, Robertson JE, Rozman C et al, Long-term survivors in chronic granulocytic

leukaemia: a study by the International CGL Prognosis Study Group. *Br J Haematol* 1994; **87:** 293–300.

55. The Italian Cooperative Study Group on Chronic Myeloid Leukemia, Long-term follow-up of the Italian trial of interferon-α versus conventional chemotherapy in chronic myeloid leukemia. *Blood* 1998; **92:** 1541–8.
56. McGlave PB, De Fabritiis P, Deisseroth A et al, Autologous transplants for chronic myelogenous leukaemia: results from eight transplant groups. *Lancet* 1994; **343:** 1486–8.
57. Coutinho LH, Brereton ML, Santos AMW et al, Evaluation of cytogenetic conversion to Ph^- haemopoiesis in long-term bone marrow culture for patients with chronic myeloid leukaemia on conventional hydroxyurea therapy, on pulse high-dose hydroxyurea and on interferon-alpha. *Br J Haematol* 1996; **93:** 869–77.
58. Petzer AL, Eaves CJ, Barnett MJ, Eaves AC, Selective expansion of primitive normal hematopoietic cells in cytokine-supplemented cultures of purified cells from patients with chronic myeloid leukemia. *Blood* 1997; **90:** 64–9.
59. Jiang X, Lopez A, Holyoake T et al, Autocrine production and action of IL-3 and granulocyte colony-stimulating factor in chronic myeloid leukemia. *Proc Natl Acad Sci USA* 1999; **96:** 12804–9.
60. Cervantes F, Pierson BA, McGlave PB et al, Autologous activated natural killer cells suppress primitive chronic myelogenous leukemia progenitors in long-term culture. *Blood* 1996; **87:** 2476–85.
61. Zhao RCH, McIvor RS, Griffin JD, Verfaillie CM, Gene therapy for chronic myelogenous leukemia (CML): a retroviral vector that renders hematopoietic progenitors methotrexate-resistant and CML progenitors functionally normal and nontumorigenic in vivo. *Blood* 1997; **90:** 4687–98.
62. Druker BJ, Tamura S, Buchdunger E et al, Effects of a selective inhibitor of the Abl tyrosine kinase on the growth of Bcr–Abl positive cells. *Nature Med* 1996; **2:** 561–6.
63. Sokal JE, Cox EB, Baccarani M et al, Prognostic discrimination in 'good-risk' chronic granulocytic leukemia. *Blood* 1984; **63:** 789–99.

28

Autografting with Ph-negative haematopoietic progenitor cells

Angelo M Carella

CONTENTS • Introduction • The general concept • Rationale for autografting • Laboratory results on stem cell mobilization • Clinical results with the in vivo technique employed by Genoa • Quantitative competitive RT-PCR in Ph-negative collections • Autografting with mobilized haematopoietic progenitor cells • Results achieved internationally with in vivo purging • Conclusions and further directions

INTRODUCTION

Allografting represents the only therapeutic procedure capable of curing chronic myeloid leukaemia (CML). Unfortunately, the majority of CML patients do not have an HLA-matched sibling donor, and matched or partially matched unrelated donor transplants are still associated with a high transplant-related mortality within the first 100 days.[1] For patients who do not have compatible donors and for older patients, therapy includes hydroxyurea, busulfan, and interferon-α (IFN-α). For patients who do not achieve haematologic and/or cytogenetic remission after IFN-α therapy, alternative treatment strategies are needed. One option is offered by autologous stem cell transplantation. This procedure has been explored with in vitro and in vivo manipulation techniques for the treatment of late chronic-phase or more advanced-phase disease, and, more recently, upfront at diagnosis.[2–6] Another approach has recently been proposed, using specific chemical inhibitors of ABL tyrosine kinase (see Chapter 32). In particular, preclinical studies with STI571 (Glivec; Gleevec) have demonstrated significant haematologic responses at higher dose levels of the drug[7,8] (see Chapter 34). In this chapter, we will focus on the results achieved with high-dose therapy followed by 'rescue' with mobilized haematopoietic progenitor cells (HPC).

THE GENERAL CONCEPT

It is conventional to assume that the acquisition of the Philadelphia chromosome (Ph) by the targeted stem cells confers on its progeny a proliferative advantage whereby the leukaemic clone expands inexorably while the proliferation of normal HPC is suppressed indefinitely. However, a number of clinical and laboratory observations imply that this interpretation may be an oversimplification. There are, for example, patients in whom leukaemic and normal HPC coexist for many years in apparently stable mosaicism. This implies that leukaemic cells do not always express a proliferative advantage over residual normal haematopoiesis, even though in other cases there is evidence that both populations may be of clonal origin and therefore part of the original leukaemic clone.[9] The first evidence for Ph-negative haematopoietic stem cells in CML was obtained by cytogenetic analysis of granulocyte–macrophage colony-forming unit (CFU-GM) colonies grown from CML marrow cells in vitro.[10] More recently, a considerable amount of data has demonstrated that partial or transient normal haematopoiesis is seen in a high proportion of patients whose marrow is studied early at diagnosis.[11–13] Evidence for the persistence of HPC in CML has been provided by the fact that Ph-negative cells are mobilized into the blood of CML patients treated with intensive chemotherapy[2,3,14] and by Ph-negative recovery of patients treated with IFN-α.[15,16]

RATIONALE FOR AUTOGRAFTING

There are at least two possible related rationales for autografting to prolong life for CML patients:

- Long-term culture-initiating cells (LTC-IC) from CML patients have shown a very poor self-maintenance capacity;[17] therefore steps that temporarily reduce to low levels the numbers of both normal and leukaemic stem cells can give a proliferative advantage to normal over leukaemic cells.
- Since it seems that the normal haematopoietic reservoir declines with time, it may be desirable to mobilize and collect peripheral HPC in order to store Ph-negative progenitors as soon after diagnosis as possible.

In vivo purging aims at the reduction of the leukaemic clone, after which normal stem cells can be harvested and used for autografting. An example of such an approach is the protocol developed by Simonsson et al,[18] and see also discussion in Chapter 10.

LABORATORY RESULTS ON STEM CELL MOBILIZATION

Peripheral HPC usually have the advantage of being harvested via leukapheresis, bypassing the need for general anaesthesia. In addition, the use of peripheral HPC results in a faster haematologic recovery compared with bone marrow transplant. In the last few years, several groups have analysed different mobilization protocols for stem cell content. Sutherland et al[19] reported the kinetics of committed and primitive HPC mobilization after chemotherapy and cytokines, and demonstrated that LTC-IC are present in these harvests. Breems et al[20] analysed the leukaphereses using the cobblestone area-forming cell (CAFC) assay and standard clonogenic assays. They demonstrated a good correlation between the numbers of colony-forming units (CFU) and different subsets of CAFC; moreover, the quality of the progenitor cell harvests, in terms of engraftment, correlated well with the numbers of mobilized HPC. Prosper et al[21] evaluated the phenotypic and functional aspects of LTC-IC, and demonstrated a 60-fold increase in LTC-IC at week 5 and a 12-fold increase in CFU after granulocyte colony-stimulating factor (G-CSF) therapy; moreover, the combination of stem cell factor (SCF) with chemotherapy and G-CSF was able to mobilize an increasing number of LTC-IC.[22] Finally, Ho et al[23] demonstrated that a pluripotent and lineage-committed $CD34^+$ subset in the leukapheresis product was mobilized by G-CSF, granulocyte–macrophage colony-stimulating factor (GM-CSF), or a combination of the two. In conclusion, these results taken together indicate that primitive as well as more mature HPC can be mobilized, depending on the mobilization protocol used.

CLINICAL RESULTS WITH THE IN VIVO TECHNIQUE EMPLOYED IN GENOA

On December 1999, 194 patients with Ph-positive CML in different phases of the disease entered our protocol. Thirty-eight patients were mobilized in blastic phase, 28 patients in accelerated phase, and 128 patients in chronic phase (Table 28.1). Sixty patients in chronic phase were in the first year of disease and had not been pretreated with IFN-α; 68 other patients had received previous IFN-α therapy and turned out to be cytogenetically refractory and/or intolerant to it. The treatment regimen for mobilization consisted of idarubicin 8 mg/m^2/day on days 1–5, cytosine arabinoside (Ara-C) 800 mg/m^2 by 2-hour infusion on days 1–5, and etoposide 150 mg/m^2/day by 2-hour infusion on days 1–3 (the ICE protocol). All the data concerning the patients pretreated with IFN-α have recently been updated.[24–26] In this chapter, we will give an update on patients in the early phase of disease and who have not previously been treated with IFN-α (Table 28.2).[14,27] Seventeen patients received the ICE protocol, and the other 43 patients were given the same drugs but for 3 days (the mini-ICE protocol). In all cases, G-CSF was given at 5–10 μg/kg from day 8 after chemotherapy. Leukaphereses were started the day on which the white blood cell (WBC) count exceeded (0.8–1) × 10^9/l and there were at least 10 CD34$^+$ cells/μl in the peripheral blood. The procedure was performed until the total

Table 28.1 Mobilization of progenitor cells in CML: 10 years of experience in Genoa (1989–1999)

Number of patients	194
Age (median)	47 years (range 21–62 years)
Phase of disease:	
Blastic phase (BP)	38 patients
Accelerated phase (AP)	28 patients
Chronic phase (CP)	68 patients
Early CP	60 patients
Procedure-related deaths	8 (4%) (BP 5; AP 2; CP 1)

Table 28.2 Patients mobilized within 12 months of diagnosis and not pretreated with IFN-α

Number of patients	60
Age (median)	46 years (range 21–62 years)
Gender	47 male; 13 female
WBC at diagnosis (median)	136 × 10^9/l (range (13–550) × 10^9/l)
Sokal index:	
Low	23 patients (38%)
Intermediate	22 patients (37%)
High	15 patients (25%)
Interval from diagnosis to mobilization (median)	2 months (range 1–12 months)
Mobilization regimen:	
ICE	17
mini-ICE	43

number of $CD34^+$ cells collected was at least 2×10^6/kg.

All patients completed the mobilization protocol, and no patient died of the procedure. Toxicity consisted of alopecia, mild mucositis, and diarrhoea, mainly in patients treated with the ICE protocol. In 5 (30%) out of 17 patients treated with the ICE protocol, grade 3 oral mucositis (WHO) and diarrhoea occurred; in contrast, only 7 (16%) out of 43 patients treated with the mini-ICE protocol experienced any non-haematologic toxicity. Cytogenetic analysis of collected peripheral HPC showed only diploid cells in 36 patients (60%) and 34% or less Ph-positive cells in 14 patients (23%). Fifty (83%) of the 60 patients had Ph-negative cells plus major cytogenetic remission (we consider a collection Ph-negative when a patient has had one or more leukaphereses that are completely diploid and contain at least 2×10^6/kg $CD34^+$ cells). Comparison of these data with those achieved in patients in late chronic phase, cytogenetically refractory to IFN-α, revealed a higher rate of complete cytogenetic remission among patients mobilized early at diagnosis (early chronic phase 36/60 (60%) versus late chronic phase 23/68 (34%)). These results were supported by the observation of significantly greater numbers of $CD34^+$ cells, CFU-GM, and LTC-IC.[28]

QUANTITATIVE COMPETITIVE RT-PCR IN Ph-NEGATIVE COLLECTIONS

The high rate of Ph-negative collections obtained with our procedure has prompted us to find a method other than cytogenetics to quantify their leukaemic content. We have been routinely monitoring the minimal residual disease in Ph-negative collections using quantitative competitive reverse-transcriptase polymerase chain reaction (QC-RT-PCR) for *BCR/ABL*.[29,30] So far, we have analysed 52 consecutive patients, 35 of them in the early phase of disease. The median follow-up of these patients was 24 months (range 3–57 months). Our main goal was to evaluate the importance of minimal residual disease in the graft as a prognostic factor for outcome after autografting. In a recent paper,[30] we have shown that a ratio *BCR/ABL* : *ABL* of less than 0.01 in the graft was strongly correlated with a longer duration of cytogenetic response in the marrow after transplant. Eleven patients who received grafts with low-level contamination showed a longer duration of response, none experienced prolonged neutropenia and/or thrombocytopenia, and nine of them had long-lasting complete or major cytogenetic remission after transplant. Figure 28.1 shows the actuarial plots relative to the duration of the cytogenetic response in 52 patients.

AUTOGRAFTING WITH MOBILIZED HAEMATOPOIETIC PROGENITOR CELLS

To date, 42 patients in early chronic phase who achieved complete or major cytogenetic remission have undergone autografting. High-dose therapy consisted of busulfan (4 mg/kg/day × 4 days) in 36 patients and a total-body irradiation (TBI)-containing regimen (idarubicin, etoposide, and single-dose TBI) in 6 patients. All patients engrafted, and no patient died of procedure. After haematopoietic recovery, all patients were treated with low doses of interleukin-2 (IL-2) (2 MU/day for 5 days every 9 weeks) and IFN-α (3 MU/day for 8 weeks): after 1 week of rest, the cycle was repeated for a total of three courses. Subsequently, the patients were maintained with IFN-α alone.[27] The median follow-ups from autografting are 32 months (range 4–91 months) and 37 months (range 19–90 months) in the previously published 30 patients[27] (Figures 28.2 and 28.3). Four patients evolved to blast crisis at 18, 29, 35, and 38 months after autografting, and died of leukaemia. The other 38 patients are alive in haematologic remission, and 14 of them are also in complete remission (11 patients) or major cytogenetic remission (3 patients) in the marrow 3–62 months after autografting.

	Chi-square	d.f.	*p*-value
Logrank (Mantel–Cox)	15.035	1	0.0001
Breslow–Gehan–Wilcoxon	18.881	1	<0.0001
Tarone–Ware	18.081	1	<0.0001
Peto–Peto–Wilcoxon	18.406	1	<0.0001
Harrington–Fleming	17.472	1	<0.0001

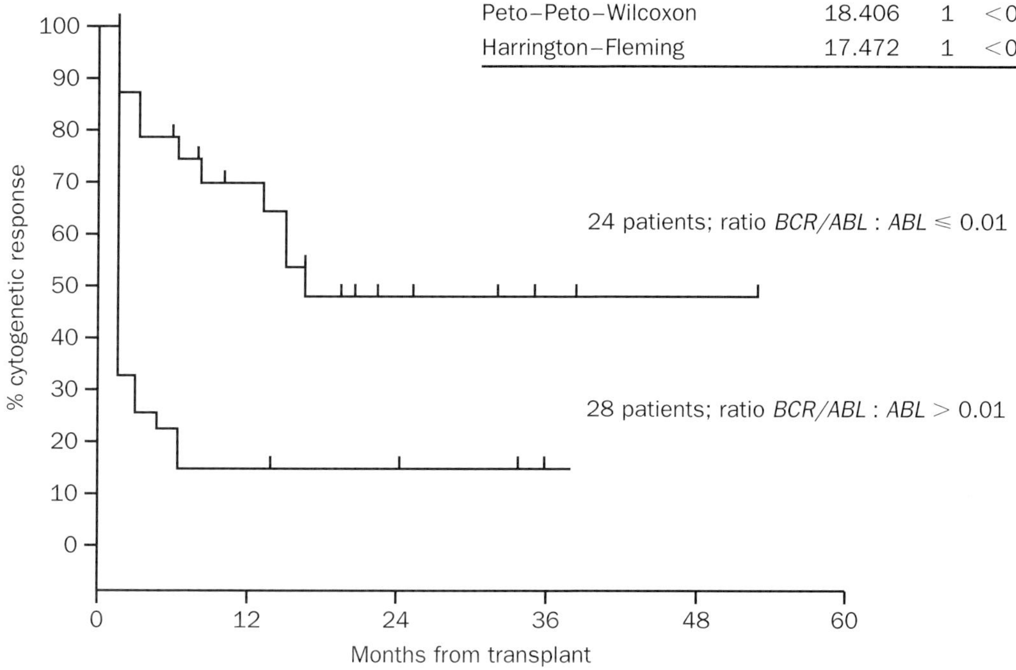

Figure 28.1 Duration of cytogenetic response after transplant according to the amount of leukaemic cells infused.

RESULTS ACHIEVED INTERNATIONALLY WITH IN VIVO PURGING

Several groups have undertaken efforts to reproduce these results and improve the mobilization protocols. Results for more than 500 patients who received this procedure are given in Table 28.3.

Kantarjian et al[31] treated 55 patients who had advanced-phase disease or were in late chronic phase but cytogenetically refractory to IFN-α and other therapies with two different mobilization protocols. Despite the refractory state of these patients, the Houston team was able to obtain 44% of leukaphereses that were completely Ph-negative (27%) or with less than 34% of Ph-positive cells (17%) (total response 44%); moreover, 29% of patients in accelerated phase achieved complete and major cytogenetic remissions on leukaphereses.

Van den Berg et al[32] evaluated 14 patients after the ICE protocol. Patients in advanced phase gave 100% Ph-positive harvests, whereas chronic-phase patients gave 100% Ph-negative leukaphereses.

Chalmers et al[33] treated 40 patients at different UK institutions with the IDAC regimen (idarubicin and Ara-C); 43% of the aphereses were 100% Ph-negative using standard cytogenetics. Subsequently, 20 patients were autografted, and 15 are alive at a median follow-up of 24 months. Fisher et al[34] investigated the fea-

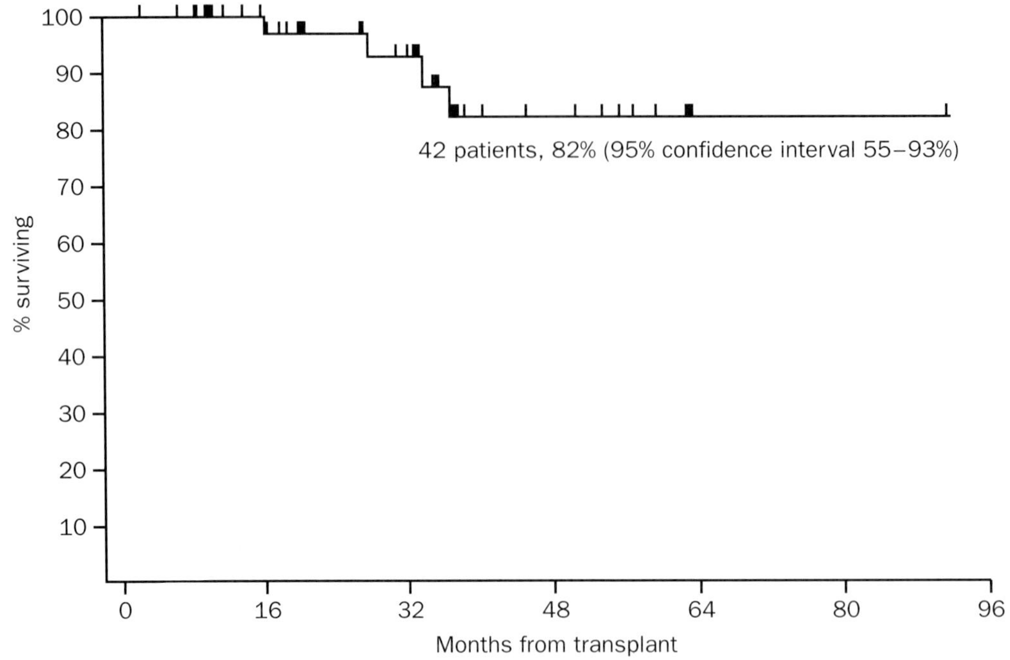

Figure 28.2 Overall survival (December 1999) of 42 patients autografted with Ph-negative or <34% Ph-positive haematopoietic progenitor cells and maintained with IFN-α.

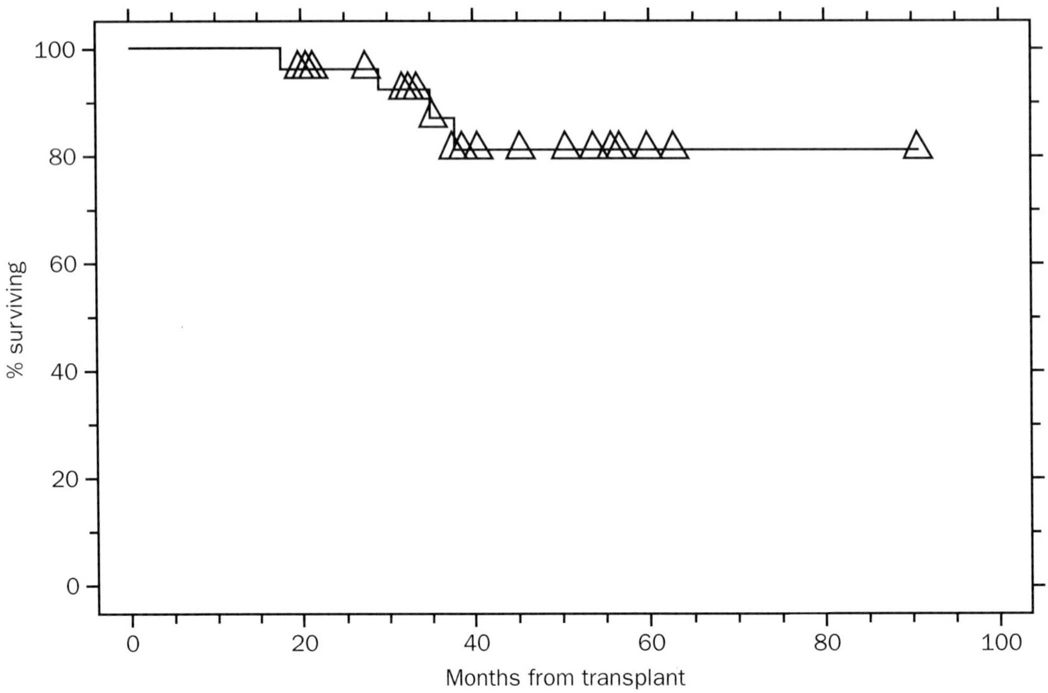

Figure 28.3 Kaplan–Meier cumulative survival plot in 30 patients (update as of December 1999 of results reported in Carella et al[27]).

Table 28.3 Haematopoietic progenitor cell mobilization and autografting in CML: international review

Authors	No. of patients (CML phase)[a]	Previous therapy[b]	Mobilization regimen[c]	PRD[d]	HPC[e]		Autografting[f]	PRD[d]	Outcome	
					CCyR	MCyR			Alive	Follow-up (months)
Carella et al (Dec. 1999)	ECP: 60	HU	ICE/mini-ICE	0	36 (60%)	14 (23%)	42	0	38	32 (4–91)
					83%					
	CP: 68	IFN/chemo*	ICE/mini-ICE	1 (1%)	23 (33%)	15 (22%)	49	2	26	40 (5–98)
					55%					
	AP/BP: 66	IFN/chemo*	ICE	7 (11%)	13 (20%)	6 (9%)	12	3	0	—
				8 (4%)	29%		105	5 (5%)		
	Total 194									
Kantarjian et al[31]	LCP: 30	IFN*	DNR–HDAC FAM	2 (3.6%)	8 (27%)	5 (17%)	NA			
					43%					
	AP: 17	IFN/chemo			3 (18%)	2 (11%)	NA			
					29%					
	BP: 8	IFN/chemo			0	0	NA			
	Total 55									
Chalmers et al[33]	ECP: 8	IFN*	IDAC	2 (5%)	6 (75%)	2 (25%)				
					100%		20	3 (15%)	15	24
	LCP: 32	IFN*	IDAC		10 (31%)	4 (12%)				
					43%					
	Total 40									
Fisher et al[34]	ECP: 10	HU	mini-ICE, ICE,	1 (2%)	18 (16%)	10 (20%)	31	0	26	12 (4–32)
	LCP: 30	IFN*	5 + 2/7 + 3		36%					
	AP/BP: 10	IFN*								
	Total 50									
Waller et al[36]	CP 17	IFN*, HU	ICE	0	29/71 (41%) aphereses negative to RT-PCR		16	0	16	18
Lennard et al[37]	CP: 29	HU	DNR/VCR/Ara-C	0	10 (33%)		ND	—	—	—
	AP: 1									
	Total 30									
Sureda et al[38]	ECP: 20	HU	mini-ICE	0	4 (22%)	9 (50%)	18	0	—	—
					72%					
Morton et al[39]	LCP: 8	IFN*/chemo	ICE	0	3 (14%)	6 (28%)	7	—	—	—
	AP: 11				42%					
	BP: 2									
	Total 21									
Johnson et al[40]	ECP: 10	IFN*/chemo	HU	0	3 (30%)	3 (30%)	7	1 (14%)	5	10 (2–22)
					60%					
	LCP: 7	IFN*/chemo	HU		3 (43%)	0				
	Total 17									
Hughes et al[41]	ECP: 21	HU	Cy	0	2 (9%)	5 (24%)	ND	—	—	—
					33%					
Carella et al[25]	LCP	IFN*	ICE/DNR/Ara-C	0	6 (21%)	4 (14%)	16	0	16	9 (3–12)
					35%					
Janssen (personal communication)	ECP: 19	HU	ICE-modified HDAC/AMSA	1	4 (21%)	11 (57%)	7	0	16	33 (25–44)
					15 (78%)					

[a] ECP, early chronic phase; CP, chronic phase; AP, accelerated phase; BP, blastic phase; LCP, late chronic phase.
[b] HU, hydroxyurea; IFN, interferon-α; * cytogenetically refractory.
[c] ICE/mini-ICE, idarubicin, Ara-C, etoposide; DNR, daunorubicin; HDAC, high-dose Ara-C; FAM, fludarabine, intermediate-dose Ara-C, mitoxantrone; IDAC, idarubicin, Ara-C; VCR, vincristine; Cy, cyclophosphamide; AMSA, amsacrine.
[d] Procedure-related deaths.
[e] Haematopoietic progenitor cell; CCyR, complete cytogenetic response; MCyR, major cytogenetic response.
[f] NA, not applicable; ND, no data.

sibility and toxicity of this procedure in patients in late chronic phase or advanced phases. Different protocols were used to mobilize haematopoietic progenitor cells (ICE, mini-ICE, and the daunorubicin-containing regimens 3 + 7 and 2 + 5). Complete and major responses were achieved in 9 out of 13 patients (69%) treated with mini-ICE and 3 out of 23 patients (13%) treated with the 3 + 7 or 2 + 5 protocol. Of 21 patients autografted, 7 achieved complete or major cytogenetic remission. Transplantation-related mortality was absent.

Heinzinger et al[35] selected Ph-negative progenitor cells that were not able to express the HLA-DR antigen. Eight patients in early chronic phase were mobilized with the ICE protocol followed by G-CSF and IL-3. The content of Ph-positive cells in the leukapheresis product as well as after $CD34^+$ enrichment and after in vitro culture was analysed with fluorescence in situ hybridization (FISH) and RT-PCR. A substantial number of peripheral haematopoietic progenitor cell samples were negative for the *BCR/ABL* mRNA rearrangement. More recently, the same group has treated 17 patients.[36] High numbers of $CD34^+$ $HLA\text{-}DR^-$ cells were obtained. Autografting of mostly Ph-negative aphereses was performed in 16 out of 17 patients after high-dose therapy. Ten patients achieved complete or major cytogenetic remission. The median follow-up after transplantation was 18 months.

Lennard et al[37] collected peripheral HPC in 30 patients after intensive chemotherapy and G-CSF. Chemotherapy was well tolerated, and progenitor cells were collected early during WBC recovery. In 10 patients, the collections showed over 75% Ph-negativity (range 79–100%), even though the aphereses gave positive results for the *BCR/ABL* transcript. Twenty-one out of 30 patients were considered to have adequate progenitor cell collections for engraftment.

Sureda et al[38] treated 20 consecutive patients with the mini-ICE regimen shortly after diagnosis. Complete cytogenetic remission on peripheral blood was observed in 25% of patients, and 50% achieved a major remission for a total of 75% of responses. After autografting, many patients did not develop febrile neutropenia, with four patients being treated on an outpatient basis. No patient died of transplant-related procedure.

Morton et al[39] treated 21 patients in advanced phase of disease with the ICE protocol and G-CSF. Despite the advanced phase of disease and the heavy pretreatment, 52% of patients (11/21) achieved a complete or major cytogenetic response on peripheral blood.

Johnson et al[40] treated 10 patients (9 in stable chronic phase and 1 in accelerated phase) with high-dose hydroxyurea (3–5 $g/m^2/day$ for 7 days) followed by 300 μg of G-CSF daily until the last day of harvesting. Five patients required admission to hospital with neutropenic fever, and four patients developed skin rash and mucositis. All aphereses were PCR-positive, but half of the patients had more than 98% normal metaphases.

A multicentre European study on advanced patients has been published.[25] The aim of this study was to evaluate the quantity and quality of mobilized progenitor cells in patients ineligible for allografting and cytogenetically refractory to IFN-α. Thirty-two patients received intensive chemotherapy and G-CSF. A total of 119 leukaphereses was performed. Out of 29 evaluable patients 6 (21%) achieved complete cytogenetic remission and 4 (14%) a major response, for a total of 35% of major responses. Sixteen patients were autografted, all of whom are alive at a median follow-up of 9 months (range 3–12 months). Despite the high-risk characteristics of this study population, Ph-negative and partially negative HPC were successfully mobilized in more than one-third of patients.

Recently, it has been investigated whether an additional cycle of intensive chemotherapy would increase the number of Ph-negative progenitors in the harvest. The authors collected HPC in 19 patients during early chronic phase following each of two consecutive cycles with the ICE-modified protocol (first cycle) and high-dose Ara-C and amsacrine (second cycle). After the first cycle, all patients showed a cytogenetic response to their graft (complete in 3 patients and major in 5); after the second cycle, 7 patients obtained complete (1) or major (6) cytogenetic remissions. Seven patients were autografted and after engraftment were maintained with IFN-α. Currently, 16 patients are alive, 50% of them with major cytogenetic remission. In conclusion, a second cycle did not appear effective in improving the Ph negativity of the HPC graft (Janssen et al, personal communication).

Finally, we can conclude that premobilization chemotherapy is able to provide preferential in vivo reduction of the Ph-positive stem cell population and to synergize the effects of G-CSF to stimulate the release of primitive Ph-negative HPC into the blood. The entire procedure is well tolerated. Nothwithstanding the different phases of disease, 13 (2%) out of 529 patients, many of whom were in advanced phase of disease and highly pretreated, died of mobilization therapy and 9 (4%) out of 237 died of autografting. In early chronic phase, the HPC collections yielded significantly more $CD34^+$ $HLA\text{-}DR^-$ cells than collections from steady-state or mobilized bone marrow.[12] Moreover, Ph-negative mobilized cells were polyclonal (X-chromosome inactivation) in the majority of patients with early chronic phase.[16] Following on from these results, an international protocol under the aegis of the Eastern Cooperative Oncology Group (ECOG), the European Group for Blood and Marrow Transplantation (EBMT), and the UK Medical Research Council (MRC) is investigating the role of autografting followed by IFN-α ± Ara-C versus IFN-α ± Ara-C alone.

CONCLUSIONS AND FUTURE DIRECTIONS

Residual normal haematopoiesis is present at diagnosis in some CML patients. During their chronic phase, the leukaemic cells can be destroyed with relative ease by therapy. Various markers exist whereby leukaemia cells can readily be recognized and quantitated, and may thus be exploited for therapeutic purposes. Recently, we have confirmed that it is possible to mobilize non-clonal HPC in other haematologic diseases with cytogenetic markers, such as Ph-positive acute lymphoblastic leukaemia and myelodysplastic syndromes.[42,43] Thus it is likely that attention in the next four years will focus on this aspect, giving more impulse to the role of autografting. From a therapeutic point of view, there seems to be general agreement that younger patients (less than 50 years old) with an HLA-identical sibling should receive an allograft. This procedure should also be offered to younger patients who are able to find a matched unrelated donor. Since it has been clearly demonstrated that the normal haematopoiesis reservoir declines with time, it may be desirable to mobilize and collect HPC in order to store Ph-negative or prevalently Ph-negative cells as soon after diagnosis as possible, when the WBC count is being controlled by hydroxyurea while the search for a matched unrelated donor proceeds. After 6–8 months, if a donor has not been found, the patient could undergo autografting with the previously stored Ph-negative progenitors followed by IFN-α therapy.

There is no doubt that tyrosine kinase inhibitors, in particular STI571, as potentially useful therapeutic agents are modifying this algorithm for CML. The unresolved questions related to STI571 are so numerous that many further studies are needed. In the mean time, autografting followed by 'rescue' with Ph-negative HPC collections remains a very good procedure to guarantee a prolongation of survival to patients mobilized and autografted early at diagnosis. Of 42 patients autografted and maintained with IFN-α, 38 (90%) are alive, with a median duration of survival from autografting of 32 months (range 4–90 months), and 14 patients maintain cytogenetic remission 4–63 months after autografting. Such results are better than those achieved by IFN-α, and are similar to the best results obtained in younger patients with allografting from an HLA-identical sibling. In the next few years, the integration of STI571 into the mobilization/autografting procedure could represent important progress in the cure of CML in patients who cannot undergo conventional allografting.

REFERENCES

1. Carella AM, Frassoni F, Melo J et al, New insights in biology and current therapeutic options for patients with chronic myelogenous leukaemia. *Haematologica* 1997; **4:** 478–95.
2. Carella AM, Gaozza E, Raffo MR et al, Therapy of acute phase chronic myelogenous leukemia with intensive chemotherapy, blood cell autotransplant and cyclosporine A. *Leukemia* 1991; **5:** 517–21.
3. Carella AM, Podestà M, Frassoni F et al, Collection of 'normal' blood repopulating cells during early hemopoietic recovery after intensive conventional chemotherapy in chronic myelogenous leukemia. *Bone Marrow Transplant* 1993; **12:** 267–71.
4. O'Brien SG, Goldman JM, Autografting in chronic myeloid leukaemia. *Blood Rev* 1994; **8:** 63–9.
5. Carella AM, Autotransplant in chronic myeloid leukemia. *Oncologist* 1998; **3:** 54–60.
6. Thjisen SFI, Schuurhuis GJ, Van Oostveen JW, Ossenkoppele GJ, Chronic myeloid leukemia from basics to bedside. *Leukemia* 1999; **13:** 1645–74.
7. Druker BJ, Tamura S, Buchdunger E et al, Effect of a selective inhibitor of the ABL tyrosine kinase on the growth of BCR–ABL positive cells. *Nature Med* 1996; **2:** 561–6.
8. Druker BJ, Talpaz M, Resta R et al, Clinical efficacy and safety on an abl specific tyrosine kinase inhibitor as target therapy for chronic myelogenous leukemia. *Blood* 1999; **94:** 368a.
9. Grand FH, Marley SB, Chase A et al, BCR/ABL-negative progenitors are enriched in the adherent fraction of CD34+ cells circulating in the blood of chronic phase chronic myeloid leukemia patients. *Leukemia* 1997; **11:** 1486–92.
10. Chervenick PA, Ellis LD, Pan SF, Human leukemic cells: in vitro growth of colonies containing the Philadelphia chromosome. *Science* 1971; **174:** 1134–6.
11. Coulombel L, Kalousek DK, Eaves CJ et al, Long-term marrow culture reveals chromosomally normal hematopoietic progenitor cells in patients with Philadelphia chromosome-positive chronic myelogenous leukemia. *N Engl J Med* 1983; **308:** 1493–8.
12. Verfaillie CM, Bhatia R, Steinbuch M et al, Comparative analysis of autografting in chronic myelogenous leukemia: effects of priming regimen and marrow or blood origin of stem cells. *Blood* 1998; **92:** 1820–31.
13. Gordon MY, Goldman JM, Cellular and molecular mechanisms in chronic myeloid leukemia: biology and treatment. *Br J Haematol* 1996; **95:** 10–20.
14. Carella AM, Cunningham I, Lerma E et al, Mobilization and transplantation of Philadelphia-negative peripheral blood progenitor cells early in chronic myelogenous leukemia. *J Clin Oncol* 1997; **15:** 1575–82.
15. Giralt S, Kantarjian H, Afar DE, The natural history of chronic myelogenous leukemia in the interferon era. *Semin Hematol* 1995; **32:** 152–8.
16. Bergamaschi G, Podestà M, Frassoni F et al, Restoration of normal polyclonal hemopoiesis in patients with chronic myeloid leukemia autografted with Ph1-negative peripheral stem cells. *Br J Haematol* 1994; **87:** 867–70.
17. Udomsakdi C, Eaves CJ, Swolin B et al, Rapid decline of chronic myloid leukemic cells in long-term culture due to a defect at the leukemic stem cell level. *Proc Natl Acad Sci USA* 1992; **89:** 6192–6.
18. Simonsson B, Oberg G, Bjoreman M et al, Intensive treatment in order to minimize the Ph-positive clone in CML. Danish–Sweden CML Group. *Bone Marrow Transplant* 1994; **17**(Suppl 3): S63–4.
19. Sutherland HJ, Eaves CJ, Lansdorp PM et al, Kinetics of committed and primitive blood progenitor mobilization after chemotherapy and growth factor treatment and their use in autotransplants. *Blood* 1996; **12:** 3808–14.
20. Breems DA, van Hennik PB, Kusadasi N et al, Individual stem cell quality in leukapheresis products is related to the number of mobilized stem cells. *Blood* 1996; **87:** 5370–8.
21. Prosper F, Stroneck D, Verfaillie CM, Phenotypic and functional characterization of long-term culture-initiating cells in peripheral blood progenitor collections of normal donors treated with granulocyte colony-stimulating factor. *Blood* 1996; **88:** 2033–42.
22. Weaver A, Ryder D, Crowther D et al, Increased numbers of long-term culture-initiating cells in the apheresis product of patients randomized to receive increasing doses of stem cell factor administrated in combination with chemotherapy and a standard dose of granulocyte colony-stimulating factor. *Blood* 1996; **88:** 3323–8.
23. Ho AD, Young D, Maruyama M et al, Pluripotent and lineage-committed CD34+ subsets in leukapheresis products mobilized by G-CSF, GM-CSF vs. a combination of both. *Exp Hematol* 1996; **24:** 1460–8.

24. Carella AM, Autografting with non-clonal mobilized hematopoietic progenitor cells in CML. *Leukemia* 2000; **14**: 954–5.
25. Carella AM, Simonsson B, Link H et al, Mobilization of Philadelphia-negative peripheral blood progenitor cells with chemotherapy and rhuG-CSF in chronic myelogenous leukaemia patients with a poor response to interferon-alpha. *Br J Haematol* 1998; **101:** 111–18.
26. Carella AM, Frassoni F, ICE, mini-ICE or high-dose hydroxyurea to mobilize Ph[1]-negative PBPC in CML. *Br J Haematol* 1996; **95:** 213–14.
27. Carella AM, Lerma E, Corsetti MT et al, Autografting with Philadelphia chromosome-negative mobilized hematopoietic progenitor cells in chronic myelogenous leukemia. *Blood* 1999; **93:** 1534–9.
28. Podestà M, Piaggio G, Frassoni F et al, Very primitive hemopoietic cells (LTC-IC) are present in Philadelphia negative cytaphereses collected during early recovery after chemotherapy for chronic myelogenous leukemia. *Bone Marrow Transplant* 1995; **16:** 549–55.
29. Corsetti MT, Lerma E, Dejana A et al, Quantitative competitive reverse transcriptase–polymerase chain reaction for BCR–ABL on Philadelphia-negative leukaphereses allows the selection of low-contaminated peripheral blood progenitor cells for autografting in chronic myelogenous leukemia. *Leukemia* 1999; **13:** 999–1008.
30. Corsetti MT, Lerma E, Dejana A et al, Cytogenetic response to autografting in chronic myelogenous leukemia correlates with the amount of BCR–ABL positive cells in the graft. *Exp Hematol* 2000; **28:** 104–11.
31. Kantarjian HM, Talpaz M, Hester J et al, Collection of peripheral blood diploid cells from chronic myelogenous leukemia patients early in the recovery phase from myelosuppression induced by intensive chemotherapy. *J Clin Oncol* 1995; **13:** 553–9.
32. Van den Berg D, Wessman M, Murray L et al, Leukemic burden in subpopulations of CD34+ cells isolated from the mobilised peripheral blood of alfa-interferon-resistant or intolerant patients with chronic myeloid leukemia. *Blood* 1996; **87:** 4348–57.
33. Chalmers EA, Franklin IM, Kelsey SM et al, Treatment of chronic myeloid leukaemia in first chronic phase with idarubicin and cytarabine: mobilization of Philadelphia-negative peripheral blood stem cells. *Br J Haematol* 1997; **96:** 627–34.
34. Fisher T, Neubauer A, Mohm J et al, Outcome of peripheral blood stem cell mobilization in advanced phases of CML is dependent on the type of chemotherapy applied. *Ann Hematol* 1998; **77:** 21–6.
35. Heinzinger M, Waller CF, Rosenstiel A et al, Quality of IL-3 and G-CSF-mobilized peripheral blood stem cells in patients with early chronic phase CML. *Leukemia* 1998; **12:** 333–9.
36. Waller CF, Heinzinger M, Rosenstiel A, Lange W, Mobilization and transplantation of Philadelphia chromosome-negative peripheral blood progenitor cells in patients with CML. *Br J Haematol* 1998; **103:** 227–34.
37. Lennard A, Storey N, Dickinson AM et al, Collection of Philadelphia-negative peripheral blood progenitor cells in unselected patients with chronic granulocytic leukaemia. Northern Regional Haematology Group. *Leukemia* 1998; **12:** 746–52.
38. Sureda A, Petit J, Brunet S et al, Mini-ICE regimen as mobilization therapy for chronic myelogenous leukaemia patients at diagnosis. *Bone Marrow Transplant* 1999; **12:** 1285–90.
39. Morton J, Mollee P, Taylor K et al, Safe mobilization of normal progenitors in advanced chronic myeloid leukemia with intensive chemotherapy and granulocyte-colony stimulating factor. *Leuk Res* 1999; **23:** 177–83.
40. Johnson RJ, Owen RG, Child JA et al, Mobilization of Philadelphia-negative peripheral blood mononuclear cells in chronic myeloid leukaemia using hydroxyurea and G-CSF (filgrastim). *Br J Haematol* 1996; **93:** 863–8.
41. Hughes TP, Grigg A, Szer J, Mobilization of predominantly Ph-chromosome negative blood progenitors using cyclophosphamide and rhuG-CSF in early chronic phase CML: correlation with Sokal prognostic index and hematological control. *Br J Haematol* 1997; **96:** 635–40.
42. Carella AM, Frassoni F, Pollicardo N et al, Philadelphia-chromosome-negative peripheral blood stem cells can be mobilized in the early phase of recovery after a myelosuppressive chemotherapy in Philadelphia-chromosome-positive acute lymphoblastic leukaemia. *Br J Haematol* 1995; **89:** 535–8.
43. Carella AM, Dejana A, Lerma E et al, In vivo mobilization of karyotypically normal peripheral blood progenitor cells in high-risk MDS, secondary or therapy-related acute myelogenous leukaemia. *Br J Haematol* 1996; **95:** 127–30.

29

Autologous hematopoietic stem cell transplantation: Experience at the University of Minnesota

Philip McGlave

CONTENTS • Introduction • Autologous transplantation with IFN-γ-purged marrow • Autologous transplantation with mobilized progenitors • NK-cell-based immunotherapy after autologous transplantation • Effects of patient characteristics and transplant conditions on survival after autologous transplantation • Discussion

INTRODUCTION

We and others have investigated the use of autologous hematopoietic stem cell transplantation (HSCT) in the treatment of chronic myeloid leukemia (CML).[1] Originally, this approach was based on the observation that benign hematopoietic stem cells coexist with their malignant counterparts in at least some CML patients.[2-5] Autologous transplant approaches included preparation with high-dose chemoradiotherapy followed by infusion of unmanipulated cells,[6] marrow cells purged ex vivo with mafosfamide,[7] recombinant human interferon-γ (IFN-γ),[8] or antisense oligodeoxynucleotides to c-*myb*,[9] and marrow cells purged by in vitro culture.[10] Other approaches included in vivo purging with single-agent or combination chemotherapy.[11,12] Prolonged survival following autologous HSCT using one of several approaches has been reported.[13] A high incidence of complete or major cytogenetic responses following autologous HSCT has also been observed.[14] In most cases, however, cytogenetic responses have not been durable, and the malignant clone has not been eradicated.[15] Efforts to capitalize on the high rate of initial major cytogenetic remission following autologous HSCT are underway. These include the use of autologous HSCT followed by recombinant IFN-α, interleukin-2 (IL-2)-based immunotherapy,[16] and, most recently, non-myeloablative allogeneic HSCT.[17]

AUTOLOGOUS TRANSPLANTATION WITH IFN-γ-PURGED MARROW

In the mid-1980s, we began to explore the in vitro growth characteristics of hematopoietic progenitor cells obtained from the marrows of patients with CML. These studies showed that CML marrow cells grown in methylcellulose hematopoietic progenitor assays contained not only Philadelphia chromosome (Ph)-positive cells, but also an unexpectedly high proportion of Ph-negative cells. Furthermore, incubation of CML marrow with IFN-γ resulted in a dose-dependent suppression of CML progenitors that was significantly greater than that observed when normal marrow was cultured under similar conditions.[18] We inferred from these experiments that incubation of CML marrow with IFN-γ on a large scale might provide selective purging of malignant progenitors while sparing a residual benign hematopoietic progenitor population. This purging technique was then combined with autologous transplantation using a standard myeloablative chemoradiotherapy approach currently being used to prepare CML patients for allogeneic HSCT.[19]

Subsequently, we performed 43 consecutive autologous transplantations using marrow treated for 36 hours ex vivo with 1000 units of IFN-γ prior to infusion (protocol 'γ purge').[8] The patient group was relatively old (median age 49 years), and consisted primarily of patients with advanced disease (AP) (19 patients), or in late chronic phase (LCP) (21 patients). Only 3 patients were transplanted in early chronic phase (chronic phase within 1 year of diagnosis) (ECP). Recipients were prepared for transplantation with a regimen consisting of cyclophosphamide (Cy), 60 mg/kg/day (days −7 and −6) and 165 cGy fractionated total-body irradiation (FTBI), given twice daily for 4 days (total dose 1320 cGy) (days −4, −3, −2, and −1) (Cy–TBI). In most cases, recombinant human IFN-α was administered as post-transplant antileukemia therapy when the absolute neutrophil count exceeded 1000/μl for 3 days without cytokine support, platelets were over 80 000/μl, and patients were red blood cell transfusion-independent. The subcutaneous IFN-α dose was 0.1×10^6 U/m^2 daily for 1 week, 0.25×10^6 U/m^2 daily for 1 week, 0.5×10^6 U/m^2 daily for 1 week, and then escalated by 0.5×10^6 U/m^2 every 2 weeks to the maximum tolerated dose.

The median proportion of Ph-positive marrow metaphases prior to transplant was 100% (range 25–100%), which fell to a median of 80% (range 0–100%) in the acute post-transplant interval (2–6 weeks following transplant). Unfortunately, the ex vivo purging approach was associated with toxicity to hematopoietic progenitors. In approximately one-third of cases thawed, untreated 'backup' autologous marrow cells were administered to treat tardy or incomplete engraftment. Moreover, 1-year follow-up demonstrated a return to primarily Ph-positive hematopoiesis in most cases. The median proportion of Ph-positive marrow metaphases in recipients evaluated at 1 year post transplant was 100% (range 25–100%), and only 4 recipients had less than 50% Ph-positive marrow metaphases. Of interest, 10 patients from this original series survive at a median of 76 months (6.3 years) from transplant (range 41–312 months). Of these 10 survivors, 9 were transplanted in chronic phase. This experience suggested to us that autologous transplantation could provide partial or complete cytogenetic remissions and perhaps increase the incidence of long-term survival. However, improved methods were needed to reduce the hematopoietic toxicity associated with ex vivo purging. Reversion to Ph positive hematopoiesis at 1 year post transplant suggested that additional, ongoing post-transplant antileukemia therapy would be useful to sustain cytogenetic remissions.

AUTOLOGOUS TRANSPLANTATION WITH MOBILIZED PROGENITORS

In subsequent laboratory-based studies, our group and others demonstrated that CD34$^+$HLA-DR$^-$ cells present in steady-state marrow of ECP CML patients were highly enriched for Ph-negative, *BCR/ABL* mRNA-negative, polyclonal primitive hematopoietic progenitors.[20,21] We reasoned that selection of such cells, coupled with autologous transplantation, might result in improved outcome. We therefore investigated methods for in vivo selection of benign primitive hematopoietic progenitors using chemotherapy and growth factor mobilization followed by autologous transplantation. This in vivo purging approach was first used widely in CML therapy by Carella et al.[22] Our initial goals were to determine the mobilization method as well as the stem cell source (marrow or blood) providing the optimal yield of benign hematopoietic progenitors in the inoculum, to determine the absolute number and clonal origin of $CD34^+HLA\text{-}DR^-$ cells in the inoculum, and to correlate priming approaches with outcome. Forty-four additional autologous transplants were performed in this trial, and results have been published.[23] Patients were prepared for transplant with Cy–TBI and received post-transplant antileukemia therapy with IFN-α as described above. Patients were treated with one of two 'intermediate' priming protocols, or with a third 'intensive' priming protocol followed by infusion of either marrow or blood as a source of HSCT.

1. The first 17 consecutive patients received bone marrow (BM) after priming with a single 'intermediate dose' of Cy ($4\,g/m^2$) and granulocyte–macrophage colony-stimulating factor (GM-CSF) ($250\,\mu g/m^2$) administered subcutaneously from day 4 after Cy until the end of 'backup' peripheral blood progenitor cell (PBPC) collection (protocol 'Cy/GM/BM').
2. Nine additional patients received peripheral blood progenitor cells (PBPC) after 'intermediate-dose' priming with Cy ($4\,g/m^2$, day 1) and granulocyte colony-stimulating factor (G-CSF) ($5\,\mu g/kg$) from day 4 until the completion of PBPC collection (protocol 'Cy/G/PB').
3. Finally, 18 patients received PBPC after 'intensive-dose' priming with Cy ($4\,g/m^2$, day 1), mitoxantrone ($4\,mg/m^2$, days 1 and 2) and cytosine arabinoside (Ara-C) ($1\,g/m^2$ twice daily, days 1 and 2), followed by G-CSF ($5\,\mu g/kg$) from day 4 until after completion of PBPC collection (protocol 'MAC/G/PB').

Neutrophil engraftment was enhanced in all three priming groups compared with our previous experience with ex vivo purging. Autologous transplant morbidity and cytogenetic responses were similar for the three priming groups. The cytogenetic status of the inoculum predicted the cytogenetic status of the marrow at 3 weeks post transplant. However, cytogenetic status of the marrow at later time points (up to 1 year post transplant) correlated with the number of Ph-negative, $CD34^+HLA\text{-}DR^-$ cells found in the inoculum. Among ECP patients, mobilized peripheral blood samples yielded more $CD34^+HLA\text{-}DR^-$ cells than resting or mobilized marrow samples. Moreover, these cells were Ph-negative and polyclonal. These data suggested to us that mobilization strategies yielding an inoculum containing large numbers of $CD34^+HLA\text{-}DR^-$ cells would be most effective in future autologous transplant trials. Current in vivo purging studies are focused on intermediate-dose priming with Cy/G/PB performed, ideally, while patients are still in ECP.

NK-CELL-BASED IMMUNOTHERAPY AFTER AUTOLOGOUS TRANSPLANTATION

In recent parallel studies, our group evaluated the use of IL-2 and natural killer (NK)-cell-based immunotherapy following autologous transplantation for CML. These clinical trials were based on a series of laboratory and clinical observations made over the last decade. In our experience, NK cells cultivated from CML patients do not contain the Ph, suggesting that they might be useful as autologous antitumor therapy.[24] Of note, autologous, IL-2-activated NK cells suppress progenitors from CML marrow significantly more than those from normal marrow, suggesting a specific antitumor effect.[25] NK cells obtained from the blood of CML patients can be expanded ex vivo to large numbers suitable for clinical trials.[26] Phase I trials suggest that subcutaneous administration of IL-2 following autologous transplant is well tolerated and results in enhanced cytotoxicity of circulating NK cells.[27] Phase I dose-escalation studies demonstrate that autologous NK cells can be safely administered intravenously post transplant at a dose of $1.75 \times 10^6/kg$. In an ongoing phase II trial, 13 CML patients have received autologous HSCT after Cy/G/PB priming followed by subcutaneous

IL-2 administration and infusion of autologous, IL-2-activated NK cells. Preliminary results suggest that the approach is well tolerated; however, efficacy is not yet evaluable. Theoretical concerns with the use of autologous NK cells as post-transplant antileukemia therapy include the possibility that as disease progresses, some NK cell clones may contain the *BCR/ABL* fusion gene and display diminished proliferative capacity and toxicity. Alternatively, coexistent, malignant myeloid cells may suppress the function of benign NK cells. Finally, the antitumor effect of autologous NK cells may be compromised by the recognition of malignant myeloid cells as 'self' through HLA class I-associated 'killer immunoglobulin receptors' (KIR) or related mechanisms.[28]

EFFECTS OF PATIENT CHARACTERISTICS AND TRANSPLANT CONDITIONS ON SURVIVAL AFTER AUTOLOGOUS TRANSPLANTATION

We have now performed 103 consecutive autologous transplants for CML at the University of Minnesota between 1988 and 1999. The median age of recipients is 49 years (range 14–64 years). The median interval from diagnosis to HSCT is 23 months. The median follow-up of survivors is 2.5 years (range 0.3–10 years). Transplants were performed using either ex vivo purging with IFN-γ (43 patients) or in vivo purging with intermediate (42 patients) or intensive (18 patients) priming chemotherapy. In the majority of cases, patients were prepared for transplant with Cy–TBI and received post-transplant antileukemia therapy with low-dose IFN-α as described above. All patients received standardized, protocol-guided care and follow-up in the University of Minnesota Inpatient BMT Unit and in the Outpatient BMT Clinic. All patients signed informed consent approved by the University of Minnesota Committee on the Use of Human Subjects in Research.

We analyzed the effect of various disease characteristics found at the time of transplant on survival for the entire group. We hypothe-

Table 29.1 Disease characteristics at transplant

Characteristic	No. of patients
Hemoglobin:	
<10 g/dl	15 (15%)
⩾10 g/dl	88 (85%)
White blood cells:	
⩽100 000/μl	100 (97%)
>100 000/μl	3 (3%)
Platelet levels:	
⩽750 000/μl	90 (87%)
>750 000/μl	13 (13%)
% basophils (bone marrow):	
⩽5%	94 (93%)
>5%	7 (7%)
% basophils (blood):	
⩽5%	64 (63%)
>5%	37 (37%)
Myelofibrosis:	
None–mild	95 (95%)
Moderate–severe	4 (4%)
% blasts:	
⩽5%	101 (98%)
>5%	2 (2%)
Post blast crisis:	
No	100 (97%)
Yes	3 (3%)
Chromosome abnormalities:[a]	
No	82 (80%)
Yes	21 (20%)
Palpable spleen:	
Yes	22 (22%)
No	79 (78%)
Missing	2

[a] Other than single Ph.

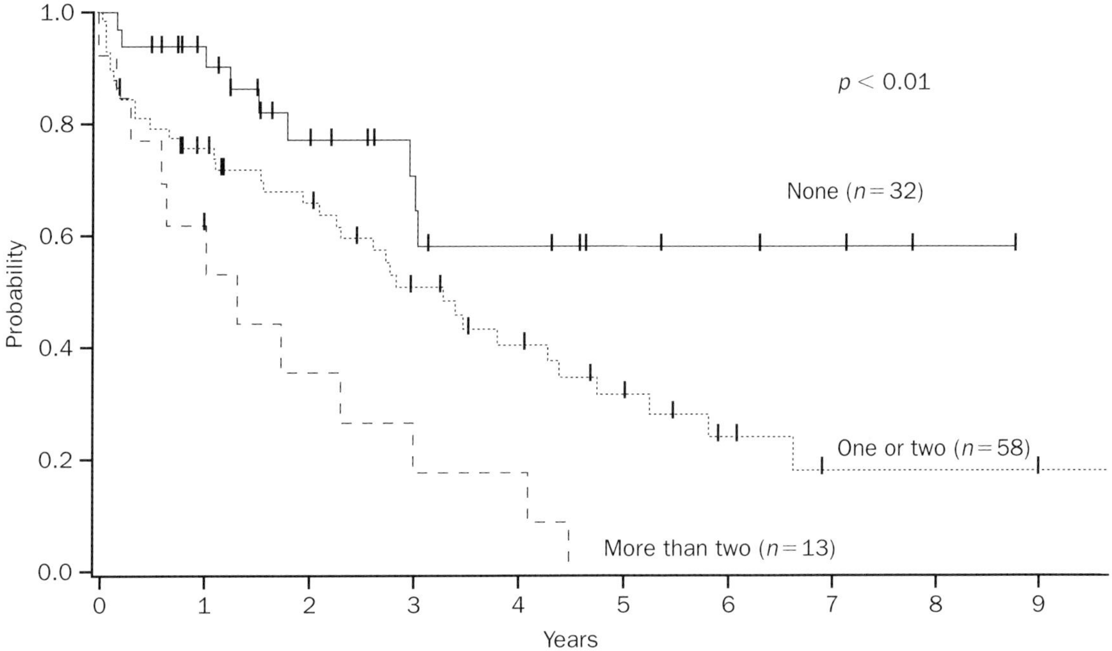

Figure 29.1 Probability of survival in recipients presenting for transplantation with no, one or two, or more than two abnormal disease characteristics at the time of transplantation.

sized that one or more of these disease characteristics might constitute risk factors useful for prognostication. These characteristics included anemia, leukocytosis or leukopenia, thrombocytosis or thrombocytopenia, marrow or blood basophilia, excess of blasts in marrow or blood, moderate or severe marrow fibrosis, palpable splenomegaly, cytogenetic abnormalities other than the standard t(9;22), and history of previous blast crisis. Patient characteristics are further defined and presented in Table 29.1. Of interest, patients with none of the above-mentioned disease characteristics at transplant had a significantly greater incidence of survival at 5 years (0.58; 95% confidence interval (CI) 0.35–0.80) than patients transplanted with one or two (0.31; 95% CI 0.17–0.46), or more than two (0) abnormal disease characteristics ($p = 0.01$) (Figure 29.1). In multivariate analysis, marrow or blood basophilia ($p < 0.01$) and the presence of marrow cytogenetic abnormalities other than the single Ph associated with a t(9;22) ($p = 0.04$) had an independent, adverse affect on survival.

As previously noted, this heterogeneous patient group received one of several transplant approaches, including use of ex vivo purged marrow, or mobilization with either relatively low-dose priming (Cy/GM/BM or Cy/G/PB) or high-dose combination chemotherapy priming (MAC/G/PB). We therefore included these and other transplant conditions and patient characteristics in our multivariate analysis. Of interest, the number of abnormal disease characteristics at transplant was the only factor that had an independent effect on the incidence of survival. Specifically, patients transplanted with no discernible abnormal disease characteristics had the best outcome. No independent effect of transplant year, interval from diagnosis to transplant, patient age or gender, preparative regimen, purging or priming approach, stem cell source (blood or marrow), or IL-2-based immunotherapy could be identified (Table 29.2).

Table 29.2 Disease characteristics affecting survival: Multivariate analysis

No. of risk factors	No. of patients	Relative risk	95% confidence interval	*p*
0	32	1.0		
1	42	2.2	1.0–4.7	0.04
2	16	2.2	0.9–5.5	0.08
>2	13	5.1	2.1–12.2	<0.01

DISCUSSION

The optimal approach to autologous HSCT therapy for CML has not yet been defined. Our experience suggests that prolonged survival can be achieved if CML patients are transplanted before characteristics indicating unstable or progressive disease appear. Such risk factors seem to have a cumulative, adverse effect on survival. We have tested ex vivo purging as well as in vivo purging with either intermediate-dose or intensive-dose priming chemotherapy. Neither purging method, choice of growth factor, nor autologous HSC source (blood or marrow) has a clear-cut effect on survival. Ex vivo purging is associated with tardy or incomplete engraftment requiring the infusion of untreated 'backup' autologous HSC. In vivo priming, particularly with intensive-dose chemotherapy, is associated with earlier engraftment, and rarely requires additional infusion of autologous HSC. Currently, we employ Cy/G/PB priming for autologous HSCT therapy of CML.

In this patient group, autologous HSCT had a predictable effect on marrow cytogenetics. Transplant was followed in many cases by a partial – even major – cytogenetic remission. However, examination of marrow cytogenetics at 1 year following autologous HSCT revealed recurrence of the Ph in most patients. We would predict that the use of more intensive ex vivo purging or in vivo priming approaches would cause dose-limiting hematopoietic or systemic toxicity without necessarily improving the incidence or persistence of cytogenetic remissions. Improvements in autologous HSCT are more likely if (i) newly diagnosed patients with minimal abnormal disease characteristics are transplanted, and (ii) the transplant is combined with additional peri- and post-transplant antileukemia therapy. It is not yet known if autologous HSCT will provide a higher incidence of major cytogenetic remissions than INF-α ± Ara-C.[29] Newly diagnosed patients are unlikely to have resistant disease or additional abnormal hematopoietic progenitor clones resistant to autologous HSCT therapy. Additional antileukemia therapy used as an adjunct to autologous HSCT might include tyrosine kinase inhibitors,[30] autologous or allogeneic NK-cell therapy,[27] subsequent allogeneic transplant with a non-myeloablative preparative regimen,[17] or chemotherapy following transplant of autologous HSC containing a 'drug resistance gene'.[31]

Investigation of promising therapy for CML is very active, and the role of autologous HSCT in the overall therapeutic approach to a given patient is not clear. Allogeneic HSCT with a related or unrelated donor can provide a high incidence of long-term disease-free survival in selected patient groups; however, morbidity and mortality are still high in unfavorable risk groups, and transplant is still limited by the availability of a suitably HLA-matched donor.[32] Therapy with IFN-α, perhaps combined with Ara-C, can produce major cytogenetic remissions and long-term survival in approximately 40–50% of newly presenting patients.[29] This approach, however, can be associated with long-term morbidity even in responding patients, is ineffective in many newly diagnosed patients, and may not be effective in previously treated or advanced patients.[33] Kinase inhibitors such as STI571 reverse abnormal intracellular signals of the BCR/ABL protein, and may have important therapeutic value. Clinical trials are underway, and early results suggest that STI571 has biological activity in CML with acceptable toxicity.[31] For further details, see Chapter 34.

At present, we are investigating the role of autologous HSCT as a 'platform' for combined-modality therapy of CML. The autologous HSCT group consists of CML patients with relatively few abnormal disease characteristics who are ineligible for allogeneic HSCT either because of poor prognostic features or unavailability of a suitable donor. Autologous HSCT is combined with post-transplant autologous or allogeneic IL-2-activated NK-cell therapy. Alternatively, selected patients will receive autologous hematopoietic progenitors transduced with a gene containing *BCR/ABL* antisense and conferring methotrexate resistance, followed by post-transplant low-dose methotrexate therapy.[31] Finally, after more information becomes available concerning the efficacy and toxicity of STI571 and related compounds, this promising agent may be incorporated into our autologous HSCT strategy.

ACKNOWLEDGEMENT

This work was supported in part by Grant CA 65493 from the US National Institutes of Health.

REFERENCES

1. Bhatia R, Verfaillie CM, Miller JS, McGlave PB, Autologous transplantation therapy for chronic myelogenous leukemia. *Blood* 1997; **89:** 2623–34.
2. Goto T, Nishikori M, Arlin A et al, Growth characteristics of leukemic and normal hematopoietic cells in Ph[1]+ chronic myelogenous leukemia and effects of intensive treatment. *Blood* 1982; **59:** 793–8.
3. Coulombel L, Kalousek DK, Eaves CJ et al, Long-term marrow culture reveals chromosomally normal hematopoietic progenitor cells in patients with Philadelphia chromosome-positive chronic myelogenous leukemia. *N Engl J Med* 1983; **308:** 1493–8.
4. Takahira H, Ideguchi H, Hirara J et al, Appearance of chromosomally normal hemopoiesis during busulfan-induced remission in a case of Ph[1] positive chronic myelogenous leukemia. *Rinsho Ketsueki* 1989; **30:** 251–5.
5. Leemhuis T, Leibowitz D, Cox G et al, Identification of BCR/ABL-negative primitive hematopoietic progenitor cells within chronic myelogenous leukemia marrow. *Blood* 1993; **81:** 801–7.
6. Haines ME, Goldman JM, Worsley AM et al, Chemotherapy and autografting for chronic granulocytic leukaemia in transformation: probable prolongation of survival for some patients. *Br J Haematol* 1984; **58:** 711–21.
7. Rizzoli V, Mangoni L, Pharmacological-mediated purging with mafosfamide in acute and chronic myeloid leukemias: the Italian Study Group. *Prog Clin Biol Res* 1990; **333:** 21–36 (discussion 37–8).
8. McGlave PB, Arthur D, Miller WJ et al, Autologous transplantation for CML using marrow treated ex vivo with recombinant human interferon gamma. *Bone Marrow Transplant* 1990; **6:** 115–20.
9. Gewirtz AM, Treatment of chronic myelogenous leukemia (CML) with c-myb antisense oligodeoxynucleotides. *Bone Marrow Transplant* 1994; **14:** S57.
10. Barnett MJ, Eaves CJ, Phillips GL et al, Autografting with cultured marrow in chronic myelogenous leukemia: results of a pilot study. *Blood* 1994; **84:** 724–32.
11. Carella AM, Podesta M, Grassoni F et al, Selective overshoot of Ph-negative blood hemopoietic cells after an intensive idarubicin-containing regimen and their repopulating capacity after reinfusion. *Stem Cells* 1993; **11:** 67–72.
12. Hughes T, Grigg A, Szer J et al, Mobilization of predominantly Philadelphia chromosome-negative blood progenitors using cyclophosphamide

and rhuG-CSF in early chronic-phase chronic myeloid leukemia: correlation with Sokal prognostic index and haematological control. *Br J Haematol* 1997; **96:** 635–40.
13. McGlave PB, De Fabritiis P, Deisseroth A et al, Autologous transplants for chronic myelogenous leukemia: results from eight transplant groups. *Lancet* 1994; **343:** 1486–8.
14. Carella A, Cunningham I, Lerma E et al, Mobilization and transplantation of Philadelphia-negative peripheral-blood progenitor cells early in chronic myelogenous leukemia. *J Clin Oncol* 1997; **15:** 1575–82.
15. Bhatia R, Forman SJ, Autologous transplantation for the treatment of chronic myelogenous leukemia. *Hematol Oncol Clin North Am* 1998; **12:** 151–72.
16. Miller JS, Innovative therapy for chronic myelogenous leukemia. *Hematol Oncol Clin North Am* 1998; **12:** 173–6.
17. Carella AM, Lerma E, Corsetti MT et al, High-intensity autotransplantation followed by reduced-intensity cytotoxic allotransplantation regimen (mini-allografting). *Blood* 1999; **94**(Suppl 1): 319a.
18. McGlave PB, Mamus S, Vilen B, Dewald G, Effect of recombinant gamma interferon on chronic myelogenous leukemia bone marrow progenitors. *Exp Hematol* 1987; **15:** 331–5.
19. McGlave PB, Arthur DC, Weisdorf D et al, Allogeneic bone marrow transplantation as treatment for accelerating chronic myelogenous leukemia. *Blood* 1984; **63:** 219–22.
20. Verfaillie CM, Miller WJ, Boylan K, McGlave PB, Selection of benign primitive hematopoietic progenitors in chronic myelogenous leukemia on the basis of HLA-DR antigen expression. *Blood* 1992; **79:** 1003–10.
21. Verfaillie CM, Bhatia R, Miller W et al, BCR/ABL-negative primitive progenitors suitable for transplantation can be selected from the marrow of most early-chronic phase but not accelerated-phase chronic myelogenous leukemia patients. *Blood* 1996; **87:** 4770–9.
22. Carella AM, Podesta M, Frassoni F et al, Collection of 'normal' blood repopulating cells during early hemopoietic recovery after intensive conventional chemotherapy in chronic myelogenous leukemia. *Bone Marrow Transplant* 1993; **12:** 267–71.
23. Verfaillie CM, Bhatia R, Steinbuch M et al, Comparative analysis of autografting in chronic myelogenous leukemia: effects of priming regimen and marrow or blood origin of stem cells. *Blood* 1998; **92:** 1820–31.
24. Verfaillie C, Kay N, Miller W, McGlave P, Adherent lymphokine activated killer cells in chronic myelogenous leukemia: a benign cell population with potent cytotoxic activity. *Blood* 1989; **74:** 793–7.
25. Cervantes F, Pierson BA, McGlave PB et al, Autologous activated natural killer cells suppress primitive chronic myelogenous leukemia progenitors in long-term culture. *Blood* 1996; **87:** 2476–85.
26. Miller JS, Klingsporn S, Lund J et al, Large scale ex vivo expansion and activation of human natural killer cells for autologous therapy. *Bone Marrow Transplant* 1994; **14:** 555–62.
27. Miller JS, Tessmer-Tuck J, Pierson BA et al, Low dose subcutaneous interleukin-2 after autologous transplantation generates sustained in vivo natural killer cell activity. *Biol Blood Marrow Transplant* 1997; **3:** 34–44.
28. Moretta A, Vitale M, Bottino C et al, p58 molecules as putative receptors for major histocompatibility complex (MHC) class I molecules in human natural killer (NK) cells. Anti-p58 antibodies reconstitute lysis of MHC class I-protected cells in NK clones displaying different specificities. *J Exp Med* 1993; **178:** 597–604.
29. Guilhot F, Chastang C, Michallet M et al, Interferon alfa-2b combined with cytarabine versus interferon alone in chronic myelogenous leukemia. French Chronic Myeloid Leukemia Study Group. *N Engl J Med* 1997; **337**: 223–9.
30. Druker BJ, Talpaz M, Resta D et al, Clinical efficacy and safety of an ABL specific tyrosine kinase inhibitor as targeted therapy for chronic myelogenous leukemia. *Blood* 1999; **94**(Suppl 1): 368a.
31. Zhao RCH, McIvor RS, Griffin JD, Verfaillie CM, Gene therapy for chronic myelogenous leukemia (CML): a retroviral vector that renders hematopoietic progenitors methotrexate-resistant and CML progenitors functionally normal and non tumorigenic in vivo. *Blood* 1997; **90**: 4687–98.
32. McGlave PB, Xiao OS, Wen W et al, Unrelated donor marrow transplantation for chronic myelogenous leukemia: nine years experience of the National Marrow Donor Program. *Blood* 2000; **95**: 2219–25.
33. Kantarjian HG, Giles FJ, O'Brien SM, Talpaz M, Clinical course and therapy of chronic myelogenous leukemia with interferon-alpha and chemotherapy. *Hematol Oncol Clin North Am* 1998; **12**: 31–80.

30

What role for autografting? A personal view

Stephen G O'Brien

CONTENTS • Introduction • What is the rationale for autografting in CML? • How and when should autografting be performed? • Is there any good evidence that autografting extends survival? • Is there a role for autografting in the era of STI571? • What might be the role of autografting in the future? • Conclusions

INTRODUCTION

The purpose of this chapter is to consider some of the broad issues involved in the use of autografting for chronic myeloid leukaemia (CML): the results of various specific approaches have been discussed in the preceding chapters. Despite the considerable experience and strenuous efforts of numerous international clinical trial groups over many years, we are unfortunately still not in a position to clearly define the role of autografting in CML, since there are no prospective randomized survival data. The major confounding factor in our efforts to assess autografting is the advent of new ways to treat CML. Perhaps more than most of the haematological malignancies, the therapeutic options available for CML patients have changed markedly in the last five years or so – and particularly over the last 18 months. The development of interferon-α (IFN-α)-containing regimens, progress in allogeneic transplantation, and the advent of STI571 (Glivec; Gleevec) have made it much more difficult to know which patients should be advised to undergo autografting, what type of autograft should be employed, and when it should be performed. In this chapter, as well as reviewing some basic concepts, I shall discuss a number of these issues, as well as considering overall management strategies.

WHAT IS THE RATIONALE FOR AUTOGRAFTING IN CML?

There is no evidence that autografting in CML 'cures' patients: the objective is to prolong survival. At first sight, it might seem illogical to autograft a patient with CML. Many initial studies used material collected at diagnosis that would have been frankly contaminated with leukaemic cells; however, even using this material, some intriguing clinical data have been derived. Subsequent clinical efforts have largely focused on using a Philadelphia chromosome (Ph)-negative autograft derived by either in vivo or in vitro purging approaches, but there are still protagonists for the 'straight' autografting approach, and overview analyses have not shown a significant difference in outcome with the various approaches.

A number of lines of evidence indicate that residual 'normal' stem cells coexist in at least some newly diagnosed CML patients.[1–3] These data are partly derived from in vitro observations: Ph-negative colonies can be found in CML patients;[4,5] clonality studies suggest the presence of Ph-negative haematopoietic progenitors.[6,7] Clinical data also support this concept, in that a number of therapeutic modalities, including high-dose chemotherapy,[8] various autografting approaches (see the preceding chapters), IFN-α and now STI571, can induce Ph-negativity. In the light of these data, there are three conceptual reasons why autografting might prolong life: if progression to transformation depends on random genetic events in primitive *BCR/ABL*-positive stem cells, any approach that reduced their number might delay transformation; steps to reduce both normal and leukaemic stem cells to a low level may favour the regeneration of normal stem cells – at least in the short term; it may be possible to develop reliable techniques for collection of and subsequent autografting with Ph-positive-depleted stem cells.[9]

HOW AND WHEN SHOULD AUTOGRAFTING BE PERFORMED?

Autografting in CML has been performed for at least 25 years, initially in blast crisis and subsequently in earlier phases of the disease. As with the introduction of many new leukaemia therapies, it was initially considered as a salvage procedure, and was gradually brought forward to earlier stages of the disease, eventually being employed in newly diagnosed patients. A variety of stem cell preparations have been evaluated, from 'straight', unmanipulated blood or marrow stem cells collected at diagnosis to the use of completely or predominantly Ph-negative cells derived by various in vitro and in vivo means. Whilst intuitively one would expect clinical results to be better using Ph-negative cells for the autograft, there are insufficient numbers of patients treated using these various approaches to allow meaningful comparison. The results from groups using Ph-negative cells are quite impressive, but it cannot be safely concluded that this is the best approach. There are also a number of technical considerations that can affect the quality of the stem cell infusion: failure of engraftment and/or microbial contamination may confound any overall survival benefit for the procedure, as has been experienced in acute myeloid leukaemia.

A variety of mobilization and pretransplant cytoreductive regimens have been employed, again perhaps suggesting that none is clearly superior. Perhaps most experience has been derived using variations on the ICE (idarabicin, cytosine arabinoside, and etoposide) regimen as piloted by the Genoa group.[10] For cytoreduction prior to the autograft, the role of irradiation, cyclophosphamide, and other agents is far from clear. Given that autografting is not performed with curative intent, a simple minimally toxic approach might seem to be the most logical, and the use of busulfan alone has recently been reported.[11]

The most appropriate patients for autografting and when during the course of their disease autografting should be done remain contentious issues. Outside large-scale trials, autografting has traditionally been considered in later-chronic-phase patients for whom an allograft is deemed inappropriate by virtue of age, medical fitness, or lack of donor, and often in whom IFN-α has proven ineffective or intolerable. Although useful pilot studies have been conducted in such groups of patients, the value of autografting in this context remains uncertain, although anecdotally impressive results have occasionally been seen. It could be argued that further pilot studies are no longer appropriate and that all patients in whom it is thought autografting might be beneficial should be entered into a large study. However, a study of this type for late-chronic-phase patients has not been established, and such patients are now increasingly being treated with STI571.

For newly diagnosed patients, the above considerations of age and allogeneic donor availability are of course important, and if it seems to patient and doctor that autografting might be useful then it is appropriate for such a patient to go into a large-scale trial, such as CML2000 (EBMT99) (Figure 30.1). This offers a consistent approach and contributes to a greater understanding of the survival question. There would seem to be little rationale in this situation for

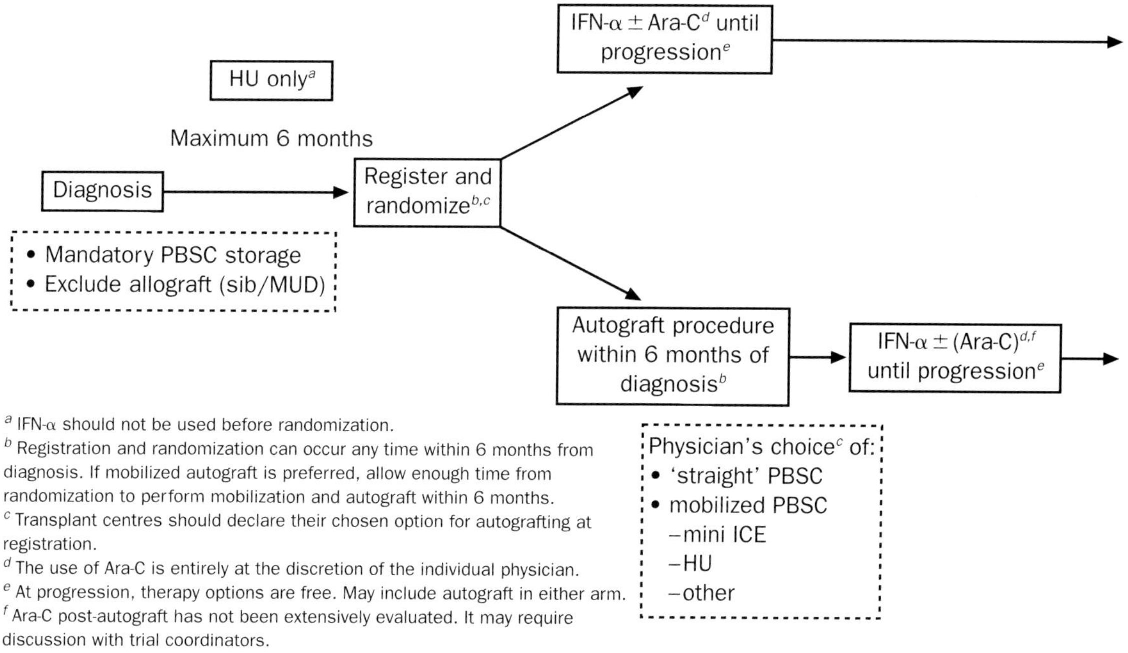

Figure 30.1 Design of the current CML2000 (EBMT 99) autografting study. *Abbreviations:* HU, hydroxyurea; IFN-α, interferon-α; Ara-C, cytosine arabinoside; PBSC, peripheral blood stem cells; sib/MUD, sibling/matched unrelated donor; ICE, idarubicin, Ara-C and etoposide.

performing an experimental autograft procedure outwith a prospective randomized trial.

IS THERE ANY GOOD EVIDENCE THAT AUTOGRAFTING EXTENDS SURVIVAL?

In short, the answer is no. Numerous single-arm studies exploring various autografting approaches have been published and some comparisons with historical patient populations have been conducted. However, such analyses are of limited value, and large-scale prospective randomised trials have proven difficult.

It is useful to consider the evolution of prospective randomized controlled trials for autografting in CML. In times where, quite rightly, there is increasing pressure on us as clinicians to have a sound evidence base for our practice, the need for well-designed and well-conducted prospective clinical trails to answer important questions has never been greater. For many years, there was little convincing evidence to support the adoption of autografting in CML into mainstream practice, although the procedure was regularly being performed. This unsatisfactory situation was addressed by a number of large trial groups, and over time a consortium evolved comprising the UK Medical Research Council (MRC) group, the European Group for Blood and Marrow Transplantation (EBMT), and the US Eastern Cooperative Oncology Group (ECOG). A trial was designed to address the question of whether autografting could improve on the survival advantage offered by IFN-α. Figure 30.1 shows the final design of this study, commonly designated CML2000 or EBMT99. The trial was carefully designed with a number of considerations in mind, not all of which were easy to reconcile. Some thought the interval prior to randomization was too short, some thought it too long; some thought the autograft must be purged, some favoured 'straight' autografting; there was divergence regarding the best mobilization regimen. Many doctors and patients found the prospect of many weeks in hospital (autograft arm) compared with outpatient treatment with self-administered injections also difficult to accept, and opted not to participate. These differences in the clinical practicalities of different treatment arms are a particular problem for any comparative transplant studies, including CML2000. Despite these difficulties, recruitment was slow but steady. And then came STI571.

IS THERE A ROLE FOR AUTOGRAFTING IN THE ERA OF STI571?

In mid 1999, the first clinical results with STI571 were made public. Even to the most cautious of observers, it was clear that this drug was set to revolutionize the treatment of CML, and a study addressing the role of autografting became even more difficult. The STI571 data continue to be impressive, although it is clear that, especially in advanced phases of CML, STI571 does not work in all patients and resistance develops in a significant number. It is worth emphasizing that STI571 has not been shown to extend survival in CML, although cytogenetic response rates are superior to those achieved historically with IFN-α. It will take at least 3–5 years for meaningful comparative survival data to accrue. The problem for autografting trials, however, is simple, and even as a vigorous supporter of such studies for many years, I cannot help but alter my views. If I were in a position where an allograft was inappropriate, IFN-α had perhaps failed, and my doctor offered me the option of either taking a few capsules of STI571 each day with little risk of serious morbidity or mortality, or participating in a study involving the prospect of many weeks in hospital going through an arduous medical procedure with a small but significant risk of serious complications, I would probably take the capsules and try to sustain the normal routines of my life despite the future uncertainties. Of course this is a simplistic analysis – not least because STI571 is not as readily available as my comments imply – but this dichotomy reflects the nature of many clinic consultations at present, and STI571 will become broadly available as a licensed medication before the end of 2001. It is still early days for this exciting new drug, but STI571 has changed the rules, and, no matter how much effort has been put into evaluating a certain treatment strategy, if the facts change then one has to adapt accordingly (Figure 30.2). I suspect for the next year or two, until the role of STI571 becomes clearer, large-scale studies of autografting in CML will simply not be viable – most patients and their doctors will want to either allograft or use STI571. However, as STI571 will not produce long-term disease control in all CML patients, it seems likely that the role of autografting will in due course be revisited.

WHAT MIGHT BE THE ROLE OF AUTOGRAFTING IN THE FUTURE?

Autografting in CML at present faces considerable problems. If there is a survival benefit, it is likely to be small – but it may be significant enough to be important: the use of tamoxifen in breast cancer is based on a marginal but significant improvement in survival that was not evident in small initial studies. Demonstrating such a benefit with sufficient power is likely to take up to 1000 randomized patients, and given that CML is a rare disease and that there are novel therapies to consider, a trial of this magnitude could theoretically take ten years to recruit. An example of the competition is the recently closed Novartis 0106 study, which is a prospective randomized comparison of STI571 monotherapy against IFN-α and cytosine arabinoside in patients within 6 months of diagnosis. This was the fastest-recruiting study in CML ever conducted, and enrolled 1106 patients in 7 months. Patient informed consent will continue to be the most decisive element of success.

Although a direct comparison of autografting versus STI571 in newly diagnosed patients is unlikely to be popular, one can conceive of a number of important autografting questions that could be valid (Table 30.1). These studies will not commence until 2002 for a variety of reasons, and the current shift towards drug therapy and away from transplantation may well affect viability until longer-term data with STI571 are available.

CONCLUSIONS

In the face of new therapeutic developments in CML, one has to be dispassionate about the efficacy and role of autografting. I, and many others, have spent many years endeavoring to define a role for this procedure, but one has to put aside any vested interests if newer and better treatments come along. Foremost in our minds should be the aim of prolonged survival for CML patients of all ages – not the vindication of a particular therapeutic approach.

Currently there is probably a role for autografting in the year 2001 where allografting is unavailable or inappropriate and/or when other therapies such as STI571 have failed. Although this may seem to be a reversion to using autografting as salvage therapy rather than 'upfront', the simple fact is that most

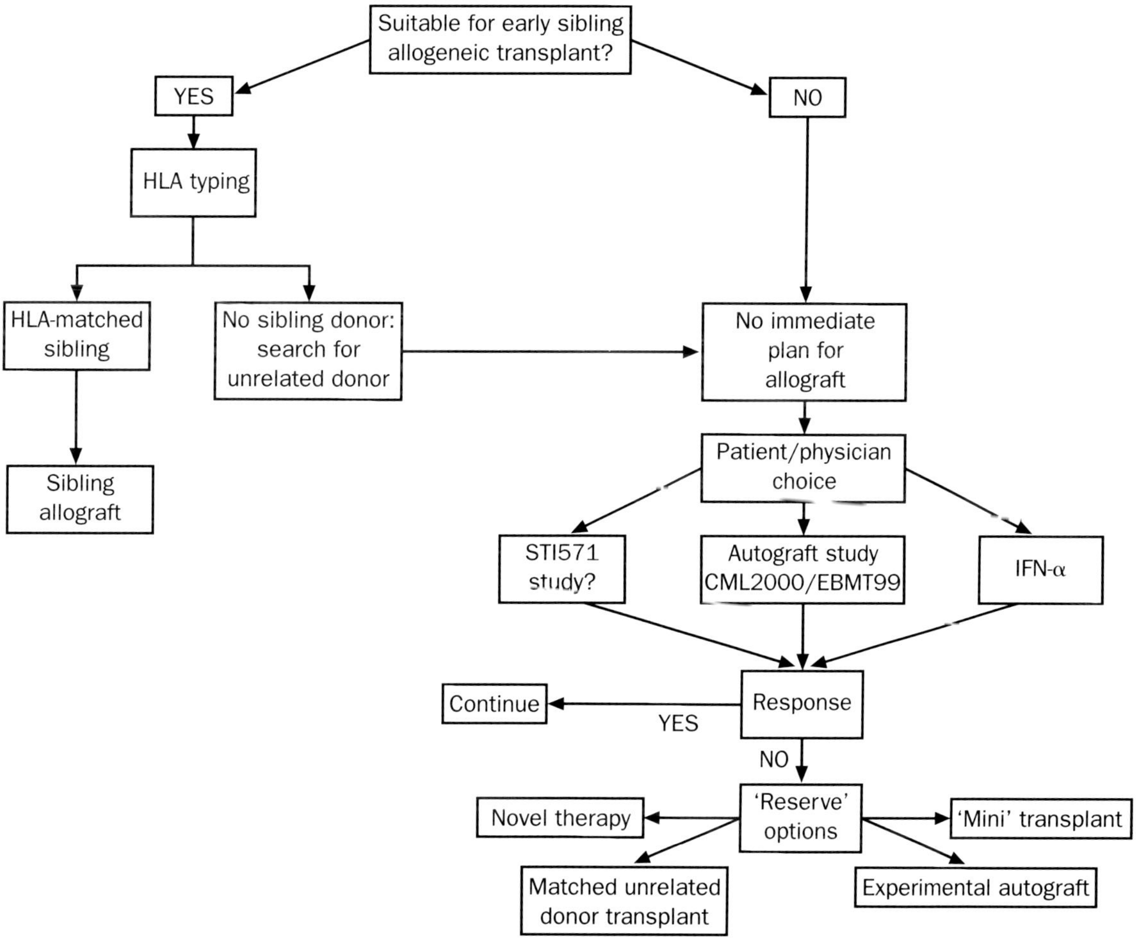

Figure 30.2 Possible role of autografting in a newly diagnosed patient with CML.

Table 30.1 Possible autografting studies in the era of STI571. The ideas are necessarily based on the premise that STI571 will become the de facto therapeutic standard for non-allografted patients. There is only one study comparing IFN-α plus cytosine arabinoside (the current 'standard') with STI571, and it seems likely from a patient acceptability point of view that all future studies will be obliged to incorporate STI571, although this might not be the ideal design from a statistical point of view

Question	Clinical context	Rationale	Comment
Can peripheral blood stem cells be harvested from patients achieving complete cytogenetic response (with or without *BCR/ABL*-negativity) with STI571. Pilot study.	Recently diagnosed and long-standing patients.	Non-leukaemic stem cells could be collected and frozen for use if/when STI571 resistance develops. Probably use granulocyte colony-stimulating factor only for mobilization.	An intriguing question that is just starting to be explored. Although Ph-negative (and possibly *BCR/ABL*-negative) stem cells can probably be collected, achieving sufficient stem cell numbers for a viable autograft will probably be difficult. Most patients with complete cytogenetic responses have hypocellular marrows and variable degrees of peripheral cytopenia.
STI571 versus autograft 'up front'. Survival study.	Patients within 6 months of diagnosis.	Perhaps assumes that STI571 is superior to IFN-α – which is yet to be proven. Evaluates survival in a homogeneous group of patients.	Likely to be unpopular with patients.
STI571 versus autograft followed by STI571 'up front'. Survival study.	Patients within 6 months of diagnosis.	Can autografting add to any benefit achieved with STI571?	Could be more acceptable to patients in that STI571 is assured. However, if STI571 monotherapy data from the Novartis 0106 trial are good, patients may not accept the additional inconvenience and potential toxicity of an autograft.
Autograft for STI571 failures. Pilot. Randomized question could be devised.	Patients at any stage.	Salvage therapy. STI571 may have altered the biology of the disease – synergistic effect?	Very few patients have been treated in this way so far.
STI571 for autograft failures	Patients at any stage.	Salvage therapy.	Effectively already being done. Many patients in the initial STI571 studies had had previously unsuccessful autografts.
High-dose STI571 cytoreduction. Pilot.	Patients at any stage.	May be of interest as a cytoreductive agent in both auto- and allografting.	Has never been tested

patients and haematologists have been voting with their feet: given the choice of a prolonged hospital stay undergoing mobilization and an autograft with some procedural risk against an oral medication with few side-effects and impressive initial results, it is not surprising that autografting studies have struggled recently. Although cost may well come into the equation as well, at the time of writing the eventual cost of STI571 is unknown. Autografting costs vary considerably and have never been comprehensively documented.

Autografting should probably continue to be evaluated – but only within the context of trials. STI571 has not yet been shown to prolong survival or 'cure' any CML patients, and the temptation to dispense with autografting altogether should be resisted: novel applications for the procedure will be defined in due course. There is correspondingly an onus on trial coordinators to ensure that trials are sufficiently imaginative and flexible to allow entry to all patients for whom it is thought that autografting may be of benefit. We live in exciting, if complex, times, and now more than ever we must carefully consider what place autografting has in the modern management of CML.

REFERENCES

1. Dunbar CE, Stewart FM, Separating the wheat from the chaff: selection of benign hematopoietic cells in chronic myeloid leukemia [editorial]. *Blood* 1992; **79:** 1107–10.
2. Eaves AC, Barnett MJ, Ponchio L et al, Differences between normal and CML stem cells: potential targets for clinical exploitation. *Stem Cells* 1998; **16**(Suppl 1): 77–83; discussion 89.
3. Petzer AL, Eaves CJ, Lansdorp PM et al, Characterization of primitive subpopulations of normal and leukemic cells present in the blood of patients with newly diagnosed as well as established chronic myeloid leukemia. *Blood* 1996; **88:** 2162–71.
4. Chervenick PA, Ellis LD, Pan SF, Lawson AL, Human leukemic cells: in vitro growth of colonies containing the Philadelphia (Ph) chromosome. *Science* 1971; **174:** 1134–6.
5. Coulombel L, Kalousek DK, Eaves CJ et al, Long-term marrow culture reveals chromosomally normal hematopoietic progenitor cells in patients with Philadelphia chromosome-positive chronic myelogenous leukemia. *N Engl J Med* 1983; **308:** 1493–8.
6. Fialkow PJ, Martin PJ, Najfeld V et al, Evidence for a multistep pathogenesis of chronic myelogenous leukemia. *Blood* 1981; **58:** 158–63.
7. Raskind WH, Ferraris AM, Najfeld V et al, Further evidence for the existence of a clonal Ph-negative stage in some cases of Ph-positive chronic myelocytic leukemia. *Leukemia* 1993; **7:** 1163–7.
8. Goto T, Nishikori M, Arlin Z et al, Growth characteristics of leukemic and normal hematopoietic cells in Ph'+ chronic myelogenous leukemia and effects of intensive treatment. *Blood* 1982; **59:** 793–808.
9. O'Brien SG, Goldman JM, Current approaches to hematopoietic stem-cell purging in chronic myeloid leukemia [editorial] *J Clin Oncol* 1995; **13:** 541–6.
10. Carella AM, Lerma E, Corsetti MT et al, Autografting with Philadelphia chromosome-negative mobilized hematopoietic progenitor cells in chronic myelogenous leukemia. *Blood* 1999; **93:** 1534–9.
11. Olavarria E, Kanfer E, Szydlo R et al, High-dose busulphan alone as cytoreduction before allogeneic or autologous stem cell transplantation for chronic myeloid leukaemia: a single-centre experience. *Br J Haematol* 2000; **108:** 769–77.

Part 5

Target-directed therapies: Chronic myeloid leukaemia as a paradigm for oncology

31

Gene therapy

Alan M Gewirtz

CONTENTS • Introduction • Targeting the *BCR/ABL* gene • Alternative gene targets in CML • Clinical experiences with antisense oligonucleotides • Introduction of exogenous genes into CML cells for therapeutic purposes • Conclusions

INTRODUCTION

Significant progress is being made in the identification of genes responsible for cell growth and malignant transformation.[1–3] With this knowledge has come a natural desire to 'translate' this information into new, 'target-specific', therapeutic strategies for the treatment of cancer. The recent development of a relatively specific biochemical inhibitor of the BCR/ABL protein tyrosine kinase in patients with chronic myeloid leukemia (CML)[4] is a stunning example of this quest (see Chapters 32 and 34). For therapies aimed directly at replacement, repair, or disabling of disease-causing genes, progress has been slower, and a success equivalent to the biochemical BCR/ABL inhibitor has yet to be achieved. The reasons for this are complex, and vary with the type of gene-directed therapy being employed. For strategies involving the use of viral vectors, issues related to efficient infection of human hematopoietic stem cells, as well as efficiency and persistence of expression of the gene cassette transferred, remain unsolved problems. The 'simpler' approach of delivering a gene-modifying nucleic acid, such as an antisense oligodeoxynucleotide or ribozyme, has also proven problematic. There are many recent reviews discussing the problems and potential of these various approaches.[5–7] This chapter will focus on the use of nucleic acid molecules, the so-called 'antisense' strategy, for treating CML, and will briefly discuss approaches employing viral vectors.

That gene expression could be modified through the use of exogenous nucleic acids derives from studies by Paterson et al,[8] who first used single-stranded DNA to inhibit translation of a complementary RNA in a cell-free system in 1977. The following year, Zamecnik and Stephenson[9] showed that a short (13-nucleotide) DNA oligonucleotide reverse-complementary in sequence (antisense) to the Rous sarcoma virus could inhibit viral replication in culture. These investigators are widely credited with having first suggested the therapeutic utility of antisense nucleic acids, and, indeed, Dr Zamecnik was recently awarded a Lasker prize in recognition of the potential importance of this work. In the mid-1980s, the existence of naturally occurring antisense RNAs and their role in regulating gene expression was demonstrated.[10–12] These observations were particularly important, because they lent credibility to the belief that 'antisense' was more than a laboratory phenomenon, and encouraged belief in the hypothesis that reverse-complementary oligonucleotides could be utilized in living cells to manipulate gene expression. These seminal papers, and the many that have followed, have stimulated the development of technologies employing nucleic acids to manipulate gene expression. Virtually all available methods rely on some type of nucleotide sequence recognition for targeting specificity, but differ in where and how they perturb the flow of genetic information. Simply stated, strategies for modulating gene expression may be thought of as being targeted to the gene itself, or its messenger RNA.

Antigene strategies focus primarily on gene targeting by homologous recombination[13] or by triple-helix-forming oligodeoxynucleotides (TFOs).[14,15] For many technical reasons, including very limited gene accessibility within the highly condensed, protein-wrapped chromosomal structure, the clinical application of these methods has not progressed rapidly. An alternative approach, using polyamides that can diffuse into the nucleus and recognize specific DNA sequences, has recently been described by Dervan and colleagues.[16] While very exciting, this methodology is still in its infancy, and its ultimate clinical utility remains unknown.

A larger body of work has focused on destabilizing mRNA. This approach, while less favorable than antigene strategies from a stoichiometric point of view, is attractive because mRNA is much more accessible. Two basic strategies have emerged for this purpose. One employs an oligonucleotide that acts as an alternate binding site, or 'decoy', for protein-stabilizing elements that normally interact with a given mRNA.[17,18] By attracting away mRNA-stabilizing protein, the decoy induces instability, and ultimately destruction, of the mRNA. The other is the more familiar, and more widely applied 'antisense' strategy. Here, a reverse-complementary (antisense) oligonucleotide is introduced into a cell in the hope that it will form Watson–Crick base pairs with the targeted gene's mRNA. Stable mRNA–oligonucleotide duplexes cannot be translated, and almost certainly initiate processes that lead to the destruction of the mRNA. Failure to synthesize the disease-causing protein is the predictable result. The oligonucleotide can be composed of DNA or RNA, and both types of molecules can be modified for stability as well as being engineered to contain inherent cleaving activity.[19,20]

TARGETING THE *BCR/ABL* GENE

Szczylik and colleagues[21] were among the first to suggest that oligonucleotides targeting *BCR/ABL* might be of therapeutic utility. They found that when primary leukemic blast cells were exposed to synthetic 18-mer oligodeoxynucleotides (ODNs) complementary to b2a2 or b3a2 *BCR/ABL* junctions, leukemic cell colony formation in vitro was significantly suppressed. In contrast, granulocyte–macrophage colony formation from normal marrow progenitors was unaffected by the same ODNs. Suppression of colony growth was reported to be sequence-specific. Finally, when equal proportions of normal marrow progenitors and blast cells were mixed, exposed to the ODNs, and assayed for residual colony formation, the majority of residual cells were normal. These findings suggested that *BCR/ABL*-targeted oligonucleotides represented a means for specifically killing CML cells. This work was followed by a number of reports from the same group, and others, which reported very similar findings.[22–28] Work in animal models appeared to confirm the utility of this approach, especially when the oligonucleotides were used in conjunction with chemotherapy.[29,30]

The results reported above have not been universally reproducible.[31–37] For example, O'Brien and colleagues[35] examined the effects of antisense oligonucleotides of various lengths, sequences, and chemistry on the proliferation of eight different cell lines – five derived from patients with CML and three from other sources. They found that phosphodiester oligonucleotides had little antiproliferative activity in their system, presumably because of degradation by nucleases present in fetal calf serum or rapid intracellular breakdown. Phosphorothioate oligonucleotides antisense –

but not sense - to the b2a2 and b3a2 breakpoints significantly inhibited the proliferation of three CML cell lines (BV173, LAMA84, and KYO1). However, the antiproliferative effect appeared to be independent of the type of breakpoint expressed by each cell line, suggesting that the inhibition was sequence-dependent but not sequence-specific. Other investigators have reported that inhibition of CML cell growth with oligonucleotides is not sequence-dependent, suggesting that an aptameric effect is responsible.[37] Pigneux and co-workers[38] very recently reported that *BCR/ABL*-targeted ODNs were non-toxic to normal cells and that specific inhibition of CML colony-forming units in culture could be achieved. Nevertheless, while colony formation was inhibited by around 60%, residual colonies in treated dishes were all *BCR/ABL*-positive.

Ribozymes have been applied against *BCR/ABL*, and appear to give rise to more specific, but still inefficient, cleavage of their target.[39–42] An apparent explanation for the controversy surrounding the ability of this breakpoint to be specifically cleaved has been reported.[43] Calculations of the local folding potential of the RNA indicated that the *BCR/ABL* fusion point sequences are not easily accessible for complementary nucleic acid hybridization.[43] The study further suggested that selective and efficient antisense sequences should be directed against the *BCR* portion neighboring the fusion point as well as the first eight nucleotides of the *ABL* sequence. To effectively inhibit this target, then, relatively high doses of oligonucleotides may be required, and these in turn may produce non-specific effects. In addition, if ribozymes with unfavorable kinetics are employed to target the sequence, inhibition is likely to be inefficient, and therefore difficult to measure.

More recently, Zhao and colleagues[44] reported a clever and apparently successful strategy for inhibiting growth of CML cells with an anti-*BCR/ABL* ribozyme delivered by a retroviral vector that also delivered a methotrexate-resistance gene. The hypothesis underlying these experiments was that transfer of a vector that combined a drug-resistance gene with anti-*BCR/ABL* antisense sequences might allow for post-transplant chemotherapy to decrease persistent disease while rendering inadvertently transduced CML stem and progenitor cells functionally normal. A retroviral vector (LasBD) that combined a methotrexate-resistance gene and antisense sequences directed at the b3a2 *BCR/ABL* breakpoint was constructed. Cells engineered to express *BCR/ABL* were transduced with LasBD and selected in methotrexate for 14 days. Expression of the antisense sequences was reported to reduce *BCR/ABL* mRNA and p210 *BCR/ABL* protein levels by 6- to 10-fold in most cells, with apparent normalization of cell growth. LasBD also rendered 20–30% of primary Philadelphia chromosome (Ph)-negative and Ph-positive $CD34^+$ cells methotrexate-resistant, and decreased *BCR/ABL* mRNA levels in methotrexate resistant Ph-positive $CD34^+$ cells by 10-fold. LasBD decreased the tumorigenicity of 32D *BCR/ABL* cells in vivo by 3–4 logs. Based on these results, the investigators concluded that the methotrexate-resistance gene in the LasBD vector could protect normal hematopoietic cells from methotrexate-mediated toxicity, whereas the antisense sequences in LasBD could suppress expression of the *BCR/ABL* gene and restore the normal function of *BCR/ABL* cDNA-containing cells. While the system described was highly constrained, these results were nonetheless very encouraging, and form the basis for a planned clinical trial.

ALTERNATIVE GENE TARGETS IN CML

While *BCR/ABL* is an obvious target for antigene therapeutics, a number of considerations suggest that it may not be as ideal a target as first considerations would suggest. It must be recalled that since anti-mRNA strategies based on the use of ODNs are transient interventions, the target has to be expressed when oligonucleotides are physically present in the cell. In addition, it is straightforward that the strategy will only be effective if the target cell fails to tolerate transient downregulation of the targeted mRNA. Recent results using the c-ABL kinase inhibitor STI571 (Glivec; Gleevec) suggest that while BCR/ABL is clearly important for CML cell proliferation, the persistence of BCR/ABL-positive cells in treated patients implies that inhibition of BCR/ABL is insufficient to kill the malignant stem cells. Accordingly, the search for additional gene targets remains of interest.

Transcription factors

c-*myb*

The c-*myb* proto-oncogene is the normal cellular homologue of v-*myb*, the transforming oncogene of the avian myeloblastosis virus (AMV) and avian leukemia virus E26. c-*myb* is a member of a family of transcription factor genes that includes at least two other highly homologous genes designated A-*myb* and B-*myb*.[45] c-*myb* is located on chromosome 6q in humans, and its predominant transcript encodes an approximately 75 kDa nuclear binding protein (Myb), which recognizes the core consensus sequence 5'-PyAAC(G/Py)G-3'.[46]

The ability of c-*myb* to transactivate genes important for hematopoietic cell proliferation,[47,48] and differentiation,[49] including c-*kit*,[50] may also play a role in its ability to transform cells. Recent work reporting that AMV's v-*myb* transactivates the homeobox gene *GBX2*, and that *GBX2* in turn mediates autocrine growth and monocytic differentiation by transactivation of myelomonocytic growth factor gene (c-*MGF*) illustrates this point.[51] Accordingly, c-*myb* is a rational target for manipulation with therapeutic intent. Clinical data with a c-*myb*-targeted oligodeoxynucleotide will be briefly discussed below.

c-*myc*

Work from Sawyers and co-workers[52,53] has suggested that in the absence of functional Myc, *BCR/ABL* is unable to transform primary mouse marrow cells. Based on these studies, Skorski et al have targeted c-*myc*[54] and *BCR/ABL* simultaneously in an effort to improve on results obtained by targeting *BCR/ABL* alone.[55] In vitro colony-forming unit assays and SCID mouse studies were conducted. The latter were of particular interest, since they represent a potentially relevant treatment model. In these studies, animals were injected with primary blast-crisis CML cells, and were then treated systematically with equal doses of phosphorothioate ODNs targeted at *BCR/ABL*, c-*myc*, or *BCR/ABL* + c-*myc*. Compared with mice treated with individual compounds, the disease process appeared to be better controlled in the group treated with both ODNs, though the animals were not cured. The authors suggested that targeting multiple cooperating oncogenes might be a useful strategy for increasing the effectiveness of oligonucleotide therapeutics.

Receptors and signaling proteins

Other potential mRNA targets for treating CML might also be envisioned. These may be found among the surface receptors and signaling proteins constitutive to hematopoietic cells. For example, we have previously suggested that the Kit receptor might serve this purpose.[56] As noted above, c-*kit* appears to be a c-*myb*-regulated gene, and downregulation of c-*kit* in hematopoietic cells is associated with induction of apoptosis, perhaps an important mechanistic component of anti-c-*myb*'s ability to kill malignant cells. Directly comparing the ability of anti-c-*myb* and anti-c-*kit* targeted oligonucleotides to inhibit the growth of leukemic cells suggests this possibility, while at the same time supporting the potential of c-*kit*-targeted oligonucleotides in the treatment of CML and other leukemias.

A newer target that may prove to be of even greater utility in patients with hematologic malignancies is the signaling protein Vav encoded by the *vav* proto-oncogene.[57,58] Vav is expressed exclusively in hematopoietic cells, where it is assumed to play a role in signaling. The importance of this role is uncertain – in part because of conflicting functional studies that have employed different strategies for abrogating *vav* gene expression in murine embryonic stem cells.[59–62] Our studies with *vav*-targeted oligonucleotides lend some support to each of the conflicting reports cited above, and imply that *vav* would be a therapeutically attractive target in CML.[63] We have found that while *vav* appears to be required for erythropoiesis in both normal and malignant hematopoietic cells, *malignant* myeloid cell growth – in particular, growth of myeloid cells derived from CML patients – does appear to be dependent on *vav* expression.[63] The rationale for *vav* as an antisense target is therefore anchored in the fact that it is differentially used in normal and malignant cells.

CLINICAL EXPERIENCES WITH ANTISENSE OLIGONUCLEOTIDES

Clinical experience with oligonucleotides has been reported by several groups. de Fabritis et al[26] treated a patient with CML in accelerated phase with autologous bone marrow transplantation. Before reinfusion, cells were purged in vitro with a 26-nucleotide phosphorothioate antisense ODN specific for the b2a2 junction. This treatment resulted in 24% and 41% reductions of granulocyte–macrophage colony-forming units (CFU-GM) and $CD34^+$ cells, respectively. The patient was successfully engrafted with the purged marrow cells after 17 and 25 days for platelets and neutrophils, respectively. Using fluorescence in situ hybridization (FISH) in interphase nuclei, some Ph-positive cells were found after the autograft. The patient was reported to be in a complete hematologic remission at 9 months post treatment. In a larger purging study carried out on eight CML patients with accelerated or second chronic-phase disease, de Fabritis and colleagues[64] reported further encouraging results. In this study, marrow mononuclear cells were treated in vitro for 24 or 72 hours with *BCR/ABL*-targeted antisense ODN. After a conditioning regimen including busulfan and etoposide, the patients were autografted with purged marrow, and all reconstituted. Evaluation of the antileukemic effect by standard cytogenetic analysis and FISH showed a complete karyotypic response in two cases and a minimal or no response in the other six. The patient autografted in second chronic phase died in blast crisis at 7 months. Of the seven patients autografted in transformation, three developed blast crisis 21–39 months after autografting, one died from unrelated complications 30 months after transplant, and three were in persistent second chronic phase 14–26 months after autografting.

Clark and colleagues have sought to improve on these results by augmenting the delivery of the oligonucleotides into cells. Antisense ODNs targeted against the breakpoint in *BCR/ABL* mRNA will specifically decrease *BCR/ABL* mRNA, provided cells are first permeabilized with streptolysin-O (SL-O). We used an 18-mer chimeric methylphosphonodiester : phosphodiester-linked (4-9-4) ODN complementary to 9 bases either side of the *BCR/ABL* junction to purge harvests ex vivo in three CML patients who remained completely Ph-positive after multiple chemotherapy courses. After $CD34^+$ cell selection and SL-O permeabilization, harvests were purged with 20 mM ODN. After purging, all individual CFU-GM colonies grown from the two b3a2 breakpoint cases remained positive for *BCR/ABL* mRNA. In contrast, all 24 colonies grown from the b2a2 breakpoint case were *BCR/ABL* mRNA-negative. Patients were conditioned with busulfan 16 mg/kg. The initial post-transplant course was uneventful, although the time to return to $0.5 \times 10^9/l$ neutrophils was slow at 25–51 days. Both chronic-phase patients remain in hematologic remission at 1724 and 1610 days, although each has cytogenetic evidence of relapse. The b2a2 accelerated-phase patient died of myeloid blast transformation at day 191. The present SL-O-facilitated ODN purging strategy appears to be without significant toxicity, and offers considerable improvements in ODN delivery to the cytosol.

After extensive preclinical development (see above), we initiated clinical trials to evaluate the effectiveness of c-*myb*-targeted oligonucleotide drugs for the treatment of CML and acute leukemias. A phosphorothioate modification of the anti-c-*myb* ODN was used as a marrow purging agent in chronic-phase or accelerated-phase CML patients. At the time of writing, we have carried out a total of 18 bone marrow autografts. The marrow employed has been purged for either 24 hours (13 patients) or 72 hours (5 patients) with the ODN. We have also carried out 20 intravenous infusions. In brief, major cytogenetic responses were observed in 5 out of 8 evaluable patients who underwent 24-hour marrow purges. Of these, 7 out of 8 are still alive up to 4 years post procedure. The 72-hour purging regimen was very effective in vitro, but was associated with a prolonged period of marrow hypoplasia. The results of these studies are being prepared for publication.

In a phase I study, a c-*myb*-targeted phosphorothioate ODN has been administered to 20 patients with blast-crisis CML or other refractory leukemias by constant intravenous infusion. Dose levels ranged between 0.3 mg/kg/day × 7 days and 2.0 mg/kg/day × 7 days. After one week of infusion, patients were 'rested' for three weeks (one cycle). If still alive, they were eligible for another cycle of treatment. Hypotension was not observed during the infusions. No consistent metabolic abnormality or coagulopathy was noted. Two patients had incidents questionably related to the study ODN (one transient renal failure, one pericarditis), but these were not observed again when the patients were re-treated at the same or higher doses. One blast-crisis CML patient received anti-c-*myb* ODN at a dose of 0.3 mg/kg/d × 7 days every 3 weeks, as well as intermittent low-dose hydroxyurea (approximately 1–2 g/day). The patient received a total of nine infusion cycles before control of her disease was lost. She survived for about 12 months with excellent quality of life. The other responses are summarized in Table 31.1.

INTRODUCTION OF EXOGENOUS GENES INTO CML CELLS FOR THERAPEUTIC PURPOSES

While the strategies discussed above demonstrate the potential utility of modifying genes directly involved in the pathogenesis of CML, a

Table 31.1 Response to anti-c-*myb* ODN infusions

Diagnosis	Number of patients	Number of cycles delivered
Refractory acute myeloid leukemia	7	2 ± 1
Blast-crisis CML	7	2.7 ± 2.9
Accelerated-phase CML	6	4.0 ± 1
	Total: 20	Mean: 2.9 ± 2

- Progressive disease (<2 cycles): 8/20 patients
- Disease 'stabilization' (>2 cycles): 12/20 patients
- 'Stabilization' with hematologic improvement: 5/20 patients

number of groups have explored the therapeutic potential of introducing into hematopoietic cells genes that might augment the host response to the CML cells and adversely affect cell proliferation. Good examples of this approach are older studies describing infection of fibroblasts with an interferon (IFN) expression gene,[65] and more recent ones that report diminished cell growth after introduction of the IFN-α gene[66,67] into hematopoietic cells. In the studies of Salesse and colleagues,[66] for example, K562 cells and $CD34^+$ CML cells were transduced with the retroviral vector LIα2SN, containing an IFN-α2 gene expression cassette. Transduction efficiencies of 50% and 85% after three and six infections, respectively, were reported. The IFN-α secretion after three and six infections was 5400 and 18 000 U/24 h/10^6 cells for unselected K562 cells, and 7000 and 290 U/24 h/10^6 cells for CML $CD34^+$ cells at days 4 and 5. The major histocompatibility complex (MHC) class I antigens were also found to be overexpressed in both K562 and CML $CD34^+$ cells after infection with LIα2SN. Proliferation in liquid culture and cloning efficiency were reported to be significantly decreased after LIα2SN treatment. Seiter and co-workers[67] reported somewhat better results using the fibronectin fragment CH-296 as an aid to transduction. They found that infected cells produced approximately 400 units of IFN-α protein compared with $CD34^+$ cells or cells transduced with empty vector. IFN-α gene-transduced $CD34^+$ cells generated similar numbers of CFU-GM colonies as compared with control $CD34^+$ cells. Engraftment of $CD34^+$ cells transduced with the IFN-α gene in NOD/SCID mice was successful for the first 30 days. Seiter et al also studied the effect of local IFN-α expression on the cellular adhesion molecules VLA-4, Mac-1, ICAM-1, and L-selectin in K562 cells and human umbilical endothelial vein cells. K562 cells transduced with the IFN-α gene expressed significantly elevated levels of VLA-4, Mac-1, and ICAM-1. Based on these results, it is also possible that other exogenously expressed targets, such as the Wilms' tumor transcription factor (WT1), might also prove immunogenic, and therefore therapeutic, if expressed in chronic-phase CML cells.[68] Strategies for improving retroviral transduction currently being developed will undoubtedly assist in this effort.[69,70]

CONCLUSIONS

Many challenges remain to be addressed before viral- or nucleic-acid-based gene therapies become a reality. Significant problems in both approaches arise from the limited ability to deliver the therapeutic agent to hematopoietic stem cells. Even when appropriately delivered, viral-based therapies will still need to solve the problem of expression of the gene delivered at satisfactory levels, and for extended periods of time. In the case of antisense drugs, efficient delivery will not solve all the problems inherent to this approach either. In order for an oligonucleotide to hybridize with its mRNA target, it must find an accessible sequence. Sequence accessibility is at least in part a function of mRNA physical structure, which is dictated in turn by internal base composition and associated proteins in the living cell. Attempts to describe the in vivo structure of RNA, in contrast to DNA, have been fraught with difficulty. Accordingly, mRNA targeting is largely a random process, accounting for many experiments where the addition of an oligonucleotide yields no effect on expression. Strategies to address this fundamental problem are presently under development.[71,72]

Those of us who care for patients with cancer are constantly reminded of the importance of work focused on the mission of making anticancer therapy less morbid, and less deadly to those unfortunate individuals who must endure it. Investigators are following many paths towards this goal, including strategies designed to interrupt the most fundamental of processes within a cell – gene expression. When this goal is finally accomplished, it will truly represent the culmination of many small steps toward a major leap in the practice of medicine in the 21st century.

ACKNOWLEDGEMENTS

This work was supported in part by grants from the US NIH and the Doris Duke Charitable Foundation.

REFERENCES

1. Varmus HE, Nobel lecture. Retroviruses and oncogenes. I. *Biosci Rep* 1990; **10:** 413–30.
2. Fearon ER, Dang CV, Cancer genetics: tumor suppressor meets oncogene. *Curr Biol* 1999; **9:** R62–5.
3. Hahn WC, Counter CM, Lundberg AS et al, Creation of human tumour cells with defined genetic elements. *Nature* 1999; **400:** 464–8.
4. Druker BJ, Lydon NB, Lessons learned from the development of an abl tyrosine kinase inhibitor for chronic myelogenous leukemia. *J Clin Invest* 2000; **105:** 3–7.
5. Heslop HE, Gene therapy of pediatric leukemia. *Clin Lab Med* 2000; **20:** 183–95.
6. Engel BC, Kohn DB, Stem cell directed gene therapy. *Front Biosci* 1999; **4:** 26–33.
7. Gewirtz AM, Sokol DL, Ratajczak MZ, Nucleic acid therapeutics: state of the art and future prospects. *Blood* 1998; **92:** 712–36.
8. Paterson BM, Roberts BE, Kuff EL, Structural gene identification and mapping by DNA–mRNA hybrid-arrested cell-free translation. *Proc Natl Acad Sci USA* 1977; **74:** 4370–4.
9. Stephenson ML, Zamecnik PC, Inhibition of Rous sarcoma viral RNA translation by a specific oligodeoxyribonucleotide. *Proc Natl Acad Sci USA* 1978; **75:** 285–8.
10. Simons RW, Kleckner N, Translational control of IS10 transposition. *Cell* 1983; **34:** 683–91.
11. Mizuno T, Chou MY, Inouye M, A unique mechanism regulating gene expression: translational inhibition by a complementary RNA transcript (micRNA). *Proc Natl Acad Sci USA* 1984; **81:** 1966–70.
12. Izant JG, Weintraub H, Inhibition of thymidine kinase gene expression by anti-sense RNA: a molecular approach to genetic analysis. *Cell* 1984; **36:** 1007–15.
13. Melton DW, Gene targeting in the mouse. *Bioessays* 1994; **16:** 633–8.
14. Helene C, Control of oncogene expression by antisense nucleic acids. *Eur J Cancer* 1994; **30A:** 1721–6.
15. Majumdar A, Khorlin A, Dyatkina N et al, Targeted gene knockout mediated by triple helix forming oligonucleotides. *Nature Genet* 1998; **20:** 212–14.
16. Kielkopf CL, Baird EE, Dervan PB, Rees DC, Structural basis for G.C recognition in the DNA minor groove. *Nature Struct Biol* 1998; **5:** 104–9.
17. Beelman CA, Parker R, Degradation of mRNA in eukaryotes. *Cell* 1995; **81:** 179–83.
18. Liebhaber SA, mRNA stability and the control of gene expression. *Nucleic Acids Symp Ser* 1997; **36:** 29–32.
19. Eckstein F, The hammerhead ribozyme. *Biochem Soc Trans* 1996; **24:** 601–4.
20. Joyce GF, Nucleic acid enzymes: playing with a fuller deck. *Proc Natl Acad Sci USA* 1998; **95:** 5845–7.
21. Szczylik C, Skorski T, Nicolaides NC et al, Selective inhibition of leukemia cell proliferation by BCR–ABL antisense oligodeoxynucleotides. *Science* 1991; **253:** 562–5.
22. Skorski T, Szczylik C, Malaguarnera L, Calabretta B, Gene-targeted specific inhibition of chronic myeloid leukemia cell growth by BCR–ABL antisense oligodeoxynucleotides. *Folia Histochem Cytobiol* 1991; **29:** 85–9.
23. Wu AG, Joshi SS, Chan WC et al, Effects of BCR–ABL antisense oligonucleotides (AS-ODN) on human chronic myeloid leukemic cells: AS-ODN as effective purging agents. *Leuk Lymphoma* 1995; **20:** 67–76.
24. de Fabritiis P, Amadori S, Calabretta B, Mandelli F, Elimination of clonogenic Philadelphia-positive cells using BCR–ABL antisense oligodeoxynucleotides. *Bone Marrow Transplant* 1993; **12:** 261–5.
25. de Fabritiis P, Skorski T, De Propris MS et al, Effect of bcr–abl oligodeoxynucleotides on the clonogenic growth of chronic myelogenous leukaemia cells. *Leukemia* 1997; **11:** 811–19.
26. de Fabritis P, Amadori S, Petti MC et al, In vitro purging with BCR–ABL antisense oligodeoxynucleotides does not prevent haematologic reconstitution after autologous bone marrow transplantation. *Leukemia* 1995; **9:** 662–4.
27. de Fabritiis P, Calabretta B, Antisense oligodeoxynucleotides for the treatment of chronic myelogenous leukemia: Are they still a promise? *Haematologica* 1995; **80:** 295–9.
28. Chasty R, Whetton A, Lucas G, A comparison of the effect of bcr/abl breakpoint specific phosphothiorate oligodeoxynucleotides on colony

formation by bcr/abl positive and negative, CD34 enriched mononuclear cell populations. *Leuk Res* 1996; **20:** 391–5.
29. Skorski T, Nieborowska-Skorska M, Barletta C et al, Highly efficient elimination of Philadelphia leukemic cells by exposure to bcr/abl antisense oligodeoxynucleotides combined with mafosfamide. *J Clin Invest* 1993; **92:** 194–202.
30. Skorski T, Nieborowska-Skorska M, Wlodarski P et al, Treatment of Philadelphia leukemia in severe combined immunodeficient mice by combination of cyclophosphamide and bcr/abl antisense oligodeoxynucleotides. *J Natl Cancer Inst* 1997; **89:** 124–33.
31. Kirkland MA, O'Brien SG, McDonald C et al, BCR–ABL antisense purging in chronic myeloid leukaemia. *Lancet* 1993; **342:** 614.
32. Maekawa T, Kimura S, Hirakawa K et al, Sequence specificity on the growth suppression and induction of apoptosis of chronic myeloid leukemia cells by BCR–ABL anti-sense oligodeoxynucleoside phosphorothioates. *Int J Cancer* 1995; **62:** 63–9.
33. Mahon FX, Belloc F, Vianes I et al, Specific antisense oligomer anti Bcr–abl junctions in chronic myeloid leukemia: a cell cycle analysis and CFU-GM study. *Leuk Lymphoma* 1995; **19:** 423–9.
34. Mahon FX, Ripoche J, Pigeonnier V et al, Inhibition of chronic myelogenous leukemia cells harboring a BCR–ABL B3A2 junction by antisense oligonucleotides targeted at the B2A2 junction. *Exp Hematol* 1995; **23:** 1606–11.
35. O'Brien SG, Kirkland MA, Melo JV et al, Antisense BCR–ABL oligomers cause non-specific inhibition of chronic myeloid leukemia cell lines. *Leukemia* 1994; **8:** 2156–62.
36. Smetsers TF, van de Locht LT, Pennings AH et al, Phosphorothioate BCR–ABL antisense oligonucleotides induce cell death, but fail to reduce cellular bcr–abl protein levels. *Leukemia* 1995; **9:** 118–30.
37. Vaerman JL, Lammineur C, Moureau P et al, BCR–ABL antisense oligodeoxyribonucleotides suppress the growth of leukemic and normal hematopoietic cells by a sequence-specific but nonantisense mechanism. *Blood* 1995; **86:** 3891–6.
38. Pigneux A, Mahon FX, Jazwiec B et al, Effect of antisense oligonucleotides on CD34$^+$ cells from chronic myeloid leukemia. *Leuk Lymphoma* 2000; **36:** 569–78.
39. Leopold LH, Shore SK, Reddy EP, Multi-unit anti-BCR–ABL ribozyme therapy in chronic myelogenous leukemia. *Leuk Lymphoma* 1996; **22:** 365–73.
40. Lange W, Daskalakis M, Finke J, Dolken G, Comparison of different ribozymes for efficient and specific cleavage of BCR/ABL related mRNAs. *FEBS Lett* 1994; **338:** 175–8.
41. Pachuk CJ, Yoon K, Moelling K, Coney LR, Selective cleavage of bcr–abl chimeric RNAs by a ribozyme targeted to non-contiguous sequences. *Nucleic Acids Res* 1994; **22:** 301–7.
42. James HA, Gibson I, The therapeutic potential of ribozymes. *Blood* 1998; **91:** 371–82.
43. Kronenwett R, Haas R, Sczakiel G, Kinetic selectivity of complementary nucleic acids: bcr–abl-directed antisense RNA and ribozymes. *J Mol Biol* 1996; **259:** 632–44.
44. Zhao RC, McIvor RS, Griffin JD, Verfaillie CM, Gene therapy for chronic myelogenous leukemia (CML): a retroviral vector that renders hematopoietic progenitors methotrexate-resistant and CML progenitors functionally normal and nontumorigenic in vivo. *Blood* 1997; **90:** 4687–98.
45. Nomura N, Takahashi M, Matsui M et al, Isolation of human cDNA clones of myb-related genes, A-myb and B-myb. *Nucleic Acids Res* 1988; **16:** 11075–89 [Erratum 1989; **17:** 1282].
46. Biedenkapp H, Borgmeyer U, Sippel AE, Klempnauer KH, Viral myb oncogene encodes a sequence-specific DNA-binding activity. *Nature* 1988; **335:** 835–7.
47. Mucenski ML, McLain K, Kier AB et al, A functional c-myb gene is required for normal murine fetal hepatic hematopoiesis. *Cell* 1991; **65:** 677–89.
48. Gewirtz AM, Calabretta B, A c-myb antisense oligodeoxynucleotide inhibits normal human hematopoiesis in vitro. *Science* 1988; **242:** 1303–6.
49. Weston K, Myb proteins in life, death and differentiation. *Curr Opin Genet Dev* 1998; **8:** 76–81.
50. Ratajczak MZ, Perrotti D, Melotti P et al, Myb and Ets proteins are candidate regulators of c-kit expression in human hematopoietic cells. *Blood* 1998; **91:** 1934–46.
51. Kowenz-Leutz E, Herr P, Niss K, Leutz A, The homeobox gene GBX2, a target of the myb oncogene, mediates autocrine growth and monocyte differentiation. *Cell* 1997; **91:** 185–95.
52. Sawyers CL, Callahan W, Witte ON, Dominant negative MYC blocks transformation by ABL oncogenes. *Cell* 1992; **70:** 901–10.
53. Afar DE, Goga A, McLaughlin J et al, Differential complementation of Bcr–Abl point mutants with c-Myc. *Science* 1994; **264:** 424–6.

54. Skorski T, Perrotti D, Nieborowska-Skorska M et al, Antileukemia effect of c-myc N3'→P5' phosphoramidate antisense oligonucleotides in vivo. *Proc Natl Acad Sci USA* 1997; **94:** 3966–71.
55. Skorski T, Nieborowska-Skorska M, Wlodarski P et al, Antisense oligodeoxynucleotide combination therapy of primary chronic myelogenous leukemia blast crisis in SCID mice. *Blood* 1996; **88:** 1005–12.
56. Ratajczak MZ, Luger SM, DeRiel K et al, Role of the KIT protooncogene in normal and malignant human hematopoiesis. *Proc Natl Acad Sci USA* 1992; **89:** 1710–14.
57. Bonnefoy-Berard N, Munshi A, Yron I et al, Vav: function and regulation in hematopoietic cell signaling. *Stem Cells* 1996; **14:** 250–68.
58. Katzav S, vav: a molecule for all haemopoiesis? *Br J Haematol* 1992; **81:** 141–4.
59. Wulf GM, Adra CN, Lim B, Inhibition of hematopoietic development from embryonic stem cells by antisense vav RNA. *EMBO J* 1993; **12:** 5065–74.
60. Zhang R, Tsai FY, Orkin SH, Hematopoietic development of vav−/− mouse embryonic stem cells. *Proc Natl Acad Sci USA* 1994; **91:** 12755–9.
61. Zhang R, Alt FW, Davidson L et al, Defective signalling through the T- and B-cell antigen receptors in lymphoid cells lacking the vav proto-oncogene. *Nature* 1995; **374**: 470–3.
62. Zmuidzinas A, Fischer KD, Lira SA et al, The vav proto-oncogene is required early in embryogenesis but not for hematopoietic development in vitro. *EMBO J* 1995; **14:** 1–11.
63. Luger SM, Ratajczak J, Ratajczak MZ et al, A functional analysis of protooncogene Vav's role in adult human hematopoiesis. *Blood* 1996; **87:** 1326–34.
64. de Fabritiis P, Petti MC, Montefusco E et al, BCR–ABL antisense oligodeoxynucleotide in vitro purging and autologous bone marrow transplantation for patients with chronic myelogenous leukemia in advanced phase. *Blood* 1998; **91:** 3156–62.
65. Ogura H, Tani K, Ozawa K et al, Implantation of genetically manipulated fibroblasts into mice as antitumor alpha-interferon therapy. *Cancer Res* 1990; **50:** 5102–6.
66. Salesse S, Moreau-Gaudry F, Pigeonnier-Lagarde V et al, Retroviral vector-mediated transfer of the interferon-alpha gene in chronic myeloid leukemia cells. *Cancer Gene Ther* 1998; **5:** 390–400.
67. Seiter K, Kancherla R, Yang L et al, Adenovirus and retrovirus mediated interferon alpha gene transfer into $CD34^+$ cells maintains regeneration capacity and enhances adhesion molecules in K562 cells. *J Invest Med* 1999; **47:** 414–24.
68. Gao L, Bellantuono I, Elsasser A et al, Selective elimination of leukemic CD34(+) progenitor cells by cytotoxic T lymphocytes specific for WT1. *Blood* 2000; **95:** 2198–203.
69. Garrett E, Garin MI, Miller AR et al, Enhanced retroviral gene transfer into CML and normal bone marrow, and CML and mobilized peripheral blood $CD34^+$ cells using the recombinant fibronectin fragment CH-296. *Br J Haematol* 1999; **107:** 401–8.
70. Liu H, Hung Y, Wissink SD, Verfaillie CM, Improved retroviral transduction of hematopoietic progenitors by combining methods to enhance virus–cell interaction. *Leukemia* 2000; **14:** 307–11.
71. Sokol DL, Zhang X, Lu P, Gewirtz AM, Real time detection of DNA.RNA hybridization in living cells. *Proc Natl Acad Sci USA* 1998; **95:** 11538–43.
72. Ho SP, Bao Y, Lesher T et al, Mapping of RNA accessible sites for antisense experiments with oligonucleotide libraries. *Nature Biotechnol* 1998; **16:** 59–63.

32

Target-directed therapies

Mikhail L Gishizky

CONTENTS • Introduction • Targeting BCR/ABL • Targeting BCR/ABL signal transduction pathways • Issues and summary

INTRODUCTION

In the past quarter century, tremendous strides have been made in our understanding of the molecular mechanisms involved in human disease. These advances have led to a dramatic change in the drug discovery paradigm within the pharmaceutical industry, which has evolved from a random screening approach to a target-driven drug discovery process. The progress made within the field of chronic myeloid leukemia (CML) is emblematic of this new paradigm, and serves as an example of how basic research is setting the stage to bring therapeutics to the bedside. As described in other chapters in this volume, many molecular entities have been identified as potential targets for therapeutic intervention. I will limit my discussion to the molecular targets and signaling pathways shown in Figure 32.1, highlighting strategies and technological advances that show promise for developing pharmaceuticals targeting BCR/ABL function and that can be applied to other molecular entities not specifically mentioned.

The identification of the Philadelphia chromosome (Ph) by Nowell and Hungerford[1] in 1960 and its characterization as a molecular hallmark of CML by Rowley[2] in 1973 ushered in the era of molecular medicine by bringing into the realm of clinical practice the use of a genetic marker for diagnosis of human disease. The cloning of the *BCR/ABL* gene as the product of Ph and the demonstration that the t(9;22)(q34;q11) translocation produced a chimeric protein containing sequences from the BCR serine–threonine kinase (chromosome 22) fused to the ABL tyrosine kinase (chromosome 9) unleashed a tremendous effort focused on understanding whether BCR/ABL played a causative role in the disease. These efforts culminated in the demonstration by several groups that expression of BCR/ABL in the bone marrow of mice induced a syndrome that recapitulates aspects of CML and Ph-positive acute lymphoblastic leukemia (ALL) (reviewed in Chapter 6). This confirmed the role of BCR/ABL as an etiologic agent in our current understanding of CML pathogenesis.

TARGETING BCR/ABL

In many ways, BCR/ABL represents an ideal target for developing therapeutics. It is expressed at high levels in leukemic cells and is absent in non-hematopoietic and normal hematopoietic cell types. The structure of the BCR/ABL protein is complex, comprising elements with enzymatic activity and distinct protein-binding domains (reviewed in Chapter 2). Three different forms of BCR/ABL have been identified – p185, p210, and p230 – which contain the same sequence derived from the c-ABL tyrosine kinase but vary in the amount of BCR sequence in the chimeric protein. p185, p210, and p230 BCR/ABL are each associated with a distinct clinical disorder – Ph-positive ALL, CML, and chronic neutrophilic leukemia, respectively – which differ in their clinical presentation and treatment.[3] In this chapter, I will focus on recent development of potential therapeutics for the treatment of CML that may or may not be transferable to other Ph-positive disorders.

The observations that proved critical in defining BCR/ABL as a target for drug discovery were the following:

- BCR/ABL exhibits elevated tyrosine kinase activity relative to endogenous c-ABL protein;
- overexpression of BCR/ABL can induce transformation of hematopoietic cells;
- tyrosine kinase activity is essential for BCR/ABL's oncogenic function;
- mice inoculated with hematopoietic cells expressing BCR/ABL protein developed leukemia.

Thus, inhibiting BCR/ABL tyrosine kinase activity or decreasing the level of BCR/ABL protein expression should have therapeutic utility.

Inhibiting BCR/ABL tyrosine kinase activity

More than a decade ago, it was demonstrated that inhibitors of tyrosine kinase activity, such as hebimycin A and erbstatin, could attenuate the growth of Ph-positive cells in vitro.[4,5] Although these compounds were non-specific and had other activities besides acting as tyrosine kinase inhibitors, the observations supported the hypothesis that inhibiting the enzymatic activity of BCR/ABL could have potential clinical benefit.

In developing tyrosine kinase inhibitors, or indeed any therapeutic agent, a number of issues must be considered:

- potency and selectivity for the target;
- the consequences of inhibiting the target (or normal counterpart) in non-diseased tissue;
- specific and non-specific toxicity;
- the physical properties of the agent (i.e. solubility, cell permeability, stability, tissue distribution, metabolism, and excretion).

The relative importance of each of these criteria varies according to the target, the type of agent, and the disease indication. Historically, cancer therapy was based on the use of non-specific inhibitors of cell proliferation that afforded relatively narrow therapeutic windows for affecting the growth of cancer cells versus normal tissue. Within the context of the new drug discovery paradigm, developing drugs with high potency and selectivity for the target would seem to be critical in terms of limiting non-specific toxic effects. In the case of CML, a highly specific inhibitor of the ABL tyrosine kinase would seem the most appropriate first-line single agent during the chronic phase of the disease. However, during progression toward blast crisis, other molecular events cooperate with or supplant the oncogenic effect of BCR/ABL. The use of agents with different modes of action, possibly in combination, or the development of agents exhibiting activity on several targets, could provide greater clinical efficacy.

Conceptually, synthetic tyrosine kinase inhibitors can be divided into two general categories: (i) inhibitors of substrate phosphorylation and (ii) ATP mimetics. The rationale for developing substrate inhibitors is the knowledge that tyrosine kinases phosphorylate different substrates. So, theoretically, compounds of this type could be very selective and inhibit phosphorylation of distinct intracellular molecules. In this manner, the inhibitor could modulate the activity of a specific signal transduction pathway while not affecting other cellular processes regulated by the kinase. The observation that substrate binds at a site distinct from the ATP-binding site within the kinase domain supported the notion that selectivity could be achieved by this approach.[6] The 'tyrphostins' represent one family of substrate phosphorylation inhibitors that exhibit selectivity among diverse tyrosine kinases (reviewed by Levitzki[7]). The tyrphostins AG957 and AG1112 can preferentially inhibit BCR/ABL kinase activity in biochemical assays with K_i values <1.0 μM.[8,9] Consistent with the mechanism of action of this family of compounds, inhibition is competitive with substrate and non-competitive with ATP. Interestingly, AG957 exhibits almost a 10-fold difference in K_i values for inhibiting p210 BCR/ABL versus c-ABL, suggesting that the fusion with BCR induces a conformational change within the kinase domain that may be exploited for further therapeutic development.[10] Treatment of the Ph-positive cell line K562 with AG1112 is not overtly toxic, but rather induces differentiation.[9] It has recently been reported that treatment of CML progenitor cells with AG957 can restore β_1-integrin-mediated adhesion and, in conjunction with anti-Fas antibody, can eliminate Ph-positive cells from CML bone marrow samples in vitro.[11,12] At present, compounds of this class have not progressed into clinical trials for CML.

Efforts to develop ATP mimetics as selective kinase inhibitors went counter to the general wisdom of the 1980s and early 1990s, which surmised that ATP mimetics would not make good drugs because: (i) the structure of the ATP-binding site in kinases is very similar, and selectivity would be difficult to achieve; (ii) many enzymes within a cell utilize ATP, and thus the drugs would have many unwanted effects; and (iii) the potency of the inhibitor would have to be very high to overcome the high concentration of ATP within the cell. The initial discovery that dianilinophthalimides and 4-phenylaminoquinazolines could act as potent and selective inhibitors of tyrosine kinase activity dispelled some of these concerns.[13,14] Subsequently numerous chemical entities that function as ATP mimetics have been reported to act as potent and selective inhibitors of kinases (reviewed by McMahon et al,[15] Stover et al,[16] and Adams and Lee[17]). Recent co-crystallization of several of these synthetic inhibitors with various protein kinases has allowed the generation of new models that explain how a chemical entity may impart specificity. Importantly, information based on the crystal structures can be used in the development of clinical drug candidates to preserve the spatial and structural entities critical for potency and selectivity of kinase inhibition while optimizing the pharmacologic and safety properties of the compound. The success of this approach is evident from the number of compounds within this class that have entered clinical trials. One such compound, STI571 (Glivec; Gleevec), is being developed for the treatment of CML.[18] STI571 preferentially inhibits a number of tyrosine kinases, including BCR/ABL, platelet-derived growth factor receptor (PDGFR) and c-Kit. STI571 has favorable physical properties, being orally bioavailable with a relative lack of toxicity. The very encouraging clinical results using STI571 are further described in Chapter 34, while there is further discussion of tyrosine kinase inhibitors in Chapter 33.

Decreasing the level of BCR/ABL expression

An alternative strategy to attenuate the effect of BCR/ABL would be to decrease the level of the activated tyrosine kinase protein being expressed. Suppression of BCR/ABL expression should reverse the phenotype, and would theoretically be curative if the expression remained suppressed or if the clone harboring the oncogene were eliminated from the population. Methods for selectively inhibiting transcription of a specific gene in mammalian cells currently do not exist. Technologies such as antisense oligonucleotides (ASOs) and ribozymes have shown mixed results in decreasing *BCR/ABL* RNA levels in vitro.

ASOs work by forming RNA–DNA hybrids, thus inhibiting translation and inducing RNase H-mediated degradation of the RNA. Although ASOs have been widely used to 'knock out' gene function in vitro, their physical properties (such as solubility), degradation, and in vivo delivery issues, along with their sequence-specific and non-antisense properties present significant challenges to their use in the clinic. Attempts to use *BCR/ABL*-directed ASOs for CML have at times produced effective yet variable results. *BCR/ABL*-specific ASOs have been shown to be effective at inhibiting colony formation and inducing apoptosis of CML cells in vitro.[19,20] Intriguingly, *BCR/ABL* ASO-induced apoptosis was not associated with an apparent decrease in the level of BCR/ABL protein.[20] This apparent incongruity underscores the difficulties one may encounter in developing ASOs as therapeutic agents. However, clinical trials using ASOs directed at *c-raf-1* have shown reductions in *c-raf-1* mRNA in patients in whom clinical benefits were observed.[21]

Ribozymes are catalytic RNA molecules with an intrinsic capacity to cleave RNA. There are several different classes of ribozymes that can be engineered to recognize specific sequences to target the RNA for degradation (reviewed by James and Gibson[22]). The chimeric structure of *BCR/ABL* RNA transcripts makes an attractive target for this approach in CML. Early studies using 'hammerhead' ribozymes demonstrated that they effectively cleaved *BCR/ABL* RNA in vitro and in cells. However, issues such as selectivity of the ribozyme and delivery of the agent to the target tissue needed to be resolved. Recent technological advances have produced ribozymes with greater selectivity and cleavage activity in cells. The modified ribozymes have been used to decrease levels of *BCR/ABL* transcript in cells, with a concomitant decrease in their ability to proliferate in the absence of growth factors.[23,24] Although these new ribozyme molecules show promise, efficient delivery of the agent to affected tissue remains an obstacle.

TARGETING BCR/ABL SIGNAL TRANSDUCTION PATHWAYS

Overexpression of BCR/ABL in hematopoietic cells can induce a range of biologic phenotypes, including cytokine-independent proliferation, protection from programmed cell death (apoptosis), and changes in cellular adhesion properties. Investigations into the molecular mechanisms responsible for these phenotypes have not succeeded in defining a specific signaling pathway or molecular target that is unique to BCR/ABL-induced transformation (reviewed in Chapter 2). Rather, the general theme emerging from such studies is that BCR/ABL activates the same signaling pathways that are utilized by cytokine and growth factor receptors that regulate differentiation and proliferation (reviewed in Chapter 4). As a consequence of its deregulated tyrosine kinase activity, BCR/ABL appears to constitutively activate these pathways, subverting the constraints imposed on normal hematopoietic cells, and resulting in a leukemic phenotype.

Ras signaling

Induction of growth-factor-independent growth and inhibition of apoptosis by BCR/ABL have been intimately linked to its ability to activate the Ras–GTPase. Expression of dominant-negative forms of Ras can block BCR/ABL-induced transformation and inhibit its anti-apoptotic function.[25,26] The molecular pathway linking BCR/ABL to Ras activation has been extensively studied. The basic framework of this process is consistent with the mechanism originally described for activation of Ras by epidermal growth factor receptor (EGFR) (reviewed by Margolis and Skolnik[27]). The basic principle involves the formation of a juxtamembrane complex comprising the SH2/SH3 domain of the adaptor protein Grb2 together with the guanine nucleotide exchange factor Sos, which associates with Ras and induces activation by enhancing GTP binding. Although the core has been defined, there appear to be at least three different mechanisms by which BCR/ABL can accomplish this (Figure 32.1).

By virtue of its chimeric structure, BCR/ABL can interact directly with the adaptor protein Grb2. The intrinsic catalytic activity of BCR/ABL phosphorylates tyrosine residue 177

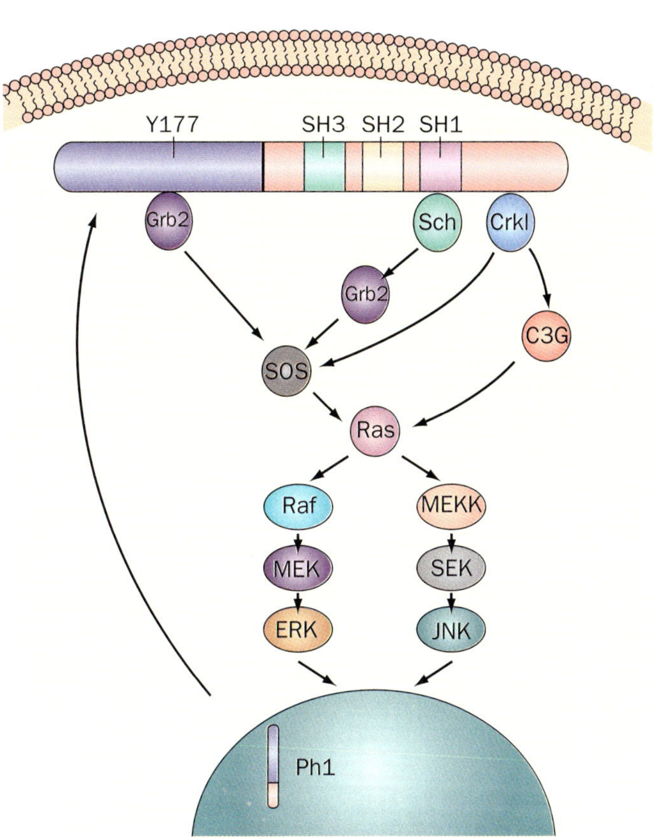

Figure 32.1 Molecular scaffold linking BCR/ABL to MAPK signal transduction cascades.

within the BCR portion of the chimera. Phosphorylated Y177 serves as a docking site for the SH2 domain of Grb2, which in turn provides a direct connection to Sos and Ras activation.[28] BCR/ABL also associates with the adaptor protein Shc.[29,30] Phosphorylation of Shc by BCR/ABL induces association with the SH2 domain of Grb2, leading to recruitment of Sos and Ras activation. Still a third potential pathway for Ras activation involves the SH2/SH3 domain of the adaptor protein Crkl – a prominent substrate of BCR/ABL in CML cells.[31] Association between Crkl and BCR/ABL is mediated through the binding of the SH3 domain of Crkl to a proline sequence within the ABL portion of the chimera.[32] The finding that Crkl also associates with the guanine nucleotide exchange proteins C3G and Sos provides other potential routes to Ras activation (reviewed by Sattler and Salgia[33]).

Although it is not clear which of the above-mentioned pathways plays the pre-eminent role in mediating Ras activation, studies indicate that inhibiting the function of the Grb2 protein may have therapeutic utility. Expression of dominant-negative Grb2 constructs in BCR/ABL-transformed and Ph-positive cell lines can reverse the transformed phenotype and induce differentiation.[34] Consistent with this observation, treatment of BCR/ABL-expressing 32D cells with a compound having the ability to disrupt the interaction between the SH2 domain of Grb2 and BCR/ABL (SU5220) can abrogate BCR/ABL-induced growth-factor-independent proliferation (G McMahon and ML Gishizky, unpublished work). Treatment with SU5220 induces a reversion of the transformed phenotype, so that cells once again require the cytokine interleukin-3 (IL-3) to sustain growth. These studies suggest that targeting Grb2 or other signal transduction molecules with compounds that inhibit protein–protein interaction may provide a viable therapeutic strategy in the future.

Many pharmaceutical companies are attempting to develop drugs that directly inhibit Ras function. There are three *ras* genes, which encode four Ras proteins. A common element critical to their function is the requirement for a post-translational lipid modification that results in their localization to the plasma membrane. These lipid modifications are catalyzed by three prenyl transferases: farnesyl transferase, geranylgeranyl transferase I and geranylgeranyl transferase II (reviewed by Zhang and Casey[35]). In the case of farnesyl transferase (FTase) the 15-carbon farnesyl moiety is transferred from farnesyl pyrophosphoate to a cysteine at the carboxyl terminus of proteins that end with CAAX sequences, where C is cysteine, A is an aliphatic amino acid, and X is any amino acid except leucine or isoleucine. Several structurally diverse inhibitors of FTase have been developed and evaluated in biologic systems (reviewed by Sebti and Hamilton[36]). These compounds effectively antagonize oncogenic Ras signaling and inhibit the growth of a broad range of human tumor cell lines in xenograft mouse models with relatively low toxicity (reviewed by Gibbs and Oliff[37] and Rowinsky et al[38]). FTase inhibitors also attenuate the growth of BCR/ABL-transformed murine hematopoietic cells and human Ph-positive cell lines in soft agar and in mice (GQ Daley, personal communication). Although FTase inhibitors are efficacious, recent studies indicate that targets other than Ras may be responsible for their antitumor activity (reviewed by Sebti and Hamilton[36]). The basis for the efficacy of these compounds is further complicated by the demonstration that treatment with FTase inhibitors can induce alternative forms of Ras prenylation via geranylgeranyl transferases.[39] Although mechanistically these compounds remain a mystery, their efficacy and relatively low toxicity in preclinical models make them viable clinical candidates with potential therapeutic utility in CML.

MAPK signaling pathways

One function of Ras is to regulate the evolutionarily conserved MAP kinase (MAPK) signaling pathways that transmit and amplify signals downstream, resulting in activation of transcription factors and other effector proteins (reviewed by Cobb[40] and Garrington and Johnson[41]). At least three different MAPK pathways exist in mammalian cells (Erk, Jnk/SAPK, and p38 kinase pathways), two of which, JnK/SAPK and Erk, have been implicated in CML (described in Chapter 2 and reviewed by Warmuth et al[42] and Raitano et al[43]). The MAPK pathways are cascades of different yet partially linked serine–threonine kinases (STKs) and dual-specificity kinases (those that phosphorylate both serine–threonine and tyrosine residues). Because many STKs function in the middle of signaling cascades, determining their exact role in disease progression is difficult. This is where the use of compounds developed by the pharmaceutical industry to act as selective inhibitors can potentially provide valuable information on the target and the signaling pathway. In the past five years, significant progress has been made in synthesizing potent and selective STK inhibitors (reviewed by Adams and Lee[17]). Mechanistically, these compounds function as inhibitors of substrate phosphorylation, as non-competitive allosteric regulators, or as ATP competitive inhibitors. As with tyrosine kinases, ATP mimetics have provided the greatest success in developing potent and selective inhibitors of STK activity, several of which have entered clinical trials. With the general acceptance of kinases as important drug discovery targets, one can expect many compounds to be identified that act as selective kinase inhibitors but for a variety of reasons do not progress through clinical development. Use of these compounds, such as the potent MEK kinase inhibitor PD98059, as research tools can provide valuable information; however, caution must be used in interpreting the results thus obtained. Continued effort in this area will undoubtedly lead to the development of STK inhibitors that may find utility in the treatment of CML.

PI3-K signaling pathway

The phosphatidylinositol 3'-kinase (PI3-K) signaling pathway has also been implicated as a mediator of BCR/ABL-induced transformation.[44] A unique feature of this pathway is that it centers on the activation of a lipid kinase. PI3-K is a heterodimeric protein composed of a regulatory subunit p85 and an enzymatic subunit p110 that functions as a phospholipid kinase. The p85 subunit is composed of an amino-terminal SH3 domain, several proline-rich binding motifs, a region with homology to BCR, and two SH2 domains at the carboxyl terminus. In addition to being responsible for the enzymatic activity that phosphorylates phosphatidylinositol-4-phosphate and phosphatidylinositol-4,5-bisphosphate, the p110 subunit contains binding sites for the p85 subunit and Ras. Activation of PI3-K triggers a signal that activates the downstream serine–threonine kinase Akt, which has been implicated as a critical element in mediating BCR/ABL-induced cell survival. Although the basic features of this pathway have been identified, critical molecular elements within the cascade still need elucidation. As with Ras, several mechanism by which BCR/ABL activates PI3-K have been proposed, involving multiple adaptor proteins and even a protein tyrosine phosphatase as a mediator (reviewed by Warmuth et al[42]). In addition, the molecular entities responsible for linking PI3-K to Akt and downstream effectors are not clear. From a therapeutic perspective, this signaling pathway presents the added challenge of developing drugs to affect lipid kinases. Compounds that inhibit PI3-K activity, such as wortmmanin and LY294002, already exist, and have been shown to be effective at inhibiting the growth of human tumor cells, including Ph-positive cell lines in vitro.[45] It remains to be seen if the extensive effort currently being applied to the development of protein kinase inhibitors will also be applied to lipid kinases or whether the protein kinase effort will serendipitously identify chemical scaffolds that may prove useful for developing inhibitors of lipid kinases.

Numerous signal transduction pathways have been implicated in BCR/ABL-induced transformation, including Jak–STAT, Crkl–Cas, Myc, I-κB–NF-κB, and others that are described in this volume and elsewhere.[33,42,43,46] This diverse list underscores both the opportunities and challenges that we face in deciding on which targets and pathways to focus our efforts in developing therapeutic agents. Because these pathways comprise families of proteins that have common biophysical properties (i.e. kinases, prenyl transferases, adaptor proteins, etc.) a platform-based drug discovery process would seem to be the most efficient way of tackling this dilemma. As noted above, the platform-based approach has been successful in developing protein kinase inhibitors, and it is hoped that it will yield similar success when applied to other classes of protein families.

ISSUES AND SUMMARY

The general consensus within the field of oncology is that cancer is a progressive disease that results from a succession of molecular changes leading to a highly malignant state. The clinical presentation of CML serves as a testament to this view of oncogenesis. The importance of *BCR/CBL* in the presentation of chronic-phase CML has been well established; however, it is not clear whether *BCR/ABL* continues to play a significant role during blast crisis. Additional cytogenetic alterations often accompany disease progression. However, no single genetic event has been consistently observed, indicating that different molecular defects can contribute to progression and produce a common pathology. This raises the obvious questions as to whether

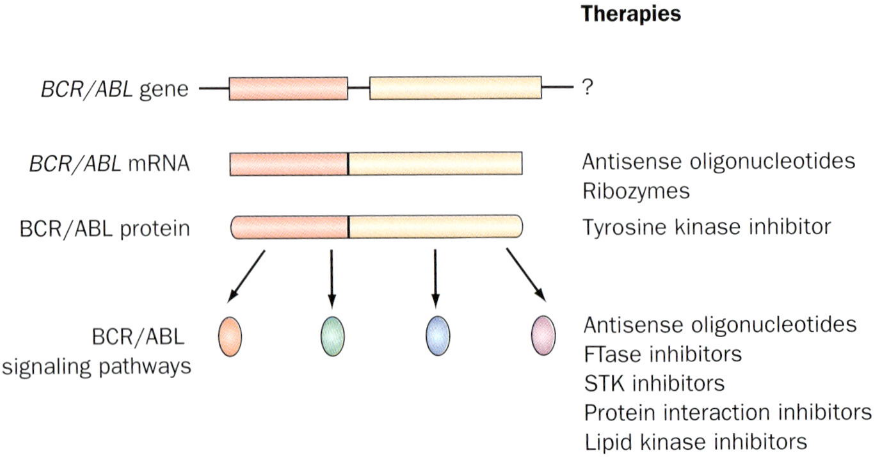

Figure 32.2 Potential future therapeutic modalities for the treatment of CML.

these secondary events supplant the requirement for BCR/ABL and whether a common molecular target can be found for intervention at this stage of the disease. The stratification of patients on the basis of secondary molecular alterations will be critical in defining the appropriate therapeutic regimen in the future. Another issue to be considered is that BCR/ABL may not be the primary etiologic agent in CML but rather a manifestation of another underlying defect. If that is the case then targeting BCR/ABL will provide only temporary clinical benefit, and a cure will only come from additional therapies or from extinguishing the diseased clone.

In a relatively short period of just over a decade, the field of CML research has progressed from cloning the product of a chromosomal translocation, *BCR/ABL*, to having a target-directed therapy demonstrating clinical benefit, namely STI571 (Glivec; Gleevec). Significant issues remain to be resolved, and it is not clear which therapy or combination of therapies will provide long-term benefit (Figure 32.2). In this regard, therapies being developed for other indications, such as those directed at inhibiting Ras or telomerase activity, or targeting Myc or p53 signaling pathways, will, in all likelihood, provide additional options for treatment of CML. Advances in the fields of biology, combinatorial chemistry, and computer science have revolutionized the drug discovery process and have established the structure–function-based paradigm in pharmaceutical development. In the future, implementation of genomic and proteomic microarray technologies will allow us to capitalize on the information resulting from sequencing of the human genome to bring forward innovative therapies for the long-term management of CML and other oncologic diseases.

ACKNOWLEDGEMENTS

I appreciate many helpful discussions with Jerry McMahon and all my colleagues at SUGEN. Thank you to Cynthia Harris for assistance in preparing the manuscript.

REFERENCES

1. Nowell PC, Hungerford DA, A minute chromosome in human chronic granulocytic leukemia. *Science* 1960; **132:** 1497.
2. Rowley JD, A new consistent chromosomal abnormality in chronic myelogenous leukemia identified by quinacrine fluorescence and Giemsa banding. *Nature* 1973; **243:** 290–1.
3. Melo JV, The diversity of BCR–ABL fusion proteins and their relationship to leukemia phenotype. *Blood* 1996; **88:** 2375–84.
4. Honma Y, Okabe-Kado J, Hozumi M et al, Induction of erythroid differentiation of K562 human leukemic cells by herbimycin A, an inhibitor of tyrosine kinase activity. *Cancer Res* 1989; **49:** 331–4.
5. Umezawa K, Imoto M, Use of erbstatin as protein-tyrosine kinase inhibitor. *Meth Enzymol* 1991; **201:** 379–85.
6. Posner I, Engel M, Levitzki A, Kinetic model of the epidermal growth factor (EGF) receptor tyrosine kinase and a possible mechanism of its activation by EGF. *J Biol Chem* 1992; **267:** 20638–47.
7. Levitzki A, Protein tyrosine kinase inhibitors as novel therapeutic agents. *Pharmacol Ther* 1999; **82:** 231–9.
8. Kaur G, Gazit A, Levitzki A et al, Tyrphostin induced growth inhibition; correlation with effect on p210bcr–abl autokinase activity in K562 chronic myelogenous leukemia. *Anticancer Drugs* 1994; **5:** 213–22.
9. Anafi M, Gazit A, Zehavi A et al, Tyrphostin-induced inhibition of p210bcr–abl tyrosine kinase activity induces K562 to differentiate. *Blood* 1993; **82:** 3524–9.
10. Anafi M, Gazit A, Gilon C et al, Selective interactions of transforming and normal abl proteins with ATP, tyrosine–copolymer substrates, and tyrphostins. *J Biol Chem* 1992; **267:** 4518–23.
11. Bhatia R, Munthe HA, Verfaillie CM, Tyrphostin AG957, a tyrosine kinase inhibitor with anti-BCR/ABL tyrosine kinase activity restores beta1 integrin-mediated adhesion and inhibitory signaling in chronic myelogenous leukemia hematopoietic progenitors. *Leukemia* 1998; **12:** 1708–17.
12. Carlo-Stella C, Regazzi E, Sammarelli G et al, Effects of the tyrosine kinase inhibitor AG957 and an anti-Fas receptor antibody on CD34(+) chronic myelogenous leukemia progenitor cells. *Blood* 1999; **93:** 3973–82.
13. Trinks U, Buchdunger E, Furet P et al, Dianilinophthalimides: potent and selective, ATP-competitive inhibitors of the EGF-receptor protein tyrosine kinase. *J Med Chem* 1994; **37:** 1015–27.
14. Fry DW, Kraker AJ, McMichael A et al, A specific inhibitor of the epidermal growth factor receptor tyrosine kinase. *Science* 1994; **265:** 1093–5.
15. McMahon G, Sun L, Liang C et al, Protein kinase inhibitors: structural determinants for target specificity. *Curr Opin Drug Disc Dev* 1998; **1:** 131–46.
16. Stover DR, Lydon NB, Nunes JJ, Recent advances in protein kinase inhibition: Current molecular scaffolds used for inhibitor synthesis. *Curr Opin Drug Disc Dev* 1999; **2:** 274–85.
17. Adams JL, Lee D, Recent progress towards the identification of selective inhibitors of serine/threonine protein kinases. *Curr Opin Drug Disc Dev* 1999; **2:** 96–109.
18. Druker, BJ, Tamura S, Buchdunger E et al, Effects of a selective inhibitor of the Abl tyrosine kinase on the growth of Bcr–Abl positive cells. *Nature Med* 1996; **2:** 561–6.
19. Szczylik C, Skorski T, Nicolaides NC et al, Selective inhibition of leukemia cell proliferation by BCR–ABL antisense oligodeoxynucleotides. *Science* 1991; **253:** 562–5.
20. Smetsers TF, van de Locht LT, Pennings AH et al, Phosphorothioate BCR–ABL antisense oligonucleotides induce cell death, but fail to reduce cellular bcr–abl protein levels. *Leukemia* 1995; **9:** 118–30.
21. O'Dwyer PJ, Stevenson JP, Gallagher M et al, c-raf-1 depletion and tumor responses in patients treated with the c-raf-1 antisense oligodeoxynucleotide ISIS 5132 (CGP 69846A). *Clin Cancer Res* 1999; **5:** 3977–82.
22. James HA, Gibson I, The therapeutic potential of ribozymes. *Blood* 1998; **91:** 371–82.
23. Kuwabara T, Warashina M, Tanabe T et al, A novel allosterically trans-activated ribozyme, the maxizyme, with exceptional specificity in vitro and in vivo. *Mol Cell* 1998; **2:** 617–27.
24. Cobaleda C, Sanchez-Garcia I, In vivo inhibition by a site-specific catalytic RNA subunit of RNase P designed against the BCR–ABL oncogenic products: a novel approach for cancer treatment. *Blood* 2000; **95:** 731–7.
25. Sawyers CL, McLaughlin J, Witte ON, Genetic requirement for Ras in the transformation of

fibroblasts and hematopoietic cells by the Bcr–Abl oncogene. *J Exp Med* 1995; **181:** 307–13.

26. Cortex D, Stoica G, Pierce JH et al, The BCR–ABL tyrosine kinase inhibits apoptosis by activating a RAS-dependent signaling pathway. *Oncogene* 1996; **13:** 2589–94.
27. Margolis B, Skolnik EY, Activation of Ras by receptor tyrosine kinases. *J Am Soc Nephrol* 1994; **5:** 1288–99.
28. Pendergast AM, Quilliam LA, Cripe LD et al, BCR–ABL-induced oncogenesis is mediated by direct interaction with the SH2 domain of the GRB-2 adaptor protein. *Cell* 1993, **8:** 175–85.
29. Tauchi T, Boswell HS, Leibowitz D et al, Coupling between p210 bcr–abl and She and Grb2 adaptor proteins in hematopoietic cells permits growth factor receptor-independent link to ras activation pathway. *J Exp Med* 1994; **179:** 167–75.
30. Puil L, Liu J, Gish G et al, Bcr–Abl oncoproteins bind directly to activators of the Ras signalling pathway. *EMBO J* 1994; **13:** 764–73.
31. ten Hoeve J, Kaartinen V, Fioretos T et al, Cellular interactions of CRKL, and SH2–SH3 adaptor protein. *Cancer Res* 1994; **54:** 2563–7.
32. Kolibaba KS, Bhat A, Heaney C et al, CRKL binding to BCR–ABL and BCR–ABL transformation. *Leuk Lymphoma* 1999; **33:** 119–26.
33. Sattler M, Salgia R, Role of the adapter protein CRKL in signal transduction of normal hematopoietic and BCR/ABL-transformed cells. *Leukemia* 1998; **12:** 637–44.
34. Gishizky ML, Cortez D, Pendergast AM, Mutant forms of growth factor-binding protein-2 reverse BCR–ABL-induced transformation. *Proc Natl Acad Sci USA* 1995; **92:** 10889–93.
35. Zhang FL, Casey PJ, Protein prenylation: molecular mechanisms and functional consequences. *Annu Rev Biochem* 1996; **65:** 241–69.
36. Sebti S, Hamilton AD, Inhibitors of prenyl transferases. *Curr Opin Oncol* 1997; **9:** 557–61.
37. Gibbs JB, Oliff A, The potential of farnesyltransferase inhibitors as cancer chemotherapeutics. *Annu Rev Pharmacol Toxicol* 1997; **37:** 143–66.
38. Rowinsky EK, Windle JJ, Von Hoff DD, Ras protein farnesyltransferase: a strategic target for anticancer therapeutic development. *J Clin Oncol* 1999; **17:** 3631–52.
39. Whyte DB, Kirschmeier P, Hockenberry TN et al, K- and N-Ras are geranylgeranylated in cells treated with farnesyl protein transferase inhibitors. *J Biol Chem* 1997; **272:** 14459–64.
40. Cobb MH, MAP kinase pathways. *Prog Biophys Mol Biol* 1999; **71:** 479–500.
41. Garrington TP, Johnson GL, Organization and regulation of mitogen-activated protein kinase signaling pathways. *Curr Opin Cell Biol* 1999; **11:** 211–18.
42. Warmuth M, Danhauser-Riedl S, Hallek M, Molecular pathogenesis of chronic myeloid leukemia: implications for new therapeutic strategies. *Ann Hematol* 1999; **78:** 49–64.
43. Raitano AB, Whang YE, Sawyers CL, Signal transduction by wild-type and leukemogenic Abl proteins. *Biochim Biophys Acta* 1997; **1333:** F201–16.
44. Skorski T, Bellacosa A, Nieborowska-Skorska M et al, Transformation of hematopoietic cells by BCR–ABL requires activation of a PI-3k/Akt-dependent pathway. *EMBO J* 1997; **16:** 6151–61.
45. Skorski T, Kanakaraj P, Nieborowska-Skorska M et al, Phosphatidylinositol-3 kinase activity is regulated by BCR/ABL and is required for the growth of Philadelphia chromosome-positive cells. *Blood* 1995; **86:** 726–36.
46. Denhardt DT, Oncogene-initiated aberrant signaling engenders the metastatic phenotype: synergistic transcription factor interactions are targets for cancer therapy. *Crit Rev Oncog* 1996; **7:** 261–91.

33

Development of kinase inhibitors

Enrica Lerma, Tao Wang, Takuma Fujii, Victor Chang, David Austin, Albert A Deisseroth

CONTENTS • Introduction and background • Differences between ABL and p210 BCR/ABL kinases • Strategies for developing ABL kinase inhibitors • Unanswered questions, and limitations of tyrosine kinase inhibitors • Future directions

INTRODUCTION AND BACKGROUND

Chronic myeloid leukemia (CML) is a disease in which the acquisition of the Philadelphia chromosome (Ph) translocation is a universal change present in all of the cells of the population of leukemia cells and in over 95% of the patients in whom the clinical phenotype of CML is present.[1] Analysis of the junction point of the fusion chromosome between chromosomes 9 and 22 has shown that a chimeric protein, p210 BCR/ABL, is generated by the chromosomal translocation.[1] Detailed comparisons of the p210 BCR/ABL protein and its normal homologue, the p145 c-ABL kinase, have indicated that this translocation changes the intracellular location of the kinase from the nucleus and plasma membrane[2] to the cytoplasmic fraction.[3] In contrast to the p145 c-ABL kinase, which induces cell cycle arrest and apoptosis when overexpressed in cells,[4] overexpression of p210 BCR/ABL generates apoptosis rescue and continuous cycling of the myeloid cell.

In the clinic, the acquisition of p210 BCR/ABL confers the phenotypes of anchorage-independent growth and genetic instability on myeloid cells.[5] The genetic instability of the cells leads to the evolution of the phenotype of the myeloid leukemia from an indolent disease characterized by elevations of the circulating myeloid cell mass to a fulminant blastic transformation in which patients die of infection and bleeding.[1]

Cell lines and animal models have been used to show that inhibition of this altered expression and function of the ABL kinase in p210 BCR/ABL is important for the transformed phenotype of these cells. Incubation of p210 BCR/ABL-positive cells with antisense oligonucleotides directed at the *BCR/ABL* mRNA inhibits growth-factor-independent growth and anchorage-independent growth.[6] Transfection of plasmid transcription units containing temperature-sensitive mutants of the ABL kinase[7] and a tetracycline-inducible *BCR/ABL* transcription unit have shown that the transformation phenotypes of growth-factor-independent growth and anchorage- independent growth can be reversibly conferred on myeloid cells.[8]

Transfection of BCR/ABL retroviral vectors into mouse bone marrow cells has created a disease that is close in phenotype to CML in the mouse animal model in which the transduced cells are transplanted into the mouse.[9] It has been more difficult to use the transgenic model for *BCR/ABL* transcription units, since the p210 BCR/ABL oncoprotein has lethal effects in utero.

The phenotypes of genetic instability and

anchorage-independent growth are thought to arise from the effect of p210 BCR/ABL on the following targets: the Ras pathway into the nucleus through the MAP kinase pathway,[10] the Ras pathway via the Akt kinase to phosphorylation of Bad, which generates high levels of free Bcl-2, the stimulation of phosphatidylinositol 3′-kinase (PI3-K), which leads to increased Bcl-2 levels through the Akt kinase and Bad phosphorylation,[11] and the activation of the SAP pathway.[12] Transdominant-negative inhibitors of SAP kinase inhibit the transforming effect of p210 BCR/ABL on myeloid cells,[12] and the transdominant-negative inhibitor of the interaction of p210 BCR/ABL and Sos via the Grb2 pathway has also been shown to suppress the transformed phenotype of p210 BCR/ABL-positive cells in fibroblasts.[13] Huettner and co-workers[8] have shown that a B-cell leukemia is reversibly induced in a mouse model by a tetracycline-inducible p190 *BCR/ABL* transcription unit and that loss of the expression of p190 *BCR/ABL* results in loss of the leukemic phenotype.[8]

Vectors carrying inhibitory peptide transcription units, based on inhibitors of the oligomerization domain[14,15] and of binding of ATP to the ATP-binding sites near the kinase site of p210 BCR/ABL,[16,17] have all led to suppression of the transformed phenotypes of p210 BCR/ABL cells. These studies have shown that the transforming activity of p210 BCR/ABL depends on the ABL kinase. This has opened the door to the development of inhibitors of this kinase as a primary way of treating the disease.

DIFFERENCES BETWEEN ABL AND p210 BCR/ABL KINASES

The p145 c-ABL protein is found in the nucleus, associated with DNA, and bound to plasma membrane proteins such as PI3-K and cytoskeletal elements such as actin,[18] whereas p210 BCR/ABL is found in the cytoplasm of the cell.[3] Overexpression of p145 c-ABL results in cell cycle arrest at the G_1/S interface, and induction of apoptosis.[4] In contrast, the expression of p210 BCR/ABL promotes continuous cell cycle progression and diminution of sensitivity to apoptosis-inducing agents.[1] The p145 c-ABL kinase is inactive unless activated by activation of DNA protein kinase by DNA-damaging agents.[19] When activated, it results in the inhibition of PI3-K,[20] whereas p210 BCR/ABL activates P13-K,[25] and is continuously active in the cytoplasm but not in the nucleus of the cell.[3,11,30] Recently, three groups have shown that the c-ABL tyrosine kinase regulates another protein, p73, which is related to p53.[21–23] Both c-ABL and p73 are part of a mismatch-repair apoptotic pathway induced by DNA-damaging agents such as cisplatin.[21] Exposure of the cell to DNA-damaging agents (cisplatin or ionizing radiation) activates c-ABL, and this results in phosphorylation of p73 at tyrosine 99 by the c-ABL tyrosine kinase.[21–23] c-ABL binds to the carboxyl terminus of p73 through the SH3 domain of c-ABL.[22,23]

p210 BCR/ABL continuously binds to and activates PI3-K through its SH2 domain,[11] whereas p145 c-ABL binds continuously to PI3-K through its SH3 domain,[20] but inhibits PI3-K only when activated by DNA-damaging agents through phosphorylation at sites distinct from that phosphorylated by p210 BCR/ABL. The autophosphorylation activity of p145 c-ABL is very focused on one site, whereas the autophosphorylation activity of p210 BCR/ABL occurs at multiple sites.[24]

STRATEGIES FOR DEVELOPING ABL KINASE INHIBITORS

Antisense oligonucleotides

Calabretta and colleagues[6] first showed that the effect of antisense oligonucleotides on colony growth of CML cells in methylcellulose was detectable in CML cells taken from blast-crisis patients. In addition, they have shown that suppression of the level of p210 BCR/ABL protein by antisense oligonucleotides directed at the *BCR/ABL* mRNA sensitizes these CML cells to the toxic effects of chemotherapy. This result was not anticipated, since it was predicted that, as the disease progressed from the initial 'chronic phase' into the terminal acute leukemic 'blastic phase', the myeloid leukemia cells would become increasingly independent of p210 BCR/ABL because of the acquisition of additional somatic mutations that would override and supplant the effect of p210 BCR/ABL. The results of Calabretta and his co-workers using the antisense approach to suppress *BCR/ABL* mRNA and the intracellular levels of p210 BCR/ABL have suggested that CML cells retain a dependence on the apoptosis-rescue function of p210 BCR/ABL, even in the blastic stage of CML. The studies summarized above suggest very strongly that inhibition of the ABL kinase should be effective in sensitizing CML cells to chemotherapy at all stages of the evolution of the disease, even in blast crisis,[6] as well as inducing apoptosis and cell cycle arrest in the earlier stages, at which time the CML cells are still dependent on p210 BCR/ABL for proliferation and survival.

Natural products that are tyrosine kinase inhibitors

One set of kinase-inhibitory compounds studied in CML includes natural products that were known to inhibit kinases in cell lines. Herbimycin as well as other natural product tyrosine kinase inhibitors have been shown to induce cell cycle arrest and suppress anchorage-independent growth in CML cells in vitro.[26] These compounds, however, are not very specific for the ABL kinase, and therefore may be too toxic because they inhibit kinases too broadly to be used meaningfully in the clinical setting for the treatment of CML.

Tyrphostins

Another class of compounds that has received attention are the tyrphostins,[27] which were modeled to bind to the substrate-binding site of the ABL kinase catalytic site. Tests of the effects of these agents in cell lines have shown that they not only induce apoptosis and cell cycle arrest of p210 BCR/ABL cells without affecting normal hematopoietic cells, but also interact synergistically with chemotherapy in inducing apoptosis of CML cells.

STI571

Brian Druker and his colleagues first reported that the tyrosine kinase inhibitor, STI571 (Glivec; Gleevec), resulted in over a 90% decrease in colony formation in methylcellulose of CML peripheral blood cells, whereas it did not reduce the plating efficiency of normal cells.[28] These studies showed a dose-dependent suppression of the growth of tumors in a human xenograft model of p210 BCR/ABL myeloid leukemia cells.

Recently, Druker reported the results of his initial phase I studies of STI571 in interferon-α (IFN-α)-resistant late chronic-phase CML patients.[29] All patients treated with over 140 mg/day exhibited a greater than 50% reduction in white blood cell count for at least 2 weeks, and all patients treated with over 300 mg/day exhibited a complete hematological response. One-third of these patients developed cytogenetic responses, which persisted for as long as 18 months. No dose-limiting side-effects were seen. See Chapter 34 for a more detailed discussion of STI571.

UNANSWERED QUESTIONS, AND POTENTIAL LIMITATIONS OF TYROSINE KINASE INHIBITORS

Why only one-third of the patients treated with STI571 developed cytogenetic responses is at present unknown. Whether this is a manifestation of the acquisition of additional somatic mutations in these patients that make the cells independent of p210 BCR/ABL, or whether it represents the evolution of resistance to the STI571 kinase inhibitor is not known. It will be important to determine the duration of the cytogenetic remissions and the percentage of individuals in whom complete or major cytogenetic remissions are generated. Ultimately, the effect of STI571 on survival will need to be tested to determine its ultimate value in therapy.

Carlo Gambacorti-Passerini of the Istituto Nazionale Tumori in Italy reported that amplification of the *BCR/ABL* gene accompanies the evolution of resistance by p210 BCR/ABL-positive cell lines during 6 months of in vitro culture in STI571. This may not be surprising when one considers the genetic instability of CML cells, and that it is already known that during the evolution to blast crisis, double Philadelphia chromosomes do evolve. In addition, it is well known that CML cells from blastic-phase patients frequently display changes at the cytogenetic level, such as trisomy 8, trisomy 13, and 17p deletions. The genetic rearrangement is revealed to be even more extensive when CML cells taken from blast-crisis patients are analyzed at a cytogenetic level using comparative genomic hybridization. The assumption is that, at a molecular level, the extent of molecular rearrangement and mutational change will be even greater when analyzed and that STI571 resistance will occur.

L Tyler Thiesing at the University of Oregon Health Sciences Center has reported that combination of STI571 with other chemotherapeutic agents such as cytosine arabinoside (Ara-C) dramatically enhances its inhibition of CML cells. It may be that the combination of chemotherapy with STI571 will prevent the evolution of resistance due to the emergence of clones of cells that are increasingly resistant to this particular kinase inhibitor.

FUTURE DIRECTIONS

Future trials with STI571

Obvious next trials include a phase II trial with STI571 alone in patients newly diagnosed. Combination of STI571 with chemotherapy (Ara-C) in late chronic-phase patients and more advanced patients is a very important issue to resolve, because these patients often have limited therapeutic options. Perhaps the use of chemotherapy and STI571 will increase the percentage of patients in whom cytogenetic remissions are generated. The use of STI571 in maintaining remissions after autologous and allogeneic transplants is also an important area for future clinical study.

New directions in the development of kinase inhibitors

The successes in developing STI571 and in utilizing analysis of protein structure in the design of low-molecular-weight inhibitors of HIV has aroused the interest of the world of drug development. Inhibitors that are selectively toxic for oncoprotein targets may soon become available. The results obtained with STI571 have been impressive, but we now know that resistance will evolve to this drug when it is used as a single agent. We do not yet know if the use of STI571 in combination with chemotherapy will be sufficient to prevent the evolution of drug resistance that is predicted by in vitro studies.

One approach is to modify the STI571 molecule. Obviously, now that X-ray crystal structure data on p210 BCR/ABL is available, the modification of STI571 could make this compound more effective as an inhibitor of CML cells.

Another approach to the prevention of resistance may be the development of inhibitors that interact with other sites of functional importance on the p210 BCR/ABL protein. This would allow the development of combinations of low-molecular-weight chemical inhibitors of p210 BCR/ABL, each of which is inhibiting the kinase at a different site. An alternative is to develop inhibitors that interact at sites independent of the catalytic domain.

Finally, the development of compounds that are inhibitors of key downstream targets of p210 BCR/ABL might be of value if such inhibition were to sensitize the CML cell to other types of therapy. An example would be inhibition of the effect of p210 BCR/ABL on PI3-K, which indirectly results in an increase in the level of Bcl-2 within the leukemic cell.

Approaches to the development of new inhibitors of p210 BCR/ABL

We have summarized above the use of the tyrphostins, which were designed to be competitive inhibitors of the binding of substrates to the ABL kinase catalytic site on p210 BCR/ABL, and STI571, which was conceived originally as a competitive inhibitor at the ATP-binding site in the catalytic domain of the ABL kinase.

Another logical approach to the development of inhibitors of the ABL kinase is to develop mimics of ATP. David Austin has proposed the development of low-molecular-weight inhibitors of p210 BCR/ABL by making mimics of either the triphosphate or the adenosine parts of the ATP molecule. Computational analyses of candidate molecular scaffolds that are coupled to adenosine have shown that these compounds have the same molecular dimensions as ATP. This molecular scaffold approach allows the development of compounds that may engage multiple local domains of the ABL catalytic domain in the neighborhood of the ATP-binding site. The strategy is to use convergent combinational synthesis to introduce structural diversity in the multiple functional groups projected by the scaffold linked to the adenosine, and then to screen the low-complexity combinatorial library thus generated with recombinant p210 BCR/ABL to identify molecules that inhibit the p210 BCR/ABL kinase at low concentrations and do so selectively.

A further approach is to choose other sites on the p210 BCR/ABL protein that are functionally important. One class of sites are points of protein–protein contact between p210 BCR/ABL and downstream targets that are important for clinically important phenotypes, such as chemotherapy resistance. The SH2 domain is the point of contact between p210 BCR/ABL and PI3-K. This contact results in the activation of PI3-K, which increases the intracellular levels of Bcl-2 through Akt-mediated phosphorylation of Bad. This pathway is widely recognized as playing a role in chemotherapy resistance. Many groups have tried to develop SH2 domain inhibitors, and have found this a difficult task. Another site is the transporter that carries p210 BCR/ABL from the nucleus into the cytoplasm.[30]

The solution of the X-ray crystal structure of p210 BCR/ABL may produce information that can be used in the design of drugs that are directed at an alternative site of action on the p210 BCR/ABL kinase and that would thereby produce an additive, if not synergistic, effect on kinase inhibition when used with STI571. This might reduce the likelihood of emergence of resistance to functional inhibitors of p210 BCR/ABL acting at a single site.

ACKNOWLEDGEMENTS

AD recognizes support from NIH NCI Grants NCI P01 CA 49639 and CA 551164, from the Bush Leukemia Research Fund, the Hull Development Fund of the Yale Cancer Center, the Donahue Foundation, and the Ensign Professorship at the Yale University School of Medicine.

REFERENCES

1. Melo JV, The diversity of BCR–ABL fusion proteins and their relationship to the leukemia phenotype. *Blood* 1996; **88:** 2375–84.
2. Wang JYJ, Kipreos ET, Differential phosphorylation of c-abl in cell cycle determined by CDC 2 and phosphatase activity. *Science* 1990; **248:** 217–20.
3. Van Etten RA, Jackson P, Baltimore D, The mouse type IV c-abl gene product is a nuclear protein, and activation of transforming ability is associated with cytoplasmic localization. *Cell* 1989; **58:** 669–78.
4. Wen ST, Jackson RK, Van Etten RA, The cytostatic function of c-abl is controlled by multiple nuclear localization signals and requires the p53 and Rb suppressor gene products. *EMBO J* 1995; **15:** 1583–95.
5. Renshaw MW, McWhirter JR, Wang JYJ, The human leukemia oncogene bcr–abl abrogates the

anchorage requirement but not the growth factor requirement for proliferation. *Mol Cell Biol* 1995; **156:** 1286–93.
6. Szczylik C, Skorski T, Nicolaides NC et al, Selective inhibition of leukemia cell proliferation by BCR–ABL antisense oligodeoxynucleotides. *Science* 1991; **253:** 562–5.
7. Carlesso N, Griffin JD, Druker BJ, Use of a temperature-sensitive mutant to define the biological effects of the p210 bcr–abl tyrosine kinase on proliferation of a factor-dependent murine myeloid cell line. *Oncogene* 1994; **9:** 149–56.
8. Huettner CS, Zhang P, Van Etten RA, Tenen DG, Reversibility of acute B-cell leukaemia induced by BCR–ABL. *Nature Genet* 2000; **24:** 57–60.
9. Daley GQ, Van Etten RA, Baltimore D, Induction of CML in mice by the p210 bcr–abl. *Science* 1990; **247:** 824–30.
10. Cortez D, Kadlec L, Pendergast AM, Structural and signaling requirements for bcr–abl mediated transformation and inhibition of apoptosis. *Mol Cell Biol* 1995; **15:** 5531–41.
11. Skorski T, Bellacosa A, Nieborowska-Skorska M, Transformation of hematopoietic cells by BCR/ABL requires activation of a PI-3K/AKT-dependent pathway. *EMBO J* 1997; **16:** 6151–61.
12. Raitano AB, Halpern JR, Hambuch TM, Sawyers CL, The bcr–abl leukemia oncogene activates Jun kinase and requires Jun for transformation. *Proc Natl Acad Sci USA* 1995; **92:** 11746–50.
13. Pendergast AM, Quilliam LA, Cripe LD et al, Bcr–abl induced oncogenesis is mediated by direct interaction with the SH2 domain of the GRB-2 adaptor protein. *Cell* 1993; **75:** 175–85.
14. McWhirter JR, Galasso DL, Wang JYJ, A coiled-coil oligomerization domain of bcr is essential for the transformation function of bcr–abl oncoproteins. *Mol Cell Biol* 1993; **13:** 7587–95.
15. Guo XYD, Cuillerot JM, Wang T et al, BCR oligomerization domain inhibits IL3 independent growth of p210 bcr–abl myeloid leukemia cells. *Oncogene* 1998; **17:** 825–33.
16. Welch PJ, Wang JYJ, Abrogation of retinoblastoma protein function by c-abl through tyrosine kinase-dependent and independent mechanisms. *Mol Cell Biol* 1995; **15:** 5542–51.
17. Guo WXD, Balague C, Wang T et al, The shift of the retinoblastoma C-box peptide from the nucleus to the cytoplasm results in inhibition of p210 bcr–abl transforming function. *Oncogene* 1999; **18:** 1589–95.
18. McWhirter JR, Wang JYJ, An actin-binding function contributes to transformation by the BCR–ABL oncoprotein of Philadelphia chromosome positive human leukemias. *EMBO J* 1993; **12:** 1533–46.
19. Kharbanda S, Ren R, Pandeyk P et al, Activation of the c-Abl tyrosine kinase in the stress response to DNA damaging agents. *Nature* 1995; **376:** 785–8.
20. Varticovski L, Daley GQ, Jackson P et al, Activation of phosphatidylinositol 3-kinase in cells expressing abl oncogene variants. *Mol Cell Biol* 1991; **11:** 1107–13.
21. Gong JG, Costanzo A, Yang HQ et al, The tyrosine kinase c-Abl regulates p73 in apoptotic response to cisplatin-induced DNA damage. *Nature* 1999; **399:** 806–9.
22. Agami R, Blandino G, Oren M, Shaul Y, Interaction of c-Abl and p73α and their collaboration to induce apoptosis. *Nature* 1999; **399:** 809–13.
23. Yuan ZM, Shioya H, Ishiko T et al, p73 is regulated by tyrosine kinase c-Abl in the apoptotic response to DNA damage. *Nature* 1999; **399:** 814–17.
24. Konopka JB, Watanabe SM, Witte ON, An alteration of the human c-Abl protein in K562 leukemia cells unmasks associated tyrosine kinase activity. *Cell* 1984; **37:** 1035–42.
25. Skorski T, Palanisamy K, Niebortowska-Skorska ML et al, Phosphatidylinositol-3 kinase activity is regulated by bcr/abl and is required for the growth of Philadelphia chromosome-positive cells. *Blood* 1995; **86:** 726–36.
26. Honma Y, Okabe-Kado J, Jozumi M et al, Induction of erythroid differentiation of K562 human leukemic cells by herbimycin A, an inhibitor of tyrosine kinase activity. *Cancer Res* 1989; **49:** 331–4.
27. Anafi M, Gazit A, Zehavi A et al, Tyrphostin-induced inhibition of p210 bcrabl tyrosine kinase activity induces K562 to differentiate. *Blood* 1993; **82:** 3524–9.
28. Druker BJ, Tamura S, Buchdunger E et al, Effects of a selective inhibitor of the ABL tyrosine kinase on the growth of BCR–ABL positive cells. *Nature Med* 1996; **2:** 561–6.
29. Druker BJ, Lydon NB, Lesson learned from the development of an abl tyrosine kinase inhibitor for chronic myelogenous leukemia. *J Clin Invest* 2000; **105:** 3–7.
30. Vigneri P, Wang JYJ, Induction of apoptosis in CML cells through nuclear entrapment of BCR–ABL tyrosine kinase. *Nature Medicine* 2001; **7:** 228–33.

34

STI571 as a therapeutic agent

Michael E O'Dwyer, Michael J Mauro, Brian J Druker

CONTENTS • BCR/ABL kinase activity as a molecular target for therapy of CML • Designing a tyrosine kinase inhibitor • Preclinical testing of STI571 • Phase I trials of STI571 • Lessons learned about BCR/ABL, and future questions • Integration of STI571 into CML treatment algorithms • Conclusions

BCR/ABL KINASE ACTIVITY AS A MOLECULAR TARGET FOR THERAPY OF CML

The BCR/ABL tyrosine kinase, generated by the Philadelphia chromosome (Ph) translocation, is present in virtually all patients with chronic myeloid leukemia (CML) and has been demonstrated to be the causative agent of CML. BCR/ABL functions as a constitutively activated tyrosine kinase, and this kinase activity is required for the transforming function of BCR/ABL.[1,2] Thus, BCR/ABL is an ideal candidate as a molecular target for a therapeutic agent, and an inhibitor of the BCR/ABL kinase would be predicted to be an effective and selective therapeutic agent for CML.

DESIGNING A TYROSINE KINASE INHIBITOR

As described in Chapter 33, by the late 1980s, synthetic, competitive inhibitors of ATP binding with some degree of specificity among tyrosine kinases had been generated.[3] Working independently, scientists at Novartis identified a lead kinase inhibitor by the time-consuming process of random screening, that is, the testing of large compound libraries for inhibition of protein kinases in vitro. In this case, the initial lead compound was a relatively weak inhibitor of protein kinase Cα (PKCα) and the platelet-derived growth factor receptor (PDGFR).[4] The activity of the initial lead compound was optimized by synthesizing a series of chemically related compounds and analyzing the relationship between structure and activity for each compound. The most potent molecules in the series were all dual inhibitors of the v-Abl and the PDGFR kinases.[5,6] STI571 (Glivec, Gleevec) emerged from these efforts as the lead compound for preclinical development. The mechanism of action of STI571 is shown schematically in Figure 34.1.

PRECLINICAL TESTING OF STI571

STI571 has been tested in a number of preclinical models, including in vitro assays of enzyme inhibition, cellular assays of proliferation, and in vivo assays of tumor formation. These studies demonstrate that STI571 inhibits all ABL kinases at submicromolar concentrations, including p210 BCR/ABL, p185 BCR/ABL, v-Abl, and the c-ABL tyrosine kinases.[7] Numerous tyrosine and serine–threonine protein kinases have been tested for inhibition by STI571, and, except for the PDGFR and the c-Kit tyrosine kinases, no others are inhibited.[7]

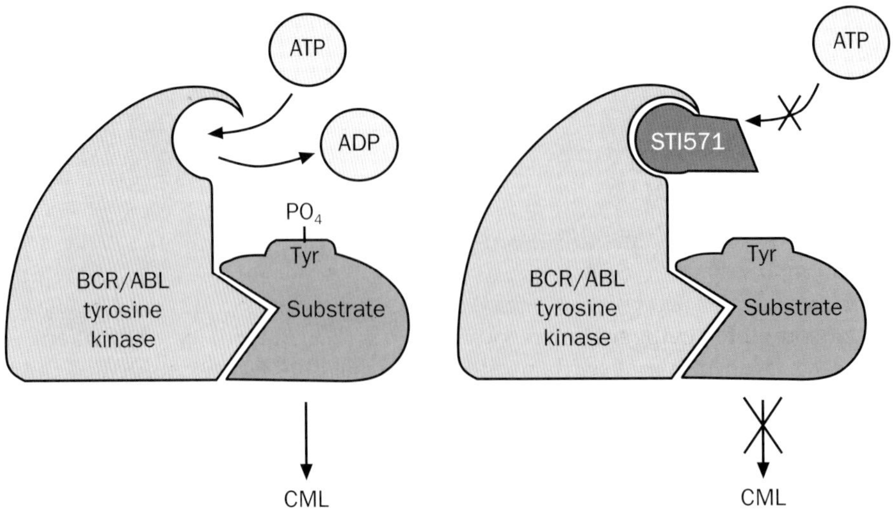

Figure 34.1 Mechanism of action of STI571. The BCR/ABL tyrosine kinase is a constitutively active kinase that functions by binding ATP and transferring phosphate from ATP to tyrosine residues on various substrates. This activity causes the excess proliferation of myeloid cells characteristic of CML. STI571 functions by blocking the binding of ATP to the BCR/ABL tyrosine kinase, thus inhibiting the activity of the kinase. In the absence of tyrosine kinase activity, substrates required for BCR/ABL function cannot be phosphorylated.

STI571, at concentrations of 1 and 10 μM, kills or inhibits the proliferation of all BCR/ABL-expressing cell lines tested to date.[7–11] In contrast, a variety of immortalized or transformed cell lines that do not express BCR/ABL are not sensitive to STI571. In colony-forming assays using CML bone marrow or peripheral blood samples, treatment with STI571 decreases the number of colonies formed, and may select for the growth of BCR/ABL-negative progenitor cells.[9,12,13] Minimal inhibition of the colony-forming potential of normal bone marrow has been observed. Similar results, showing selective depletion of BCR/ABL-positive cells, have been observed in long-term marrow cultures.[14] Thus, STI571 appears to be selectively toxic to cells expressing the constitutively active BCR/ABL protein tyrosine kinase. Studies in mice also showed that STI571 had in vivo activity against BCR/ABL-expressing cells. Initial experiments inhibited, but did not eradicate BCR/ABL-expressing tumors.[12] However, subsequent experiments showed that continuous exposure to STI571 was necessary to eradicate the tumors, suggesting that this would be important for optimal antileukemic effects.[15]

Early pharmacokinetic studies in rats and dogs demonstrated that bioactive concentrations are readily achieved in the circulation with an oral formulation of STI571.

PHASE I TRIALS OF STI571

Based on the efficacy of STI571 in a variety of preclinical models and an acceptable animal toxicology profile, phase I clinical trials were begun in June 1998. The initial study was a dose-escalation study designed to establish the maximum tolerated dose (MTD), with a secondary endpoint of clinical efficacy. Patients were eligible if they were in the chronic phase of CML and had failed therapy with interferon-α (IFN-α). STI571 was administered as a once-daily oral therapy, and no other cytoreductive agents were allowed. Once doses of 300 mg or greater were reached, all 31 patients on treatment for at least 4 weeks achieved a complete hematological response.[16] Responses were typically seen within the first 3 weeks of therapy and have been maintained in all patients for up to 8 months. At an STI571 dose of 300 mg or greater, cytogenetic responses were seen within 5 months in 14 of 31 (45%) patients, with 10% achieving a complete cytogenetic response. Side-effects have been minimal, with no dose-limiting toxicities encountered. Grade 2 and 3 myelosuppression was observed at a dose of 300 mg or greater in 21% and 8% of patients, respectively.[16] The myelosuppression might be consistent with a therapeutic effect, as the Ph-positive clone contributes the majority of hematopoiesis in these patients. Pharmacokinetic studies showed that at a dose of 300 mg or greater, plasma levels equivalent to the predicted, effective, in vitro level of 1 μM were achieved. The half-life of STI571 is 13–16 hours, which is sufficiently long to permit once-daily dosing.[17] Although the follow-up on this group of patients is relatively short, these data indicate that an ABL-specific tyrosine kinase inhibitor has significant activity in CML, even in IFN-α-refractory patients.

Given the effectiveness of STI571 in chronic-phase patients who had failed IFN-α, the phase I studies were expanded to include CML patients in myeloid and lymphoid blast crisis and patients with relapsed or refractory Ph-positive acute lymphoblastic leukemia (ALL). Patients have been treated with daily doses of 300–1000 mg of STI571. Of 38 patients with myeloid blast crisis, 21 (55%) responded to therapy, defined by a decrease in percentage of marrow blasts to less than 15%, and 9 (27%) completely cleared their marrows of blasts (<5%). Of 20 patients with lymphoid-phenotype disease, CML in lymphoid blast crisis, or Ph-positive ALL, 14 (70%) responded, with 4 (20%) completely clearing their marrow of blasts. Unfortunately, all but one of the lymphoid-phenotype patients have relapsed between days 45 and 117. However, 7 (18%) of the 38 myeloid blast-crisis patients continue to be maintained in remission on STI571, with follow-up ranging from 101 to 349 days.[18] Thus, STI571 has significant single-agent activity in BCR/ABL-positive acute leukemias, but resistance to STI571 can occur – at least in more advanced stages. However, these studies demonstrate that, in the majority of cases, the leukemic clone in BCR/ABL-positive acute leukemias, including CML blast crisis, remains at least partially dependent on BCR/ABL kinase activity for survival.

LESSONS LEARNED ABOUT BCR/ABL, AND FUTURE QUESTIONS

The success of STI571 as a therapeutic agent for CML answers several questions about CML biology, but leaves many more to be addressed. The most important issue that this clinical trial has demonstrated is that the BCR/ABL tyrosine kinase, as predicted from animal models, is critical to the development of CML. However, it has not yet been possible to determine the primary mechanism of action of BCR/ABL or the kinase inhibitor. That is, the question remains as to whether BCR/ABL induces proliferation or whether it protects cells from apoptotic cell death. In the former case, it is possible that STI571 would simply prevent proliferation of the leukemic clone without eliminating it. Even in this scenario, it is possible that cytogenetic responses would be observed. Presumably, with the inhibition of BCR/ABL kinase activity, the leukemic clone would be subjected to normal marrow regulatory influences and would be eliminated at the end of the progenitor cell's natural lifespan. It is also likely that normal hematopoietic progenitors might regain a proliferative advantage or that progression to blast crisis could be delayed or avoided. If BCR/ABL protects from apoptotic cell death, it is possible that treatment with a kinase inhibitor could eliminate the leukemic clone.

The activity in blast-crisis patients demonstrates that the leukemic clone remains at least partially dependent on BCR/ABL kinase activity for survival. However, these trials also point out that resistance to STI571 as a single agent is a reality. Several publications examining cell lines that express BCR/ABL have shown that *BCR/ABL* gene amplification is one of several potential mechanisms of resistance.[19–21] BCR/ABL is known to render cells resistant to chemotherapeutic agents, although the mechanism of resistance remains unclear.[22,23] Preliminary in vitro evidence demonstrates that treatment of cells expressing BCR/ABL with STI571 reverses this chemotherapy resistance.[24] Further, additive or even synergistic antiproliferative effects between STI571 and other antileukemic agents, including IFN-α and cytosine arabinoside (Ara-C), have been observed.[24] Such studies provide a strong rationale for combining STI571 with other active agents, both in advanced disease and in chronic-phase patients.

The optimal use of STI571 has yet to be defined. There are ongoing phase II studies using STI571 as a single agent in CML patients refractory to, or intolerant of, IFN-α, and in patients in accelerated phase or blast crisis. These studies will provide valuable information regarding the effectiveness and safety profile of STI571 in a larger cohort of patients, and will allow a determination of the durability of responses. A phase III randomized study, comparing STI571 with IFN-α plus Ara-C in newly diagnosed patients, is currently in progress. STI571 will likely be tried in a variety of CML patient populations, including patients relapsing after stem cell transplantation (SCT), as an adjunct to autologous SCT, and possibly as an in vitro purging agent for autologous SCT. However, as with most antineoplastic agents, it is likely that the best responses to STI571 will be observed early in the course of the disease. It is even conceivable that in early chronic-phase patients, BCR/ABL may be the sole molecular abnormality and that STI571 alone could eradicate the malignant clone. Additional tasks for the future will be studies aimed at predicting response to this molecularly targeted agent and ultimately combining STI571 with agents directed against pathways mediating resistance to STI571.

INTEGRATION OF STI571 INTO CML TREATMENT ALGORITHMS

The rapid success of STI571 has already rendered many CML treatment algorithms obsolete. As the duration of follow-up is relatively short, predictions regarding the potential use of STI57I range widely. However, at present, allogeneic SCT remains the only treatment known to cure CML in a large percentage of cases. As is it unknown whether initial treatment with STI571 will compromise the outcome of transplantation, it is difficult to know whether it is advisable to delay transplantation for a trial of STI571 in a younger patient. In the absence of firm data, individual decisions regarding the choice and timing of transplantation will continue to depend on factors such as patient age, availability of a well-matched donor, individual prognostic factors, and, of course, patient preference. For patients who are not candidates for transplantation, STI571, at least on the basis of the early studies, is an attractive alternative.

CONCLUSIONS

STI571 is an example of a rationally designed, molecularly targeted therapy based on a specific abnormality present in a human malignancy. Clinical trials with STI571 confirm the essential role of BCR/ABL tyrosine kinase activity in CML. STI571 is a promising new therapy for CML, and its development represents a new paradigm in cancer drug development.

REFERENCES

1. Lugo TG, Pendergast AM, Muller AJ, Witte ON, Tyrosine kinase activity and transformation potency of bcr–abl oncogene products. *Science* 1990; **247:** 1079–82.
2. Oda T, Tamura S, Matsuguchi T et al, The SH2 domain of Abl is not required for factor independent growth induced by Bcr–Abl in a murine myeloid cell line. *Leukemia* 1995; **9:** 295–301.

3. Yaish P, Gazit A, Gilon C, Levitzki A, Blocking of EGF-dependent cell proliferation by EGF receptor kinase inhibitors. *Science* 1988; **242:** 933–5.
4. Zimmermann J, Caravatti G, Mett H et al, Phenylamino-pyrimidine (PAP) derivatives: a new class of potent and selective inhibitors of protein kinase C (PKC). *Arch Pharm* 1996; **329:** 371–6.
5. Buchdunger E, Zimmermann J, Mett H et al, Selective inhibition of the platelet-derived growth factor signal transduction pathway by a protein-tyrosine kinase inhibitor of the 2-phenylaminopyrimidine class. *Proc Natl Acad Sci USA* 1995; **92:** 2558–62.
6. Buchdunger E, Zimmermann J, Mett H et al, Inhibition of the Abl protein-tyrosine kinase in vitro and in vivo by a 2-phenylaminopyrimidine derivative. *Cancer Res* 1996; **56:** 100–4.
7. Druker BJ, Lydon NB, Lessons learned from the development of an abl tyrosine kinase inhibitor for chronic myelogenous leukemia. *J Clin Invest* 2000; **105:** 3–7.
8. Carroll M, Ohno-Jones S, Tamura S et al, CGP 57148, a tyrosine kinase inhibitor, inhibits the growth of cells expressing BCR–ABL, TEL–ABL and TEL–PDGFR fusion proteins. *Blood* 1997; **90:** 4947–52.
9. Deininger MW, Goldman JM, Lydon N, Melo JV, The tyrosine kinase inhibitor CGP57148B selectively inhibits the growth of BCR–ABL-positive cells. *Blood* 1997; **90:** 3691–8.
10. Beran M, Cao X, Estrov Z et al, Selective inhibition of cell proliferation and BCR–ABL phosphorylation in acute lymphoblastic leukemia cells expressing Mr 190,000 BCR–ABL protein by a tyrosine kinase inhibitor (CGP-57148). *Clin Cancer Res* 1998; **4:** 1661–72.
11. Gambacorti-Passerini C, le Coutre P, Mologni L et al, Inhibition of the ABL kinase activity blocks the proliferation of BCR/ABL+ leukemic cells and induces apoptosis. *Blood Cells Mol Dis* 1997; **23:** 380–94.
12. Druker BJ, Tamura S, Buchdunger E et al, Effects of a selective inhibitor of the ABL tyrosine kinase on the growth of BCR–ABL positive cells. *Nature Med* 1996; **2:** 561–6.
13. Marley SB, Deininger MW, Davidson RJ et al, The tyrosine kinase inhibitor STI571, like interferon-alpha, preferentially reduces the capacity for amplification of granulocyte–macrophage progenitors from patients with chronic myeloid leukemia. *Exp Hematol* 2000; **28:** 551–7.
14. Kasper B, Fruehauf S, Schiedlmeier B et al, Favorable therapeutic index of a p210(BCR–ABL)-specific tyrosine kinase inhibitor; activity on lineage-committed and primitive chronic myelogenous leukemia progenitors. *Cancer Chemother Pharmacol* 1999; **44:** 433–8.
15. le Coutre P, Mologni L, Cleris L et al, In vivo eradication of human BCR/ABL-positive leukemia cells with an ABL kinase inhibitor. *J Natl Cancer Inst* 1999; **91:** 163–8.
16. Druker BJ, Talpaz M, Resta D et al, Clinical efficacy and safety of an Abl specific tyrosine kinase inhibitor as targeted therapy for chronic myelogenous leukemia. *Blood* 1999; **94:** 368a.
17. Peng B, Hayes M, Druker B et al, Clinical pharmacokinetics and pharmacodynamics of STI571 in a phase 1 trial in chronic myelogenous leukemia (CML) patients. *Proc Am Assoc Cancer Res* 2000; **41:** 256a.
18. Druker BJ, Sawyers CL, Kantarjian H et al, Activity of a specific inhibitor of the BCR-ABL tyrosine kinase in the blast crisis of chronic myeloid leukemia and acute lymphoblastic leukemia with the Philadelphia chromosome. *N Engl J Med* 2001; **344:** 1038–42.
19. Weisberg E, Griffin JD, Mechanism of resistance to the ABL tyrosine kinase inhibitor STI571 in BCR/ABL-transformed hematopoietic cell lines. *Blood* 2000; **95:** 3498–505.
20. Mahon FX, Deininger MW, Schultheis B et al, Selection and characterization of BCR–ABL positive cell lines with differential sensitivity to the tyrosine kinase inhibitor STI571: diverse mechanisms of resistance. *Blood* 2000; **96:** 1070–9.
21. le Coutre P, Tassi E, Varella-Garcia M et al, Induction of resistance to the Abelson inhibitor STI571 in human leukemic cells through gene amplification. *Blood* 2000; **95:** 1758–66.
22. Bedi A, Zehnbauer BA, Barber JP et al, Inhibition of apoptosis by BCR–ABL in chronic myeloid leukemia. *Blood* 1994; **83:** 2038–44.
23. Nishii K, Kabarowski JH, Gibbons DL et al, ts BCR–ABL kinase activation confers increased resistance to genotoxic damage via cell cycle block. *Oncogene* 1996; **13:** 2225–34.
24. Thiesing JT, Ohno-Jones S, Kolibaba KS, Druker BJ, Efficacy of an Abl tyrosine kinase inhibitor in conjunction with other anti-leukemic agents against Bcr–Abl positive cells. *Blood* 2000; **96:** 3195–9.

35

Immunotherapeutic strategies

Kathleen NS Cathcart, Javier Pinilla, David A Scheinberg

CONTENTS • Introduction • MHC-restricted T-cell effectors • BCR/ABL-specific peptide targets • Dendritic cells and ex vivo T-cell priming • MHC-unrestricted effectors • Monoclonal antibodies • Conclusions

INTRODUCTION

Chronic myeloid leukemia (CML) is a pluripotent stem cell disorder characterized by the presence of the Philadelphia chromosome which is formed by the translocation of chromosomes 9 and 22. The disease is characterized by progression from a subacute chronic phase to a rapidly lethal blastic phase. Chemotherapeutic strategies may reduce tumor burden in CML, but are not curative. Allogeneic bone marrow transplantation (BMT) remains the treatment of choice for those patients of appropriate age and with a suitable HLA-matched donor, and has been associated with prolonged disease-free survival in the majority of those patients who survive the peritransplant period. Unfortunately, many patients with CML are unable to receive a BMT, due to age, comorbidity, or lack of an available donor. The use of immunomodulators such as interferon-α (IFN-α) forms the mainstay of treatment for those patients who do not undergo BMT. The search for other treatment modalities has resulted in renewed interest in immunotherapeutic strategies for the disease.

Clinical observations have provided evidence that the immune system plays an integral role in the biology and therapy of CML. Unmodified BMT is associated with a significant incidence of acute and chronic graft-versus-host disease (GVHD); attempts to reduce this risk have centered around T-cell depletion (TCD) of the donor graft. TCD allogeneic grafts have been associated with a marked reduction of GVHD, as well as an increased risk for myeloid leukemia relapse.[1–5] It is known that patients who develop GVHD following BMT have a lower incidence of leukemia relapse, suggesting that T cells responsible for this alloreactive effect may also have antileukemia activity.[6,7] Alloreactive T-cell action may not completely explain the relationship between the graft-versus-leukemia (GVL) and GVHD effects, since it has been observed that allogeneic transplants are associated with a lower relapse rate than syngeneic transplants, even in the absence of overt GVHD.[8,9] Kolb et al[10] were the first to report that infusions of donor leukocytes from the donors of patients with CML who relapsed following an unmodified allogeneic transplant could induce durable remissions. This chapter will not focus on donor leukocyte infusions as immunotherapy for relapsed CML post allogeneic transplant, but rather will describe other specific immunotherapeutic strategies under investigation. These include vaccines, specific T cells, and antibodies (Table 35.1).

Table 35.1 Immunotherapeutic strategies in CML

Approach	Advantages	Disadvantages
Donor leukocytes	Effective; safer than second BMT	Requires donor; lethal risks
Allogeneic BMT	Effective; proven record	Toxic, often lethal; requires donor
Vaccines	Controlled specificity; potentially non-toxic	Unproven and largely untested; potency unknown
Monoclonal antibodies	Relatively safe; controlled dosing; effect stops	Poor antigen selections; variable potency

MHC-RESTRICTED T-CELL EFFECTORS

As already mentioned, CML is characterized by the presence of the Philadelphia chromosome (Ph) in the leukemic cells of all CML patients. Ph represents a translocation in which the c-*ABL* oncogene has moved from chromosome 9 into the major breakpoint cluster region (M-*bcr*) within the *BCR* gene on chromosome 22, resulting in a chimeric *BCR/ABL* gene.[11–13] The fused gene encodes an 8.5 kb chimeric mRNA,[14,15] which is translated into a 210 kDa protein. This p210 BCR/ABL protein shows tyrosine kinase activity and is uniquely present in the leukemic cells of CML patients.[17] The breakpoint in the *BCR* gene occurs either between *BCR* exons 2 (b2) and 3 (b3) or alternatively between *BCR* exons 3 (b3) and 4 (b4). Therefore, in the mature *BCR/ABL* mRNA, either b2 or b3 is spliced to *ABL* exon a2, which results in two alternative chimeric p210 BCR/ABL proteins comprising either the b2a2 or the b3a2 junction.[18] The two different amino acid sequences at the point of this junction represent unique tumor-specific determinants (Tables 35.2 and 35.3). Previous work[19] has shown that these two joining determinants are exposed on the p210 BCR/ABL molecule in an immunogenic fashion and that the BCR/ABL joining region can elicit specific antibody.

T-cell recognition of antigen requires two interactions between the peptide and cells. First, peptide must bind to major histocompatibility complex (MHC) molecules with high affinity, and, second, T cells must be capable of recognizing the peptide–MHC complex on the target cell. In a murine model, MHC class II-restricted T cells were induced in vivo by a b3a2 breakpoint-derived peptide.[20] Subsequently, in vitro immunization of human T cells with a similar peptide resulted in a b3a2 peptide-specific HLA-DRB1*1501-restricted $CD4^+$ cell line.[21] Additionally, ten Bosch et al[22] have shown that a 17-amino-acid peptide spanning the b3a2 breakpoint junction can be presented by DRB1*0401 molecules, and that these MHC class II-restricted cell lines could recognize DRB1*0401- and b3a2-expressing CML blasts. These data give support to the theory that the b3a2 breakpoint oncogene can be processed and presented by MHC class II molecules of leukemic cells.

Oettel et al[23] have used BCR/ABL-positive EBV–lymphoblastoid cell lines (EBV–LCLs) to stimulate HLA-disparate mononuclear cells to produce BCR/ABL-specific T cells. Unfortunately, these T cells lost their specificity in culture and began to kill BCR/ABL-negative EBV–LCLs. Faber et al[24] were able to generate $CD4^+$ T-cell clones using irradiated CML cells

Table 35.2 Possible protein targets for T cells in CML

BCR/ABL-related
b3a2 peptides
b2a2 peptides
e1a2 peptides
Differentiation antigens
WT1
Proteinase-3
Myeloperoxidase
Minor histocompatibility antigens
CD33
p53 and Ras
Non-specific mixtures
CML whole-cell extracts
CML-derived dendritic cells

Table 35.3 Selected peptide sequences showing potential as CML immunogens

BCR/ABL b3a2
KQSSKALQR
ATGFKQSSK
GFKQSSKAL
HSATGFKQSSK
BCR/ABL b2a2
IPLTINKEEALQRPVAS
BCR/ABL e1a2
···DGEGAFHGDAEALQRPVASDF···
Proteinase-3
VLQELNVTV

incubated with HLA-identical mononuclear cells. $CD8^+$ cells with enhanced lytic activity were seen with the addition of IFN-α, but these T cells did not specifically lyse host myeloid leukemia cells. Proliferative activity was not assessed. Serody et al[25] were able to produce $CD4^+$ cytotoxic and proliferative T-cell clones from normal donors that lysed or proliferated HLA-matched myeloid cells. Donor peripheral blood mononuclear cells (PBMC) were incubated with irradiated myeloid tumor cells, and the resultant T-cell lines were cloned in the presence of cytokines (either interleukin (IL)-2, IL-2 plus IL-7 and IL-12, or IL-7 and IL-12). The majority of clones isolated did not show either lytic or proliferative activity; however, a subset of clones did demonstrate effector activity. The combination of IL-2, IL-7, and IL-12 enhanced the recovery of tumor-specific T-cell clones. As virtually all of the clones showed proliferative activity in response to patient myeloid cells, but not to corresponding EBV–LCLs, the authors concluded that BCR/ABL fusion peptides are not likely to be the recognized antigen. Rather, they suggested that the clones are recognizing early myeloid proteins.

It has been shown that cytotoxic T-lymphocyte (CTL) lines can be generated against CML cell populations in HLA-identical sibling pairs.[26,27] Irradiated leukemic cells were used as antigen sources to normal donor PBMC responder cells. MHC class II-restricted $CD4^+$ clones were established from these lines; however, differential recognition of leukemic cells versus normal lymphocytes from the same patient was not always demonstrated.[26] Other work was able to demonstrate leukemia-specific lysis by HLA-matched donor-derived CTL lines,[27] forming the basis behind a therapeutic trial of leukemia-reactive CTL.[28] These cell lines were generated from the HLA-identical donor of a patient who relapsed with accelerated phase of CML after allogeneic stem cell transplant. Cell lines were found that lysed the leukemic cells of the patient, inhibited the growth of leukemic progenitor cells, and did not respond to non-leukemic patient cells or donor lymphocytes. Cytolytic activity could be inhibited by the addition of anti-CD4 and anti-HLA-DR antibodies, but was not affected by anti-CD8 or anti-HLA class I antibodies. Three ex vivo expanded cell lines were later infused into the patient, with the resultant eradication of disease as measured by karyotyping, fluorescence in situ hybridization (FISH), molecular analysis of *BCR/ABL* mRNA, and chimerism studies. Progenitor cell inhibitor lymphocyte precursor (PCILp) frequency analysis correlated with clinical response. Chronic skin GVHD was increased approximately 200 days post first CTL infusion. Although the described donor–recipient pair was an allogeneic match, it is likely that the generated CTL were directed against minor histocompatibility antigens with restricted tissue distribution rather than CML-specific antigens.

Papadopoulos et al[29] have taken another approach and characterized the native self-peptide repertoire of CML blast cells. They identified high-copy-number autoantigens naturally processed and bound to HLA-A2, HLA-B, and HLA-DR molecules, including those whose parent proteins are involved in malignant transformation, signal transduction, and protein kinase activity. Other peptides found were derived from proteins involved in myeloid effector functions, including cathepsin G and proteinase-3. Proteinase-3 is a primary granule protein expressed in myeloid cells. CTL lines from healthy donors were developed to the HLA-A2.1-restricted self-peptide PR-1 derived from proteinase-3,[30] and had the ability to lyse myeloid leukemia cells. Further work showed that these CTL could inhibit granulocyte–macrophage colony-forming units (CFU-GM) from normal and leukemic donors.[31] The PR-1-peptide specific T cells exhibited preferential inhibition of leukemic CFU-GM based on relative overexpression of cytoplasmic proteinase-3 in the tumor cells versus normal cells. Molldrem et al[32] have also shown that a PR1-HLA-A2.1 tetramer can be used to select CTL from normal donors that preferentially lyse CML cells. These data provide the rationale for peptide-specific adoptive immunotherapy in patients with myeloid malignancies.

BCR/ABL-SPECIFIC PEPTIDE TARGETS

The use of T-cell infusions in patients with Ph-positive leukemic cells post allogeneic transplant provides evidence of the power of alloreactive T cells to eradicate CML cells.[33] CML-derived fusion proteins have been shown to bind human MHC class I molecules,[34] and peptides that bind to HLA class I may be capable of T-lymphocyte stimulation.[20] The ability of CML-derived BCR/ABL fusion proteins to bind to purified MHC class I molecules has been investigated by Bocchia et al.[35] A total of 76 possible peptide sequences spanning 8, 9, 10, or 11 amino acids of the b2a2 and b3a2 junctional regions of BCR/ABL proteins were analyzed for motifs with potential to bind to HLA-A1, -A2.1, -A3.2, -A11, -A24 and HLA-B7, -B8, and -B27. Based on their sequences alone, 21 BCR/ABL peptides of 8, 9, or 10 amino acids in length were predicted to have the potential of binding one or more class I molecules. Six of 11 b3a2 peptides displayed significant binding affinities for both HLA-A3.2 and -A11. None of the 10 peptides belonging to the b2a2 breakpoint showed high or intermediate affinity for any of the purified HLA class I molecules used in the binding assay.

The ability of these peptides to induce specific class I-restricted CTL in vitro in HLA-matched healthy donors was then evaluated.[34] In four out of four HLA-A3 donors tested, CML-A3/A11 peptide-specific CTL were induced that killed an allogeneic HLA-A3-matched peptide-pulsed leukemia cell line. In two of three HLA-A3 donors, the CML-A3/A11 peptide was able to induce killing of autologous and allogeneic HLA-matched peptide-pulsed PBMC. The CML-A3 peptide induced peptide-specific CTL in one of the four HLA-A3 donors tested. In related work, Greco et al[36] evaluated nonamers spanning the b2a2 and b3a2 fusion points for their ability to bind HLA class I and to elicit specific $CD8^+$ T-cell responses in vitro. An HLA class I α-chain refolding assay was used to test for peptide binding, and specific binding to HLA-A3.2 of two b3a2-derived peptides was demonstrated.

Bocchia et al[35] have also reported HLA class I-specific binding of these two peptides – one peptide binding to HLA-A3.2, and the other binding to HLA-A11. As neither of these peptides contained the expected HLA-A3 binding motifs, testing of modifications of the primary anchor residues was also pursued. The binding affinities for these modified peptides were variable, with both increases and decreases compared with the parent compound affinities noted. The junction peptides were also tested for their ability to induce CTL responses in HLA-A3 patients with CML. Class I-specific lysis was verified by anti-HLA class I antibody inhibition. Peripheral blood lymphocytes from non-responding patients were stimulated multiple times with autologous peptide-pulsed T-cell blasts, with CTL responses then detectable in two of six cell lines tested. One of these samples also showed a response to an anchor-residue-modified peptide. While these data support the concept that the T-cell repertoire may include precursors specific for exogenously modified peptides, they are unlikely to be sufficiently primed in vivo by the lower-affinity parent peptide to induce significant cytolytic responses without additional ex vivo priming and expansion. These data[34] provide the first evidence of a cytolytic human immune response against CML *BCR/ABL* oncogene-derived peptides, and affords the rationale for developing peptide-based vaccines to generate specific T-cell populations in vivo.

MacIntyre et al[37] investigated the specificity of HLA class II type on the T-cell proliferative responses of normal donor PBMC stimulated with a 21-amino-acid b3a2 fusion peptide. The investigators found that there was a high incidence of $CD4^+$ responses to this peptide, with 50 of 54 donors responding over controls. No consistent association with particular HLA types was seen. Bhatia and McGlave[38] have analyzed T cells cultured from the bone marrow of CML patients for their ability to suppress autologous hematopoietic progenitors. Patient bone marrow mononuclear cells were initially stimulated with phytohemagglutinin (PHA), then cultured in the presence of recombinant IL-2. This resulted in selective expansion of both $CD4^+$ and $CD8^+$ cells, and these lymphocytes demonstrated $CD4^+$-mediated suppression of autologous progenitor cells. Normal bone marrow T cells cultured in a similar fashion did not suppress autologous hematopoietic progenitors, providing evidence for the enhanced susceptibility of tumor cells to autologous T lymphocytes.

A phase I dose-escalation trial was designed to evaluate the safety and immunogenicity of b3a2-derived CML breakpoint peptides when administered to patients with chronic-phase disease.[39] Twelve patients (29–73 years old, also receiving IFN-α hydroxyurea) were vaccinated with a preparation of four peptides of 9–10 amino acids in length, and a 25-amino-acid peptide symmetrically spanning the fusion point and capable of eliciting a MHC class II response in vitro. Cohorts of three patients received escalating doses of peptides mixed with the adjuvant QS-21 in five subcutaneous injections over a 10-week period. At study midpoint and/or 2 weeks after the last vaccination, three of six patients treated at the two highest dose levels of vaccine (500 μg or 1500 μg total peptides) generated peptide-specific T-cell proliferative responses or delayed-type hypersensitivity responses, or both. One patient maintained a response for more than five months after all vaccinations were completed. CTL were not identified. Significant adverse effects were not seen. This study shows that a BCR/ABL-derived peptide vaccine can be safely administered to patients with chronic-phase CML, and can elicit a specific immune response. An additional HLA-A2.1-binding peptide with CD8-mediated cytolytic activity has been identified,[40] and a phase II trial incorporating this peptide and the previously studied peptides is currently ongoing (KNS Cathcart, J Pinilla, and DA Scheinberg, unpublished).

DENDRITIC CELLS AND EX VIVO T-CELL PRIMING

Dendritic cells (DC) are potent antigen-presenting cells (APC) capable of priming primary and secondary $CD4^+$ and $CD8^+$ T-cell responses.[41] DC can induce CTL to respond to tumor antigens,[42,43] even without $CD4^+$-mediated help.[44,45] Eibl et al[46] have shown that Ph-positive DC can be generated from PBMC of CML patients. These DC were then used to generate a CTL line. A clone from this line exhibited specific recognition of Ph-positive cells, and did not lyse HLA-identical, Ph-negative PBMC from a healthy donor. Choudhury et al[47] have also generated DC of leukemic origin from peripheral blood cells of patients with CML, have used these to stimulate autologous T cells in the presence of IL-2, and have shown increased cytotoxicity of DC-stimulated T cells versus IL-2-expanded T cells against autologous targets. T-cell subtype separation experiments showed that this activity was mainly due to $CD8^+$ T cells. Weakly cytolytic $CD4^+$ cells have been recognized to secrete soluble factors that can inhibit leukemia cell growth,[48] and Choudhury et al[47] demonstrated that culture supernatant from $CD4^+$ but not $CD8^+$ DC-stimulated T cells inhibited autologous CML cell colony growth. Additionally, leukemic DC-stimulated T cells were able to lyse autologous CML targets, but had little cytolytic activity against autologous IFN-α-induced remission-state bone marrow mononuclear cells in two patients.

An HLA-DR1-restricted $CD4^+$ T-cell line has been generated from normal donor PBMC, and has shown responses to two b3a2-derived fusion peptides 11 and 12 amino acids in length.[49] Presentation by peptide-pulsed DC was more efficient than by other APC. The T-cell line had significant proliferative responses to a b3a2-containing CML PBMC lysate or to K562 cell lysates containing b3a2, but not to lysates derived from b2a2-containing cells. These data confirm that peptide-specific T cells can recognize leukemia cell targets. Nieda et al[50] have investigated the ability of normal donor PBMC-derived DC primed with a 16-amino-acid b3a2-derived peptide to generate $CD8^+$ cytotoxic normal donor T cells, and have demonstrated b3a2-specific lysis of peripheral blood CML cells. Cytotoxicity was likely not due to alloreactivity, since PHA-stimulated peripheral blood CML blasts were not lysed. Recognition of MHC class I molecules was shown; however, cytotoxicity was not HLA-restricted. This study shows that $CD8^+$ lymphocytes specific for BCR/ABL are present in normal individuals, and that these cells retain their antigen specificity and cytotoxic ability during in vitro expansion. Osman et al[51] have also generated b3a2-specific normal donor DC by priming with a 12-amino-acid breakpoint junction peptide. Both $CD4^+$ and $CD8^+$ T-lymphocyte effector responses were seen against target cells cultured from the HLA-identical CML patient siblings of the normal donors. The peptide-pulsed DC-primed T cells had significantly greater cytokine activity than non-pulsed DC-primed lymphocytes. These data suggest that ex vivo expansion of BCR/ABL-specific lymphocytes could potentially be used to augment CML-specific cytotoxicity and separate GVL from GVHD in donor leukocyte infusions post allogeneic BMT.

MHC-UNRESTRICTED EFFECTORS

MHC-unrestricted effector cells may also contribute to the antileukemic effects of donor cells against CML cells. Natural killer (NK) cells are a subset of PBMC that can be distinguished from T and B lymphocytes by surface markers, and which can mediate cytotoxicity without the need for antigen processing or presentation by MHC molecules.[52,53] Verfaillie et al[54] have demonstrated that non-malignant hematopoietic progenitors in CML can be distinguished by a $CD34^+$ HLA-DR phenotype, and further work has shown that NK cells are derived from these progenitors.[55] IL-2 induces rapid NK-cell activation and proliferation,[56] and IL-2-activated NK-cell activity has been demonstrated in patients with acute myeloid leukemia (AML).[57–59] Linomide, an immunomodulator that can increase IL-2 production and induce proliferation of NK cells in mice,[60] has recently been demonstrated to augment NK- and T-cell number and function post autologous transplantation.[61] Condiotti et al[62] have found linomide to potentiate proliferation of T and NK cells in normal donors, and have postulated a role for immunomodulator-mediated adoptive immunotherapy post allogeneic transplantation.

To test the impact of IL-2-responsive effectors on CML, Verma et al[63] have assessed the impact of IL-2 on long-term bone marrow culture of Ph-positive bone marrow cells. Addition of IL-2 to these cultures led to the disappearance of Ph-positive metaphases after 10 days in culture; bone marrow cells cultured under similar conditions but without the addition of IL-2 did not show a significant decrease in Ph-positivity. Additional data by Cervantes et al[64] offers evidence that IL-2-activated NK cells can suppress malignant hematopoiesis in long-term bone marrow cultures of CML cells, but that activated NK cells do not suppress normal hematopoiesis in normal donors. Miller et al[65] have reported the safety and efficacy of low-dose subcutaneous IL-2 administration to activate NK activity in 12 patients who had received autologous transplants for CML. Increases in circulating NK cells were seen in patients who received at least 28 days of IL-2 therapy. Cytolytic function against the CML target cell line K562 was increased, and lytic function against the NK-resistant cell line Raji could be enhanced after in vivo IL-2-primed NK cells were activated ex vivo with high-dose IL-2.

NK cells may play a role in the efficacy of IFN-α in the treatment of CML,[66] and increased NK activity after BMT has been described.[67]

MONOCLONAL ANTIBODIES

Monoclonal antibody (mAb)-based therapies are ideally suited to the treatment of leukemia because of the well-characterized immunophenotypes of the hematopoietic cell lineages, allowing for selective mAb binding to neoplastic cells (Tables 35.4 and 35.5). In addition, the

Table 35.4 Possible targets of monoclonal antibodies in CML

CD33 (p67)
CD13 (aminopeptidase-N)
Lewis X (carbohydrate antigen)
HLA-DR (and variant molecules)
CD45 (for broad leuko-ablation)

Table 35.5 Different strategies for use of monoclonal antibodies in CML

Approach	Advantages	Disadvantages
Native antibodies	Simple; relatively safe and specific	Low potency; best for residual leukemia
Radioimmunoablation (using ^{90}Y-IgG or ^{131}I-IgG)	Potent; effective	Requires BMT donor or stem cell rescue
Immunotoxin	Selective and potent	Untested
Alpha-radioimmunotherapy ^{213}Bi-IgG	Selective and potent	Probably best for residual leukemia

neoplastic cells in the blood and marrow are readily accessible to the infused agent. CD33 is an antigen present on early myeloid cells (CFU-GM and erythroid burst-forming units (BFU-E)) and most myeloid leukemias, and is not present on stem cells.

M195 is a mouse IgG2a reactive with CD33 that is rapidly internalized into target cells after binding. An early clinical trial demonstrated that M195 specifically targeted the bone marrow in patients with myeloid leukemias and could provoke human anti-mouse antibodies (HAMA) even in severely immunosuppressed, heavily pretreated patients.[68] M195 does not efficiently activate cellular cytotoxicity or complement, and clinical responses were not seen. Silla et al[69] have shown that NK-mediated cytotoxicity of myeloid leukemia cells can be augmented through the use of an immunoconjugate of anti-CD16 and anti-CD33; CD16 corresponds to the FcγRIII expressed by NK cells.

A subsequent phase I trial used iodine-131-labeled M195 (^{131}I-M195) in patients with relapsed or refractory myeloid leukemias (AML, blastic myelodysplastic syndrome (MDS), and blastic CML), and showed that leukemic cytoreduction could be achieved in the majority of patients, with 8 of 24 patients achieving sufficient myeloablation to proceed to bone marrow transplant.[70] HAMA responses were noted in 37% of patients evaluated, and the retreatment of two patients with HAMA resulted in rapid clearance of the antibody without toxicity. Jurcic et al (reference 71 and unpublished work) have used ^{131}I-M195 and ^{131}I-HuM195 (HuM195 is a humanized antibody – see below) as part of an allogeneic BMT preparative regimen in patients with relapsed or refractory myeloid leukemias. Fourteen of 30 patients received transplants for CML (10 patients underwent a first BMT for accelerated or myeloblastic disease, and 4 patients underwent a second BMT for relapsed chronic-phase or accelerated disease). Thirteen of the patients achieved complete remission of disease; 3 of these relapsed from 3–22 months post transplant, 2 patients died of liver toxicity, and 9 patients died of infection.

A humanized M195 antibody construct (HuM195) has been developed that retains the murine CDR-binding sites, but contains human constant and framework regions.[72] In contrast to the parent antibody, HuM195 has the ability to mediate antibody-dependent cellular cytotoxicity (ADCC) against leukemia targets in vitro.[73] Theoretically, these antibodies would be less immunogenic than murine anti-CD33, and repeated cycles of therapy would not be complicated by HAMA responses. Subsequent trial results supported this hypothesis,[74] and supersaturating doses of HuM195 have shown antileukemic activity in patients with myeloid leukemias.[75,76] Preclinical studies have shown that effector cells exhibit enhanced ADCC when they have been incubated with IL-2. Based on these data, 14 patients with relapsed or refractory AML or MDS were treated with sequential HuM195 and IL-2 infusions. Two patients demonstrated significant reductions in blast counts, and one patient achieved complete remission.[77]

^{131}I-M195 has been used as part of pretransplant myeloablative therapy, and has shown antileukemic activity.[71] The use of ^{131}I-anti-CD33 constructs is hindered by several factors, however. The hypervariable regions contain large numbers of tyrosine residues, and radiolabeling at high specific activities results in decreased biological activity.[78] Therefore, multiple infusions of the conjugate agent are needed to deliver sufficient radiation doses to the marrow. Therapy at high ^{131}I doses requires patient isolation, has the potential to expose hospital staff to significant radiation, and poses a radioactive waste hazard due to this isotope's relatively long half-life (8 days). These issues make such therapy cumbersome, and the gamma-emission range of the isotope makes it difficult to utilize this approach outside the context of transplantation.

The use of radioisotopes with shorter emission ranges can circumvent the need for patient isolation and can reduce radiation exposure to health care personnel. Beta particles can destroy target cells without antigen–antibody complex internalization, and because of their range may kill antigen-negative cells in close proximity to targets. Yttrium-90-labeled HuM195 (^{90}Y-HuM195) is currently under evaluation in a phase I trial.[79] Fourteen patients with relapsed or refractory AML received 0.1–0.3 mCi/kg of ^{90}Y-HuM195 as a single dose. Nine of 13 evaluable patients had reductions in bone marrow blasts, with all three patients treated at the highest dose level achieving marrow aplasia without evidence of residual leukemia 2–4 weeks after treatment. These data suggest that ^{90}Y-HuM195 may be useful as part of a pretransplant myeloablative conditioning regimen.

Alpha-particle-emitting radioimmunoconjugates may also have a role to play in the therapy of myeloid leukemias. Alpha particles have high linear energy transfer and a 50–80 μm range, and are thus unlikely to significantly affect normal bystander cells. The alpha-particle-emitting isotopes bismuth-212 (^{212}Bi), ^{213}Bi, and astatine-211 (^{211}At) have demonstrated antitumor effects in preclinical work.[80] A clinical trial of ^{213}Bi-HuM195 in patients with advanced myeloid malignancies demonstrated an antitumor effect, with 13 of 18 patients showing decreased bone marrow blasts.[81] Additionally, the absorbed-dose ratios between marrow, liver, and spleen and the whole body were 1000–10 000 times greater with ^{213}Bi-HuM195 than had been seen with ^{131}I- and ^{90}Y-radioimmunoconjugates. This suggests that targeted alpha-particle therapy will be useful in patients with minimal or reduced disease.

Antibody–drug conjugates have also been investigated for use in the treatment of myeloid leukemias. Immunotoxins are proteins constructed by covalently linking or genetically fusing a monoclonal antibody to a toxic molecule.[82] These novel agents are thus able to target specific cell populations. Both ricin and gelonin toxins have been conjugated to anti-CD33 antibodies, and have demonstrated antileukemic activity in vitro[83–85] or in vivo in murine leukemia models.[86] A clinical trial of CMA-676, a conjugate of a humanized anti-CD33 antibody linked to the cytotoxic agent calicheamicin, demonstrated antileukemic effects in 38% of patients with relapsed AML treated with a single course of therapy.[87] Immunotoxins may prove useful in the treatment of myeloid leukemias, both in vivo and in bone marrow purging ex vivo.

CONCLUSIONS

The first evidence of the importance of the immune system in the control of CML was gathered from the clinical associations between GVHD and GVL effects post allogeneic transplantation. Subsequent investigation has sought to characterize the effector cells responsible for these effects; there is now substantial evidence that diverse T-cell subsets account for the observed differential effects. Moreover, the unique expression of the Philadelphia chromosome in the leukemic cells of patients with CML offers the opportunity for the development of tumor-specific immunotherapeutic strategies. CML peptide vaccine strategies, adoptive immunotherapy strategies, and myeloid-specific antibody strategies have all shown promising results, and, to varying degrees, may become acceptable treatment options for this disease in the future. Interest in the effector cell populations responsible for antileukemic effects have identified both MHC-restricted and MHC-unrestricted CML-directed mediators, and radioimmunoconjugates and monoclonal-antibody–immunotoxin compounds have a potential role to play in CML therapy. Immunotherapy will undoubtedly play an important role in future treatment schemes for patients with CML and other cancers.

REFERENCES

1. Goldman JM, Gale RP, Horowitz MM et al, Bone marrow transplantation for chronic myelogenous leukemia in chronic phase. Increased risk for relapse associated with T-cell depletion. *Ann Intern Med* 1988; **108:** 806–14.
2. Apperley JR, Mauro FR, Goldman JM et al, Bone marrow transplantation for chronic myeloid leukemia in chronic phase: importance of a

graft-versus-leukemia effect. *Br J Haematol* 1988; **69:** 239–45.

3. Horowitz MM, Gale RP, Sondel OM et al, Graft-versus-leukemia reactions after bone marrow transplantation. *Blood* 1990; **75:** 555–62.
4. Marmont AM, Horowitz MM, Gale RP et al, T-cell depletion of HLA-identical transplants in leukemia. *Blood* 1991; **78:** 2120–30.
5. Antin JH, Graft-versus-leukemia: no longer an epiphenomenon. *Blood* 1993; **82:** 2273–7.
6. Weiden OL, Flourney N, Thomas ED et al, Antileukemic effect of graft-versus-host disease in human recipients of allogeneic-marrow graft. *N Engl J Med* 1979; **300:** 1068–73.
7. Weiden PL, Sullivan KM, Flourney N et al, Antileukemic effect of chronic graft-versus-host disease: contribution to improved survival after allogeneic marrow transplantation. *N Engl J Med* 1981; **304:** 1529–33.
8. Fefer A, Sullivan KM, Weiden P et al, Graft versus leukemia effect in man: the relapse rate of acute leukemia is lower after allogenic than after syngeneic transplantation. *Prog Clin Biol Res* 1987; **244:** 401–8.
9. Gale RP, Horowitz MM, Asta RC et al, Identical-twin bone marrow transplants for leukemia. *Ann Intern Med* 1994; **120:** 646–52.
10. Kolb HJ, Mittermuller J, Clemm C et al, Donor leukocyte transfusions for treatment of recurrent chronic myelogenous leukemia in marrow transplant patients. *Blood* 1990; **76:** 2462–5.
11. Rowley JD, A new consistent chromosomal abnormality in chronic myelogenous leukemia, identified by quinacrine fluorescence and Giemsa staining. *Nature* 1973; **243:** 290–3.
12. de Klein A, Guerts van Kessel A, Grosveld G et al, A cellular oncogene is translocated to the Philadelphia chromosome in chronic myelocytic leukemia. *Nature* 1982; **300:** 765–7.
13. Heisterkamp N, Stephenson JR, Groffen J et al, Localization of the c-abl oncogene adjacent to a translocation breakpoint in chronic myelocytic leukemia. *Nature* 1983; **306:** 239–42.
14. Shtivelman E, Lifshitz B, Gale RP, Canaani E, Fused transcript of abl and bcr genes in chronic myelogenous leukemia. *Nature* 1985; **15:** 550–4.
15. Grosveld G, Verwoerd T, van Agthoven T et al, The chronic myelocytic cell line K562 contains a breakpoint in bcr and produces a chimeric *bcr–abl* chimeric transcript. *Mol Cell Biol* 1986; **6:** 607–16.
16. Ben-Neriah Y, Daley GQ, Mes-Massan AM et al, The chronic myelogenous leukemia-specific P210 protein is the product of the bcr/abl hybrid gene. *Science* 1986; **233:** 212–14.
17. Kloetzer W, Kurzrock R, Smith L et al, The human cellular abl gene product in the chronic myelogenous leukemia cell line K562 has associated tyrosine kinase activity. *Virology* 1985; **140:** 230–8.
18. Shtivelman E, Lifshitz B, Gale RP et al, Alternative splicing of RNAs transcribed from the human abl gene and from the bcr–abl fused gene. *Cell* 1986; **47:** 277–84.
19. van Denderen J, Hermans A, Meeuwsen T et al, Antibody recognition of the tumor specific bcr–abl joining region in chronic myeloid leukemia. *J Exp Med* 1989; **169:** 87–98.
20. Chen W, Peace DJ, Rovira DK et al, T-cell immunity to the joining region of $p210^{BCR-ABL}$ protein. *Proc Natl Acad Sci USA* 1992; **89:** 1468–72.
21. ten Bosch GJA, Toornvliet AC, Friede T et al, Recognition of peptides corresponding to the joining region of $p210^{BCR-ABL}$ by human T cells. *Leukemia* 1995; **9:** 1344–8.
22. ten Bosch GJA, Joosten AM, Kessler JH et al, Recognition of bcr–abl positive leukemic blasts by human $CD4^+$ T cells elicited by primary in vitro immunization with a bcr–abl breakpoint peptide. *Blood* 1996; **88:** 3522–7.
23. Oettel KR, Wesly OH, Albertini MR et al, T-cell clones able to selectively destroy Philadelphia chromosome-bearing (Ph1+) human leukemia lines can also recognize Ph1− cells from the same patient. *Blood* 1994; **83:** 3390–402.
24. Faber LM, van-Luxemburg-Heijs SAP, Rijnbeek M et al, Minor histocompatibility antigen-specific, leukemia-reactive cytotoxic T cell clones can be generated in vitro without in vivo priming using chronic myeloid leukemia cells as stimulators in the presence of α-interferon. *Biol Blood Marrow Transplant* 1996; **2:** 31–6.
25. Serody JS, Brecher ME, Dent G et al, A method for the production of CD4+ chronic myelogenous leukemia-specific allogeneic T lymphocytes. *Cancer Res* 1997; **57:** 1547–53.
26. Faber LM, van Luxemburg-Heijs SA, Veenhof WF et al, Generation of CD4+ cytotoxic T-lymphocyte clones from a patient with severe graft-versus-host disease after allogeneic bone marrow transplantation: implications for graft-versus-leukemia reactivity. *Blood* 1995; **86:** 2821–8.
27. Falkenburg JH, Faber LM, van den Elshout M et

al, Generation of donor-derived antileukemic cytotoxic T-lymphocyte responses for treatment of relapsed leukemia after allogeneic HLA-identical bone marrow transplantation. *J Immunother* 1993; **14:** 305–9.

28. Falkenburg JHF, Wafelman AR, Joosten P et al, Complete remission of accelerated phase chronic myeloid leukemia by treatment with leukemia-reactive cytotoxic T lymphocytes. *Blood* 1999; **94:** 1201–8.
29. Papadopoulos KP, Suciu-Foca N, Hesdorffer CS et al, Naturally processed tissue- and differentiation stage-specific autologous peptides bound by HLA class I and II molecules of chronic myeloid leukemia blasts. *Blood* 1997; **90:** 4938–46.
30. Molldrem J, Dermime S, Parker K et al, Targeted T-cell therapy for human leukemia: cytotoxic T lymphocytes specific for a peptide derived from proteinase 3 preferentially lyse human myeloid leukemia cells. *Blood* 1996; **88:** 2450–7.
31. Molldrem JJ, Clave E, Jiang YZ et al, Cytotoxic T lymphocytes specific for a nonpolymorphic proteinase 3 peptide preferentially inhibit chronic myeloid leukemia colony-forming units. *Blood* 1997; **90:** 2529–34.
32. Molldrem JJ, Lee PP, Wang C et al, A PR1-human leukocyte antigen-A2 tetramer can be used to isolate low-frequency cytotoxic T lymphocytes from healthy donors that selectively lyse chronic myelogenous leukemia. *Cancer Res* 1999; **59:** 2675–81.
33. MacKinnon S, Papadopoulos EB, Carabisi MH et al, Adoptive immunotherapy evaluating escalating doses of donor leucocytes for relapse of chronic myeloid leukemia after bone marrow transplantation: separation of graft-versus-leukemia responses from graft-versus-host disease. *Blood* 1995; **86:** 1261–8.
34. Bocchia M, Korontsvit T, Xu Q et al, Specific human cellular immunity to bcr–abl oncogene-derived peptides. *Blood* 1996; **87:** 3587–92.
35. Bocchia M, Wentworth PA, Southwood S et al, Specific binding of leukemia oncogene fusion protein peptides to HLA class I molecules. *Blood* 1995; **85:** 2680–4.
36. Greco G, Fruci D, Accapezzato D et al, Two bcr–abl junction peptides bind HLA-A3 molecules and allow specific induction of human cytotoxic T lymphocytes. *Leukemia* 1996; **10:** 693–9.
37. MacIntyre AR, Christmas SE, Clark RE, The influence of class II HLA type on the lymphoproliferative response of normal donors to a bcr–abl fusion peptide. *Exp Hematol* 1996; **24:** 1307–11.
38. Bhatia R, McGlave PB, T lymphocytes cultured from chronic myelogenous leukemia bone marrow suppress autologous hematopoetic progenitors. *Leukemia* 1995; **9:** 1006–12.
39. Scheinberg DA, Cathcart KN, Korontsvit TA et al, BCR–ABL breakpoint derived oncogene fusion peptide vaccines generate specific immune responses in patients with chronic myelogenous leukemia (CML). *Proc Am Soc Clin Oncol* 1999; **18:** Abst 1665.
40. Yotnda P, Firat H, Garcia-Pons F et al, T cell response against the chimeric p210 BCR–ABL protein in patients with chronic myelogenous leukemia. *J Clin Invest* 1998; **101:** 2290–6.
41. Steinman RM, The dendritic cell system and its role in immunogenicity. *Annu Rev Immunol* 1991; **9:** 271–96.
42. Cohen PJ, Cohen PA, Rosenberg SA et al, Murine epidermal Langerhans cells and splenic dendritic cells present tumor-associated antigens to primed T cells. *Eur J Immunol* 1994; **24:** 315–19.
43. Flamand V, Sornasse T, Thielemans K et al, Murine dendritic cells pulsed *in vitro* with tumor antigen induce tumor resistance in vivo. *Eur J Immunol* 1994; **24:** 605–10.
44. Inaba K, Young JW, Steinman RM, Direct activation of $CD8^+$ cytotoxic T lymphocytes by dendritic cells. *J Exp Med* 1987; **166:** 182–94.
45. Young JW, Steinman RM, Dendritic cells stimulate primary human cytolytic lymphocyte responses in the absence of $CD4^+$ helper T cells. *J Exp Med* 1990; **171:** 1315–18.
46. Eibl B, Ebner S, Duba C et al, Dendritic cells generated from blood precursors of chronic myelogenous leukemia patients carry the Philadelphia chromosome translocation and can induce a CML-specific primary cytotoxic T-cell response. *Genes, Chromosomes, Cancer* 1997; **20:** 215–23.
47. Choudhury A, Gajewski JL, Liang JC et al, Use of leukemic dendritic cells for the generation of antileukemic cellular cytotoxicity against Philadelphia chromosome-positive chronic myelogenous leukemia. *Blood* 1997; **84:** 1133–42.
48. Jiang YZ, Barrett AJ, Cellular and cytokine-mediated effects of CD4-positive lymphocyte lines generated in vitro against chronic myelogenous leukemia. *Exp Hematol* 1995; **23:** 1167–72.
49. Mannering SI, McKenzie JL, Fearnley DB, Hart DNJ, HLA-DR1-restricted bcr–abl (b3a2)-specific

CD4+ T lymphocytes respond to dendritic cells pulsed with b3a2 peptide and antigen-presenting cells exposed to b3a2 containing cell lysates. *Blood* 1997; **90:** 290–7.
50. Nieda M, Nicol A, Kikuchi A et al, Dendritic cells stimulate the expansion of bcr–abl specific CD8+ T cells with cytotoxic activity against leukemic cells from patients with chronic myeloid leukemia. *Blood* 1998; **91:** 977–83.
51. Osman Y, Takahashi M, Aheng Z et al, Generation of bcr–abl specific cytotoxic T-lymphocytes by using dendritic cells pulsed with brc–abl (b3a2) peptide: its applicability for donor leukocyte transfusions in marrow grafted CML patients. *Leukemia* 1999; **13:** 166–74.
52. Trinchieri G, Biology of natural killer cells. *Adv Immunol* 1989; **47:** 187–376.
53. Herberman RB, Nunn ME, Holden HT et al, Natural cytotoxic reactivity of mouse lymphoid cells against syngeneic and allogeneic tumors. II. Characterization of effector cells. *Int J Cancer* 1975; **16:** 230–9.
54. Verfaillie CM, Miller WJ, Boylan K, McGlave PB, Selection of benign primitive hematopoietic progenitors in chronic myelogenous leukemia on the basis of HLA-DR antigen expression. *Blood* 1992; **79:** 1003–10.
55. Miller JS, Verfaillie C, McGlave PB, The generation of human natural killer cells from CD34+/DR− primitive progenitors in long-term bone marrow culture. *Blood* 1992; **80:** 2182–7.
56. Ortaldo JR, Mason A, Overton R, Lymphokine-activated killer cells. Analysis of progenitors and effectors. *J Exp Med* 1986; **164:** 1193–205.
57. Hauch M, Gazzola M, Small T et al, Antileukemia potential of interleukin-2 activated natural killer cells after bone marrow transplantation for chronic myelogenous leukemia. *Blood* 1990; **75:** 2250–62.
58. Maraninchi D, Blaise D, Viens P et al, High-dose recombinant interleukin-2 and acute myeloid leukemias in relapse. *Blood* 1991; **78:** 2181–7.
59. Soiffer RJ, Murray C, Cochran K et al, Clinical and immunologic effects of prolonged infusion of low-dose recombinant interleukin-2 after autologous and T-cell-depleted allogeneic bone marrow transplantation. *Blood* 1992; **79:** 517–26.
60. Kalland T, Alm G, Stalhandske T, Augmentation of mouse natural killer cell activity by LS2616, a new immunomodulator. *J Immunol* 1985; **134:** 3956–61.
61. Bengtsson M, Simonsson B, Carlsson K et al, Stimulation of NK cell, T cell and monocyte functions by the novel immunomodulator linomide after autologous bone marrow transplantation. *Transplantation* 1992; **53:** 882–8.
62. Condiotti R, Slavin S, Barak V, Nagler A, The novel immunomodulator, linomide, stimulates interleukin-2-induced human natural killer (NK) cell and PHA-stimulated T cell proliferation from normal donors. *Leuk Res* 1996; **20:** 57–63.
63. Verma UN, Bagg A, Brown E et al, Interleukin-2 activation of human bone marrow in long-term cultures: an effective strategy for purging and generation of anti-tumor cytotoxic effectors. *Bone Marrow Transplant* 1996; **13:** 115–23.
64. Cervantes F, Pierson BA, McGlave PB et al, Autologous activated natural killer cells suppress primitive chronic myelogenous leukemia progenitors in long-term culture. *Blood* 1996; **87:** 2476–85.
65. Miller JS, Tessmer-Tuck J, Pierson BA et al, Low-dose subcutaneous interleukin-2 after autologous transplantation generates sustained in vivo natural killer cell activity. *Biol Blood Marrow Transplant* 1997; **3:** 34–44.
66. Herberman RB, Ortaldo JR, Rubenstein M, Pestka S, Augmentation of natural and antibody-dependent cell-mediated cytotoxicity by pure human leukocyte interferon. *J Clin Immunol* 1981; **1:** 149–53.
67. Higuchi CM, Thompson JA, Cox T et al, Lymphokine-activated killer function following autologous bone marrow transplantation for refractory hematological malignancies. *Cancer Res* 1989; **49:** 5509–13.
68. Scheinberg DA, Lovett D, Divgi CR et al, A phase I trial of monoclonal antibody M195 in acute myelogenous leukemia: specific bone marrow targeting and internalization of radionuclide. *J Clin Oncol* 1991; **9:** 478–90.
69. Silla LM, Chen J, Zhong RK et al, Potentiation of lysis of leukaemia cells by a bispecific antibody CD33 and CD16 (Fc gamma RIII) expressed by human natural killer (NK) cells. *Br J Haematol* 1995; **89:** 712–18.
70. Schwartz MA, Lovett DR, Redner A et al, Dose-escalation trial of M195 labeled with iodine 131 for cytoreduction and marrow ablation in relapsed or refractory myeloid leukemias. *J Clin Oncol* 1993; **11:** 294–303.
71. Jurcic JG, Caron PC, Nikula TK et al, Radiolabeled anti-CD33 monoclonal antibody M195 for myeloid leukemias. *Cancer Res* 1995; **55** (Suppl): 5908s–10s.

72. Co MS, Avdalovic NM, Caron PC et al, Chimeric and humanized antibodies with specificity for the CD33 antigen. *J Immunol* 1991; **148:** 1149–54.
73. Caron OC, Co MS, Bull MK et al, Biological and immunological features of humanized M195 (anti CD33) monoclonal antibodies. *Cancer Res* 1992; **52:** 6761–7.
74. Caron PC, Jurcic JG, Scott AM et al, A phase 1B trial of humanized monoclonal antibody M195 (anti-CD33) in myeloid leukemia: specific targeting without immunogenicity. *Blood* 1994; **7:** 1760–8.
75. Caron PC, Dumont L, Scheinberg DA, Supersaturating infusional humanized anti-CD33 monoclonal antibody HuM195 in myelogenous leukemia. *Clin Cancer Res* 1998; **4:** 1421–8.
76. Feldman E, Kalaycio M, Schulman P et al, Humanized monoclonal anti-CD33 antibody HuM195 in the treatment of relapsed/refractory acute myelogenous leukemia: preliminary report of a phase II study. *Proc Am Soc Clin Oncol* 1999; **18:** 4a.
77. Kossman SE, Scheinberg DA, Jurcic JG et al, A phase I trial of humanized monoclonal antibody HuM195 (anti-CD33) with low dose interleukin-2 (IL-2) in acute myelogenous leukemia. *Clin Cancer Res* 1999; **5:** 2748–55.
78. Nikula T, Bocchia M, Curcio MJ et al, Impact of the high tyrosine fraction in complementarity determining regions: measured and predicted effects of radioiodination of IgG immunoreactivity. *Mol Immunol* 1995; **32:** 865–72.
79. Jurcic JG, Divgi CR, McDevitt MR et al, Potential for myeloablation with yttrium-90-labeled HuM195 (anti-CD33): a phase I trial in advanced myeloid malignancies. *Blood* 1998; **92:** 613a.
80. McDevitt MR, Sgouros G, Finn RD et al, Radioimmunotherapy with alpha-emitting nuclides. *Eur J Nucl Med* 1998; **25:** 1341–51.
81. Jurcic JG, McDevitt MR, Sgouros G et al, Phase I trial of targeted alpha-particle therapy for myeloid leukemia with bismuth-213-HuM195 (anti-CD33). *Proc Am Soc Clin Oncol* 1999; **18:** 7a.
82. Hertler AA, Frankel AE, Immunotoxins: a clinical review of their use in the treatment of malignancies. *J Clin Oncol* 1989; **7:** 1932–42.
83. Roy DC, Griffen JD, Belvin M et al, Anti-MY9-blocked ricin: an immunotoxin for selective targeting of acute myeloid leukemia cells. *Blood* 1991; **77:** 2404–12.
84. McGraw KJ, Rosenblum MG, Cheung L, Scheinberg DA, Characterization of murine and humanized anti-CD33, gelonin immunotoxins reactive against myeloid leukemias. *Cancer Immunol Immunother* 1994; **39:** 367–74.
85. Pagliaro LC, Liu B, Munker R et al, Humanized M195 monoclonal antibody conjugated to recombinant gelonin: an anti-CD33 immunotoxin with antileukemic activity. *Clin Cancer Res* 1998; **4:** 1971–6.
86. Xu Y, Xu Q, Rosenblum MG, Scheinberg DA, Antileukemic activity of recombinant humanized M195-gelonin immunotoxin in nude mice. *Leukemia* 1996; **10:** 321–6.
87. Sievers E, Larson RA, Estey E et al, Preliminary results of the efficacy and safety of CMA-676 in patients with AML. *Proc Am Soc Clin Oncol* 1999; **18:** 7a.

Index

Note: page numbers in **bold** denote figures and tables

Abelson murine leukaemia virus (A-MLV), v-*abl* oncogene 19
ABL, exon–intron structure 341
ABL sequences, role 25–7
ABL tyrosine kinase inhibitors 175–6, 495–500
ABL-derived oncogene, genomic history 3–6
acute lymphoblastic leukaemia (ALL), p185 BCR/ABL protein 20
adhesion proteins
  alterations 49
  regulation 139–40
Akt kinase, PI3-K–Akt signalling pathway 30–1, 496
allogeneic SC/BMT
  see also allogeneic SCT, HLA-identical sibling
  advanced stage patient 268–9
  alternative donors (VUDs) 323–37
    numbers **324**
  biology 273–5
  vs blood-derived SC (PBSCT) 265, 292–4, 309
    see also cord blood
  conditioning regimens
    myeloablative 277–9
    non-myeloablative 279–81
    reduced-intensity 280–1
  determinants 274
  donor selection 241–50
  long-term follow-up 401–9
  malignancies, secondary 409, **410**
  monitoring *BCR/ABL*-positive cells 339–51
    chimerism analysis 349–51
    cytogenetics 339–40
    FISH 340
    quantitative PCR 344–9
    RT-PCR 343–4
    screening mRNA transcripts 343
    Southern blot analysis 340–2
    Western blot analysis 342
  mortality 325–9
    engraftment failure 325–6
    GVHD 326–8
    infections 329
  newly diagnosed patient 266–9
    algorithms **267–9**
    trial of conventional therapy 266–7
  non-malignant complications 409–13
    avascular necrosis of bone 412
    infertility 412–13
    ophthalmologic 411–12
    thyroid abnormalities 410–11
  optimization strategies **275**, 277–9
  PBSC boosts 293
  pretreatment
    intensive chemotherapy 188
    interferon-α 173–4
  principles 251–2
  prognostic factors 262–70
    at relapse 258–9
    CMV serostatus 265
    depletion of donor mononuclear T-cells 265
    pretreatment with IFN 255, 265
    reduced-intensity-conditioning 266
  relapse 329–31, 385–9
  risk analysis 252–62
    disease-specific factors 252–6
    donor–transplant factors 256–7
    gender of recipient 256, 304, 333
    outcomes **254**
    patient factors 256
    score 257–8
  survival
    OS and DFS 331–4
    prediction 264–5
  T-cell depletion 281–2
    donor mononuclear cells 265
    mechanisms of graft failure 274–5
  VUDs 323–37
  see also mortality; relapse; T–cell depletion
allogeneic SCT, HLA-identical sibling 303–21
  assessing donor 304–5
  assessing recipient 305–7
  conditioning regimens 307–8
  donor lymphocyte infusion (DLI) 315–16
  graft-vs-leukaemia (GVL) effect 313, 329–30
  GVHD prophylaxis 309–10
  HLA typing 304
  management of splenomegaly 308
  minimal residual disease 313–14
  prognosis 312
  relapse
    donor cell relapse 315
    family mismatched transplant 330
    haematologic 313–14
    molecular/cytogenetic 313–14
    treatment 315–16
  results
    numbers **324**
    transplant in chronic/advanced phase 305–6, 310–11
  source of stem cells 308–9
  survival, randomized studies **295**
  T-cell depletion **310**
alpha particles, radioimmunoconjugates 515
American Society of Hematology, establishment of evidence-based guidelines (EB-CPGs) 225
AML, p185 BCR/ABL protein 20
animal models
  Ph-positive leukaemia 101–31
  see also murine models
anthracyclines 307
anti-c-*myb*, c-*myc* proto-oncogenes 478
antibodies, T-cell depleting 280
antigen-presenting cells (APCs)
  dendritic cells 392
  GVL effect 372
  see also dendritic cells
antigens
  BCR/ABL protein as antigen 375–6
  leukaemia-specific 392
  targets for immune responses to CML **375**
  see also histocompatibility antigens
antiproliferative drugs, with DLI 390–1
antisense oligodeoxynucleotides (ASOs) 476, 479–80, 487–8
  inhibition of ABL kinase 496–7
apoptosis
  control by IFN-α 139
  p145 c-ABL kinase, normal activity 496
Ara-C *see* cytarabine
ASCT *see* autografting

astatine-211 radioimmunoconjugates 515
ATP mimetics, tyrosine kinase inhibitors 486–7, 499
autografting
algorithm **469**
bone marrow cells 422
choice of HPC 422
chronic phase 421–7, 466
cultured bone marrow 431–44
long-term culture 432–3
Manchester study 436–9
Vancouver studies 433–6
disease status at transplant **460**
effect on survival 460–3
future prospects 465–72
mobilized HPC 446, 448–9, 458–9
NK cell-based immunotherapy 459–60
Ph-negative HPC 445–56
phase of disease, European (EBMT) experience 421–7, **467**
rationale 446, 473–4
and STI571 (Glivec), clinical trials, possible studies **470**
and survival 467–8
toxicity and post-SCT therapy 425–6
University of Minnesota 457–64
unmanipulated SCs 421–30, **423**
avascular necrosis of bone, complication of allogeneic BMT 412
avian myeloblastosis virus (AMV) 478

B7-1/B7-2 372
B-cell acute lymphoblastic leukaemia (B-ALL)
characteristics 101
Ph-positive 102
in vitro correlate 101
B-lymphoid leukaemia, in p190 *BCR/ABL* transgenic mice 109–10
BCR (breakpoint cluster region) gene
BCR ratio, defined 342
genomic history 4–6
intron–extron organization 4–5
M-*bcr*, m-*bcr* and *μ-bcr* 4, 20, **21**, 340–1
schema **5**
size 4
see also BCR/ABL oncogene
BCR protein 6–12
C2 domain 10–11
Dbl homology domain 9–10
XPB/ERCC protein 10
function 6–11
GAP domain 10–11
Grb2- and Grb10-binding sites 8–9
N-terminal oligomerization domain 6–7
Pleckstrin homology domain 10
sequences, role 24–5
serine/threonine kinase 7
sizes 6
structure **21**
tyrosine phosphorylation 7–8
whole, *in vivo* 11
bcr-null mutant mouse 11–12
BCR/ABL oncogene 3–18
activation
incidence 20
oligomerization and localization 63
BCR/ABL-positive cells, residual disease analysis 339–51
breakpoints
p185/p190, p210 and p230 transcripts 20, **21**, 508
peptide sequences **509**
cause of generation 6
and CNL 20
cytokine production, lymphoid progenitors (BaF/3 cells) 60–1
cytokine receptor signalling 55–72
fusion point sequences 477
generation 6
lack of *in vitro* model of CML 102
lethal effect on embryogenesis 108–9
murine models
embryonic stem-cell-based approaches 112–14
p190 110, 112, 122–3
p210 111, 117–19, 122
p230 forms 122–3
see also BCR/ABL transgenic mice
in pathogenesis of chronic-phase CML 58–9
reciprocal translocation product 4
signalling, mimicry of cytokine receptor signalling 62–3
signalling pathways, abnormal integrin function 47–50
structure 3–6, **21**
targeted oligodeoxynucleotides 477
targeting 476–7
ts-p210, switching 59
BCR/ABL protein
actin-binding activity 10
activity 4
as antigen 375–6
assays for BCR/ABL translocation 22–3
BCR/ABL-transformed HC lines, Ph-positive murine leukaemia 105–7
cytokine-dependent cell lines, transformation 60
decreasing level of expression 487–8
domain function and signalling 19–40
haematological malignancies 20
haematopoiesis, suppression by INF-α 140
inhibitor *see* STI571 (Glivec; Gleevec)
leukaemia-specific antigens 392
normal homologue (p145 c-ABL kinase) 495
p185/p190 5, 20–2
p210 (classical) 4–5, 20–2
breakpoints (b2, b3 and b4) 508
peptides **509**
p230 5, 20–2
properties 101
SH2 domain, Grb2- and Grb10-binding sites 8–9
SH3 domain, leukaemogenicity 123
signal transduction pathways 488–91
MAPK 490–1
PI3-K 491
Ras 488–90
signalling pathways downstream 27–33, **48**
Hck and Fes tyrosine kinases 33
Jak–STAT pathway 31–2
PI3-K–Akt pathway 30–1
Rac-GTP-ase 32
Ras pathway 27–30
SHIP1 and SHIP2 33
transcription factors 32
targeting 485–8
tyrosine kinase targets **28**, 486–9
transformation assays, murine BM cells 58
ultimate oncoprotein 65–6
variant sequences (b2a2, b3a2 and e1a2) 375
BCR/ABL transgenic mice
conditional transgenic systems 114–16
double, tTA expression 115
induction of leukaemia 110–11
and myeloid leukaemia 111–12
Ph-positive leukaemia 107–16
transgenes, promoters and diseases **109**
BCR/ABL-induced leukaemias
human, p190, p210, p230 forms 19–22, 122, **341**
murine 20–2
translocations 19–20
BCR/v-*abl* transgene, lymphoid malignancies 108
bismuth-212 radioimmunoconjugates 515
blood-derived SC
leukapheresis 309
vs marrow SC 265, 309
PBSCs, identical siblings 280
peripheral blood mononuclear cells (PBMC) 509–11
see also cord blood; peripheral blood stem cells (PBSC)
bone, avascular necrosis, complication of allogeneic BMT 412
bone marrow
cultured, autografting 431–44
syngeneic identical-twin donors 311–12
bone marrow retroviral *BCR/ABL* transduction/transplantation

models 116–24
advantages/disadvantages 121–2
induction of CML-like disease 119
p210 *BCR/ABL* malignancies 117–19, 122
pathophysiology of CML 122–3
schema **116**
studies (oncogenes, and diseases) **109**
target cells 120–1
bone marrow transplantation *see* allogeneic SCT
breakpoint cluster region gene *see BCR*
busulfan 182–3, 277
autografting, post-SCT therapy 425–6
and cyclophosphamide (BuCy2) 277, 308
long-term follow-up 404
pretreatment for BMT 255
superiority of hydroxyurea 227

C2 domain 10–11
c-*ABL*, genomic history 3–6
c-ABL protein, structure **21**
c-BCR protein, structure **21**
c-*myb*, c-*myc* proto-oncogenes 478
calicheamicin 515
Campath MAb, T-cell depletion 310
Cas 49
cataracts, complications of allogeneic BMT 411–12
cathepsin G 510
CD3, downregulation 140
CD4$^+$, and INF-α 140–1
CD8$^+$
cytotoxic/suppressor T-cells 389
depletion 377, 389
and INF-α, CML patients 141
CD25$^+$ (IL-2), T-cell depletion 390
CD28, downregulation 140
CD33$^+$, CD45 MAbs 308
CD34$^+$
cell dose, transplant outcome 376
engraftment 459, 481
LIa2SN infection 481
ODN purging 479
PBSCT 288–9
Ph$^{+/-}$, LasBD 477
SCID/NOD mice 394
selection 281
T-cell depletion 296
CD34$^{+/-}$ populations
growth factor mRNAs **89**
IL-3 and G-CSF 91
CD95, Fas-induced apoptosis 139
CD, *see also* T-cells
Cdc42 50
Cdk inhibitors 138
cell cycle, control by INF-alpha 138–9
censoring events, survival (LFS) times **360**
chemotherapy 181–90
aims 181
effect on BM morphology 169
vs IFN-α 154–9, 165–80
dose–response 167
non-randomized trials 165–6
randomized trials 154–9, 166–7
with IFN-α **158**, 161, 168, 191–204
intensive 184–8
drug combinations **186**
drug list **185**
palliative/symptomatic 182–4
drug list **182**
chimerism analysis
mixed chimerism persistence, GVL effect 371
residual disease analysis 349–51
chronic myeloid leukaemia
CFCs, factor-independent growth 88–9
characteristics 101
Chronic Leukemia Working Committee (IBMTR) recommendations 362–4
chronic phase
deregulated haematopoiesis 82–92
malignant clone structure 73–82
cure definitions 263–4
cytokine production, autocrine and paracrine 61, 86–91
granulocytes, chronic-phase malignant clone structure 73–82
lack of *in vitro* correlate 101
latency period 82
myeloid colony formation 57
pathogenesis, autocrine mechanisms 87
Ph-positive 102
primitive leukaemic cells, factor-independent expansion **87**
prognostic factors, CMV serostatus 265
prognostic scores 211–12
extraction and validation **209**
treatment
BMT vs INF 226
evidence-based guidelines (EB-CPGs) 225–37
goals 181
immunotherapy 392–5, 507–19
see also BCR/ABL-induced leukaemia; progenitor cells; relapse; remission; response to therapy; survival; *specific treatments*; target-directed therapies
classification and regression tree (CART) 210
clinical trial(s)
acute/chronic GVHD **292**
allogeneic SC/BMT, new diagnosis, trial of conventional therapy 266–7
autografting 421–7, 457–64
and STI571 (Glivec; Gleevec) **470**
chemotherapy, randomized trials 154–9, 166–7
CPFP 169, 213–22
cultured bone marrow 431–44
GVL effect, vaccine trials 378
IFN-α therapy
with chemotherapy 153–4, 161, 168, 196–201
non-randomized trials 165–6
randomized trials 152–4, **156–7**
methodology 206–11
PBSCT vs BMT 293–4
prognostic scores 211–12
protocol 206
STI571 (Glivec) 468–71, **470**, 502–3
Clinimacs system, TCD 296
CMA-676 515
CML Collaborative Prognostic Factors Project (CPFP) 169, 213–22
cobblestone area-forming assay (CAFA) 446
colony-forming cells (CFC), proliferation 85
conditioning regimens, allogeneic BMT 275–81, 307–8
cord blood transplantation (CBT) 246–8
Crkl activation 47–8
Crkl adaptor 137
CXCR4 274
cyclophosphamide 277
autografting, post-SCT therapy 425–6
and busulfan (BuCy2) 277, 308, 404
and TBI (CyTBI) 307, **404**
cytarabine (Ara-C) **158**, 161, 168, 182, 184
with INF **158**, 161, 168, 191–204
observational studies 193–6
toxicity and compliance 201
with mitoxantrone 459
rationale for use in CML 191–3
with STI571 (Glivec; Gleevec) 498
cytarabine octaphosphate (YNK01) 201–3
cytogenetics
relapse, allogeneic HLA-identical sibling BMT 313–14
residual disease analysis 339–40
response
complete response 170–3
current criteria, response to therapy **358**
partial, post STI571 (Glivec; Gleevec) therapy 497–8
STI571 (Glivec; Gleevec) treatment 497
cytokine receptor signalling 55–72
and *BCR/ABL* signalling **62**
complementation by BCR/ABL 60–1
intrinsic cell defects in MPDs 56–7
mimicry by *BCR/ABL* 62–3
Ras signalling pathway activation 63–4
and *BCR/ABL* oncogene 63–4

cytomegalovirus (CMV)
disease, in alloSCT 329
serostatus, prognosis of allogeneic HLA-identical SCT 305
cytotoxic T cells 140, 372, 377–8, 389, 393
generation against CML cells in sibling pairs 509–10

dendritic cells
b3a2 priming 512
and *ex vivo* T-cell priming 512
leukaemia-specific 392
dianilinophthalamides 487
donor lymphocyte infusion (DLI) 280, 282, 385–99
administration 388
with antiproliferative drugs 390–1
effective dose 389
efficacy 386
ganciclovir, HSV-Tk suicide genes 377
GVL effect 371
HLA-identical sibling transplantation 315–16
with immune modulators 391
optimization 376
post T-cell depletion, pre-emptive treatment of relapse 377
response 386–8, **387**
durability 389
with steroids 391
T-cell depletion, CD8-depleted 389
targets 391–2
treatment of relapse 359–60
donor selection 241–50
algorithm **247**
alloreactivity 371
assessment, allogeneic HLA-identical BMT 304–5
HLA typing, matched donors 246–8
non-HLA factors 248–9
PBSCT 287–8
volunteer unrelated donors (VUDs) 323–34
drug testing, cell-line based murine models 107

E2F1 138
embryogenesis, lethal effect of *BCR/ABL* oncogene 108–9
erbstatin 486
European (EBMT) Group, autografting
chronic phase 421–7
design **467**
followed by IFN/Ara-C regimens 453
evidence-based guidelines (EB-CPGs) 225–37
defined 225–6

F-actin binding 47
FACS, LTC-IC turnover, cell isolation, FACS 83, **84**
farnesyl transferase (FTase) 490
Fas ligand
CD95-induced apoptosis 139
CML cells 372, 373
fertility, and allogeneic BMT 412–13
fludarabine 279
fluorescence *in situ* hybridization (FISH)
hypermetaphase FISH 340, 358
residual disease analysis 340
fluorescence-activated cell sorting (FACS) 83–4
Fyn (Src family kinases) 137

G-CSF
and myeloablative treatment 452, 459
PBSCT pre-treatment 248, 288–9, 293, 446
ganciclovir, herpes simplex (HSV-Tk) suicide genes 377
gelonin 515
gender of SCT donor, and survival times 256, 304, 333
gene therapy 475–84
alternative targets 477–9
receptors and signalling proteins 478–9
transcription factors 478
antigene strategies 476
exogenous genes into CML cells 480–1
targeting *BCR/ABL* oncogene 476–7
Genoa, autografting with Ph-negative HPC 445–56
Gleevec *see* STI571
Glivec *see* STI571
GM-CSF
antisense oligodeoxynucleotides 476, 479–80
and IFN-α 139, 140
post autografting 426
stem cell mobilization 446, 458–9
graft-vs-host disease 326–8
acute GVHD 290–1, 326–7
and alternative donors 291–2
chronic GVHD 291, 327
family mismatched donor transplants 327–8
HLA disparity, role 328
prophylaxis 294, 296, 309–10
treatment 389–91
graft-vs-leukaemia (GVL) effect 313, 329–31, 369–83
amplifying GVL responses 378–9
antileukaemic potential, factors **370**
clinical basis 369–72
disease status 371
and DLI 371
donor alloreactivity 371
historical aspects 369
HLA disparity 370–1
immunologic mechanisms 372–6
mixed chimerism persistence 371
optimizing post allogeneic SCT 376–7
PBSCT 292–4
risk factors 244
separating from GVH 377–8
T-cell depletion 371
vaccine trials 378
granulocytes, production in CML 73–82
granzymes 372
Grb2- and Grb10-binding sites 8–9
GTPase-activating protein (GAP) domain 10–11

haematologic relapse *see* relapse
haematopoiesis
autonomous, intrinsic cell defects in cytokine receptor signalling, MPDs 56–7
deregulated, mechanisms in chronic phase 82–92
expression of BCR/ABL, cytokine-independent proliferation and survival 57–9
malignant, control by INF-α 140–2
reconstitution 288–9
haematopoietic progenitor cells
abnormal adhesion 41–54
CD44 42–3
signalling 43–4
abnormal expansion 57–8
abnormal migration onto fibronectin 44
autografting 445–56
choice 422
biology, homing model 273–4
changes associated with disease progression 92–4
chronic-phase CML
deregulated haematopoiesis 82–92
malignant clone structure 73–82
dynamics 73–100
changes associated with disease progression 92–4
chronic-phase deregulated haematopoiesis 82–92
chronic-phase malignant clone structure 73–82
growth regulation **42**
integrin-mediated adhesion to fibronectin 42
LFA-3 43
mobilization and autografting 446, 458–9, **451**
phosphatidylinositol-linked receptor 43
proliferation inhibitors 85–6
proliferation and survival 57–9
quiescent subpopulation 82–5
selectins 43
summary and future questions 92–4
HAMA (human anti-mouse antibodies) 514

Hardy–Zuckerman-2 feline sarcoma virus (HZ2-FSV), v-*abl* oncogene 19
herbimycin 486, 497
herpes simplex (HSV-Tk), suicide genes 377
histocompatibility antigens
major (MHC) 390
IFN-α-induced 141
MHC-restricted T-cell effectors 508–10
minor (mHA) 242, 373, **375**, 391–2
disparity, GVL effect 370–1
disparity, role in GVHD 328
myeloid-specific 373
HIV inhibitors 498
HLA typing 241–8, 304
alleles **242**, 243–6
HLA-A2.1 511
HLA-A3 392
HLA-B8 392
HLA-DR1 512
HLA-DR 452, 459
HLA-DRB1 392
autoantigens 510
class I and II serologic specialities **242**
CTL generation against CML cells in HLA-identical sibling pairs 509–10
current techniques **244**
effect on post-transplant survival **245**
HLA-identical sibling transplantation 315–16
matched donors 246–8
see also bone marrow transplantation, HLA-identical; donor selection
HLA-identical sibling BMT 303–21
see also allogeneic SCT, HLA-identical
homoharringtonine 182, 184
HuM195 514
human anti-mouse antibodies (HAMA) 514
hydroxyurea 182, 183–4
with interferon-alpha 153–4
pretreatment for BMT 255
superiority, vs busulfan 227

I-κB inhibitor, and NF-κB 139
IBMTR Survey
Chronic Leukemia Working Committee recommendations 362–4
long-term outcome, post alloSCT 402–5
IFN regulatory factors (IRFs) 136
imatinib mesylate *see* STI571 (Glivec; Gleevec)
immune haemolytic anaemia (IHE), DLI 391
immune modulators, with DLI 391
immunodeficient mice, transplantation of CML cells, Ph-positive leukaemia 103–5
immunologic mechanisms
GVL effect 372–6
tumour escape 373
immunotherapies
BCR/ABL-specific peptide targets 510–11
dendritic cells and *ex vivo* T cell priming 512
MHC-restricted T-cell effectors 508–10
new trends 392–5
target-directed 507–19
list **508**
immunotoxins 515
infertility, complication of allogeneic BMT 412–13
integrin receptor function in CML cells 45–7
abnormal affinity 47
abnormalities **46**
alternative splicing 47
BCR/ABL gene 45
cytoskeletal interactions 45–7
integrin-mediated adhesion to fibronectin 42
interferon(s) 135–48
genes and proteins 135–6
INF-α receptor 136
integrin-mediated adhesion of CML progenitors 44–5, **46**
ISRE recognition site 137
signal transduction 136–8
types I and II **136**
interferon-α
control of cell growth 138–40
apoptosis 139
cell cycle 138–9
effects on haemopoietic progenitors 139–40
effects on immune system **141**
induction of PKR and RNaseL 139
growth control of malignant haematopoiesis 140–2
post autografting *see also* autografting
signal transduction 136–8
interferon-α receptor 136
interferon-α therapy 149–64
with Ara-C **158**, 161, 168, 191–204
toxicity and compliance 201
vs chemotherapy 154–9, 165–80
chimerism analysis 349–51
clinical resistance
lymphoma/melanoma 142
molecular mechanisms 142–3
use of STI571 (Glivec; Gleevec) 497
complete cytogenetic response 170–3
effect on BM morphology 169
observational studies 227
with Ara-C 193–6
pegylated 175
post autografting 425–6
pretreatment with
prior to allogeneic BMT 173–4, 265
prior to chemotherapy 187
prognostic risk groups, impact on response to IFN-α 169–70
randomized trials 152–4, **156–7**
with chemotherapy 153–4, 161, 168, 196–201
vs chemotherapy 154–9
high-dose vs low-dose 159–61
with IFN-γ 153
various dosages 152–3
residual disease analysis 345–51
cytogenetics 345–6
RT-PCR 346–9
response to therapy
outcomes **151**
prediction 174–5
variables 150–2
with signal transduction inhibitors 175–6
toxicities 150, 159
interferon-γ
immunomodulatory functions 140, 141
myeloablative therapy pre autografting 457–8
randomized trials, with INF-α 153
interleukin(s)
IL-2
$CD25^+$ cells, selective depletion 390
effect of IFN-α 140
IL-3
autocrine IL-3/G-CSF loop **90**
CFU-GM responses 57
in PV 56–7
withdrawal, ts-p210 59
IRFs (IFN-regulatory factors) 136
ISGF3 (IFN-stimulated gene factor-3) 136–7, 142
Isolex300i system, TCD 296

JAB 142
jack-knife techniqe 208
Jak–STAT signalling pathway 31–2, 136–7, 142
activation 64–5
Janus non-receptor tyrosine kinases (Jaks) 64, 136, 142

kinase inhibitors *see* tyrosine kinase inhibitors
Kit receptor 478

LasBD, retroviral vector 477
leukaemia-free survival (LFS) *see* survival
LIa2SN 481
LightCycler PCR technology 347
long-term culture (LTC), bone marrow cells, autografting 432–3
long-term culture-initiating cells (LTC-IC) 438
turnover, cell isolation, FACS 83, **84**
and various CFCs **86**

long-term repopulating totipotent stem cells (LTRC-ML) **76**, 86
lymphoid malignancies, *BCR*/v-*abl* transgene 108
lymphoma, resistance to INF-α therapy 142

M195, humanized MAb 514
macrophage inflammatory protein-1α 43
malignant haematopoiesis, control by INF-α 140–2
malignant transformation mechanism 65–6
Manchester study, autografting, cultured bone marrow 436–9
MAPK signal transduction pathways
 BCR/ABL 490–1, 495
 link to *BCR/ABL* **489**
me/me murine models 137–8
melanocyte-specific antigens 393
melanoma, resistance to INF-alpha therapy 142
melanoma-specific CTL 393
melphalan, autografting, post SCT therapy 425–6
methotrexate, post SCT 289
mHA, MHC *see* histocompatibility antigens
MHC, *see also* histocompatibility antigens, major (MHC) 390
MHC-restricted T-cell effectors 508–10
Minnesota, autografting 457–64
mitoxantrone 459
molecular mechanisms, resistance to IFN-α 142–3
molecular relapse
 allogeneic HLA-identical sibling BMT 313–14
 time for treatment 390
monoclonal antibodies 513–15
 in CML **513**
 humanized M195 (HuM195) 514
 targets **513**
mortality, IBMTR Survey, post alloSCT 402–5
mRNA
 destabilization 476
 sensitization of CML cells to chemotherapy 496–7
 transcripts, residual disease analysis 343
mRNA-oligodeoxynucleotide duplexes 476
murine models, Ph-positive leukaemia 101–31
 bcr-null mutant mouse 11–12
 BCR/ABL transgenic mice 107–16
 BCR/ABL-induced leukaemias 23
 BM transformation assays 58
 me/me 137–8
 propagation of BCR/ABL-transformed haematopoietic cell lines 105–7
 retroviral BM transduction/transplantation models of leukaemia 116–24
 severe combined immunodeficiency (SCID) mice 103–4, 373, 394
 xenotransplantation of CML cells into immunodeficient mice 103–5
mycophenolate mofetil/cyclosporine, GVHD prophylaxis 294
myeloablative therapy 446
 conditioning regimens, allogeneic BMT 275–81, 307–8
 in vivo results 449–53
 INF-γ, pre autografting 457–8
 iodine-131-M195 514
 pre autografting with cultured marrow 431
myeloid-specific antigens 373
myeloproliferative diseases (MPDs), cytokine receptor signalling 55–72

NF-κB, and I-κB inhibitor 139
NK-cell-based immunotherapy 459–60
NK cells, INF-α effects **142**
NOD/SCID murine assay 104–5, 394
non-myeloablative stem cell transplants (NMT) 376–7

2,5-OA synthetase 139, 142
oligodeoxynucleotides (ODNs)
 18-mer 476–7
 anti-c-*myb* 480
 phosphodiester-linked 479
 phosphorothioate, c-*myb*-targeted 480
 sequence-specific probing 244
 triple-helix-forming (TFOs) 476
 see also antisense oligodeoxynucleotides (ASOs)
oncogenesis, BCR/ABL transgenic mice 107–8
ophthalmologic complications, allogeneic BMT 411–12
outcomes
 allogeneic BMT **254**, 402–9
 CD34+ cell dose 376
 definition of variables 207
 response to therapy, INF-α **151**
 see also relapse; response to therapy

p15, *p16* genes, resistance to IFN-α 142
p48 (IFN-regulatory factor) 136
 p48ISGF3 142
p53
 inactivation 66
 murine models of p210 *BCR/ABL* 123
p73, phosphorylation 496
p145 c-ABL kinase
 normal homologue of BCR/ABL 495–6
 overexpression 496
p210 (p190, p230) *see BCR/ABL* oncogene; BCR/ABL protein
paxillin 49
PCR *see* polymerase chain reaction
peptides
 analogue peptides 390
 b3a2 fusion peptides, stimulation of CML cells 511
 BCR/ABL-specific targets 510–11
 potential as CML immunogens **509**
perforin 373
peripheral blood mononuclear cells (PBMC)
 peptide-induced killing 510–11
 stimulation with b3a2 fusion peptides 511
 T cell lines 509
peripheral blood stem cell transplantation (PBSCT) 287–302
 vs allogeneic BMT 265, 292–4, 309
 autografting, unmanipulated cells 421–30
 vs BMT 293–4, 422
 CD34 antigen 288
 G-CSF pre-treatment 248, 288–9, 293
 graft engineering and component therapy 295–6
 harvesting 287–8
 lymphocyte recovery post 289
 non-myeloablative stem cell transplants (NMT) 376–7
 prognostic factors, reduced-intensity-conditioning 294–5
 stem cell dose 376
peripheral HPC, harvesting 446
pharmaceutical inhibitors of BCR/ABL 485–94
4-phenylaminoquinazolines 487
Philadelphia (Ph) chromosome
 genomic history 3, 445–6, 507–8
 translocation event, *BCR/ABL* oncogene/protein forms 19–20
 see also BCR/ABL protein
Philadelphia-negative SCs 446
Philadelphia-positive leukaemia, animal models 101–31
phosphatidylinositol (PI)
 activation 64–5, 496
 PI3-K signal transduction pathways, BCR/ABL 491
 PI3-K–Akt signalling pathway 30–1, 496
 signalling 49–50
phosphatidylinositol-linked receptor, progenitor cells 43
phospholipid scramblase-1 (PLSCR-1) 139
PKR, induction, control by interferon-alpha 139
Pleckstrin homology domain 10
polycythemia vera (PV), erythroid colonies from BM, IL-3 effects 56–7

polymerase chain reaction (PCR)
LightCycler technology 347
monitoring response to therapy 360–1
multiplex PCR 343
as predictor of relapse **361**
quantitative PCR 344–9
real-time PCR 346–9
residual disease analysis 344–9
RT-PCR 343–4
competitive (QC-RT-PCR), Ph⁻ collections 448
nested 343–4
TaqMan 348
PR-1, proteinase-3 141, 510
progenitor cell inhibitor lymphocyte precursor (PCILp) 510
progenitor cells *see* haematopoietic progenitor cells
prognostic factors 205–23
CPFP 169, 213–22
time-dependent (TDPFs) 210–11
prognostic scores in CML 211–12
New CML score 213–22
calculation 213
vs Sokal score 213–22
proteinase-3 510
PR-1 141
purging *see* myeloablative therapy

Rac 50
Rac-GTP-ase signalling pathway 32
Raf activation 63–4
ras genes 490
Ras signalling pathway 27–30, 496
activation, mitogenesis 63–4
BCR/ABL 488–90
Rb, inactivation 66
receptors, and signalling proteins, gene therapy 478–9
reference-strand conformation analysis 244
relapse 357–64, 401–17
cytogenetic/haematologic 313–14, 362
indicators 385–6
interventions, relevance of monitoring 359–60
late 401–17
molecular 362–3
PCR as predictor **361**
post transplant 329–31
cellular therapy 363–4
HLA-identical sibling 315
pre-emptive treatment with T-cell depletion 377
TCD allografts 296
treatment 385–9
donor lymphocyte infusion (DLI) 359–60
see also outcomes
remission
complete cytogenetic response, post IFN-α therapy 170–3
molecular 362–3
partial cytogenetic response, post STI571 (Glivec; Gleevec) therapy 497–8
residual disease, residual disease analysis 339–51
residual normal (Ph-negative) cells 431
response to therapy 357–64
current criteria 359
cytogenetic response **358**
haematologic response **358**
INF-α **151**
prediction 174–5
variables 150–2
PCR monitoring 360–1
see also outcomes; *specific therapies*
retroviral BM transduction/transplantation models of *BCR/ABL*-induced leukaemia 116–24
retroviral vectors
LasBD 477
LIa2SN 481
transfection vs transgenes 495–6
Rho 50
ribozymes 477, 488
ricin 515
RNaseL, control by interferon-α 139

S-phase cells, labelling methods 82–3
SDF-1 274
selective T-cell depletion *see* T-cell depletion
sequence-specific oligonucleotide probing 244
sequence-specific primers 244
serostatus, prognosis of CML after SCT 265
severe combined immunodeficiency (SCID) mice 103–4, 373
SCID/NOD mice, CD34⁺ 104, 394
transplantation of chronic phase CML cells 103–4
transplantation of CML blast-crisis cells 103
SH2 domain, BCR/ABL protein
Grb2- and Grb10-binding sites 8–9
protein-tyrosine phosphatases (SHPTPs) 137–8
SU5220 489
SH3 domain, leukaemogenicity 123
SHPTPs 137–8
signal transducer and activator of transcription (STAT) 64–5
Jak-STAT signalling pathway 31–2
signal transduction inhibitors
ABL tyrosine kinase 175–6
with interferon-α 175–6
see also STI-571 (Glivec)
signal transduction pathways, BCR/ABL 488–91
signalling proteins, gene therapy 478–9
Sokal score 262
vs New CML score, prognostic indictors in CML 213–22
risk groups, distribution **216**
Southern blot analysis, residual disease analysis 340–2
Spectratyping 372
splenectomy 308
splenomegaly, management 308
Src family kinases 137
see also SH2, SH3 domains
STAT proteins 136–8, 141
and IFN-α 141
STAT–STAT homo/heterodimers 136
see also Jak–STATs
stem cell (steel) factor 140, 274
see also cord blood; haematopoietic progenitor cells; peripheral blood stem cells
steroids, with DLI 391
STI571 (Glivec; Gleevec) 176, 234, 501–6
with Ara-C 498
clinical trials 468–71
phase I 502–3
possible studies **470**, 503–4
resistance 504
CML treatment algorithms 504
evolution of resistance 498
future trials 468
implications for trials 468
INF-α-resistant CML patients 497
mechanism of action **502**
modification 498
oral administration 502
preclinical testing 501–2
and survival 468–9
streptolysin-O 479
suicide genes, insertion into T cells 377
survival
and autografting 467–8
autografting, and disease status at transplant 460–3
disease status affecting **460**
multivariate analysis **462**
prediction
allogeneic BMT 264–5, 331–4
conventional therapy 262–3
survival (LFS) times
age and gender 256, 304, 333
assessment, recommendations 363–4
censoring events **360**
current leukaemia-free survival 363
disease phase 331–2
OS and DFS 331–4
prior chemotherapy 333–4
regimens compared **406**
stratified for therapy and risk group **221**
syngeneic BMT, identical-twin donors 311–12

T cells
in CML, possible protein targets **509**

T cells *continued*
CTLs 372, 377
allo-restricted 393
anti-CML 509–10
BCR/ABL-positive 140
leukaemia-specific, adoptive transfer 378
melanoma-specific 393
ex vivo priming, and dendritic cells 512
insertion of suicide genes 377
precursors, GVL effect 371
recognition of CML 372–3
see also CD factors
T-cell depletion 281–2
Campath MAb 310
CD8+ 377, 389
CD25+ (IL-2) 390
CD34+ selection 296
depleting antibodies 280
donor mononuclear cells 265
prognosis of BMT 265
drawbacks 295–6
GVL effect 371
mechanisms of graft failure 274–5
Mega-TCD 296
methods 281–2
pre-emptive treatment of relapse 377
results 282
selective depletion 377–8
T-cell effectors, MHC-restricted 508–10
T-cell receptors
Spectratyping 372
Vβ families 372
selection 378
TaqMan probes **348**
target-directed therapies 473–519
ABL tyrosine kinase inhibitors 495–500
gene therapy 475–84
immunotherapies 507–19
novel pharmaceutical inhibitors of BCR/ABL 485–94
STI571 (Glivec; Gleevec) 501–6
see also specific therapies
TEL/ABL chimeric oncogene 19
telomerase, maintenance of telomeres 66
telomere length, indicator of mitotic history 84–5
tetracycline-regulated transactivator (tTA), BCR/ABL transgene **115**
thrombopoietin, TPO-induced megakaryopoiesis 139
thymic irradiation 280
[^{3}H]thymidine, (suicide) labeling of S-phase cells 83
thyroid abnormalities, allogeneic BMT 410–11
time-dependent prognostic factors (TDPFs) 210–11
total-body irradiation (TBI) 276–7, 303
and cyclophosphamide 307, **404**
low TBI-based conditioning 279–80
transcription factors, alternative targets in gene therapy 478
transformation assays, murine BM cells 58
transforming growth factor-beta (TGF-β)
inhibition of LTC-IC **86**
secretion 140
transgenes, promoters and diseases **109**
transgenic mice, BCR/ABL 107–16
transplantation of CML cells, immunodeficient mice, Ph-positive leukaemia 103–5
transplantation tolerance 385
triple helix-forming oligodeoxynucleotides (TFOs) 476
tumour escape 373
tyrosine kinase inhibitors
ATP mimetics 486–7, 499
development, new directions 498
naturally occurring 497
synthetic 486–7
targeting BCR/ABL protein **28**, 486–9
tyrphostins 487, 497
see also STI571 (Glivec; Gleevec)

v-*abl* oncogene
of Abelson murine leukaemia virus (A-MLV) 19
of Hardy–Zuckerman-2 feline sarcoma virus (HZ2-FSV) 19
transformation of murine BM cells 58
v-*abl/BCR* transgene, lymphoid malignancies 108
v-*myb*, AMV 478
vaccines, trials 378–9
validation 208–9
cross-sample 211–15
Vancouver studies, autografting, cultured bone marrow 433–6
vav proto-oncogene 478–9
VCAM-1 140, 274
VLA-4 273–4
volunteer unrelated donors (VUDs) 323–34

Western blot analysis, residual disease analysis 342
Wilms' tumour antigen 1 (WT1) 393–5, 481

XPB/ERCC protein 7
BCR Dbl homology domain 10

Y177 489
YNK01 *see* cytarabine octaphosphate
yttrium-90-labelled HuM195 515